W0111284

METHODS
IN PHARMACOLOGY

Volume 4A
Renal Pharmacology

General Editor: **Arnold Schwartz**
Baylor College of Medicine, Houston, Texas

Volume 1
Edited by   **Arnold Schwartz**

Volume 2: PHYSICAL METHODS
Edited by   **Colin F. Chignell**

Volume 3: SMOOTH MUSCLE
Edited by   **Edwin E. Daniel** and **David M. Paton**

Volume 4A: RENAL PHARMACOLOGY
Edited by   **Manuel Martinez-Maldonado**

A Continuation Order Plan is available for this series. A continuation order will bring delivery of each new volume immediately upon publication. Volumes are billed only upon actual shipment. For further information please contact the publisher.

METHODS IN PHARMACOLOGY

Volume 4A
Renal Pharmacology

Edited by
Manuel Martinez-Maldonado
*University of Puerto Rico School of Medicine
and Veterans Administration Center
San Juan, Puerto Rico*

PLENUM PRESS • NEW YORK AND LONDON

Library of Congress Catalog Card Number 74-34441
ISBN-13: 978-1-4615-8893-1   e-ISBN-13: 978-1-4615-8891-7
DOI: 10.1007/978-1-4615-8891-7

© 1976 Plenum Press, New York
Softcover reprint of the hardcover 1st edition 1976

A Division of Plenum Publishing Corporation
227 West 17th Street, New York, N.Y. 10011

All rights reserved

No part of this book may be reproduced, stored in a retrieval system, or transmitted,
in any form or by any means, electronic, mechanical, photocopying, microfilming,
recording, or otherwise, without written permission from the Publisher

Preface

In the years since Homer Smith did his pioneering work in renal physiology, interest in the kidney has grown steadily and robustly. That this wondrously designed machine—in addition to its filtering, secreting, and reabsorptive functions—can serve as an important endocrine organ has made it the investigative concern of researchers from a variety of disciplines. Not surprisingly in this era of molecular biology, attempts have been made to understand the orderly functions of the kidney in biochemical and molecular terms, and this has led to the steady entry of renal physiologists and pharmacologists into these areas. Because renal physiology is the foundation on which renal pharmacology is based, this volume has been directed toward describing and interpreting the interrelationships of these two disciplines and their relation to the biochemistry and biophysics of the kidney. Accordingly, extensive critical discussions of the current knowledge of mechanisms affected by pharmacological agents, in addition to descriptions of methods, have been included herein. Not accidentally, stress is placed on the physiological, pharmacological, and biochemical effect of diuretics. In a specific sense the drugs in this group are true "renal drugs." The scope of the material included on diuretics is wide enough that this book should be of value to almost anyone involved in their use, from the clinician to the cell biologist.

Because enzyme systems in the kidney may determine to a great extent the responses to drugs (whether aimed directly at the kidney or not), chapters have been devoted to the Na^+, K^+-ATPase and adenylate cyclase systems. Detailed analyses of the renal mechanisms responsible for handling organic acids and bases are also included. Perhaps one of the most novel roles of the kidney is its function in the metabolism of vitamin D: this is covered in the present work from the particular point of view of the action of the vitamin and its metabolites on renal function.

Some aspects of specific methodology have been omitted in each chapter because they are to be covered in a subsequent volume. Nevertheless, we hope that familiarization with the material in this tome will form the base for those embarking on the study of renal function. We hope that it will be of value to the medical and postgraduate student as well as to the investigator in the field.

The contributors have provided concise, lucid chapters and if the volume is successful in furthering the knowledge in the field, the credit is theirs. It has been a great pleasure to have had them in this collaboration, which has been successful enough to lead to a subsequent volume. The content of the volume, however, has been entirely of my choosing and I am responsible for any omissions or failings.

The unfailing help given by my secretary, Ms. Consuelo Lopez, in all aspects of the preparation of this volume, is deeply appreciated. Thanks are also due to Ms. Lucy Medina and Mrs. Dinah Mercado for their help with proofreading and indexing.

San Juan   MANUEL MARTINEZ-MALDONADO

Contributors

ARNOLD M. CHONKO
Division of Nephrology
Department of Medicine
University of Kansas Medical Center
Kansas City, Kansas

JACK W. COBURN
Medical and Research Service
Veterans Administration Wadsworth Hospital
Center
and Department of Medicine
UCLA School of Medicine
Los Angeles, California

THOMAS P. DOUSA
Department of Physiology and Biophysics
and Division of Nephrology,
Department of Medicine
Mayo Clinic and Mayo Foundation
Department of Medicine and of Physiology
Mayo Medical School
Rochester, Minnesota

GARABED EKNOYAN
Department of Medicine
Baylor College of Medicine
and Veterans Administration Hospital
Houston, Texas

GEORGE M. FANELLI, JR.
Merck Institute for Therapeutic Research
West Point, Pennsylvania

GERHARD GIEBISCH
Department of Physiology
Yale University School of Medicine
New Haven, Connecticut

JARED J. GRANTHAM
Division of Nephrology,
Department of Medicine
University of Kansas Medical Center
Kansas City, Kansas

SAULO KLAHR
Renal Division, Department of Medicine
Washington University School of Medicine
St. Louis, Missouri

FRANKLYN G. KNOX
Department of Physiology and Biophysics
Mayo Clinic
Rochester, Minnesota

GERHARD MALNIC
Department of Physiology
Instituto de Ciências Biomédicas
University of São Paulo
São Paulo, Brazil

GARY R. MARCHAND
Department of Physiology and Biophysics
Mayo Clinic
Rochester, Minnesota

MANUEL MARTINEZ-MALDONADO
Departments of Medicine and Physiology
University of Puerto Rico School of Medicine
and Veterans Administration Center
San Juan, Puerto Rico

SHAUL G. MASSRY
Department of Medicine
Los Angeles County—USC Medical Center
Los Angeles, California

BARBARA R. RENNICK
Department of Pharmacology and
Therapeutics
Medical School, State University of New
York
Buffalo, New York

ROBERT L. SALTZMAN
Medical and Research Service
Veterans Administration Wadsworth Hospital
Center
and Department of Medicine
UCLA School of Medicine
Los Angeles, California

ARNOLD SCHWARTZ
Department of Cell Biophysics
Baylor College of Medicine
Houston, Texas

WADI N. SUKI
Department of Medicine
Baylor College of Medicine
and The Methodist Hospital
Houston, Texas

JORGE TORRETTI
Department of Pharmacology
State University of New York
Upstate Medical Center
Syracuse, New York

I. M. WEINER
Department of Pharmacology
State University of New York
Upstate Medical Center
Syracuse, New York

Contents

III   METABOLISM

IV   ORGANIC ACID

I

Bicarbonate

Chapter **1**

Determination of Renal Bicarbonate Reabsorption by Micropuncture

Gerhard Malnic

Department of Physiology, Instituto de Ciências Biomédicas
University of São Paulo, São Paulo, Brazil

I. INTRODUCTION

Among the processes leading to urinary acidification, bicarbonate reabsorption is quantitatively by far the most important. In man, at a plasma bicarbonate level of 25 mM and a glomerular filtration rate (GFR) of 120 ml/min, 3 mmol of this ion are filtered per minute and are almost entirely reabsorbed by the renal tubules at a urinary pH of 6 or below. This rate of reabsorption represents a sizable fraction of total salt and water transport by the kidney and by far exceeds the rate of titratable acidity formation as well as ammonia production. According to Smith (1951), a normal man excretes about 30 mmol of titratable acid, and 30–50 mmol of ammonia per day; this compares to a level of more than 4000 mmol of bicarbonate reabsorbed per day, largely exceeding even the combined amount of titratable acid and ammonia excreted in chronically acidotic subjects, which may reach levels of the order of 500–700 mmol/day.

A. Homeostatic Role of Bicarbonate Reabsorption

The role of variations of bicarbonate reabsorption in the regulation of acid–base equilibrium is well known. The increase in bicarbonate plasma levels found in metabolic alkalosis after loading with bicarbonate leads to a marked urinary elimination of this ion, originally attributed to the existence of a *Tm* for bicarbonate reabsorption. However, more recent studies have shown that a

3

great part of this urinary loss of bicarbonate is a result of inhibition of this ion's reabsorption due to extracellular volume (ECV) expansion, since when bicarbonate plasma levels were increased with minimal expansion, reabsorption continued to increase proportionally to the filtered load (Purkerson et al., 1969; Kurtzman, 1970a; Garella et al., 1972). During respiratory alterations of acid–base equilibrium, bicarbonate reabsorption is increased (in acidosis) or decreased (in alkalosis), leading to the maintenance of acid–base homeostasis. Classically, it has been assumed that these variations are due to the regulation of the H^+ ion secretory mechanism by the cellular level of pCO_2 (Pitts, 1952). More recently, the role of alterations in effective ECV in the modulation of these respiratory variations of bicarbonate reabsorption has been stressed by a number of authors (Kurtzman, 1970a,b; Waring et al., 1974). They showed that a high pCO_2 acts in great part by inducing vasodilatation and reduction of the effective ECV, thereby enhancing bicarbonate reabsorption, while the opposite is found at a low pCO_2.

In metabolic acidosis, overall bicarbonate reabsorption is complete, which could be attributed either to the decreased filtered load or to an enhanced acidification mechanism, as will be discussed below. Finally, any process causing renal loss of bicarbonate, e.g., the chronic administration of acetazolamide, is bound to lead to a metabolic acidosis.

Bicarbonate reabsorption may be even more important than as judged by its role in the maintenance of acid–base equilibrium and in the reabsorption of a corresponding fraction of filtered fluid. Recent work has shown that active reabsorption of sodium bicarbonate, whatever its mechanism, appears to be an important factor in overall salt and water reabsorption in the proximal tubule, creating chloride concentration gradients which might sustain passive NaCl and water reabsorption (Rector et al., 1966; Froemter et al., 1973; Barratt et al., 1974). Furthermore, an electrogenic transport of H^+ or HCO_3^- ions might be partly responsible for the lumen-positive transtubular potential difference which is found in the final portion of the mammalian proximal tubule (Barratt et al., 1974; Froemter and Gessner, 1974) and appears to participate in the PD measured in the collecting duct (Stoner et al., 1974); this PD is one of the driving forces of NaCl reabsorption. Bicarbonate may have still another important relation with proximal tubular salt and water transport. Ullrich et al. (1971), as well as Maude (1974), have shown that the presence of bicarbonate in peritubular capillaries in physiological concentrations is important for the maintenance of a normal rate of fluid reabsorption as measured by the Gertz (1963) split-droplet method. This finding may be related to the function of bicarbonate as a buffer anion, since it can be substituted by other anions like glycodiazine and sulfamerazine. A similar effect has been observed in other epithelia like the toad bladder (Gonzalez et al., 1969; Singer et al., 1969, 1970). The described role of bicarbonate in proximal salt and water transfer is still not completely understood, and more data will have to be gathered to gain a better insight into the proposed mechanisms. However, these findings indicate that the importance of bicarbonate reabsorption very likely transcends its role in acid–base equilibrium.

B. Some Basic Properties of the Bicarbonate/CO_2 Buffer System

The mechanism of bicarbonate reabsorption has been studied extensively by a considerable number of investigators; in spite of this fact, this mechanism has not been conclusively elucidated, especially since, due to the particular characteristics of the bicarbonate/CO_2 buffer, several mechanisms of luminal removal of this molecule can be envisaged leading to the same end result, that is, removal of luminal bicarbonate and its transfer to peritubular capillary blood. Figure 1 summarizes some of the more important mechanisms that may lead to bicarbonate reabsorption. Bicarbonate could be transported as such, that is, in ionic form, from tubular lumen across the cell to peritubular capillaries; this process would lead to luminal acidification, since the numerator of the salt/acid ratio in the Henderson–Hasselbalch equation would be reduced:

$$pH = pK + \log [HCO_3^-]/[H_2CO_3 + CO_2] \tag{1}$$

As a first approximation, it can be assumed that the concentration of acid ($H_2CO_3 + CO_2$) remains approximately constant, since it depends mostly on the systemic pCO_2. According to the equilibria occurring within the bicarbonate/

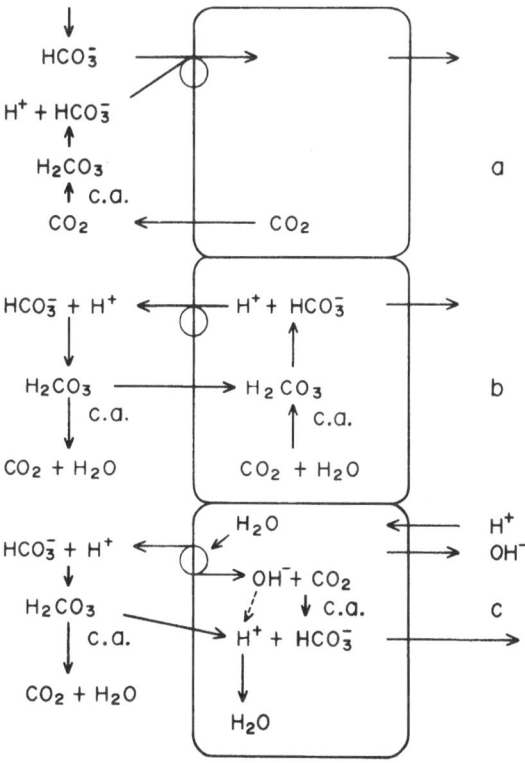

Figure 1. Schematic representation of mechanisms of bicarbonate reabsorption. (a) Bicarbonate reabsorption as such; (b) and (c) bicarbonate reabsorption by H^+ ion secretion.

CO_2 system:

$$CO_2 + H_2O \underset{k_{-1}}{\overset{k_1}{\rightleftharpoons}} H_2CO_3 \underset{k'_{-1}}{\overset{k'_1}{\rightleftharpoons}} H^+ + HCO_3^- \qquad (2)$$

the removal of bicarbonate will reduce the concentrations of the components situated to its left in the equation, except if the CO_2 concentration is immediately replenished by diffusion from capillaries and if rapid equilibrium within Eq. (2) should occur. The velocity of the first step (hydration of CO_2 and dehydration of carbonic acid) is, however, limited when not catalyzed by the enzyme carbonic anhydrase; in such conditions a lower-than-equilibrium concentration of carbonic acid could be found in the tubular lumen, leading to an alkaline disequilibrium pH (Rector, 1973). The origin of such a disequilibrium pH is clarified by an analysis of the reaction kinetics of the bicarbonate buffer system. The rate coefficients for this reaction have been measured by different methods and have been discussed elsewhere (Kern, 1960; Maren, 1967). In general, it has been found that the rates of the dissociation of carbonic acid in reaction (2) are very much faster than those for hydration of CO_2. Recent data indicate that the rate coefficient k_1, for CO_2 hydration, is of the order of 0.15 sec^{-1} at 37°C, while the coefficient k_{-1} for carbonic acid dehydration has a value of 49 sec^{-1} (Magid and Turbeck, 1968; Garg and Maren, 1972). The ratio between these two values, giving the equilibrium constant of this reaction, is of the order of 330, indicating that at equilibrium 330 times more CO_2 than H_2CO_3 will be present in a reaction mixture. This proportion is considered in the commonly used form of the Henderson–Hasselbalch equation, when a pK value of 6.1 is used. In several experimental situations, the proportion of CO_2 to H_2CO_3 may be altered, maintaining practically the same total amount of (H_2CO_3 + CO_2), but the amount of acid (H_2CO_3) in this total may be different. In this situation the equilibrium form of the Henderson–Hasselbalch equation, where a pK of 6.1 is used, will not lead to a correct value of pH on the basis of the actual concentrations of HCO_3^- and (CO_2 + H_2CO_3); when H_2CO_3 is below its equilibrium value, the pH thus calculated will be more alkaline than the measured value (alkaline disequilibrium pH); similarly, in the presence of a concentration of H_2CO_3 which is higher than expected at equilibrium, the measured pH will be lower than that calculated by Eq. (1) (acid disequilibrium pH). Under these conditions, however, the Henderson–Hasselbalch equation can be applied when only the H_2CO_3 concentration is introduced into the denominator, using the pK of 3.57 for carbonic acid given by Gibbons and Edsall (1963).

   Another form by which bicarbonate could be reabsorbed is a mechanism involving H^+ ion secretion by the tubular cell, schematically indicated in Figure 1b. According to this mechanism, the secreted H^+ ions react with filtered bicarbonate in the tubular lumen and decompose it, via carbonic acid formation, into CO_2 and water. Bicarbonate originating in the cell by the hydration of CO_2 is simultaneously transferred towards the peritubular capillary. By this means, a bicarbonate ion can be effectively transferred from lumen to blood; however, the ions disappearing from the lumen and being added to blood are not identical in this case. Since carbonic acid is formed in the lumen, the rate of its formation could exceed that of its uncatalyzed dehydration at the prevailing luminal carbonic acid concentration. This dehydration depends on the luminal acid concentration according to the following relation:

$$\dot{V}_{H_2CO_3} = k_{-1} \cdot [H_2CO_3] \tag{3}$$

where $\dot{V}_{H_2CO_3}$ is the rate of dehydration of luminal carbonic acid, k_{-1} is the dehydration rate coefficient, and $[H_2CO_3]$ the luminal acid concentration. When the rate of cellular H^+ ion secretion is high, the rate of dehydration of the formed carbonic acid must increase; it can do so only by an elevation of its luminal concentration, reaching a higher level than that corresponding to its equilibrium with CO_2; this constitutes the origin of an acid disequilibrium pH. As will be described below, the investigation of a disequilibrium pH is an important tool for the elucidation of bicarbonate transfer mechanisms.

Pitts and Alexander (1945) have shown that in phosphate-loaded dogs, much more acid phosphate is excreted than is filtered, implying that anion reabsorption cannot account for urinary acidification. On the basis of these studies, it is clear that hydrogen ion secretion is an important mechanism of urinary acidification; however, the existence of concomitant bicarbonate transport as such is more difficult to evaluate. As proposed by Menaker (1948) for the kidney and by Brodsky and Schilb (1967) for turtle bladder, diffusion of metabolic CO_2 into the lumen, hydration to carbonic acid, dissociation, and selective transport of bicarbonate back to the cell would be equivalent to H ion secretion.

In the following, some of the methods and experimental procedures developed to study these and other problems related to bicarbonate transport in the kidney will be discussed.

II. METHODS FOR THE MEASUREMENT OF BICARBONATE CONCENTRATIONS IN MICROPUNCTURE

A. The Use of the Henderson–Hasselbalch Equation

Since no direct method for the detection and determination of bicarbonate has been available until very recently, most investigators studying this ion have resorted to the application of the Henderson–Hasselbalch equation, by which bicarbonate concentrations can be obtained if the pH and pCO$_2$ of a fluid sample are known. The pH of a tubular fluid sample can be determined by means of pH microelectrodes and is measured in general after preequilibration of the sample with a known pCO$_2$. Several types of pH-sensitive microelectrodes have been used for this purpose, capable both of measuring hydrogen ion concentration of collected samples *in vitro*, and luminal pH *in vivo*.

1. Measurement of pH by Microelectrodes

The Quinhydrone Microelectrode. The first pH-sensitive microelectrode used in kidney micropuncture was the quinhydrone microelectrode, by means of which Montgomery and Pierce (1937) were able to measure pH of tubular fluid obtained from frog and *Necturus* renal tubules, showing that in these amphibia urinary acidification started only in distal tubular segments. This concept was for some time extended also to mammals, in which only the work of Gottschalk *et al.* (1960) and of Giebisch *et al.* (1960), using the same microelectrode, demonstrated proximal tubular acidification. pH measurement by this electrode is based on the measurement of the potential of a cell summarized as (Ives and Janz, 1961):

$$H_2 \ (P = 1 \text{ atm}), \ Pt|HCl, \ M \ | \ HCl, \ M, \ Q, \ QH_2|Pt \qquad (4)$$

The right half-cell is the quinhydrone electrode, composed of a very dilute solution of a mixture of quinone (Q) and hydroquinone (QH_2), in a medium containing a certain concentration of acid, the potential being measured via a platinum (or gold) wire. The relevant reaction is the reduction of quinone to hydroquinone, which can be expressed in the following way:

$$Q + 2H^+ + 2e^- \rightleftharpoons QH_2 \qquad (5)$$

The electrode potential, in terms of the activities (a) of the reaction components, will be:

$$E = E_0 + \frac{RT}{2F} \ln \frac{a_Q \cdot (a_H)^2}{a_{QH_2}} = E_0 + \frac{RT}{2F} \ln \frac{a_Q}{a_{QH_2}} + \frac{RT}{F} \ln a_H \qquad (6)$$

This relation shows that the electrode potential will be a function of hydrogen ion concentration if the factor including the quinone/hydroquinone concentrations is constant. In practice, these two substances form a compound containing equal proportions of them, $Q \cdot QH_2$, called quinhydrone. This compound forms sparingly soluble crystals which, in contact with the solution to be measured, form a very dilute solution containing equal proportions of Q and QH_2, such that the corresponding term of Eq. (6) tends to vanish. In the micropuncture technique, a thin platinum wire covered with quinhydrone crystals is introduced into a collection micropipet, as shown in Figure 2a. Pierce and Montgomery (1935) and Montgomery and Pierce (1937) filled the pipet with mercury, but later authors used mineral oil preequilibrated with a known pCO_2 for this purpose (Gottschalk *et al.*, 1960; Giebisch *et al.*, 1960). In this way, the microelectrode measures fluid pH outside the tubule, at known pCO_2, since tubular fluid has to be collected into the micropipet; the measured pH, an equilibrium pH since equilibration of the reaction of the bicarbonate buffer is practically complete within a few tenths of a second, can be used to calculate the bicarbonate concentrations of the tubular fluid. The measured pH will be equal to tubular pH, however, only if the pCO_2 of the mineral oil is equal to that of the tubular lumen, and in the absence of a luminal disequilibrium pH.

The Glass Microelectrode. Glass electrodes have displaced most other

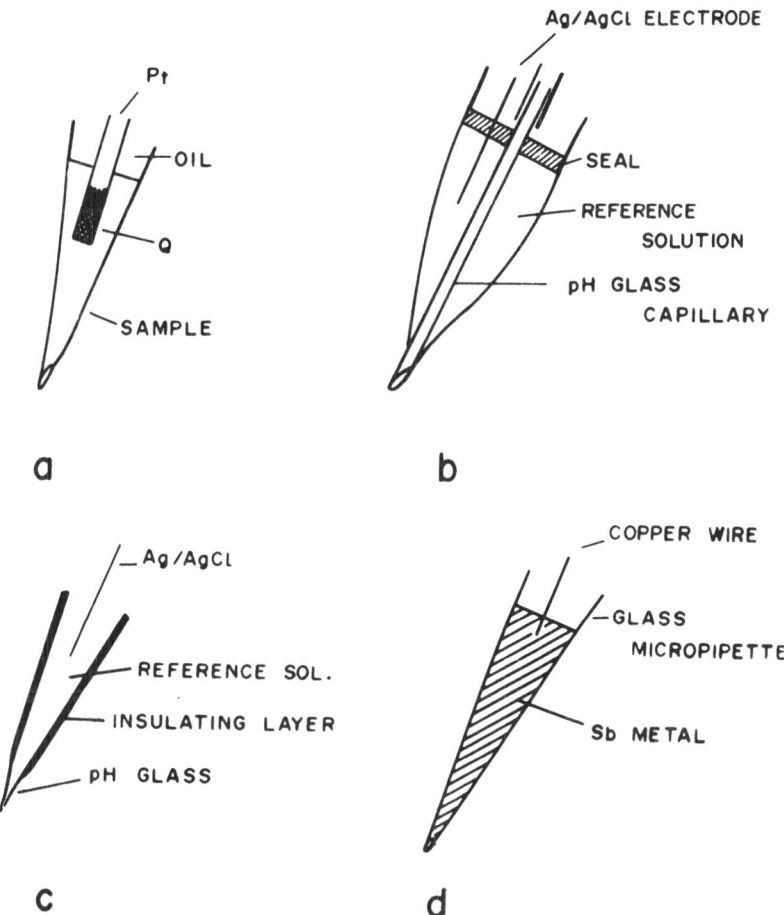

Figure 2. Microelectrodes for renal tubular pH and HCO_3^- determination, (a) quinhydrone electrode; (b) capillary glass electrode; (c) spear-type glass electrode; (d) antimony electrode.

H^+-ion-sensitive electrodes in general chemical work due to their considerable reliability as well as insensitivity to most of the interfering substances that commonly affect electrodes where electron-transfer processes occur, that is, for instance, to oxidizing and reducing substances. The origin of the potential differences in this electrode system is not entirely understood. Several theories are available, including the occurrence of permeability phenomena in glass and of surface phenomena like adsorption (Ives and Janz, 1961). Presently the most favored view holds that the glass-electrode potential is a result of the exchange characteristics of the glass, being a combination of diffusion and phase-boundary potentials (Eisenman, 1967). The glass-electrode system can be represented as:

$$Pt, H_2 = 1 \ atm, \ |HCl \ M|sol \ x|glass|HCl \ 0.1 \ M|AgCl|Ag \qquad (7)$$

where the right half-cell corresponds to a glass electrode filled with an acid reference solution, electrical contact being made by means of a silver/silver chloride electrode. The electrode potential of the glass-electrode system is given by a Nernst-type equation of the following form:

$$E = E_0 + \frac{RT}{F} \ln(H) = E_0 - \frac{2.303\ RT}{F} pH \qquad (8)$$

Since the pioneering work of Caldwell (1954), who introduced microglass electrodes for intracellular pH measurement, several types of such electrodes have been used in biological work. In kidney micropuncture, both spear-type electrodes and capillary aspiration electrodes have been used. Spear-type electrodes were introduced by Rector et al. (1965) and by Carter et al. (1967), who succeeded in overcoming the most challenging difficulties in their preparation. One of the major problems encountered in the preparation of these microelectrodes was their efficient insulation up to the last 5–20 μm, since only the very tip of the microelectrode should be pH-sensitive. This was accomplished by covering the original glass capillaries with a ceramic glaze, which renders the glass impermeable to H^+ ions, and recedes for the desired distance during the process of drawing out the glass (Carter et al., 1967) (Figure 2). The adequacy of this procedure was then tested by the procedure depicted in Figure 3, in which an agar/buffer mixture covered by a thin latex film is punctured by the electrode, and a different buffer is then applied to the latex-covered surface. Only those electrodes not responding to this application are considered satisfactorily insulated. The glass employed to produce these electrodes is normally Corning No. 0150 pH-sensitive glass. Such electrodes have a resistance of 10^9–10^{10} Ω and can be filled with a dilute reference solution or with distilled water, the necessary conductivity being achieved by the ions leached out of the glass during a period of several days. Carter et al. (1967) have described the manufacture of double-barreled microelectrodes, one barrel made of pH-sensitive glass, and the other of regular, nonsensitive glass in the form of a reference electrode, permitting one to read pH differentially and so eliminating the interference with an electrical-potential difference across a cell or epithelial membrane, without the necessity of a double impalement. More recently,

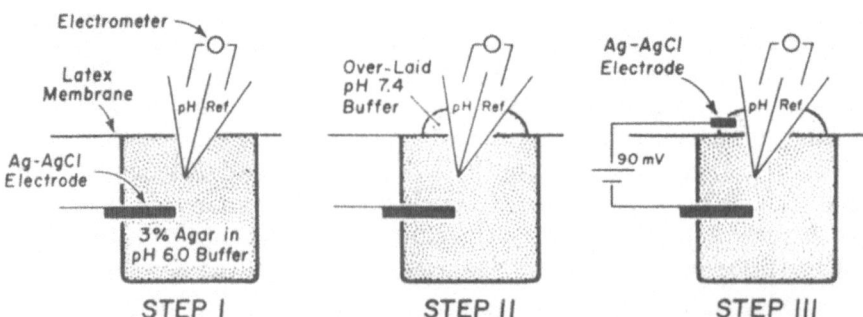

Figure 3. System for the verification of adequate insulation of double-barreled pH glass microelectrodes. The presence of an overlaid buffer above the latex membrane (step 11) or of a voltage pulse (step III) should not change the measured pH. (From Carter et al., 1967).

Thomas (1974) proposed the use of recessed-tip pH-sensitive glass microelectrodes, where the pH-sensitive glass is included within a Ling–Gerard-type glass microelectrode and is thus perfectly insulated. The fluid between the pH-sensitive glass and the tip of the electrode must equilibrate with the measured fluid, which causes a relatively slow response. However, it was shown that for the measurement of an equilibrium pH, this electrode proved quite dependable and accurate, reaching stable readings within a few minutes.

Capillary aspiration glass microelectrodes have also been used especially for bicarbonate determinations, where the measurement of an intraluminal disequilibrium pH is not intended. They were introduced into kidney micropuncture by Khuri *et al.* (1967, 1968, 1973) and modified by Uhlich *et al.* (1968) and Stackelberg (1970). A schematic drawing of an electrode as used by these authors is given in Figure 2. It consists essentially of a thin pH-sensitive glass capillary mounted inside a larger collection micropipet which is impaled into the tubule, permitting one to draw up tubular fluid into the sensitive glass segment. The reference solution of the electrode is introduced between the thin glass capillary and the outer collection pipet. A similar design was described by Levine (1971, 1972) and used by Levine and Nash (1973) for tubular bicarbonate measurements under different experimental conditions. These microelectrodes do not permit the measurement of a luminal disequilibrium pH, since, as pointed out above, the equilibrium of reaction (2) is reached in a very short time. Taking a dehydration rate coefficient (without catalysis) of carbonic acid of 15 sec^{-1} at 25°C (Maren, 1967) and since the $t_{1/2}$ of a reaction is equal to ln $(2/k)$, the half-time of the approach of this reaction to its equilibrium level will be 4.6×10^{-2} sec, showing that this equilibrium will be reached outside the tubule before any reading can be taken (Malnic and Vieira, 1972). On the other hand, for the measurement of the pH of collected fluid samples preequilibrated at a known pCO_2, that is, for the calculation of bicarbonate concentrations, these microelectrodes have proved to be of considerable value.

The Antimony Microelectrode. Antimony electrodes have been used in the past because of their simple and sturdy construction for both industrial and for biological applications. They have been replaced more recently by glass electrodes which have greater long-range stability, as well as lower sensitivity to interfering substances. However, for micropuncture antimony electrodes present several advantages. Their construction is relatively simple: antimony is melted in a quartz tube and drawn up into a 0.8-mm (O.D.) Pyrex glass tube and, after cooling, drawn out first by hand over a small flame, and then in a microforge. Finally, the tip is bevelled by grinding to a diameter of 5–10 μm. In this way, the antimony is contained entirely in a glass casing except at the tip, where grinding frees the active surface of the microelectrodes (see Figure 2). In this way, there are no difficulties in the insulation of the pH-sensitive surface of this microelectrode (Malnic and Vieira, 1972).

The half-cell corresponding to the antimony electrode in an H_2-electrode system can be summarized as follows:

$$\text{Pt, } H_2 = 1 \text{ atm} | \text{HCl M} | \text{sol x} | Sb_2O_3 | Sb \tag{9}$$

The antimony electrode is a metal/metal oxide electrode. On its surface, a layer of antimony oxide (Sb_2O_3) is formed, which in contact with water yields the following reaction:

$$Sb_2O_3 + 3H_2O \rightleftharpoons 2Sb(OH)_3 \rightleftharpoons 2Sb^{3+} + 6OH^- \qquad (10)$$

The solubility product of antimony hydroxide, a sparingly soluble compound, is given by

$$k_s = a_{Sb} \cdot a_{OH}^3 \qquad (11)$$

For water, we can write the following relation:

$$k_w = a_H \cdot a_{OH} \qquad (12)$$

Combining Eqs. (11) and (12), we have

$$a_{Sb} = (k_s / k_w^3) \cdot a_H^3 \qquad (13)$$

On the other hand, the Nernst relation between metallic antimony and antimony ions is given by

$$E = E_0 + \frac{RT}{3F} \cdot \ln a_{Sb} \qquad (14)$$

Introducing Eq. (13) into this relation and incorporating the constants into E_0, we get

$$E = E_0' + \frac{RT}{F} \cdot \ln a_H, \quad \text{or} \quad E = E_0' - \frac{2.303RT}{F} \cdot pH \qquad (15)$$

Being a metal/metal oxide electrode, the antimony microelectrode is sensitive to changes in pO_2. However, within the limits of pO_2 changes found in biological systems, that is, between the oxygen tensions of arterial and venous blood, this effect was shown to be negligible (Vieira and Malnic, 1968). Another possible source of error referred to in the literature is related to voltage changes during movement of the fluid being measured. It was, however, shown that the flow rates found within renal tubules are about an order of magnitude too low to lead to detectable errors due to this effect.

Between pH 4 and 7, a relation of about 55 mV per pH unit is found. However, above pH 7, this relation falls to about 40 mV per pH unit (Vieira and Malnic, 1968). The influence of several interfering substances has been reported in the literature. Besides oxidizing and reducing substances (Ives and Janz, 1961), recently attention has been called to the effect of the anions prevailing in the measured solutions. Karlmark and Sohtell (1973) as well as Puschett and Zurbach (1974) have shown that in bicarbonate-containing systems the antimony microelectrode may give lower readings, by 0.13 to 0.18 pH units, than the theoretical or glass-electrode values. Other authors have not encountered such deviations (Kunau, 1972). We had not detected such differences in our original paper (Vieira and Malnic, 1968), but found a difference of 0.065 units, significantly below the values measured with glass macroelectrodes, in another series of measurements (Malnic *et al.*, 1974). In the described experiments, the electrodes were standardized mostly with phosphate buffers. Green and Giebisch (1974) showed that these differences occurred when calibration and experimental solutions were of different composition with respect to their major anions, and that when standards with lower phosphate concentrations were used the observed deviations in pH readings tended to vanish. Therefore, it appears important for the calibration of antimony microelectrodes to use buffer solutions whose composition is as similar as practicable to the solutions being measured.

The more important applications of the antimony microelectrode in kidney micropuncture are summarized in Figure 4. For free-flow *in situ* pH measure-

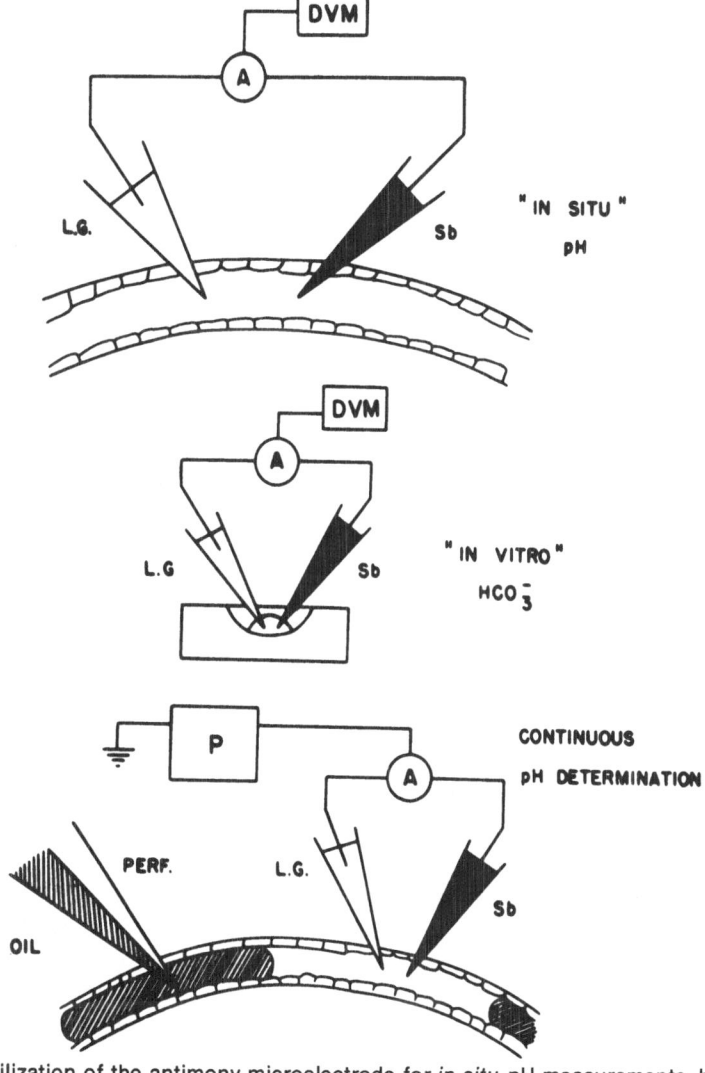

Figure 4. Utilization of the antimony microelectrode for *in situ* pH measurements, bicarbonate determination, and continuous recording of pH changes during stopped-flow microperfusion. (From Malnic and Vieira, 1972).

ments, the tubules are impaled by an Sb and a Ling–Gerard reference electrode and the pH measured differentially. In rat proximal tubule the measurement against an extratubular electrode is possible due to the low transtubular PDs normally found in this structure (Froemter and Gessner, 1974). For determinations of bicarbonate concentrations, collected fluid samples are equilibrated with mineral oil balanced with a known pCO_2, and pH is measured differentially *in vitro*. Finally, continuous luminal pH measurements can be performed during stopped-flow microperfusion experiments, as will be discussed below.

2. *Determination of Tubular* pCO_2.

In the discussion about the origin of a disequilibrium pH in the renal tubule, it was shown that an increase of both carbonic acid and CO_2 concentrations above their equilibrium levels would lead to an acid disequilibrium pH, since these two compounds make up the denominator of the buffer ratio in the Henderson–Hasselbalch equation (Eq. 1). It is thus conceivable that a disequilibrium pH measured in the tubular lumen might be due also to a disequilibrium pCO_2, that is, that the CO_2 formed in the tubular lumen by reaction between the secreted H ion and the filtered bicarbonate might not reach immediate equilibrium with plasma pCO_2. Should the tubular wall have a finite permeability to CO_2, a transtubular CO_2 gradient could be established. Kinetic measurements of the acidification of air-preequilibrated buffer solutions injected into the tubular lumen due to equilibration with tissue pCO_2 have shown that the half-time of this equilibration was of the order of 0.5–1.5 sec, being significantly increased after acetazolamide administration (Malnic and Mello Aires, 1971). Using these values, it was possible to show that a pCO_2 gradient of at least 10 mm Hg could be expected in control rats, and of 60 mm Hg after acetazolamide (Malnic *et al.*, 1974). A valid method for the determination of tubular pCO_2 is that employed by Uhlich *et al.* (1968) for papillary structures, in which the tubular sample is transferred anaerobically into a glass capillary micropipet, where pH is measured presumably at chemical equilibrium without loss of CO_2. This sample is then equilibrated with gases at different known pCO_2, the pH is measured, and from such an equilibration curve the original *in situ* pCO_2 can be calculated. These authors obtained 10 mm Hg higher collecting duct and vasa recta pCO_2 than measured simultaneously in the renal artery in a control situation. Karlmark and Davidson (1974) tried to evaluate tubular pCO_2 by collecting tubular fluid into mercury-filled micropipets, measuring the pH of these samples at several different pCO_2 values in a gas equilibration chamber under mineral oil, and interpolating the *in situ* pH measured with antimony microelectrodes. They obtained by this means early proximal pCO_2 values of up to 80 mm Hg, considerably higher than plasma levels, in control rats; these levels decreased to plasma levels in later proximal segments. However, the authors indicate that these values are calculated ascribing the whole disequilibrium pH to the disequilibrium pCO_2, assuming equilibrium concentrations of carbonic acid, an assumption that is not warranted by their method. This discussion shows that only a more direct measurement of luminal pCO_2 will permit the evaluation of the participation of an elevated pCO_2 in the establishment of a tubular disequilibrium pH. Recently, Caflisch and Carter (1974) described a pCO_2-sensitive microelectrode which appears to be adequate for intratubular measurements. This microelectrode consists of a double-barreled pH/reference glass microelectrode introduced into a collection pipet with a 10-μm tip. The pH–electrode system is immersed in a bicarbonate-containing solution, separated from the medium to be measured by a Teflon wax/oil mixture of 5–10 μm thickness introduced into the tip of the micropipet, which is permeable only to CO_2 and not to H^+ ions. This system appears to work adequately in artificial solutions and in rat blood. At the present time, however, measurements of tubular fluid with such a system are not available.

B. The Use of HCO_3^--Sensitive Microelectrodes

Recently, Khuri *et al.* (1974a,b) have measured intracellular bicarbonate concentrations by means of ion-exchange microelectrodes sensitive to bicarbonate. This method permits the direct estimation of bicarbonate ion activities in biological solutions, independently of an application of the Henderson–Hasselbalch equation. The authors use double-barreled glass microelectrodes with total tip diameter of less than 1 μm, the reference barrel being filled with a 3 M KCl or NaCl solution. The bicarbonate-sensitive barrel is first siliconized and then filled with a 3:1:6 mixture of tri-*n*-octylpropylammonium chloride, octanol, and trifluoroacetyl—*p*-butyl benzene, which is water insoluble. Electrical contact is made by Ag/AgCl electrodes in each barrel. These electrodes had a selectivity of 50:1 with respect to bicarbonate–chloride, and even better with respect to phosphate. They were sensitive to OH^- ions, but only above pH 8. They were also sensitive to the pCO_2 level of the measured medium, a reason why the authors used the same pCO_2 for their standards and for their biological preparation.

With these microelectrodes a mean intracellular bicarbonate concentration of 4.4 mM was obtained in frog muscle, and of 12.6 mM in rat skeletal muscle (Khuri *et al.*, 1974b). In *Necturus* proximal tubular cells a value of 11.1 mM was found (Khuri *et al.*, 1974a). Assuming that cell pCO_2 was near the venous pCO_2 level, these authors calculated an intracellular pH of 7–7.1 in muscle, and of 7.44 in *Necturus* proximal tubular cell. These values are compatible with a considerable number of experimental determinations of muscular pH (Waddell and Bates, 1969) and with cell pH calculated for separated renal tubules of the dog *in vitro* (Struyvenberg *et al.*, 1968). They are, however, higher than the data obtained by Carter *et al.* (1967), who found a cell pH in rat skeletal muscle of the order of 6.0. The intracellular bicarbonate levels measured by means of the described microelectrodes are considerably higher than expected from the electrical PD and Donnan equilibrium, indicating either active H^+ movement out of the cell or HCO_3^- movement into the cell; furthermore, this relation shows that there is an electrochemical driving force for extrusion of bicarbonate out of the cell, which could participate in the transfer of bicarbonate from cell to interstitium.

III. MICROPUNCTURE TECHNIQUES FOR THE STUDY OF BICARBONATE REABSORPTION

A. Cortical Free-Flow Collections: Fractional Bicarbonate Reabsorption Along the Nephron

Bicarbonate reabsorption along the nephron can be studied by collection of tubular fluid samples, equilibration of these samples with mineral oil at a known pCO_2, and measurement of their pH and inulin concentration. Fractional reabsorption can be obtained relating bicarbonate TF/P with inulin TF/P ratios in different nephron segments. Gottschalk *et al.* (1960) measured equilibrium pH in the proximal tubule by means of quinhydrone microelectrodes and showed a progressive decline of these values along the studied segment (see Figure 5). These data demonstrated an extensive reabsorption of bicarbonate along the proximal tubule in the presence of a fractional volume reabsorption of about two thirds of the filtered load; they were confirmed by Giebisch *et al.* (1960) and by Clapp *et al.* (1963a). Giebisch *et al.* (1960) observed that this fall in pH was markedly enhanced during respiratory acidosis. Studies on the dog by Clapp *et al.* (1963b) and by Bernstein and Clapp (1968), on the other hand, demonstrated that proximal tubular bicarbonate concentrations were only slightly or not at all reduced below plasma values, suggesting that in these animals acidification did not start until the distal tubules, where significant reductions in bicarbonate concentrations were found. These authors showed, however, that the proximal

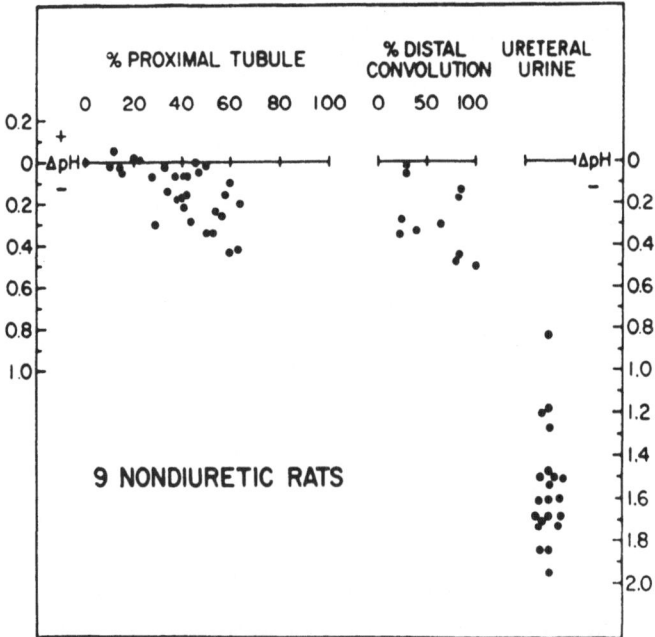

Figure 5. Acidification in rat cortical nephron as measured by microquinhydrone electrodes. pH differences with respect to blood are given. (From Gottschalk *et al.*, 1960).

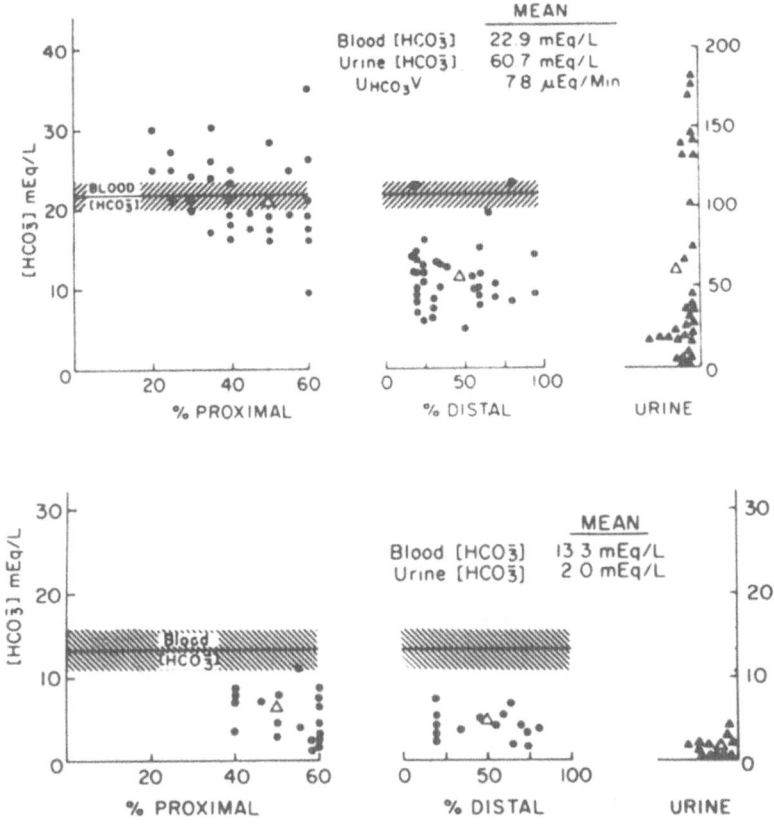

Figure 6. Bicarbonate concentrations in dog cortical nephrons, measured by microquinhydrone electrodes. Upper diagram, control dog. Lower diagram, dog submitted to NH₄Cl acidosis. (From Bernstein and Clapp, 1968).

tubule of the dog is capable of acidifying the urine when the animal is subjected to metabolic acidosis by administration of ammonium chloride (see Figure 6).

In situ determinations of proximal tubular pH by means of the glass microelectrode by Rector *et al.* (1965) have likewise shown significant acidification along the proximal tubule of the rat, as have studies by antimony microelectrodes from our laboratory (Vieira and Malnic, 1968). The latter studies have, however, failed to show the progressive fall in pH characteristic of the measurements with quinhydrone microelectrodes. This might be due to the presence of a disequilibrium pH in early segments of the proximal tubule because of disequilibrium concentrations of either CO_2 or H_2CO_3. Such a phenomenon would lead to lower pH values in early proximal tubular segments than found by quinhydrone microelectrodes; the higher bicarbonate concentrations found at this site could support a higher rate of bicarbonate reabsorption, leading to higher pCO_2 and/or H_2CO_3 concentrations. Such an explanation is supported by the data of Karlmark and Davidson (1974) who found a marked decrease of bicarbonate concentrations along the proximal tubule, while *in situ* pH variation along this segment was much less evident. At the same time, they found an acid disequilibrium pH in early proximal samples which was ascribed to an elevated pCO_2.

Bicarbonate concentrations as well as fractional reabsorption of this ion along the nephron have been studied in a variety of experimental situations. Table I shows bicarbonate concentrations in plasma, proximal and distal tubular fluid, and in final urine in rats undergoing different alterations of acid–base equilibrium. In control conditions, the lowest bicarbonate concentrations are found in the final urine, indicating an important role of the collecting duct in acidifying the urine. This function, in spite of its relevance in terms of the

Table I. Bicarbonate Concentrations along the Nephron in Different Experimental Conditions (mM)

Experiment	Plasma	Proximal	Distal	Urine	El.[a]	Reference[b]
Rat						
Control	26.6	7.5	—	—	Q	1
	26.3	7.9	5.8	—	Q	2
	25.7	8.4	6.3,8.1	3.9	Sb	3, 4
	26.0	5.04	—	—	Sb	5
	28.0	14	—	—	G	6
	23.3	12–4	—	—	Sb	7
Resp. acidosis	31.3	9.7	—	—	G	8
	27.4	15.1	5.8	9.4	Sb	4
Metab. acidosis	9.6	3.7	3.4	1.4	Sb	4
	15.0	3.3	—	—	G	6
Resp. alkalosis	18.0	16.5	10.7	10.4	Sb	4
Metab. alkalosis	38.5	57.8	—	200	Q	1
	34.4	25.1	—	—	Q	10
	45.2	34.6	57.3	252	Sb	4, 9
Low Cl, K	38.7	17.4	5.7	—	Q	2
	40.6	35.5	33.0	46.3	Sb	9
Low K	37.2	17.8	2.0	1.0	Q	1
	34.6	14.3	—	—	Q	10
Diamox	28.5	26.6	74.0	—	Sb	3
Benzolamide	21.6	17.0	—	—	Sb	5
Dog						
Control	22.9	21.1	11.5	60.7	Q	11
Metab. acidosis	13.3	5.3	4.4	2.0	Q	11
Metab. alkalosis	27.5	45.9	28.6	108.6	Q	11

[a] Electrodes: Q, quinhydrone; G, glass; Sb, antimony.
[b] References: 1 Rector *et al.* (1964); 2, Bank and Aynedjian (1965); 3, Vieira and Malnic (1968); 4, Malnic *et al.* (1972a); 5, Kunau (1972); 6, Levine and Nash (1973); 7, Karlmark and Davidson (1974); 8, Levine (1971); 9, Mello Aires and Malnic (1972); 10, Kunau *et al.* (1968); 11, Bernstein and Clapp (1968).

transepithelial concentration gradients produced, is of lesser importance with respect to the absolute amount of bicarbonate reabsorbed, since the volume reaching this segment is only a small fraction of the filtered load. Direct studies on the collecting duct have confirmed its participation in the acidifying process (Ullrich and Eigler, 1958).

As shown on Table I, respiratory acidosis leads to somewhat increased proximal, but reduced distal, bicarbonate concentrations. In Table II, fractional bicarbonate reabsorption along the nephron in the same experimental groups is summarized. Bicarbonate reabsorption is not very markedly affected by respiratory acidosis in control rats. However, the data of Levine (1971) and of Malnic *et al.* (1972a) show that after moderate bicarbonate loading, an enhancement of proximal and distal bicarbonate reabsorption may become apparent. During respiratory alkalosis (hyperventilation), on the other hand, both conventional free-flow collections, as listed in Tables I and II, as well as recollection micropuncture experiments (Malnic *et al.*, 1972a) showed considerable increases in tubular bicarbonate concentrations and reductions in fractional segmental reabsorption. During acute metabolic alkalosis, bicarbonate levels are likewise increased along the nephron, but to a considerably greater extent, reaching higher levels in the distal tubule than in plasma. In hypochloremic alkalosis, where in spite of the alkalosis a large fraction of the filtered bicarbonate is reabsorbed, and the alteration of the acid–base derangement can only be corrected by chloride administration (Atkins and Schwartz, 1962), proximal reabsorption is lower than in controls, but is largely compensated by an increase in reabsorption up to the early distal tubule, probably along the straight descending section of the proximal tubule. Reabsorption along more distal segments is also increased; final urinary bicarbonate elimination is higher than in

Table II. Bicarbonate Reabsorption along the Nephron (% of Filtered Load)

Group	Filtered load (μmol/min/kg)	Reabsorption (%)					Ref.[a]
		Proximal	Loop	Distal	Collecting Duct	Total	
Control	215	86.5	1.9	8.9	2.4	99.68	1
	233	86.3	—	—	—	—	2
	230	68	—	—	—	—	3
Resp. acidosis	191	72.7	20.7	4.1	2.3	99.78	1
Metab. acidosis	51	85.5	5.3	4.1	4.7	99.64	1
	81	85.0	—	—	—	—	3
Resp. alkalosis	153	61.0	17.3	11.4	8.4	98.13	1
Metab. alkalosis	212	55.0	7.6	18.0	—	77.5	4
Low Cl, K	216	61.1	18.1	10.8	5.9	96.1	4
Diamox	120	41.0	0.04	34.0	17.6	92.6	5
Benzolamide	180	48.7	—	—	—	—	2

[a] References: 1, Malnic *et al.* (1972a); 2, Kunau (1972); 3, Levine and Nash (1973); 4, Mello Aires and Malnic (1972); 5, Vieira and Malnic (1968).

controls, but markedly lower than that found during acute alkalosis at similar filtered loads, explaining the bicarbonate retention characteristic of this experimental situation (Mello Aires and Malnic, 1972).

Another experimental situation leading to marked increases in renal tubular bicarbonate concentrations, as well as enhanced overall excretion of this ion, is that following the administration of a carbonic anhydrase inhibitor, like acetazolamide (Clapp *et al.*, 1963a; Vieira and Malnic, 1968) or benzolamide (Rector *et al.*, 1965; Kunau, 1972). A more detailed discussion about the mechanisms involved in the inhibition of bicarbonate reabsorption by these drugs will be given below.

In Tables I and II data referring to bicarbonate reabsorption in conditions of metabolic acidosis are also given. Very low bicarbonate concentrations are found along the nephron, but overall fractional bicarbonate excretion is not much different from controls leading, however, to a low rate of excretion of this ion due to its considerably reduced filtered load. Thus, absolute reabsorption rates are decreased in all nephron segments. Levine and Nash (1973) have shown that this decreased reabsorptive rate is not due only to the low segmental load, but also, at least in the proximal tubule, to a decreased reabsorptive capacity, since chronically acidotic rats with an acute compensation of plasma bicarbonate levels by bicarbonate infusion still showed significantly reduced fractional bicarbonate reabsorption in this tubular segment with respect to controls.

Several studies of bicarbonate reabsorption in proximal tubule of potassium-deficient rats are available (Rector *et al.*, 1964; Bank and Aynedjian, 1965; Kunau *et al.*, 1968). Late proximal bicarbonate concentrations are in general equal to or higher than in control rats (see Table I). However, when rats at similar plasma bicarbonate levels, obtained by venous bicarbonate infusion, are compared to the depleted animals, it was shown that the latter are able to reduce proximal bicarbonate concentrations to a greater extent (for instance, to 8.2 mEq/liter against 22.0 in alkalotic controls, as found by Kunau *et al.*, 1968) than non-potassium-depleted alkalotic controls. This finding has led to the view that the alkalosis of hypokalemia is due to an enhanced bicarbonate reabsorption especially along the proximal tubule. The stimulation of bicarbonate reabsorption, on the other hand, has been ascribed to increased H^+ ion secretion consequent to the intracellular acidosis characteristic of the states of potassium depletion (Adler *et al.*, 1972).

B. Bicarbonate in the Renal Medulla

Relatively little is known about the acidification occurring in the medullary segments of the nephron. The collecting duct is the segment capable of establishing the highest H^+ ion gradients along the nephron, since cortical distal tubules rarely show an *in situ* pH lower than 6, while final urine can reach values as low as 4.5. Ullrich and Eigler (1958) have shown that the papillary collecting duct is able to contribute to urinary acidification, the pH of fluid collected at different levels showing progressively lower values toward the papillary tip.

Uhlich *et al.* (1968) measured the pH of vasa recta and collecting ducts by means of capillary glass microelectrodes, and calculated bicarbonate concentrations and pCO_2 values from these measurements (see p. 14). They found that bicarbonate in vasa recta did not differ from arterial blood in control conditions, suggesting that this ion did not normally participate in the concentrating mechanism of the renal papilla. Vasa recta bicarbonate increased only after considerable elevations of collecting duct bicarbonate concentrations resulting from bicarbonate loading or acetazolamide administration. On the other hand, the pCO_2 calculated from their pH measurements, which are performed at chemical equilibrium, was about 10 mm Hg higher than arterial pCO_2. This difference increased after bicarbonate loading and acetazolamide administration in both vasa recta and collecting ducts and was abolished after carbonic anhydrase infusion, suggesting that a disequilibrium concentration of CO_2 may be generated at this site, probably by H^+ ion secretion along the collecting ducts.

C. Stopped-Flow Microperfusion: A Kinetic Approach

The development by Gertz (1963) of the split-droplet method to measure the sodium-reabsorbing capacity of the tubular epithelium independently of the filtered load of this ion brought considerable progress to the knowledge about the mechanisms and characteristics of sodium and water transport in this structure. We have tried to apply a related method for the evaluation of the acidifying capacity of the tubular wall, isolating between castor oil columns a droplet of fluid containing an alkaline buffer, for instance sodium bicarbonate, in variable proportions with sodium chloride, at a total sodium concentration near the equilibrium level for this ion (approx. 100 m*M*) and adding raffinose to maintain isotonicity and to reduce the rate of volume reabsorption. As shown in Figure 4, an antimony microelectrode is impaled in the fluid column, permitting one to record pH changes during this perfusion (Malnic and Mello Aires, 1971). In Figure 7 a schematic drawing of a curve obtained by this method is shown. First the luminal free-flow pH is recorded; upon start of the perfusion, the detected pH rises to alkaline levels, but as soon as the fluid column is blocked by injection of oil, acidification starts and tends progressively to the luminal equilibrium pH. The portion of the curve obtained after blocking the fluid column is used to calculate bicarbonate concentration changes during the process of tubular acidification. This is done assuming equilibrium with the animal's pCO_2, using the measured pH and applying the Henderson–Hasselbalch equation. When air-equilibrated solutions are injected into the tubular lumen, only the later parts of the curve are actually equilibrated with the animal's pCO_2. The corresponding points fall on a straight line, corresponding in this semilogarithmic plot to an exponential decline of bicarbonate concentrations. The first portion of the graph shows a deviation of the calculated bicarbonate concentrations from this exponential; these concentrations are artifactually high due to the lower pCO_2 of the perfusate at this time. However, using the pH values and the actual bicarbonate concentrations, assumed to fall on the line extrapolated to zero along the exponential of the later points, the

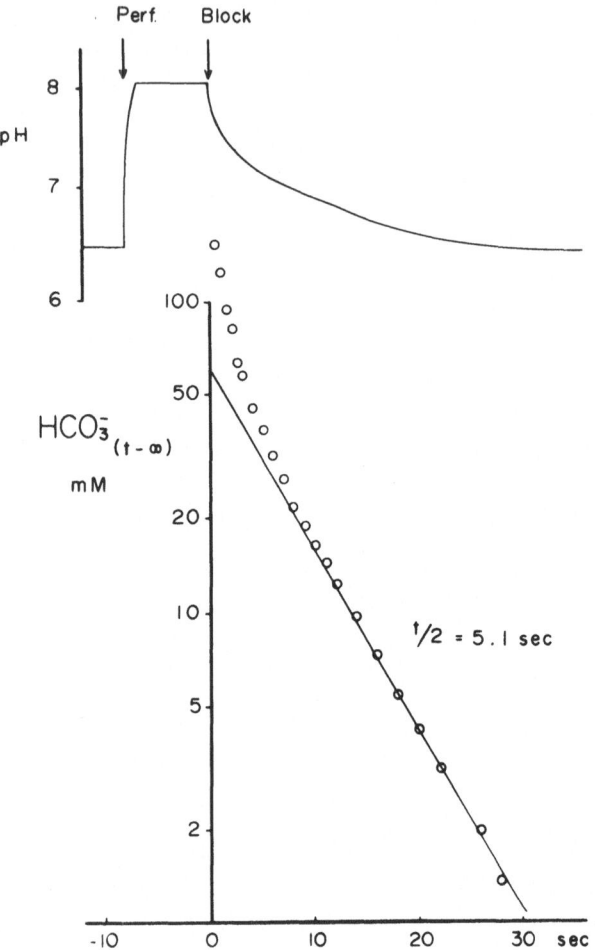

Figure 7. Acidification during stopped-flow microperfusion with 100 mM NaHCO$_3$/100 mM raffinose solution. Upper drawing, record of pH changes during perfusion, measured with antimony microelectrode. Lower graph, bicarbonate concentrations calculated from luminal pH and the rat's pCO$_2$, plotted against time in seconds. (From Malnic *et al.*, 1974.)

instantaneous carbonic acid concentrations can be calculated. Their approach to the steady-state level, supposedly equal to plasma H$_2$CO$_3$, is a measure of the rate of equilibration of the injected perfusate with blood pCO$_2$. This rate has a half-time of 0.5–1.5 sec (Malnic and Mello Aires, 1971). It can be shown that these rates of equilibration are about one order of magnitude slower than the uncatalyzed rate of formation of H$_2$CO$_3$ from CO$_2$, indicating that they probably depend on the permeability of the tubular wall to CO$_2$ and not on the hydration of CO$_2$ after its diffusion into the lumen. An interesting observation is the considerable delay of this equilibration after administration of acetazolamide, when half-times increase to about 4 sec, indicating that carbonic anhydrase may participate in the diffusion of CO$_2$ across the tubular epithelium. This is not unexpected, since *in vitro* experiments have shown that the presence of protein molecules (hemoglobin, albumin), in spite of presenting an additional resistance to CO_2 diffusion, may facilitate this process (Gros and Moll, 1971, 1974); furthermore, the presence of carbonic anhydrase was shown to facilitate CO_2 transfer across thin fluid layers, an effect which is reversed by acetazolamide (Enns, 1967; Gros and Moll, 1974).

The participation of CO_2 equilibration during the first seconds of perfusion in the described microperfusion experiments (see Figure 7) is supported by the finding of a single exponential for bicarbonate concentrations from the start of the perfusion when these solutions are preequilibrated at a pCO_2 similar to that of the experimental animal. On the other hand, an inverse deviation of the points of this first phase is found when the perfusate is preequilibrated at a pCO_2 higher than that of blood.

The slower fall in bicarbonate concentrations found after completion of the CO_2 equilibration period appears to be related to the process of bicarbonate reabsorption. The half-times for this reabsorption, of the order of 4–5 sec, are of the same order of magnitude when the perfusate is made up of 25 mM $NaHCO_3$/ 75 mM NaCl or of 100 mM $NaHCO_3$, suggesting that passive diffusion of $NaHCO_3$ out of the tubule should not be of major importance for this reabsorptive process (Malnic and Mello Aires, 1971). The exponential fall in bicarbonate concentrations suggests a direct proportionality between the rate of bicarbonate reabsorption and the luminal concentration:

$$- \frac{d[HCO_3]}{dt} = k([HCO_3]_t - [HCO_3]_\infty) \qquad (16)$$

where k is a rate coefficient and the effective bicarbonate concentration that drives the reabsorption is the difference between the instantaneous (t) concentration and the steady-state level (∞).

If acidification is viewed solely as an H^+ ion secretory process, the following two-compartment analysis can be applied (Malnic and Giebisch, 1972):

$$\frac{dS_1}{dt} = -k_{12}S_1 + k_{21}S_2 \qquad (17)$$

where S_1 is the luminal H^+ ion content, S_2 the cellular (or extraluminal) H^+ ion content, and k_{12} and k_{21} are rate coefficients for H^+ ion transfer between these compartments. Assuming that acid flow into the lumen depends only on the conditions of the cellular compartment (S_2), being constant during a given perfusion, Eq. (17) can be solved yielding

$$S_1 = S_{1\infty} - S_{1\infty}e^{-k_{12}t} \qquad (18)$$

According to this relation, the rate of change of S_1 depends essentially on k_{12}, the rate coefficient for passive flow of H from lumen to the extraluminal space, a parameter therefore related to tubular H^+ ion permeability (Malnic et al., 1976).

Another form of viewing the kinetics of bicarbonate reabsorption would be to consider only bicarbonate movements, whatever their actual mechanism. If B_1

is the luminal bicarbonate concentration and B_2 that in an extraluminal compartment, the following analysis could be made:

$$\frac{dB_1}{dt} = -k'_{12}B_1 - (k''_{12}B_1 - k_{21}B_2) \tag{20}$$

where k'_{12} is a rate coefficient related to active bicarbonate transport from 1 to 2, whatever its mechanism, k''_{12} is the coefficient describing passive flow of bicarbonate from 1 to 2, and k_{21} describes passive flow from 2 to 1, implying that $k_{21}B_2$ is constant. This equation leads to the following relation:

$$B_1 - B_{1\,\infty} = (B_{1\,0} - B_{1\,\infty})e^{-k_{12}t} \tag{21}$$

where $k_{12} = k'_{12} + k''_{12}$, that is, the experimentally measured rate coefficient is a composite of active and passive coefficients, probably with a marked predominance of that related to the active movement, since there are electrophysiological and other lines of evidence that passive permeability of the tubular epithelium to bicarbonate ions is finite, but low (Bank and Aynedjian, 1967; Froemter et al., 1971; Boulpaep and Seely, 1971). This coefficient may therefore be related to bicarbonate transport as such, or to H ion secretion, or to both. This treatment would imply, in opposition to the previous one, that the active transport rate should be variable and proportional to the luminal bicarbonate concentration or that the rate of H^+ ion secretion should be proportional to the gradient against which it proceeds.

Equation (16) gives, when adjusted for the geometrical situation in the renal tubule, the net flux across the tubular epithelium. When the luminal bicarbonate concentration varies with time, this flux will also vary, and reabsorptive flow of bicarbonate will be maximal at $t = 0$, the time at which a high concentration of this ion is introduced into the tubular lumen. The flux at this time is probably much greater than that due to passive back-flux, as indicated above, being thus an approximation of the unidirectional outflux of bicarbonate. It is given by the following relation:

$$\Phi_{HCO_3} = k_{12}([HCO_3^-]_0 - [HCO_3^-]_\infty)\frac{r}{2} \tag{22}$$

where r is the tubular radius. This flux is given in nEq/sec/cm² tubular wall.

In Table III, kinetic data relating to bicarbonate reabsorption are given for several experimental situations. Steady-state pH and bicarbonate concentrations, rate coefficients, bicarbonate disappearance half-times (= ln $2/k$), and maximal ($t = 0$) bicarbonate reabsorptive fluxes are shown, for proximal and distal tubules. In control rats, proximal reabsorption of bicarbonate at the employed tubular concentration of 100 mM is of the order of that for sodium (9 nEq/sec cm², according to Gertz, 1963). Bicarbonate reabsorption is depressed under the present stopped-flow microperfusion conditions in acetazolamide-infused animals because of both a reduced rate coefficient and a higher steady-state bicarbonate concentration, indicating a reduced capacity to maintain

Table III. Parameters of Kinetic Analysis of Bicarbonate Reabsorption in Microperfusion Experiments during Different Experimental Conditions[a]

Experiment	Location[b]	pH_∞	$HCO_{3\infty}^-$ (mM)	$t^{1/2}$ (sec)	k_{12} (sec^{-1})	$\Phi\ HCO_3^-$ (nmol/ cm^2/sec)
Control	P	6.21	1.73	5.2	0.135	9.92
	E D	6.95	11.6	3.8	0.183	10.1
	L D	6.60	4.44	5.0	0.139	8.31
Diamox	P	6.83	7.10	8.1	0.085	5.95
	E D	6.85	10.8	25.8	0.027	1.50
	L D	6.93	10.6	17.9	0.039	2.16
15% CO_2	P	5.83	1.61	3.5	0.198	14.7
	E D	6.44	7.05	22.4	0.031	1.82
	L D	6.07	2.98	18.7	0.037	2.26
Metab. acidosis	P	5.92	0.54	9.5	0.073	5.45
	E D	6.15	0.90	18.9	0.037	2.27
	L D	6.20	1.22	12.8	0.054	3.34
Metab. acidosis + Diamox	P	6.42	2.10	17.9	0.039	2.84
	E D	6.30	1.71	29.9	0.023	1.42
	L D	6.18	1.44	18.2	0.038	2.35

[a] Data from Malnic and Mello Aires (1971), Mello Aires and Malnic (1975), Malnic *et al.* (1976).
[b] P: proximal; E D: early distal; L D: late distal. For explanation of parameters, see text.

bicarbonate concentration gradients, and a slower rate of attainment of these gradients, both in proximal and distal tubule.

In respiratory acidosis by breathing of 15% CO_2, proximal bicarbonate reabsorption is enhanced mostly due to an increase in the rate coefficient. In the distal tubule bicarbonate reabsorptive rates are depressed but maximal attainable gradients are maintained or even higher than in controls, suggesting, as in metabolic acidosis, a lowered permeability of distal tubular wall to H^+ ions. These findings are compatible with a mainly proximal effect of high CO_2, establishing high pH and HCO_3^- gradients that are maintained in the distal tubule due to its lowered permeability to acid, that is, to H and/or buffer anions.

In metabolic acidosis, the established gradients are even higher than in controls, but the rate coefficients are lower. This indicates that at lower net reabsorptive rates of bicarbonate, higher pH and bicarbonate gradients can be established, suggesting the occurrence of lower passive permeabilities to H ions in this group.

It is well known that the effect of acetazolamide on bicarbonate excretion is considerably impaired in acidotic animals, but that a significant effect on titratable acidity is still found after phosphate loading (Maren, 1956; Brodsky and Satran, 1959). In the present microperfusion experiments, however, not only phosphate, but also bicarbonate reabsorption, is reduced with respect to the acidotic controls in both proximal and distal tubules when acetazolamide is given to these rats. This finding may indicate that the described absence of a bicarbonate effect of carbonic anhydrase inhibition could be related to the marked fall of buffer load to these tubular segments, while after phosphate loading the buffer load is markedly enhanced, sustaining a sizable rate of H^+ ion secretion, which is in part dependent on the catalytic process.

IV. THE MECHANISM OF BICARBONATE REABSORPTION

A. Bicarbonate Reabsorption

1. Studies in the Mammalian Kidney

As discussed above, it is not easy to distinguish acidification by reabsorption of bicarbonate ions as such from that effected by H^+ ion secretion. The work of Pitts and Alexander (1945) had shown the necessity for H ion secretion along the nephron to explain acidification in phosphate loaded dogs. This finding, however, does not exclude the possibility that, besides H^+ ion secretion, a fraction of the filtered bicarbonate might be reabsorbed by a more or less specific anion transport pathway. The evidence favoring bicarbonate reabsorption as such comes in part from pharmacological studies in the mammalian kidney, from studies on acidification in fish kidney, and from experiments in isolated acidifying membranes *in vitro* like the turtle bladder. The experiments in dog kidney are well summarized by Maren (1967, 1969). His argument is based essentially on the effect of potent carbonic anhydrase inhibitors, like acetazolamide, benzolamide (CL 11,366), ethoxzolamide, and methazolamide on renal bicarbonate excretion, assuming practically total inhibition of the catalyzing action of carbonic anhydrase. Since the administration of these drugs only leads to the reduction of bicarbonate reabsorption by some 30–40%, it is believed that the remainder of the reabsorption of bicarbonate is not related to renal cellular H ion formation catalyzed by carbonic anhydrase, but to uncatalyzed H ion generation and to bicarbonate reabsorption as such.

Experimental results and related calculations obtained by Maren (1967) in the dog by clearance methods are shown in Table IV. It can be noted that in control dogs about 67% of bicarbonate reabsorption is attributed to a H_2O/CO_2 independent system, that is, to bicarbonate transport as such. The latter quantity is calculated from the difference between total acidification, (bicarbonate reabsorption plus titratable acid formation plus ammonia excretion) minus the catalyzed and uncatalyzed H ion secretion. The total acidification is an experimental quantity; catalyzed H ion secretion is obtained from the difference between acidification in control and acetazolamide-treated animals. Uncatalyzed H ion secretion, on the other hand, was not obtained from data in animal experiments, but evaluated from the kinetics of the CO_2 hydration reaction *in vitro*. The rate coefficient k_1 of the reaction given in Eq. (2) can be used when

Table IV. Bicarbonate Reabsorption in Dog Kidney: Data Calculated from Clearance Experiments[a]

	Tubular acidification[b]		
	μmol/min	mmol/liter/sec	Total (%)
1. Filtered HCO_3^-	800	1.34	
2. Reabsorbed, control	800	1.34	
3. Reabsorbed, Diamox	650	1.08	
4. TA + NH_4^+, control[c]	20	0.03	
5. TA + NH_4^+, Diamox[c]	0	0	
6. Total, HCO_3^- + H^-	820	1.37	100
7. V_{unc}	100	0.17	12
8. V_{cat}	170	0.28	21
9. Remainder[d]	550	0.92	67

[a] Data from Maren (1967); second column recalculated considering a tubular fluid volume of 10 ml/dog, rendering the data comparable to those of Table VI.
[b] Tubular acidification in μmol/min/dog, or mmol/sec/liter tubular fluid.
[c] TA: titratable acidity.
[d] Remainder: bicarbonate reabsorption outside $CO_2 - H^+$ system: 9 = 6 − (7 + 8).

the adequate volume adjustments are made. Maren (1967) used a k_1 rate coefficient of 0.045 sec^{-1} and a tubular cellular volume of 30 ml:

$$V_{unc_1} = k_1 \times \text{Vol} \times (CO_2)$$
$$= 0.045 \times 60 \text{ min}^{-1} \times 0.030 \text{ liter} \times 1.2 \text{ m}M \cong 100 \ \mu\text{mol/min} \quad (23)$$

However, more recent data on the mechanism of the catalysis effected by carbonic anhydrase indicate that the reaction

$$CO_2 + OH^- \underset{k_{-2}}{\overset{k_2}{\rightleftharpoons}} HCO_3^- \quad (24)$$

might actually be the catalyzed step, since there is evidence that carbonic anhydrase has a site for OH^-, which reacts directly with CO_2 giving HCO_3^- (Davis, 1958; Kernohan, 1964; Maren, 1974). The dissociation of water by a redox pump, probably at the luminal cell membrane, would lead to the extrusion of H^+ toward the tubular lumen, and to accumulation of OH^- at the cellular surface of the membrane. In this way, a sufficiently alkaline medium would be available for this reaction to proceed, since it predominates over the hydration of CO_2 only at a pH of above 10; between pH 8 and 10 both mechanisms are important (Kern, 1960). The second-order rate constant, k_2, is of the order of 20,000 M^{-1} sec^{-1} at 37°C (Sirs, 1958; Maren, 1974). Thus, the uncatalyzed rate would be

$$V_{unc_2} = k_2(CO_2)(OH^-) = 20,000 \times 1.2 \times 10^{-5} = 0.24 \text{ mmol/liter/sec} \quad (25)$$

Here, a 10^{-5} M concentration of OH^- is assumed. This assumption, of course, is based on the amount of H^+ ions which is supposed to be secreted, every H^+ ion corresponding to an OH^- ion added to the cellular side of the luminal membrane.

As a first approximation, it could be assumed that an effective OH^- concentration similar to luminal H^+ ion concentration, volume by volume, should exist in the cell. This, of course, would depend on the buffering capacity of both media; the concentration would be equal only if also the respective buffering capacity should be equivalent; this assumption is obviously not warranted. Using a volume of 10 ml of tubular fluid in the kidneys of a dog, the volume assumed to correspond to the OH^- concentration of 10^{-5} M, Maren (1974) obtained a rate of V_{unc} of 144 μmol/min, which is not far from the value given in Table IV. These considerations indicate very clearly that an evaluation of the absolute rate of V_{unc} is prone to several uncertainties and depends on a number of assumptions related to the reactions of greatest importance for the generation of H^+ or the neutralization of OH^-: the volume of the compartments partaking in these reactions; the buffer capacity of the same compartments, leading to the final H^+ or OH^- concentrations; the intracellular or subcellular CO_2 concentration relevant to these reactions; and the accepted values for the rate coefficients under the actual experimental conditions.

2. Studies in Fish Kidney

Renal function of sea-water fish has contributed some interesting information on mechanisms of urinary acidification. Elasmobranchs of the genus *Squalus* and *Raja* have a rather fixed urinary pH of the order of 5.8 (Smith, 1939). On the other hand, no renal carbonic anhydrase was detected in dogfish (*Squalus acanthias*) kidney by Hodler *et al.* (1955). According to Maren (1974), total acidification of this fish is much lower than that found in mammals, the sum of bicarbonate reabsorption and acid excretion being of the order of 3 μmol/min, while V_{unc} in this species may be of the order of half of this value. However, as was shown by Boylan *et al.* (1973), bicarbonate infusion can raise bicarbonate reabsorption in a practically unlimited way, maintaining the same low urinary pH in spite of the bicarbonate loading which may lead to an overall reabsorptive rate of up to 25 μmol/min. According to the above argument, this additional reabsorptive capacity should be ascribed to bicarbonate transport as such. A recent paper by Deetjen and Maren (1973) discusses microperfusion experiments in *Raja* measuring rates of acidification by timing the color change of bromcresol purple (BCP), an indicator which changes color from dark purple (alkaline) to yellow (acid) with a pK of 6.2. They observed that the rate of acidification using BCP as buffer was constant at different buffer concentrations, that is, at increasing buffer concentrations the time for color change increased. The same happened when phosphate buffer was added to the perfusate; however, the addition of 5–12 mM $NaHCO_3$ to the original 1 mM BCP did not lead to significant changes in the time for color change, indicating that the rate of bicarbonate reabsorption was much faster than the simultaneously occurring rate of acidification of BCP. This finding suggested that bicarbonate was reabsorbed by a different mechanism than H^+ ion secretion in this species, probably by anionic bicarbonate transport. Maren (1967, 1974) suggests that this mechanism is phylogenetically older and the most important one in lower vertebrates, where a less flexible acidification mechanism with fixed acid urine pH is prevalent. In mammals, where renal carbonic anhydrase is abundant, the more flexible H^+ ion secretory mechanism, which may permit larger variation in urinary acidification, attains importance at the side of the more primitive mechanism.

3. Competition with Other Anions

There is some evidence that under certain experimental conditions there may occur some degree of competition between bicarbonate and other anions. This has been described for maleate, which inhibits bicarbonate reabsorption in dog and rat (Gmaj et al., 1972). Maleate has no carbonic anhydrase-inhibiting activity and does not affect the transport of chloride. A relation studied quite extensively is that between phosphate and bicarbonate transport. It has been observed that metabolic alkalosis and bicarbonate loading inhibit phosphate reabsorption; this has been ascribed to the predominance of alkaline phosphate at an alkaline pH, a salt that appears to be less transported than the acid phosphate (Malvin and Lotspeich, 1956; Fulop and Brazeau, 1968; Bank et al., 1974). However, it was also observed that acetazolamide inhibits phosphate reabsorption (Fulop and Brazeau, 1968; Beck and Goldberg, 1973) and that this drug probably does not act by alkalizing the tubular fluid, since after its administration proximal tubular fluid presents a higher bicarbonate concentration, but its pH is in the normal range due to the considerable disequilibrium pH found under such conditions (Rector et al., 1965; Vieira and Malnic, 1968). Such findings suggest that phosphate transport in the proximal tubule might be impaired by competition with bicarbonate or, alternatively, that both predominance of alkaline phosphate and a direct effect of acetazolamide on phosphate transport might reduce reabsorption of this ionic species.

B. Hydrogen Ion Secretion

1. Evidence from Membranes Studied in Vitro

A recent review provides an extensive discussion of studies on acidification by the turtle bladder and other similar epithelia in vitro (Steinmetz, 1974). Such studies have provided a wealth of data, as yet not available from the mammalian kidney, which throw light on many aspects of the mechanisms of acidification in an epithelial structure. We are going to concentrate here mainly on the aspects significant for the problem of the mechanism of bicarbonate transport, that is, of bicarbonate reabsorption as such vs. H^+ ion secretion.

This argument was initially investigated by Schilb and Brodsky (1966, 1972) measuring pH and total CO_2 in mucosal and serosal medium of turtle bladder sacs, the latter by the manometric method, and calculating pCO_2 via the

Henderson–Hasselbalch equation. These authors found that the pCO_2 of the mucosal medium depended on the initial poise of the buffer system, but that under favorable conditions a lower mucosal than serosal pCO_2, compatible with anionic bicarbonate transport, could be demonstrated. However, Green *et al.* (1970) and Frazier and Vanatta (1972), using pCO_2 electrodes, showed that mucosal pCO_2 was consistently higher than serosal pCO_2 during the mucosal acidification process, even at relatively low mucosal and high serosal bicarbonate levels, a condition favoring the demonstration of mucosal pCO_2 changes according to Schilb and Brodsky (1972). A more thorough investigation of pCO_2 changes and of the role of metabolic CO_2 in the acidification process was performed by Schwartz *et al.* (1974) (see Table V).

Besides pCO_2 gradients, these authors studied the possibility of acidification in a bicarbonate- and CO_2-free medium due to metabolic CO_2 diffusion into a stationary layer on the mucosal surface of the bladder, where, with the catalysis of membrane-bound carbonic anhydrase, this molecule would be hydrated dissociating subsequently into H^+ and HCO_3^- ions. The latter would be reabsorbed, leaving the former to acidify the mucosal medium even in the absence of exogenous bicarbonate and CO_2. This mechanism, proposed by Menaker (1948) and by Brodsky and Schilb (1967), depends on an adequate

Table V. pCO_2 Gradients across Turtle Bladder *in Vitro* in Presence of High Rates of Mucosal Acidification[a]

Solution[b]	Initial pH	Final pH	Final − initial Δ pH	Final pCO_2 (mm Hg)	Δ pCO_2, M–S (mm Hg)
M	6.30	5.24	−1.06	57.1	4.2
S	7.18			52.9	
M	6.54	5.92	−0.62	55.8	2.9
S	7.20	.		52.9	
M	6.35	5.13	−1.22	59.1	6.3
S	7.20			52.8	
M	6.47	5.25	−1.22	57.8	7.6
S	7.18			50.2	
M	6.57	5.20	−1.37	74.2	23.6
S	7.20			50.6	
M	6.58	6.04	−0.54	64.4	14.1
S	7.17			50.3	
M	6.57	5.58	−0.99	56.3	6.0
S	7.18			50.3	
M	6.54	6.16	−0.38	60.8	10.3
S	7.15			50.5	
Mean ± S.E.		5.56	−0.92		9.4
		0.15	0.13		2.1
P					<0.01

[a] Taken from Schwartz *et al.* (1974).
[b] pCO_2 measurements performed by Severinghaus-type pCO_2 electrode. Mucosal (M) Ringer's solution: 4 mM HCO_3^-; Serosal (S) solution: 20 mM HCO_3^-, equilibrated with 7% CO_2 in O_2.

magnitude of metabolic CO_2 production, as well as on its diffusion from cell into the adjacent bathing media. Schwartz *et al.* (1974) showed that one third of the metabolic CO_2 appeared in the mucosal, and two thirds in the serosal medium. For the occurrence of mucosal acidification via diffusion of metabolic CO_2 and bicarbonate transport, a considerable rate of CO_2 transfer into the mucosal medium is necessary. Therefore, the serosal membrane should be considerably less permeable to CO_2 than the mucosal membrane, a proposition for which no evidence is available; this would not be necessary for the model of acidification based on H ion secretion.

Schwartz *et al.* (1974) also investigated the role of a hypothetic stationary layer in which the hydration of CO_2 could take place, measuring acidification in the presence and absence of vigorous stirring. Compatible with the H^+ secretion hypothesis, acidification increased after stirring, a procedure which should impair the reabsorption of bicarbonate formed in the vicinity of the mucosal border. Likewise, a poorly diffusible carbonic anhydrase inhibitor (CL 11,366) failed to inhibit acidification when added to the mucosal side and had a marked effect after addition to the serosal medium, showing that catalysis of CO_2 hydration in the mucosal compartment should not be of importance for the acidification mechanism in this preparation. Studies of this problem in rabbit gallbladder by Sullivan and Berndt (1973a,b) likewise showed that the metabolically produced CO_2 could not account for the observed rate of acidification by the bicarbonate transport mechanism.

The foregoing discussion suggests, therefore, that acidification by isolated epithelia *in vitro* most probably proceeds via H^+ ion secretion; however, the possibility that bicarbonate transport as such might participate in acidification of a minor fraction of the total observed rate cannot be eliminated on the basis of the analyzed evidence.

2. Evidence from Mammalian Kidney

As discussed above, the finding of a disequilibrium pH in distal tubule and in all studied segments after carbonic anhydrase inhibition has been taken as a major point of evidence in favor of tubular H^+ ion secretion (Rector *et al.*, 1965; Vieira and Malnic, 1968). Figure 8 shows the considerable magnitude of the difference between *in situ* and equilibrium pH as measured by means of antimony microelectrodes in proximal and distal tubules of acetazolamide-infused rats. This phenomenon is certainly a most definite indication of the existence of H^+ ion secretion by the tubular wall, more direct than the original evidence of Pitts and Alexander (1945) based on a greater excretion of acid phosphate in phosphate-loaded dogs, than could be explained by reabsorption of the alkaline salt. However, it does not by itself indicate that all bicarbonate reabsorption should proceed by this mechanism. On the basis of the kinetics of the uncatalyzed dehydration of carbonic acid, an attempt can be made to compare the observed luminal carbonic acid concentration to that expected on the basis of a decomposition of the filtered bicarbonate by the secreted H^+ ions. The actual luminal carbonic acid concentration can be calculated by means of

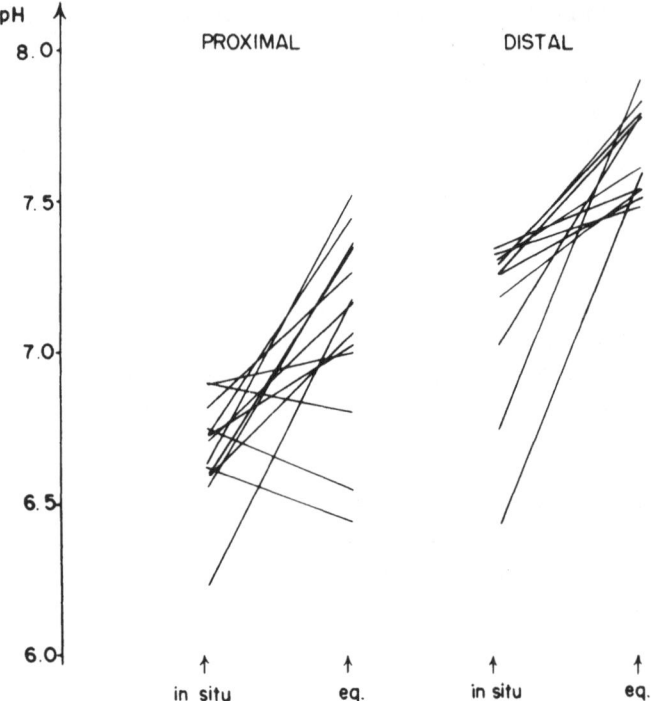

Figure 8. The acid disequilibrium pH in cortical tubules of the acetazolamide-infused rat. Ordinate, luminal pH. The disequilibrium pH is the difference between equilibrium and *in situ* pH. (From Vieira and Malnic, 1968).

the Henderson–Hasselbalch equation, using the pK for carbonic acid of 3.57, the luminal *in situ* pH, and the luminal bicarbonate concentration measured after collection of a sample of tubular fluid and its equilibration at a known pCO_2. A value of 25 μEq/liter is obtained in this way in proximal tubules of acetazolamide-treated rats (Vieira and Malnic, 1968). The carbonic acid concentration expected from the reaction of secreted H^+ ions with filtered bicarbonate can be calculated from Eq. (3):

$$[H_2CO_3] = \frac{\dot{V}_{H_2CO_3}}{k_{-1}} = \frac{\dot{V}_{HCO_3^-}}{k_{-1}} \tag{26}$$

The rate of dehydration of H_2CO_3 should be equal to that of bicarbonate reabsorption ($\dot{V}_{HCO_3^-}$) if all bicarbonate were reabsorbed by reaction with H^+ ions. A value of 46 μEq/min/kg can be used for proximal tubular bicarbonate reabsorption in the acetazolamide-infused rat (Vieira and Malnic, 1968), and a value of 49 sec^{-1} or 2940 min^{-1} for the dehydration rate coefficient (Garg and Maren, 1972). Assuming a proximal tubular volume of 1 ml/kg rat, we have

$$[H_2CO_3] = \frac{46 \ \mu\text{Eq/min/kg}}{1 \times 10^{-3} \ \text{liter/kg/2940/min}} = 15.7 \ \mu\text{Eq/liter}$$

Rector (1973), using a somewhat different method of calculation based on the same principles, obtained a value of the order of 20 μEq/liter. Considering the assumptions made for this calculation, these values are rather similar to the measured luminal carbonic acid concentration; thus, the magnitude of the luminal carbonic acid concentration, which is considerably higher than the plasma level (5 μEq/liter), suggests that a considerable proportion of bicarbonate reabsorption proceeds via H^+ ion secretion even after carbonic anhydrase inhibition. This view is compatible with the data of Rector *et al.* (1960), showing that bicarbonate reabsorption remains sensitive to blood pCO_2 after carbonic anhydrase inhibition. In spite of the fact that an increased blood CO_2 level could stimulate bicarbonate reabsorption as such by some unknown mechanism, this finding suggests that even after acetazolamide CO_2-mediated H^+ ion generation is important, although it still may not be exclusive.

Recent kinetic data obtained by the stopped-flow microperfusion technique may clarify some of these points. As summarized in Table VI, proximal tubules were perfused with bicarbonate-containing solutions, whereby the rate of bicarbonate reabsorption was evaluated independently of the filtered load. The tubules were also perfused with phosphate buffer-containing solutions; the rate of acidification of the latter perfusate provided a measurement of H^+ ion secretion (Malnic *et al.*, 1976). As explained above, the maximal net rate of acidification can be calculated at time zero, that is, after introduction of the alkaline perfusate into the tubular lumen. In Table VI, such rates are given in mmol/liter/sec (Malnic and Mello Aires, 1971; Malnic *et al.*, 1972b):

$$V_{H^+} = k_{H^+}(H_2PO_4^-)_\infty; \quad V_{HCO_3^-} = k_{HCO_3^-}[(HCO_3^-{}_0) - (HCO_3^-{}_\infty)] \quad (27)$$

where k_{H^+} and $k_{HCO_3^-}$ are the acidification rate coefficients measured during phosphate and bicarbonate microperfusion, respectively.

By this method, the overall rate of bicarbonate reabsorption is measured

Table VI. Mechanism of Proximal Tubular Acidification as Studied by Microperfusion Kinetics[a,b]

	Control		Metabolic acidosis	
Experiment	mmol/liter/sec	%	mmol/liter/sec	%
1. Total HCO_3^- reabsorbed	13.3	100	7.26	100
2. After Diamox	7.9	59.3	3.82	52.5
3. V_{unc}[c]	1.75	13.1	3.83	52.8
4. V_{cat} (1 − 2)	5.40	40.6	3.44	47.5
5. Remainder (2 − 3)	6.15	46.2	0	0
6. Total H^+ (3 + 4)	7.15	53.8	7.27	100

[a] Data from Malnic *et al.* (1976).
[b] HCO_3^- and H^+ flow rates in mM/liter tubular fluid/sec.
[c] V_{unc}: uncatalyzed H^+ ion generation and secretion, measured during phosphate perfusion in Diamox-treated rats.

during perfusion with 100 mM bicarbonate, that of H$^+$ ion secretion during perfusion with 100 mM alkaline phosphate. V_{cat}, bicarbonate reabsorption mediated by catalyzed H$^+$ ion generation is the difference between total HCO$_3^-$ reabsorption and that measured after carbonic anhydrase inhibition; V_{unc}, the noncatalyzed rate of H$^+$ ion generation, is evaluated by the rate of acidification of luminal phosphate buffer after inhibition of carbonic anhydrase by acetazolamide. Assuming that the observed rates of bicarbonate and H ion transport are limited under the described experimental conditions only by the inherent capacities of the respective transport and H$^+$ ion-generating systems, a comparison between these experimental rates may yield some information about the relative importance of H$^+$ ion secretion and ionic bicarbonate transport in the overall rate of bicarbonate reabsorption. Thus, subtracting the uncatalyzed rate of H$^+$ ion generation and secretion from the rate of bicarbonate reabsorption measured after acetazolamide administration, a fraction of the reabsorption of this ion is obtained which cannot be explained by H$^+$ ion secretion, possibly representing bicarbonate transport as such. As seen in Table VI, this fraction corresponds to 46% of the total proximal bicarbonate reabsorption in control rats, the remainder being mediated by H$^+$ ion secretion. However, this fraction may include an unspecified proportion of H$^+$ ion secretion due to carbonic acid recycling, as proposed by Rector (1973). According to this hypothesis, carbonic acid could return from lumen to cell by nonionic diffusion, especially after inhibition of carbonic anhydrase, where luminal carbonic acid concentration is enhanced. In the cell, this acid could dissociate, generating H$^+$ ions independently of catalysis by carbonic anhydrase. This process would increase item 2 of Table VI, participating therefore in item 5, the fraction of bicarbonate reabsorption apparently independent of H$^+$ ion secretion. The described methodology does not permit one to distinguish between bicarbonate transport as such and carbonic acid recirculation; both processes, however, are independent of *de novo* H$^+$ ion generation.

It is interesting to compare the proximal data obtained in control rats with those found in rats with chronic metabolic acidosis. In this case, the overall bicarbonate reabsorptive rate is decreased, but the uncatalyzed rate of H$^+$ ion generation appears to be elevated, being practically equal to the rate of bicarbonate reabsorption after carbonic anhydrase inhibition. Consequently, the portion of bicarbonate reabsorption entitled remainder in Table VI falls to zero, indicating that during metabolic acidosis H$^+$ ion generation may be sufficient to account for the entirety of bicarbonate reabsorption, which is reduced in absolute amounts not only in these microperfusion experiments, but also in free-flow conditions, since the filtered load of this ion is markedly reduced (Malnic *et al.*, 1972a; Levine and Nash, 1973). This reasoning, on the other hand, is no proof that H$^+$ ion generation independent bicarbonate reabsorption does not occur in metabolic acidosis, but only that it is not necessary to account for this reabsorption.

In the same way as discussed in the section on bicarbonate reabsorption as such, the possible rate of uncatalyzed H$^+$ ion generation can be calculated for tubular epithelium by means of the Eqs. (2) and (24), and the equations:

$$V_{unc\ 1} = k_1 \cdot CO_2 = 0.15\ sec^{-1} \times 1.35\ mM = 0.20\ mmol/liter/sec$$

and

$$V_{unc\ 2} = k_2 \cdot (CO_2) \cdot (OH^-)$$
$$= (20,000\ M^{-1} \cdot sec^{-1}) \cdot 1.35\ mM \cdot 10^{-5}\ M = 0.27\ mmol/liter/sec$$

The reaction involving CO_2 hydration (k_1) will participate in H^+ ion generation in the presence of an active H^+ ion pump from cell to lumen or of a CO_2 concentration gradient. These reactions would give a total V_{unc} of 0.47, which compares with the V_{unc} given in Table VI, measured in acetazolamide-treated rats undergoing tubular perfusion with phosphate buffer. As stressed above, these calculations involve several serious uncertainties, including the cellular OH^- concentration and the volume involved in these reactions. If it is assumed that the cell volume where these reactions occur is twice the tubular volume into which H^+ ions are secreted, the calculated V_{unc} can be doubled. Furthermore, if the contribution of H^+ ions from peritubular fluid to the cell H^+ ion pool is also considered (or, what is equivalent, a peritubular neutralization of OH^- ions generated in the cell is considered), the effective volume participating in the described reactions can still be increased. The latter possibility is supported by experiments in which the importance of peritubular pH for tubular H^+ ion secretion is shown, elevation of capillary pH to 8 practically abolishing acidification (Mello Aires and Malnic, 1975). These considerations indicate that the theoretically expected V_{unc} appears to be of the order of magnitude of the experimentally measured value in control animals. In metabolic acidosis, where the measured V_{unc} is considerably higher, an increased H^+ ion generation may be due to increased OH^- levels in the vicinity of the water-splitting membrane. The foregoing discussion shows that more precise experimental discrimination of the mechanisms involved in bicarbonate reabsorption is possible by means of micropuncture methodology, reaching some details that have hitherto been accessible only to theoretical speculation.

V. DRUGS AND BICARBONATE REABSORPTION

A. Carbonic Anhydrase Inhibitors

The chemistry and kinetic aspects of the interaction of carbonic anhydrase inhibitors with this enzyme have been expertly reviewed by Bar (1963) and Maren (1967, 1969). These studies have shown that at commonly used doses of the drug (about 5–20 mg/kg in the case of acetazolamide), inhibition of the enzyme is greater than 99.5%, leading to a maximal effect on processes related to carbonic anhydrase catalysis. There has been some argument as to the localization of carbonic anhydrase in kidney cells. Both chemical (Maren and Ellison, 1967) and histochemical studies (Haeusler, 1958; Loennerholm, 1971) have shown that the highest carbonic anhydrase concentration is found in cell cytoplasm or supernatant, especially in the proximal tubule, but also in the distal tubule. Haeusler (1958) as well as Leder (1967), Hansson (1968), and Loenner-holm (1971, 1973) have found carbonic anhydrase in proximal brush border, an enzyme fraction that has been thought to be involved in luminal carbonic acid dehydration (Rector *et al.*, 1965). However, doubts have been raised about the specificity of this histochemical detection of the enzyme in membrane fractions (Fand *et al.*, 1959; Muther, 1972). Randall and Maren (1972) have not been able to find carbonic anhydrase bound to red cell membranes, but Maren and Ellison (1967) have found a microsomal enzyme with different characteristics from that found in the supernatant in rat and dog kidney cells. The membrane-bound enzyme was shown to be less sensitive to drug inhibition than the supernatant one, but the authors indicated that in spite of this finding its inhibition should still be more than 99% at acetazolamide doses of 5 mg/kg. Based on these and other studies, Maren (1967) considers the possibility that some carbonic anhydrase escaping inhibition might be responsible for the residual bicarbonate reabsorption after drug administration highly unlikely.

In Table VII several characteristics of a number of sulfonamide carbonic anhydrase inhibitors are given. Enzyme inhibition is thought to occur by formation of a complex between enzyme (E) and inhibitor (I):

$$E_0 + I_0 \rightleftharpoons EI \rightleftharpoons E_f + I_f \qquad (28)$$

where E_0 is the tissue enzyme concentration before inhibition (about 10 μM in kidney cortex according to Maren, 1969), I_0 total tissue inhibitor concentration, EI the concentration of the complex, and E_f and I_f free enzyme and inhibitor concentrations. The dissociation of the complex will give

$$EI \rightleftharpoons E_f + I_f \qquad (29)$$

Table VII. Carbonic Anhydrase Inhibition by Different Sulfonamide Drugs: Dose for 50% Maximal Renal Effect[a]

Drug	K_I [b] ($M \times 10^7$)	k_d [c] (hr^{-1})	Dose for I_{50} [d] (mg/kg)	I_f [e] (μmol/kg)	i [f]
Sulfanilamide	57	42	1000	2300	0.9976
Acetazolamide	0.6	9	2	24	0.9975
Methazolamide	0.6	130	3	15	0.9960
Ethoxzolamide	0.02	>200	0.8	0.5	0.9960
Benzolamide (CL 11,366)	0.05	13	0.15	2	0.9975

[a] Data from Maren (1969).
[b] K_I: dissociation constant of enzyme–inhibitor complex.
[c] k_d: rate coefficient for diffusion from saline into dog red blood cell.
[d] I_{50}: drug concentration in tissue for 50% inhibition.
[e] I_f: free drug concentration in renal cortex.
[f] i: fractional inhibition of enzyme.

Thus, the dissociation constant of the complex will be given by

$$K_I = \frac{(E_f)\cdot(I_f)}{EI} = \frac{(E_0 - EI)(I_0 - EI)}{EI} \tag{30}$$

where $E_f = E_0 - EI$ and $I_f = I_0 - EI$.
The fractional inhibition of the enzyme will be

$$i = \frac{EI}{E_0}$$

Besides dissociation constants of the enzyme–inhibitor complex, Table VII shows rate coefficients for diffusion of the inhibitor from saline into dog red blood cells, which indicate that biological cell membranes are considerably less permeable to acetazolamide and benzolamide than to the other listed drugs. The table also gives drug doses necessary to obtain tissue concentrations leading to a 50% maximal renal effect (I_{50}), and the fractional enzyme inhibition obtained by such doses (i). In spite of the necessity for very different levels of these drugs to obtain a similar effect, the latter is achieved at a similar fractional inhibition of the enzyme. Below a fractional inhibition of about 0.99 practically no renal action is observed, while complete inhibition is found at a fractional inhibition of 0.9995–0.9998, which is achieved at a dose of 10–20 mg/kg in the dog.

The effect of carbonic anhydrase inhibition on the tubular reabsorption of bicarbonate was studied by a number of investigators in free-flow micropuncture experiments. Clapp *et al.* (1963a) found marked increases in pH, as measured by microquinhydrone electrodes, and bicarbonate concentrations in proximal tubule of the rat. They found TF/P ratios above 1 in most of their samples, obtaining values of up to 2.8 at a plasma bicarbonate level of 20–25 mM. Bernstein and Clapp (1968), studying the dog kidney, found a proximal mean bicarbonate of 28.8 mM after acetazolamide and a distal level of 31.9 mM, using similar methods. Vieira and Malnic (1968), using antimony microelectrodes, found, respectively, 26.6 and 74.0 mM bicarbonate in acetazolamide-infused rats. The fractional and absolute proximal tubular bicarbonate reabsorption is markedly depressed in the proximal tubule and in Henle's loop, as seen in Table II, while in the distal tubule and in collecting duct bicarbonate reabsorption is actually enhanced, probably due to the increased load reaching these segments.

Kunau (1972) studied the effect of benzolamide (CL 11,366) on the reabsorption of fluid and bicarbonate in proximal tubule of the rat and found marked increases in bicarbonate after administration of 2 and 20 mg/kg, reaching a mean level of 17 mM at the higher dosage. The drug had also a significant effect on proximal fluid reabsorption as evaluated by inulin TF/P ratios, which fell from about 2.5 to 1.5 after drug administration. Chloride TF/P ratios show a reciprocal behavior to bicarbonate; they fall from a ratio of 1.2–1.3 in controls to about 1.05 according the studies of Malnic *et al.* (1970) and Kunau (1972). Weinstein (1968), on the other hand, found greater reductions in chloride concentrations in rat proximal tubule after acetazolamide administration. According to his report, chloride TF/P ratios fell to 0.92, indicating a more marked increase in proximal bicarbonate concentrations in the rats.

Some aspects concerning the mechanism of action of carbonic anhydrase inhibition on renal tubular H^+ ion generation have been discussed above. The method of stopped-flow microperfusion of tubular segments with concomitant recording of pH changes was used to study alterations in the kinetics of bicarbonate reabsorption under the action of acetazolamide; examples of results obtained during perfusion of proximal and distal tubules are shown in Figure 9. In both tubular segments, steady-state pH and bicarbonate concentrations are significantly altered, bicarbonate concentrations rising from 3.5 mM in control proximal tubule to 7.1 mM after acetazolamide (Malnic and Mello Aires, 1971) and from 4.4 to 10.6 mM in late distal tubule. In early distal segments concentrations of 11–12 mM bicarbonate are found both in controls and after carbonic anhydrase inhibition (Malnic *et al.*, 1976). Besides these differences in steady-state concentrations, significant differences were found in the acidification half-times, as shown in Figure 9. In both proximal and distal tubule, these half-times are markedly increased, indicating that the steady-state pH levels are reached much slower than in controls. According to the described kinetics, this modification could be due to a decreased permeability of the tubular epithelium to H ions, or to a reduction in the bicarbonate transporting mechanism. Whatever the cause of the increased half-times, they correspond to a decreased net rate of bicarbonate reabsorption. This mechanism is different from that found in metabolic alkalosis, where the steady-state pH level is also markedly

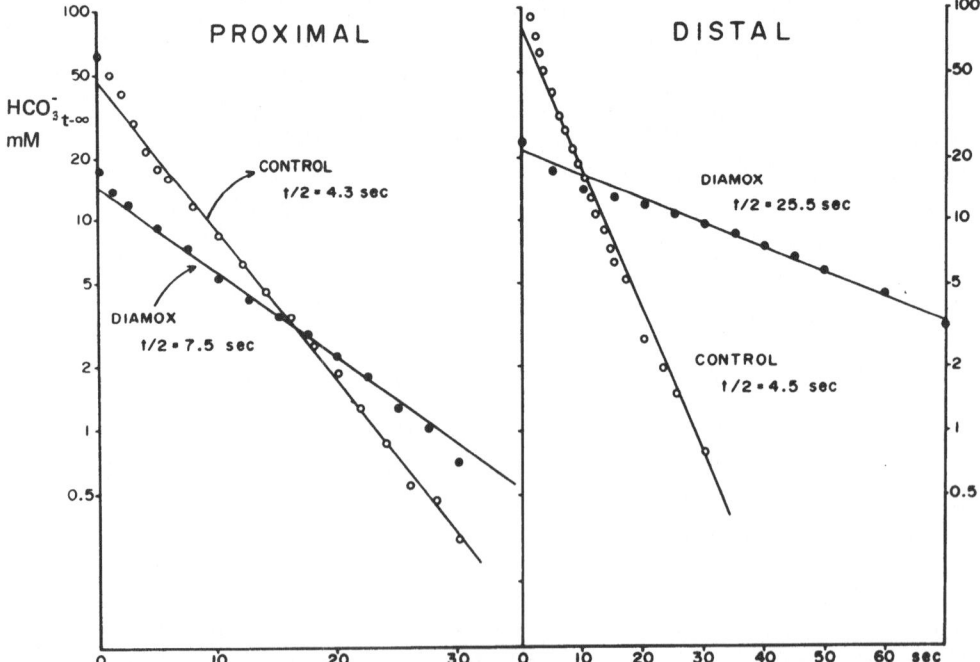

Figure 9. The effect of Diamox on the kinetics of bicarbonate reabsorption in cortical tubules of the rat. Microperfusion with 5% CO_2 preequilibrated solutions of 100 mM NaHCO$_3$/100 mM raffinose. Bicarbonate concentrations at time t minus steady-state levels are plotted against time in seconds.

increased, but where no significant alterations in acidification half-times are found (Malnic *et al.*, 1972b). In terms of the pump-leak model, these differences can be explained by supposing that in metabolic alkalosis H^+ ion secretion is reduced but constant and tubular H ion permeability unaltered, while after acetazolamide both a reduced H^+ ion secretion and permeability have to be assumed.

B. Other Drugs

Besides carbonic anhydrase inhibitors, some other drugs have been reported to have some effect on urinary acidification; such effects, however, appear to be mostly secondary to their action on sodium excretion. Thus, drugs like furosemide and ethacrynic acid, which cause massive natriuresis, have been found to acidify the urine, possibly due to the increased distal load of sodium (Suki *et al.*, 1965; Van Ypersele and Morales-Barria, 1969). In consequence, bicarbonate excretion is also reduced. Chronic administration of these drugs may in this way lead to hypochloremic alkalosis, since predominant NaCl excretion and bicarbonate reabsorption lead to decreases of extracellular fluid chloride concentrations and increases in bicarbonate levels (Mello Aires and Malnic, 1972; Cohen, 1970). On the other hand, Lehmann (1970) reported a decrease in bicarbonate reabsorption by the perfused frog kidney after administration of the cardiac glycoside, convallatoxin.

Amiloride has also been reported to impair urinary acidification (Baer *et al.*, 1967; Guignard and Peters, 1970). The latter authors attribute this effect to the fall in distal transtubular PD that is caused by this drug according to the findings of Duarte *et al.* (1971). A study by Stoner *et al.* (1974) on the effect of amiloride on ion transport in the cortical collecting duct has shown that this drug affects active Na^+ and K^+ transport, reverting the normal lumen-negative PD of -30—-40 mV to $+5$ mV. The latter PD was attributed to electrogenic H^+ ion transport into the lumen, since it was reduced by acetazolamide and low CO_2, suggesting that amiloride does not affect H^+ (or HCO_3^-) transport directly in this structure.

ACKNOWLEDGMENTS

Work from the authors laboratory has been supported by Fundação de Amparo a Pesquisa do Est. S. Paulo.

The concepts presented in this paper have greatly benefited from discussions with Drs. G. Giebisch and T. H. Maren.

REFERENCES

Adler, S., Zett, B., and Anderson, B. 1972. The effect of acute potassium depletion on muscle cell pH in vitro. *Kidney Int., 2:*159.

Atkins, L., and Schwartz, W. B. 1962. Factors governing correction of the alkalosis associated with potassium deficiency; the critical role of chloride in the recovery process. *J. Clin. Invest.*, *41:*218.

Baer, J. E., Jones, C. B., Spitzer, S. A., and Russo, H. F. 1967. The potassium-sparing and natriuretic activity of *N*-amidino-3,5-diamino-6-chloropyrazine carboxamide hydrochloride dihydrate (amiloride hydrochloride). *J. Pharmacol. Exp. Ther.*, *157:*472.

Bank, N., and Aynedjian, H. S. 1965. A micropuncture study of renal bicarbonate and chloride reabsorption in hypokalaemic alkalosis. *Clin. Sci.*, *29:*159.

Bank, N., and Aynedjian, H. S. 1967. A microperfusion study of bicarbonate accumulation in the proximal tubule of the rat kidney. *J. Clin. Invest.*, *46:*95.

Bank, N., Aynedjian, H. S., and Weinstein, S. W. 1974. A microperfusion study of phosphate reabsorption by the rat proximal renal tubule. Effect of parathyroid hormone. *J. Clin. Invest.*, *54:*1040.

Bar, D. 1963. Inhibiteurs de l'anhydrase carbonique. *Actualités Pharmacol.*, *15:*1.

Barratt, L. J., Rector, F. C., Kokko, J. P., and Seldin, D. W. 1974. Factors governing the transepithelial potential difference across the proximal tubule of the rat kidney. *J. Clin. Invest.* *53:*454.

Beck, L. H., and Goldberg, M. 1973. Effects of acetazolamide and parathyroidectomy on renal transport of sodium, calcium and phosphate. *Am. J. Physiol.*, *224:*1136.

Bernstein, B. A., and Clapp, J. R. 1968. Micropuncture study of bicarbonate reabsorption by the dog nephron. *Am. J. Physiol.*, *214:*251.

Boulpaep, E. L., and Seely, J. F. 1971. Electrophysiology of proximal and distal tubules in the autoperfused dog kidney. *Am. J. Physiol.*, *221:*1084.

Boylan, J. W., Antkowiak, D. E., and Calkins, J. 1973. Maximum rates of bicarbonate reabsorption by the dogfish kidney. *Bull. Mt Desert Island Biol. Lab.*, *13:*17.

Brodsky, W. A., and Satran, R. 1959. Comparison of effects of acidosis and alkalosis on the renal action of Diamox. *Am. J. Physiol.*, *197:*585.

Brodsky, W. A., and Schilb, T. P. 1967. Mechanism of acidification in turtle bladder. *Fed. Proc.*, *26:*1314.

Caflisch, C. R. and Carter, N. W. 1974. A micro pCO_2 electrode. *Anal. Biochem.*, *60:*252.

Caldwell, P. C. 1954. An investigation of the intracellular pH of crab muscle fibers by means of micro-glass and micro-tungsten electrodes. *J. Physiol.*, *126:*169.

Carter, N. W., Rector, F. C., Campion, D. S., and Seldin, D. W. 1967. Measurement of intracellular pH with glass microelectrodes. *Fed. Proc.*, *26:*1322.

Clapp, J. R., Watson, J. F., and Berliner, R. W. 1963a. Effect of carbonic anhydrase inhibition on proximal tubular bicarbonate reabsorption. *Am. J. Physiol.*, *205:*693.

Clapp, J. R., Watson, J. F., and Berliner, R. W. 1963b. Osmolality, bicarbonate concentration, and water reabsorption in proximal tubule of the dog nephron. *Am. J. Physiol.*, *205:*273.

Cohen, J. J. 1970. Selective Cl^- retention in repair of metabolic alkalosis without increasing filtered load. *Am. J. Physiol.*, *218:*165.

Davis, R. P. 1958. The kinetics of the reaction of human erythocyte carbonic anhydrase. Basic mechanism and effect of electrolytes on enzyme activity. *J. Am. Chem. Soc.*, *60:*5209.

Deetjen, P. and Maren, T. H. 1973. The dissociation between renal HCO_3^- reabsorption and H^+ secretion in the skate, *Raja erinacea, Pfluegers Arch.*, *346:*25.

Duarte, C. G., Chomety, F., and Giebisch, G. 1971. Effect of amiloride, ouabain, and furosemide on distal tubular function in the rat. *Am. J. Physiol.*, *221:*632.

Eisenman, G. 1967. The origin of the glass-electrode potential. In: *Glass Electrodes for Hydrogen and other Cations*, pp. 133–173. Ed. by Eisenman, G. Marcel Dekker, New York.

Enns, T. 1967. Facilitation by carbonic anhydrase of carbon dioxide transport. *Science, 155:*44.

Fand, S. B., Levine, H. J., and Erwin, H. L. A. 1959. A reappraisal of the histochemical method for carbonic anhydrase. *J. Histochem. Cytochem.*, *7:*27.

Frazier, L. W. and Vanatta, J. C. 1972. Mechanism of acidification of the mucosal fluid by the toad urinary bladder. *Biochim. Biophys. Acta, 290:*168.

Froemter, E. and Gessner, K. 1974. Free-flow potential profile along rat kidney proximal tubule. *Pfluegers Arch., 351:*69.

Froemter, E., Mueller, C. W., and Wick, T. 1971. Permeability properties of the proximal tubular epithelium of the rat kidney studied with electrophysiological methods. In: *Electrophysiology of Epithelial Cells*, pp. 119–146. Ed. by Giebisch, G. Schattauer, Stuttgart.

Froemter, E., Rumrich, G., and Ullrich, K. J. 1973. Phenomenologic description of Na^+, Cl^-, and HCO_3^- absorption from proximal tubules of the rat kidney. *Pfluegers Arch., 343:*189.

Fulop, M. and Brazeau, P. 1968. The phosphaturic effect of sodium bicarbonate and acetazolamide in dogs. *J. Clin. Invest., 47:*983.

Garella, S., Chazan, J. A., Bar-Khayim, Y., and Cohen, J. J. 1972. Isolated effect of increased ECF volume on HCO_3 and Cl reabsorption in the dog. *Am. J. Physiol., 222:*1138.

Garg, L. C. and Maren, T. H. 1972. The rates of hydration of carbon dioxide and dehydration of carbonic acid at 37°, *Biochim. Biophys. Acta, 261:*70.

Gertz, K. H. 1963. Transtubulaere Natriumchloridfluesse und Permeabilitaet fuer Nichtelektrolyte im proximalen und distalen Konvolut der Rattenniere. *Pfluegers Arch., 276:*336.

Gibbons, B. H. and Edsall, J. T. 1963. Rate of hydration of carbon dioxide and dehydration at 25°C. *J. Biol. Chem., 238:*3501.

Giebisch, G., Windhager, E. E., and Pitts, R. F. 1960. Mechanism of urinary acidification. In: *Biology of Pyelonephritis*, pp. 277–287. Ed. by Metcoff, J. Little Brown, Boston.

Gmaj, P., Hoppe, A., Angielski, S., and Rogulski, J. 1972. Acid–base behavior of the kidney in maleate-treated rats. *Am. J. Physiol., 222:*1182.

Gonzalez, C. F., Shamoo, Y. E., and Brodsky, W. A. 1969. The accelerating effect of serosal HCO_3^- on Na^+ transport in short-circuited turtle bladders. *Biochim. Biophys. Acta, 193:*403.

Gottschalk, C. W., Lassiter, W. E., and Mylle, M. 1960. Localization of urine acidification in the mammalian kidney. *Am. J. Physiol., 198:*581.

Green, R. and Giebisch, G. 1974. Some problems with the antimony microelectrode. In: *Ion Selective Microelectrodes*, pp. 43–53. Ed. by Berman, H. J. and Hebert, N. C. Plenum Press, New York.

Green, H. H., Steinmetz, P. R., and Frazier, H. S. 1970. Evidence for proton transport by turtle bladder in presence of ambient bicarbonate. *Am. J. Physiol., 218:*845.

Gros, G. and Moll, W. 1971. The diffusion of carbon dioxide in erythrocytes and hemoglobin solutions. *Pfluegers Arch., 324:*249.

Gros, G. and Moll, W. 1974. Facilitated diffusion of CO_2 across albumin solutions. *J. Gen. Physiol., 64:*356.

Guignard, J. P. and Peters, G. 1970. Effects of triamterene and amiloride on urinary acidification and potassium excretion in the rat. *Eur. J. Pharmacol., 10:*255.

Haeusler, G. 1958. Zur Technik und Spezifitaet des histochemischen Carboanhydrasenachweises im Modellversuch und in Gewebsschnitten von Rattennieren. *Histochemie, 1:*29.

Hansson, H. P. J. 1968. Histochemical demonstration of carbonic anhydrase activity in some epithelia noted for active transport. *Acta Physiol. Scand., 73:*427.

Hodler, J., Heinemann, H. O., Fischman, A. P., and Smith, H. W. 1955. Urine pH and carbonic anhydrase activity in the marine dogfish. *Am. J. Physiol., 138:*155.

Ives, D. J. G. and Janz, G. J. 1961. *Reference Electrodes, Theory and Practice*, Academic Press, New York.

Karlmark, B. and Davidson, B. G. 1974. Titratable acid, PCO_2, bicarbonate and ammonium ions along the rat proximal tubule. *Acta Physiol. Scand., 91:*243.

Karlmark, B. and Sohtell, M. 1973. The determination of bicarbonate in nanoliter samples. *Anal. Biochem., 53:*1.

Kern, D. M. 1960. The hydration of carbon dioxide. *J. Chem. Educ., 37:*14.

Kernohan, J. C. 1964. The activity of bovine carbonic anhydrase in imidazole buffers. *Biochim. Biophys. Acta, 81:*346.

Khuri, R. N., Agulian, S. K., Oelert, H., and Harik, R. I. 1967. A single unit pH glass ultramicroelectrode. *Pfluegers Arch., 294:*291.

Khuri, R. N., Agulian, S. K., and Harik, R. I. 1968. Internal capillary glass microelectrodes with a glass seal for pH, sodium and potassium. *Pfluegers Arch., 301:*182.

Khuri, R. N., Agulian, S. K., and Aklanjian, D. A. 1973. A single unit microelectrode with a glass seal and a microhole. *Pfluegers Arch., 345:*265.

Khuri, R. N., Agulian, S. R., Bogharian, K., Nassar, R., and Wise, W. 1974a. Intracellular bicarbonate in single cells of Necturus kidney proximal tubule. *Pfluegers Arch., 349:*295.

Khuri, R. N., Bogharian, K. K., and Agulian, S. K. 1974b. Intracellular bicarbonate in single skeletal muscle fibers. *Pfluegers Arch., 349:*285.

Kunau, R. T. 1972. The influence of the carbonic anhydrase inhibitor, benzolamide (CL-11,366) on the reabsorption of chloride, sodium and bicarbonate in the proximal tubule of the rat. *J. Clin. Invest., 51:*294.

Kunau, R. T., Frick, A., Rector, F. C., and Seldin, D. W. 1968. Micropuncture study of the proximal tubular factors responsible for the maintenance of alkalosis during potassium deficiency in the rat. *Clin. Sci., 34:*223.

Kurtzman, N. A. 1970a. Regulation of renal bicarbonate reabsorption by extracellular volume. *J. Clin. Invest., 49:*586.

Kurtzman, N. A. 1970b. Relationship of extracellular volume and CO_2 tension to renal bicarbonate reabsorption. *Am. J. Physiol., 219:*1299.

Leder, O. 1967. Die intracellulaere Verteilung der Carboanhydrase in der Niere von Ratten und Maeusen. *Pfluegers Arch., 297:*54.

Lehmann, H. D. 1970. Der Einfluss von Acetazolamid und Convallatoxin auf die Bikarbonat-Resorption der kuenstlich perfundierten Froschniere. *Z. Vergl. Physiol., 69:*163.

Levine, D. Z. 1971. Effect of acute hypercapnia on proximal tubular water and bicarbonate reabsorption. *Am. J. Physiol., 221:*1164.

Levine, D. Z. 1972. Measurement of tubular fluid bicarbonate concentration by the cuvette-type glass micro pH electrode. *Yale J. Biol. Med., 45:*368.

Levine, D. Z. and Nash, L. A. 1973. Effect of chronic NH_4Cl acidosis on proximal tubular H_2O and HCO_3 reabsorption. *Am. J. Physiol., 225:*380.

Loennerholm, G. 1971. Histochemical demonstration of carbonic anhydrase activity in the rat kidney. *Acta Physiol. Scand., 81:*433.

Loennerholm, G. 1973. Histochemical demonstration of carbonic anhydrase activity in the human kidney. *Acta Physiol. Scand., 88:*455.

Magid, E. and Turbeck, B. O. 1968. The rates of spontaneous hydration of CO_2 and the reciprocal reaction in neutral aqueous solutions between 0° and 38°C, *Biochim. Biophys. Acta, 165:*515.

Malnic, G. and Giebisch, G. 1972. Mechanism of renal hydrogen ion secretion. *Kidney Int., 1:*280.

Malnic, G. and Mello Aires, M. 1971. Kinetic study of bicarbonate reabsorption in proximal tubule of the rat. *Am. J. Physiol., 220:*1759.

Malnic, G. and Vieira, F. L. 1972. The antimony microelectrode in kidney micropuncture. *Yale J. Biol. Med., 45:*356.

Malnic, G., Mello Aires, M., and Vieira, F. L. 1970. Chloride excretion in single nephrons of rat kidney during alterations of acid–base equilibrium. *Am. J. Physiol., 218:*20.

Malnic, G., Mello Aires, M., and Giebisch, G. 1972a. Micropuncture study of renal tubular hydrogen ion transport in the rat. *Am. J. Physiol., 222:*147.

Malnic, G., Mello Aires, M., de Mello, G. B., and Giebisch, G. 1972b. Acidification of phosphate buffer in cortical tubules of rat kidney. *Pfluegers Arch., 331:*275.

Malnic, G., Mello Aires, M., and Cassola, A. C. 1974. Kinetic analysis of renal tubular acidification by antimony microelectrodes. In: *Ion Selective Microelectrodes,* pp. 89–108. Ed. by Berman, H. J. and Hebert, N. C. Plenum Press, New York.

Malnic, G., Mello Aires, M., de Mello, G. B., and Giebisch, G. 1976. Some kinetic aspects of hydrogen ion secretion in cortical tubules of the rat kidney (submitted to *J. Physiol.*).

Malvin, R. L. and Lotspeich, W. D. 1956. Relation between tubular transport of inorganic phosphate and bicarbonate in the dog. *Am. J. Physiol., 187:*51.

Maren, T. H. 1956. Carbonic anhydrase inhibition. The effects of metabolic acidosis on the response to Diamox. *Bull. Johns Hopkins Hosp., 98:*159.

Maren, T. H. 1967. Carbonic anhydrase: Chemistry, physiology and inhibition. *Physiol. Rev., 47:*595.

Maren, T. H. 1969. Renal carbonic anhydrase and the pharmacology of sulfonamide inhibitors. In: *Handbuch der Experimentellen Pharmakologie,* Vol. 24, pp. 195–256. Ed. by Herken, H. Springer, Berlin.

Maren, T. H. 1974. Chemistry of the renal reabsorption of bicarbonate. *Can. J. Physiol. Pharmacol., 52:*1041.

Maren, T. H. and Ellison, A. C. 1967. A study of renal carbonic anhydrase. *Mol. Pharmacol., 3:*503.

Maude, D. L. 1974. The role of bicarbonate in proximal tubular sodium chloride transport. *Kidney Int., 5:*253.

Mello Aires, M. and Malnic, G. 1972. Micropuncture study of acidification during hypochloremic alkalosis in the rat. *Pfluegers Arch., 331:*13.

Mello Aires, M. and Malnic, G. 1975. Role of peritubular pH and pCO_2 in renal tubular acidification. *Am. J. Physiol., 228:*1766.

Menaker, W. 1948. Buffer equilibria and reabsorption in the production of urinary acidity. *Am. J. Physiol., 154:*174.

Montgomery, H. and Pierce, J. A. 1937. The site of acidification of the urine within the renal tubule in amphibia. *Am. J. Physiol. 118:*144.

Muther, T. F. 1972. A critical evaluation of the histochemical methods for carbonic anhydrase. *J. Histochem. Cytochem., 20:*319.

Pierce, J. A. and Montgomery, H. 1935. A microquinhydrone electrode: Its application to the determination of the pH of glomerular urine of *Necturus. J. Biol. Chem., 110:*763.

Pitts, R. F. 1952/53. Mechanisms for stabilizing the alkaline reserves of the body. *Harvey Lect., 48:*172.

Pitts, R. F. and Alexander, R. S. 1945. The nature of the renal tubular mechanism for acidifying the urine. *Am. J. Physiol., 144:*239.

Purkerson, M. L., Lubowitz, H., White, R. W., and Bricker, N. S. 1969. On the influence of extracellular fluid volume expansion on bicarbonate reabsorption in the rat. *J. Clin. Invest., 48:*1754.

Puschett, J. B. and Zurbach, P. E. 1974. Re-evaluation of microelectrode methodology for the "in vitro" determination of pH and bicarbonate. *Kidney Int., 6:*81.

Randall, R. and Maren, T. H. 1972. Absence of carbonic anhydrase in red cell membranes. *Biochim. Biophys. Acta, 268:*730.

Rector, F. C. 1973. Acidification of the urine. In: *Handbook of Physiology*, Section 8, pp. 431–454. Ed. by Orloff, J. and Berliner, R. W. American Physiological Society, Washington, D.C.

Rector, F. C., Seldin, D. W., Roberts, A. D., and Smith, J. S. 1960. The role of plasma CO_2 tension and carbonic anhydrase activity in the renal reabsorption of bicarbonate. *J. Clin. Invest., 39:*1706.

Rector, F. C., Bloomer, H. A., and Seldin, D. W. 1964. Effect of potassium deficiency on the reabsorption of bicarbonate in the proximal tubule of the rat kidney. *J. Clin. Invest., 43:*1976.

Rector, F. C., Carter, N. W., and Seldin, D. W. 1965. The mechanism of bicarbonate reabsorption in the proximal and distal tubules of the kidney. *J. Clin. Invest., 44:*278.

Rector, F. C., Martinez-Maldonado, M., Brunner, F., and Seldin, D. W. 1966. Evidence for passive reabsorption of NaCl in proximal tubule of rat kidney. *J. Clin. Invest., 45:*1060.

Schilb, T. P. and Brodsky, W. A. 1966. Acidification of mucosal fluid by transport of bicarbonate ion in turtle bladders. *Am. J. Physiol., 210:*917.

Schilb, T. P. and Brodsky, W. A. 1972. CO_2 gradients and acidification by transport of HCO_3 in turtle bladders. *Am. J. Physiol., 222:*272.

Schwartz, J. H., Finn, J. T., Vaughan, G., and Steinmetz, P. R. 1974. Distribution of metabolic CO_2 and the transported ion species in acidification by turtle bladder. *Am. J. Physiol., 226:*283.

Singer, I., Sharp, G. W. G., and Civan, M. M. 1969. The effect of propionate and other organic anions on sodium transport across toad bladder. *Biochim. Biophys. Acta, 193:*430.

Singer, I., Civan, M. M., and Sharp, G. W. G. 1970. Mode of action of propionate in toad bladder. *Am. J. Physiol., 219:*1273.

Sirs, J. A. 1958. Electrometric stopped flow measurements of rapid reactions in solution. Conductivity measurements. *Trans. Faraday Soc., 54:*201.

Smith, W. W. 1939. The excretion of phosphate in the dogfish, *Squalus acanthias. J. Cell. Comp. Physiol., 14:*95.

Smith, H. W. 1951. *The Kidney. Structure and Function in Health and Disease*. Oxford Univ. Press, New York.

Stackelberg, W. F. 1970. A 0,1 nanoliter glass capillary electrode. *Pfluegers Arch., 321:*274.

Steinmetz, P. R. 1974. Cellular mechanisms of urinary acidification. *Physiol. Rev., 54:*890.

Stoner, L. C., Burg, M. R., and Orloff, J. 1974. Ion transport in cortical collecting tubule: effect of amiloride. *Am. J. Physiol., 227:*453.

Struyvenberg, A., Morrison, R. B., and Relman, A. S. 1968. Acid–base behavior of separated canine renal tubule cells. *Am. J. Physiol., 214:*1155.

Suki, W., Rector, F. C., and Seldin, D. W. 1965. The site of action of furosemide and other sulfonamide diuretics in the dog. *J. Clin. Invest., 44:*1458.

Sullivan, B. and Berndt, W. O. 1973a. Transport by isolated rabbit gallbladders in phosphate-buffered solutions. *Am. J. Physiol., 225:*838.

Sullivan, B. and Berndt, W. O. 1973b. Transport by isolated rabbit gall-bladders in bicarbonate-buffered solutions. *Am. J. Physiol., 225:*845.

Thomas, R. C. 1974. Intracellular pH of snail neurones measured with a new pH-sensitive glass micro-electrode. *J. Physiol., 238:*159.

Uhlich, E., Baldamus, C. A., and Ullrich, K. J. 1968. Verhalten von CO_2 Druck und Bicarbonat im Gegenstromsystem des Nierenmarks. *Pfluegers Arch., 303:*31.

Ullrich, K. J. and Eigler, F. W. 1958. Sekretion von Wasserstoffionen in den Sammelrohren der Saeugetierniere. *Pfluegers Arch., 267:*491.

Ullrich, K. J., Radtke, H. W., and Rumrich, G. 1971. The role of bicarbonate and other buffers on isotonic fluid absorption in the proximal convolution of the rat kidney. *Pfluegers Arch., 330:*149.

Van Ypersele, C. and Morales-Barria, J. 1969. The influence of dietary sodium and potassium intake on the genesis of furosemide induced alkalosis. *Clin. Sci., 37:*859.

Vieira, F. L. and Malnic, G. 1968. Hydrogen ion secretion by rat renal cortical tubules as studied by an antimony microelectrode. *Am. J. Physiol., 214:*710.

Waddell, W. J. and Bates, R. G. 1969. Intracellular pH. *Physiol. Rev., 49:*285.

Waring, D. W., Sullivan, L. P., Mayhew, D. A., and Tucker, J. M. 1974. A study of factors affecting renal bicarbonate reabsorption. *Am. J. Physiol., 226:*1392.

Weinstein, S. W. 1968. Micropuncture studies of the effects of acetazolamide on nephron function in the rat. *Am. J. Physiol., 214:*222.

II
Diuretics

Chapter **2**

The Use of the Isolated Tubule Preparation for the Investigation of Diuretics

Arnold M. Chonko and Jared J. Grantham

Division of Nephrology, Department of Medicine
University of Kansas Medical Center, Kansas City, Kansas

I. INTRODUCTION

Diuretics were discovered and used effectively in the clinic long before investigators in this century pondered their site and mechanism of action. Calomel (mercurous chloride) was combined with digitalis in the mid-nineteenth century ("Guy's Hospital Pill") and used with some success in the treatment of "dropsy." The potent diuretic properties of the antisyphilitic organomercurials were accidently discovered and used in the 1920s for the treatment of edematous conditions (reviewed by Vogl, 1950). Effective tools for definitive study of the mechanism of urine formation were not available until Richards and his associates (Richards and Schmidt, 1924) introduced the micropuncture method.

It was not until the fifth decade of this century, after the accidental discovery of the diuretic effect of sulfa derivatives that meaningful attempts were made to uncover the site of diuretic action. The evidence for the role of countercurrent multiplication in renal medulla and papilla in the concentration and dilution of urine, and especially the discovery that dilute urine was produced in the ascending portion of Henle's loop, opened the door to a number of important insights into the locus of diuretic action (Hargitay and Kuhn, 1951; Wirz *et al.,* 1951; Gottschalk and Mylle, 1959; Gottschalk, 1961). Suki and his colleagues (1965) and Goldberg and co-workers (1964) measured free water formation, an estimate of "loop" sodium chloride transport in clearance studies, and implicated the loop of Henle as the nephron segment primarily receptive to the action of the potent diuretics furosemide and ethacrynic acid. The antikali-uretic effect of amiloride and triamterene was interpreted to indicate a more distal tubular site of action for these drugs (reviewed by Seldin and Rector, 1973). Measurements of the changes in urinary phosphate and bicarbonate implicated the proximal tubule as the site of action for acetazolamide and other carbonic anhydrase inhibitors (reviewed by Goldberg *et al.*, 1973). Micropunc-ture studies by a number of investigators were interpreted to indicate that many of the diuretics disrupted sodium chloride transport in the ascending limb of the loop of Henle—mannitol (Seely and Dirks, 1969), organomercurials (Clapp and Robinson, 1968; Evanson *et al.*, 1972), furosemide (Dirks and Seely, 1970), and chlorothiazide (Clapp and Robinson, 1968). By contrast, amiloride (Duarte *et al.*, 1971) appeared to interfere with electrolyte transport primarily in the distal tubule.

Although the site of nephronal action of diuretics is reasonably well defined, the mechanism of diuretic action has been difficult to adduce by micropuncture and clearance techniques. Consequently, to define the nature of diuretic action, *in vitro* model systems have been used including toad bladders (Ferguson, 1966; Bentley, 1968; Sullivan *et al.*, 1971), renal cortical slices (Schmidt and Dubach, 1970), and renal homogenates (Hook and Williamson, 1965b; Duggan and Noll, 1972). Important concepts have derived from *in vitro* studies of transport regarding the mechanism of action of ADH (Koefoed-Johnsen and Ussing, 1953; Hays and Leaf, 1962) and the relation between renal metabolism and transmem-brane electrolyte transport (see Chapters 4 and 6). But in the final analysis anuran membranes are not simple analogs of the distal mammalian nephron (DiBona *et al.*, 1969), and interpretation of data obtained from renal slices or tubule suspensions is complicated by the fact that primarily peritubular mem-brane transport is studied, since the tubule lumens are generally collapsed in these preparations. Frustrated by the slice and suspension methods of inquiry, Burg *et al.* (1966) developed a technique for isolating and perfusing individual segments of mammalian nephrons. In the remainder of this chapter we will review some of the technical aspects of this method together with a considera-tion of the information that has been derived regarding the site and mechanism of diuretic action in nephron segments.

II. GENERAL FEATURES OF THE *IN VITRO* MICROPERFUSION METHOD

The New Zealand white rabbit has been used most extensively for these studies, although *in vitro* microperfusion has been successfully performed with tubules dissected from flounder (Burg and Weller, 1969), snake (Dantzler, 1974), and human fetal tissue (Abramow and Dratwa, 1974). To conduct an experiment the animals (2–3 kg) are sacrificed, the kidney quickly removed, and a thin (2 mm) saggital section taken and immediately immersed in rabbit serum at 4°C. This serum is equilibrated with 95% oxygen and 5% carbon dioxide and adjusted to an osmolality of 290 mOsm/kg. The slice is teased apart with fine-tipped forceps under direct visualization through a binocular microscope (10–90×). Dissection of viable tissue is an important step to the successful use of this method. The tubule is touched only at the ends and excessive traction avoided. A segment of appropriate length (usually 1–3 mm) is transferred in a small volume of serum to a thermostatically controlled incubation chamber which is mounted over an inverted microscope. The tubule is observed for damage at high magnification (100–400×). We have established several criteria that must be met prior to using a tubule for study (Table I). If the basement membrane is ruptured at any point along the tubule, the dissection has been too rough. Narrowing or abrupt constriction in the diameter of the tubule implies overzealous stretching in the course of dissection. The presence of large vacuoles or opacified areas in the tubule suggests that the metabolic machinery of the cells has been damaged. Two additional observations can be made regarding the viability of the tubule. Normal tubules reabsorb fluid at 37°C. Consequently, any lumen present at the time of transfer to the bathing chamber should disappear within a few minutes after warming. With proximal straight tubules we use another helpful indicator. These tubules normally secrete p-aminohippurate (PAH) into the tubule lumen to the extent that fluid is obligated as well (Grantham *et al.*, 1974). If lumen expansion does not occur within 5–10 min after the addition of $10^{-4} M$ PAH to the bath (37°C), metabolism of the cells may have been compromised by the dissection.

To perfuse a suitable tubule, a glass micropipet (holding pipet) is maneuvered so that one end of the tubule is engaged by gentle suction. A concentrically mounted pipet (perfusion pipet) is then inserted into the tubule lumen (Figure 1). The other end of the tubule is then gently sucked into another micropipet (collecting pipet). Either a microsyringe pump or simple hydrostatic pressure is used to propel perfusion fluid through the tubule lumen into the collecting pipet where it accumulates beneath an oil column. The oil (Sylgard 184, Dow Corning Corp., Midland, Michigan) prevents evaporation but provides no significant resistance to flow. A wide range of relatively stable rates of

Table I. Criteria for Selecting a Tubule for Microperfusion

I. Nonperfused tubule
 A. Outer tubular contour is smooth.
 B. Outer tubular diameter is relatively uniform.
 C. Large vacuoles or opacified areas are absent.
 D. Tubule lumen disappears after warming to 37°C.
 E. Fluid is secreted into the lumen (proximal straight tubule) at 37°C after the addition of $10^{-4} M$ PAH to bath.
II. After initial trial perfusion of tubule
 A. Cells are present over entire length of epithelium so that exposed areas of basement membrane do not exist.
 B. Cells are of normal size and shape without large vacuoles.
 C. Brush border of tubule epithelium is intact.
 D. Nuclei are basally oriented (proximal tubule and cortical collecting tubule).
 E. Proximal tubule lumens collapse completely upon lowering of perfusion pressure to zero.

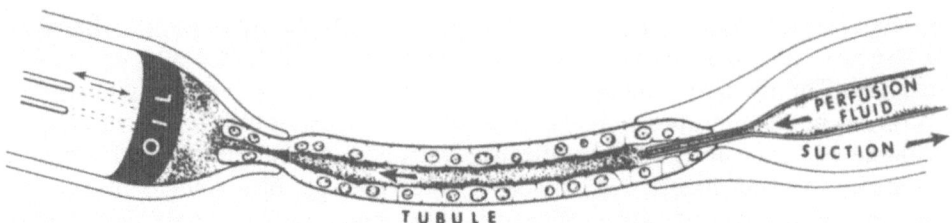

Figure 1. Arrangement for perfusing kidney tubules. A three compartment analysis of transport (bathing fluid, tissue, and luminal fluid) is possible with this perfusion arrangement. (From Burg and Orloff, 1968.)

outflow can be obtained. All the accumulated fluid is collected at periodic intervals by inserting a narrow calibrated pipet through the oil column in the collecting pipet. To approximate the *in vivo* situation (glomerular filtration), an isotonic ultrafiltrate of rabbit serum is perfused while the tubule is immersed in a bath of rabbit serum. The tubule length is measured with a micrometer in the microscope eyepiece. The absolute volume reabsorption is determined (nl/mm/ min) from the change in concentration in the collected fluid of an impermeant marker ([3H]inulin, [14C]inulin, [125I]iothalamate). Leaks around the perfusion pipet or through the tubular epithelium are detected from the appearance of the volume marker in the external bath.

In a modification of this arrangement which eliminates the need for isotopes, the distal end of the tubule is occluded (Figure 2) and the movement of an oil drop contained within the shank of the perfusion pipet is used to calculate the absolute volume reabsorption (or volume secretion, Grantham *et al.*, 1972).

Upon perfusion of the segment additional criteria must be fulfilled before the tubule is accepted for study (Table I). Cells should uniformly line the basement membrane. Swelling or absence of individual cells implies rough handling in dissection. In proximal segments the brush border is an excellent guide to the integrity of the preparation. The brush border is easily seen at 200– 400× magnification. Absence of brush border on a large number of cells may indicate that initial perfusion was too vigorous. Nuclei of most segments are oriented toward the base of the cells (the cortical ascending limb is an exception). When cells die the nucleus is often extruded into the lumen. Finally, an easy test of viability in proximal segments involves the lowering of perfusion pressure to zero, whereupon the lumen should collapse completely at 37°C.

The *in vitro* microperfusion method has several advantages that enhance its suitability for the study of transport processes. The extratubular environment (oxygen content, temperature, pH, oncotic and hydrostatic forces, and osmotic regulation) can be rigorously controlled. The constituents of the perfusate or the bathing fluid can be varied in the midst of an experiment while tubular flow and the integrity of the tubular epithelium remain undisturbed. This cannot be done easily with micropuncture techniques since the epithelium may be damaged at the site of puncture, and contamination during fluid aspiration (retrograde contamination) is a constant hazard (Rector *et al.*, 1966; Brenner *et al.*, 1969a).

The transtubule electrical potential difference and transtubule resistance are

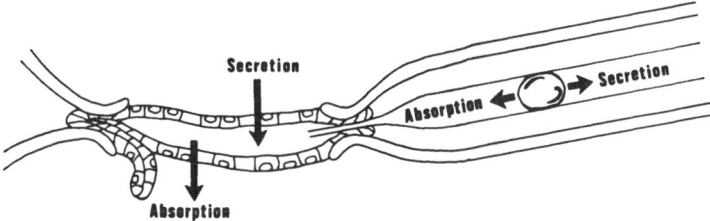

Figure 2. Modified arrangement for perfusing kidney tubules in which the distal end of the tubule is occluded. Transtubular fluid absorption (or secretion) was determined from the rate of movement of the oil drop in the perfusion pipet. (From Welling and Grantham, 1972.)

measured in isolated perfused tubules by modifying the perfusion scheme (Figure 1). Microelectrodes are inserted within the lumen of the tubule. The transtubule (lumen to bath) potential difference (Burg and Orloff, 1970; Kokko and Rector, 1971) and the segmental epithelial resistance can be measured simultaneously in this manner (Helman *et al.*, 1971; Lutz *et al.*, 1973).

The reflection coefficient for sodium chloride (or other substance) (Kokko *et al.*, 1971; Shafer and Andreoli, 1972) is determined by placing an impermeant substance such as raffinose in the bathing medium and measuring the increased volume flux out of the tubule as compared to that elicited with an equimolar concentration of sodium chloride. Similar techniques are used to calculate the osmotic permeability coefficient to water (L_p) for a given segment. Since the polarity of the tubular membrane is maintained during microperfusion and the tubular fluid, bathing fluid, and the tubule epithelium may be recovered for analysis, a three-component model of transport (lumen fluid, cell, bath fluid) can be derived for any substance which can be isotopically or microanalytically quantified (Tune *et al.*, 1969; Tune and Burg, 1971). The explicit analysis of the transport "steps" is a powerful attribute of the *in vitro* microperfusion method.

Nearly all of the individual segments of the rabbit nephron have been isolated and satisfactorily perfused. A perusal of the published data (Table II) regarding the functional characteristics for some of these segments substantiates that the rabbit nephron is heterogeneous functionally, as well as structurally. A detailed review of segmental function is beyond the scope of this presentation, but several points merit comment. First of all, the general features of each nephron segment with regard to solute and solvent permeability and transport are reasonably consistent among different observers. More specifically, the proximal tubule has a low transmembrane resistance (Lutz *et al.*, 1973), a low transmembrane potential difference (Burg and Orloff, 1970), a low reflection coefficient for sodium chloride (Kokko *et al.*, 1971), and reabsorbs fluid isotonically in the range of 1.1–1.5 nl/mm/min (Burg and Orloff, 1968; Imai and Kokko, 1972; Grantham *et al.*, 1972; Hamburger *et al.*, 1974). Chonko and associates (1974) recently observed by classical micropuncture methodology that absolute reabsorption of fluid in the rabbit proximal tubule was 1.6 nl/mm/min, on the average. This observation provides important support for the view that the proximal tubule *in vitro* reflects the basic transport properties of the segment *in vivo*.

Table II. Segmental Characteristics of the Rabbit Nephron

| | Proximal tubule | | Loop of Henle | | | Collecting tubule | |
	Convoluted	Straight	Descending limb	Ascending limb — Medullary	Ascending limb — Cortical	Cortical and medullary	Papillary
A. Transport							
1. Net fluid absorption (nl/mm/min)	1.18 (Burg and Orloff, 1968) 1.24–1.59 (Kokko et al., 1971) 0.75–1.18 (Imai and Kokko, 1972) 0.92–1.20 (Grantham et al., 1972) 1.10 (Hamburger et al., 1974)	0.42 (Burg and Orloff, 1968) 0.30 (Grantham et al., 1972) 0.53 (Hamburger et al., 1974)	0.0 (Kokko, 1970)	0.0 (Rocha and Kokko, 1973)		0.01 (Grantham et al., 1970)	
2. Limiting Na difference (mEq/liter)	34 (Kokko et al., 1971)			31 (Rocha and Kokko, 1973)	75–100 (Burg and Green, 1973a)	136 (Grantham et al., 1970)	
B. Electrical							
3. Transtubule potential (mV)	−4.0 (Burg and Orloff, 1970) −6.0 (Kokko, 1973) −4.0 (Lutz et al., 1973)	−2.0 (Lutz et al., 1973)	0.0 (Kokko, 1970)	+7 (Rocha and Kokko, 1973)	+7 (Burg and Green, 1973a)	−21.0–67.0 (Grantham et al., 1970) −11.0 (Helman et al., 1971) −35.0 (Stoner et al., 1974)	
4. Transtubule resistance (ohm cm)	964 (Lutz et al., 1973)	1188 (Lutz et al., 1973)			3430 (Burg and Green, 1973a)	13.8×10^4 (Helman et al., 1971)	

C. Permeability

5. Reflection coefficient					
σ NaCl	0.69 (Kokko et al., 1971)	0.96 (Kokko, 1970)		1.0 (Schafer and Andreoli, 1972)	.74 (Rocha and Kokko, 1974)
σ Urea	0.91 (Kokko, 1972b)	0.95 (Kokko, 1972b)		1.0 (Schafer and Andreoli, 1972)	
6. Permeability					
P_{Na} (cm/sec)	9.3×10^{-5} (Kokko et al., 1971)	1.6×10^{-5} (Kokko, 1970)	6.3×10^{-5} (Rocha and Kokko, 1973)	0.08×10^{-5} (Stoner et al., 1974)	
P urea (cm/sec)	5.3×10^{-5} (Kokko, 1972b)	1.5×10^{-5} (Kokko, 1972b)	0 (Rocha and Kokko, 1974)	$1.0 \rightarrow 1.2 \times 10^{-5}$ (Grantham and Burg, 1966)	$2.2 \rightarrow 2.4 \times 10^{-5}$ (Rocha and Kokko, 1974)
(0 ADH → +ADH)				$0.3 \rightarrow 0.3 \times 10^{-5}$ (Rocha and Kokko, 1974)	
				$0.2 \rightarrow 0.2 \times 10^{-5}$ (Grantham and Orloff, 1968)	
Lp (cm/sec atmos.)	$2.9\text{--}6.3 \times 10^{-5}$ (Kokko et al., 1971)	17×10^{-5} (Kokko, 1972b)	0 (Rocha and Kokko, 1973)	$0.2 \rightarrow 1.5 \times 10^{-5}$ (Grantham and Orloff, 1968)	$0.0 \rightarrow 0.5 \times 10^{-5}$ (Rocha and Kokko, 1974)
			7.9×10^{-7} (Burg and Green, 1973a)		
(0 ADH → +ADH)				$0.0 \rightarrow 1.1 \times 10^{-5}$ (Schafer and Andreoli, 1972)	
$P_{D\ H_2O}$ (cm/sec)				$38 \rightarrow 98 \times 10^{-5}$ (Grantham and Burg, 1966)	$40 \rightarrow 57 \times 10^{-5}$ (Rocha and Kokko, 1974)
(0 ADH → +ADH)				$40 \rightarrow 77 \times 10^{-5}$ (Burg et al., 1970)	
				$47 \rightarrow 142 \times 10^{-5}$ (Schaferd and Andreoli, 1972)	

The cortical collecting tubule has a relatively high transmembrane resistance (Helman *et al.*, 1971) and potential difference (Grantham *et al.*, 1970), an extremely low stationary-state tubular sodium concentration (flow less than 0.5 nl/min; Grantham *et al.*, 1970), and reabsorbs a small volume of fluid (0.01 nl/mm/min; Grantham *et al.*, 1970). The collecting tubule is unique in another important regard, for in this segment water permeability is dramatically increased by vasopressin (Grantham and Burg, 1966).

Evidently isolated proximal tubules absorb a relatively large quantity of solute against a low chemical gradient, whereas cortical collecting tubules transport relatively small amounts of electrolyte against a steep chemical gradient. These observations are consonant with the generally accepted view that the proximal tubule is relatively "leaky," whereas the distal nephron is relatively "tight."

The low permeability to water of the isolated ascending limb of the loop of Henle (Rocha and Kokko, 1973; Burg and Green, 1973a) is further evidence for the existence of a countercurrent multiplier system for urinary concentration and dilution in the mammalian kidney.

III. THE USE OF *IN VITRO* MICROPERFUSION TO EVALUATE DIURETIC ACTION

A. Proximal Tubule

In order to assess the effects of diuretic drugs on the proximal tubule from the perspective of the microperfusion technique, it is important to consider some of the nondiuretic factors which have been shown to influence net fluid absorption. The temperature of the bathing medium, the presence or absence of certain organic solutes in the perfusate, and the oncotic effect of serum proteins are factors which have an important influence on the maximal rate of net fluid absorption in the proximal tubule. There are anatomic considerations as well. Burg and Orloff (1968) demonstrated that the magnitude of fluid absorption in the microperfused proximal tubule differed between the convoluted and straight portions of this nephron segment. They also observed that net fluid transport was exquisitely temperature sensitive. At 37°C the proximal convoluted tubule reabsorbed fluid at approximately 1.18 nl/mm/min, while the proximal straight segment did so at approximately 0.42 nl/mm/min. With a reduction in bath temperature to 13°C, fluid transport ceased in the proximal convoluted segment. The reversibility of the hypothermic effect was interpreted to indicate that fluid transport was dependent on metabolism. Several investigators (Kokko *et al.*, 1971; Grantham *et al.*, 1972; Hamburger *et al.*, 1974) have since confirmed the presence of functional heterogeneity within the proximal tubule in regards to net fluid transport. Grantham (1973) found also that hypothermia elicited a proportional reduction of transport in the proximal straight segment as well as in the convoluted segment (lowering bath temperature to 25°C resulted in a 50% reduction in net fluid transport in both segments). Moreover, this investigator has found that net fluid secretion by the proximal straight tubule, as initiated by the addition of p-aminohippurate to the bath, was exquisitely sensitive to the effect of hypothermia (Grantham *et al.*, 1974). Therefore, investigations of transport parameters utilizing the *in vitro* microperfusion method should be conducted at a reasonably constant temperature. By convention, 37°C has been selected in most microperfusion laboratories. Indeed, an important advantage of the microperfusion technique, in contrast to the renal slice or suspension techniques, is that at 37°C the segments probably transport solutes at rates closer to the *in vivo* condition.

Burg and Orloff (1968) also noted that net fluid transport by perfused convoluted tubules was inhibited by the addition of low concentrations ($10^{-5}\,M$) of strophanthidin to the bath. Subsequently, inhibition with ouabain was also observed in perfused proximal straight tubules (Grantham, 1973) and cortical collecting tubules (Grantham *et al.*, 1970), a finding that is consonant with the generally accepted notion that net fluid absorption in microperfused tubules *in vitro* is coupled to the active transport of solute. The relative unimportance of transtubule hydrostatic pressure in the absorption of solute and water has been illustrated convincingly by Burg and Orloff (1968) and Grantham and associates (1972; Figure 3). An important derivative of these experiments was the observation that net fluid absorption was independent of the diameter of the tubule lumen. Stated in a different way, so-called "glomerulotubular balance" was not an intrinsic functional characteristic of the tubular epithelium but was related to factors extrinsic to the tubule. Lewy and Windhager (1968) and Brenner and his colleagues (1969a,b), on the basis of micropuncture studies *in situ*, suggested that the balance of Starling forces across the renal peritubular capillary influenced the control of net proximal tubule fluid absorption. It is the changes in peritubular protein concentration in consequence of perturbations in the filtration fraction that are largely responsible for the "balance" between filtration and

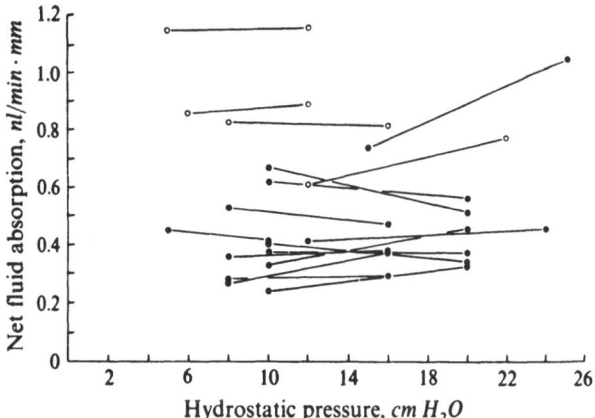

Figure 3. Lack of effect of increased luminal hydrostatic pressure on net fluid absorption of proximal convoluted tubules. Open circles, tubules bathed in 6% bovine serum albumin (BSA)—Ringer's solution; closed circles, tubules bathed in 0.3% BSA—Ringer's. (From Grantham *et al.*, 1972.)

absorption *in vivo*. Microperfusion studies by Imai and Kokko (1972, 1974) and Grantham and associates (1972) have verified the importance of the peritubular protein concentration upon net fluid reabsorption in both segments of the proximal tubule. In contrast to *in vivo* micropuncture studies, however, the oncotic effects of protein were dissociated from changes in peritubular hydrostatic pressure, extratubular interstitial volume, and renal blood flow, since the normal capillary relationship to the tubules had been disrupted. In the study by Imai and Kokko (1972), reduction of protein content in the bath from 6.4 g/100 ml to 0.0 g/100 ml caused a 38% decrease in net volume flux. Grantham and associates (1972) used a different method of perfusion (Figure 2) and found similar results. A reduction in the bath protein concentration to 0.3 g/100 ml caused net fluid absorption to decrease 40% in both proximal convoluted and straight tubules. Imai and Kokko interpreted their results in the context of studies by Welling and Grantham (1972) in which it was shown that an oncotic pressure gradient could be generated across the isolated tubular basement membrane. It was suggested that the oncotic effects of the bath protein were exerted directly across the tubular basement membrane without necessary interposition of a capillary bed and thereby acted to alter the rate of "back-leak" of reabsorbate through the extracellular pathways between tubular cells (Imai and Kokko, 1972).

The importance of transtubule oncotic pressure gradients was reexamined by Green and associates (1974) in the rat by microperfusion. The results strongly support the findings of the isolated tubule studies and indicate that the oncotic effect of proteins is mediated at the basolateral side of the tubule cells, and not across the full extent of the tubule wall.

This does not mean, however, that the passive movement of fluid across the isolated microperfused tubule in response to osmotic forces is insignificant. The osmotic water permeability of the proximal tubule is sufficiently high that small changes in the osmolality of the bath may cause a serious error in the estimation of the "active" solute absorption. On a practical point it is emphasized that evaporation occurs from the bathing chamber at 37°C to a significant extent. Accordingly, the osmolality of the bathing medium should be monitored carefully in the course of *in vitro* microperfusion studies. This complicating factor is especially troublesome when using perfusion rates greater than 10 nl/min (Kokko, 1972a).

The isolated, perfused proximal convoluted tubule has a mean transtubule potential of approximately -4.0 mV (Burg and Orloff, 1970; Kokko and Rector, 1971; Imai and Kokko, 1972; Lutz *et al.*, 1973) when bathed in rabbit serum with both ends properly insulated with the liquid dielectric Sylgard (Dow Corning Corp., Midland, Michigan). As with net fluid transport, the transmembrane potential is temperature dependent (Kokko and Rector, 1971). Elevation of temperature to 47°C caused an irreversible loss of the transtubule potential (Kokko and Rector, 1971), whereas ouabain (10^{-5} M) in the bath caused a reversible depression of potential difference (Burg and Orloff, 1970; Kokko and Rector, 1971; Lutz *et al.*, 1973). On the basis of these observations it was concluded that the transtubule potential was related to the transport activity of the tubule and was not the consequence of diffusion or streaming potentials. Since Kokko and associates (1971) had observed a limiting concentration gradient for sodium of 35 mEq/liter, it was reasonable to infer that the "active" transport of sodium was responsible for the generation of the proximal tubule potential. In the course of examining the relation between sodium transport and transtubular potential more critically, evidence was found to indicate that lumen negativity did not necessarily reflect an active transport potential. Kokko and Rector (1971), for example, found that if the perfusion rate was decreased to less than 2 nl/min, the transtubule potential decreased toward zero. This raised the possibility that the potential difference and possibly net fluid transport were dependent on essential luminal substrates which were depleted at low perfusion rates. Subsequently, it was found that removal of glucose, alanine, and bicarbonate from the perfusate decreased the potential difference (Kokko, 1973). The precise interrelationship among organic solute transport, potential difference, and net fluid transport, however, was not defined since net fluid flux had not been measured under those conditions. The influence of organic substrates on net fluid absorption and transtubule potential has been examined recently by Cardinal and associates (1975). Net fluid absorption decreased 30% and transtubule potential decreased toward zero when glucose and amino acids and most of the bicarbonate were removed from the perfusate. Net fluid absorption decreased 50% and the transtubule potential became slightly positive when all substrates were removed from the perfusate. Ouabain (10^{-5} M) added to the bath inhibited net fluid absorption further and had no effect on potential difference. From these observations it is reasonable to conclude that there is not a predictable relationship between net fluid absorption and transtubule potential. Burg and his associates (personal communication) have found similar results with the substrates previously examined (glucose, alanine, bicarbonate) and with additional organic substrates tested in the perfusate (citrate, lactate, cycloleucine, α-methyl-D-glucoside). At this juncture, there is little evidence to indicate that lumen negativity reflects an active transport potential, but there is good evidence that organic solutes increase net fluid absorption from the luminal side of the membrane. The mechanism by which this is accomplished is not clear.

There is a paucity of data available on the effect of diuretic agents on the proximal tubule as evaluated by *in vitro* microperfusion. In the only published study devoted to the action of these drugs on the proximal tubule per se, Grantham (1973) used a modified perfusion arrangement (Figure 2) and examined the effects of acetazolamide, chlorothiazide, furosemide, and theophylline on proximal convoluted and proximal straight tubules. The data from this study are summarized in Figure 4. It is apparent that at relatively low concentrations in the bath (10^{-4} M), each diuretic caused a significant reduction in net fluid absorption in both convoluted and straight proximal tubules. Inhibition occurred in several minutes. Net absorption decreased to a relatively stable value over the course of 10 min. The same pattern of inhibition followed the addition of ouabain (10^{-5} M) to the bath, but this agent was more potent than any of the other drugs examined since fluid absorption fell nearly to zero. That the inhibition of fluid absorption obtained with each diuretic was not the result of a nonspecific or

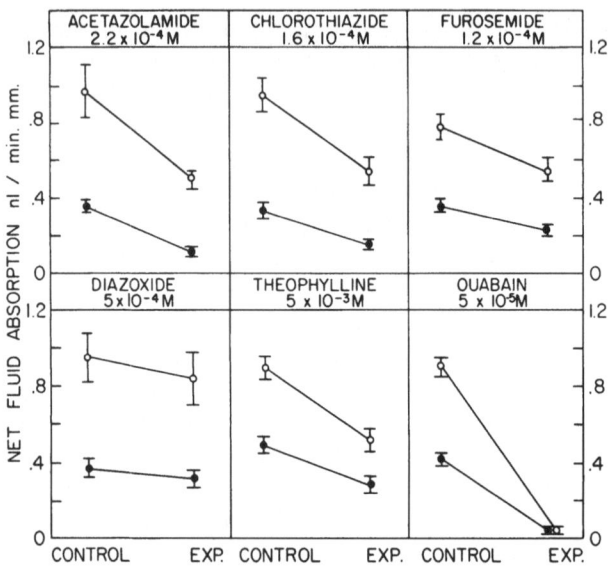

Figure 4. Depressive effect of four diuretic drugs on net fluid absorption in perfused proximal convoluted (open circles) and straight tubules (closed circles). The changes obtained with acetazolamide, chlorothiazide, furosemide, and theophylline (and ouabain) were significant. Diazoxide did not significantly depress net fluid absorption in either proximal tubular segment.

"toxic" effect was suggested by several additional observations. First, the effect of each diuretic was reversible to a significant extent when the bath was replaced with fresh rabbit serum. Secondly, tubules perfused for over 60 min had stable rates of fluid absorption (PCT 1.0 nl/mm/min; PST 0.4 nl/mm/min). Since the diuretic experiments were completed within 30–45 min of the start of perfusion, it was improbable that spontaneous variations in absorption or an unrelated factor such as depletion of organic solute (i.e., glucose) from the perfusate accounted for the effects noted with the diuretic drugs. Finally, diazoxide, a nondiuretic sulfonamide derivative, *in vivo* failed to elicit a significant reduction in fluid absorption in either segment when added to the bath at a concentration two- to threefold greater than acetazolamide, chlorothiazide, and furosemide.

Although these studies indicate the potentiality for diuretic effect in the proximal tubule, no incisive data were derived concerning the mechanism of action of the diuretics. There were two important defects in the experimental design of the study. First, the luminal fluid was not collected and analyzed (Figure 2). Second, since the diuretics were not added to the perfusate, their effect on the luminal side could not be assessed. Recently, Burg and associates (1973) have examined the effects of furosemide on proximal convoluted tubules perfused in the conventional manner (Figure 1). Furosemide in the perfusate (10^{-4} M) had no detectable effect on net fluid absorption. Nor was inhibition of fluid absorption detected in a few studies in which 10^{-3} M furosemide was added to the bath. Since the studies by Burg and his group (1973) were performed at flow rates in excess of 10 nl/min, a small but significant effect of the diuretic could have been overlooked. On the other hand, the method employed by Grantham (1973) is extraordinarily sensitive to inhibitors of fluid transport, since it does not rely on the measurement of nonabsorbable volume markers. Although a significant luminal concentration of furosemide (10^{-4} M) had no effect on net fluid transport at higher perfusion rates, this does not preclude the possibility that higher luminal or cellular concentrations may have been obtained in the "low-flow" experiments by Grantham (1973). Acetazolamide, chlorothiazide, and furosemide are all sulfonamide derivatives and possess some degree of carbonic anhydrase inhibitory activity (Baer and Beyer, 1966). High cellular concentrations of these agents may have inhibited the enzyme and mediated the decrease in net fluid absorption observed in the slow flow studies. Alternatively, since all of these agents are organic acids, they may be secreted into the lumen of the slowly perfused proximal tubule sufficiently to act as impermeant solutes and thereby retard net fluid transport.

Acetazolamide (Radtke et al., 1972), chlorthalidone (Holzgreve, 1969), and furosemide (Rector et al., 1966; Radtke et al., 1972) inhibit the "intrinsic reabsorptive capacity" of the proximal convoluted tubule as measured by the Gertz technique in situ. It should be emphasized that these studies were conducted under "split-drop" micropuncture conditions in which oil blocks prevented the flow of glomerular filtration through the proximal tubule. The split-drop micropuncture method is similar in many respects to the method used by Grantham (1973). Moreover, the results of the two methods are remarkably similar, in that sulfonamide derivatives inhibited net fluid absorption to a significant extent.

The results of "free-flow" micropuncture studies of the proximal tubule are less clearcut. Some investigators found that furosemide and certain thiazides increased fractional reabsorption in the proximal tubule (Dirks et al., 1966; Bennett et al., 1968; Knox et al., 1969), while others observed that these agents and ethacrynic acid decreased fractional reabsorption (Brenner et al., 1969a; Morgan et al., 1970, Clapp et al., 1971; Burke et al., 1972). In retrospect, the differences obtained relate mainly to the extent of extracellular volume depletion induced in these studies. If replacement of urinary losses induced by the diuretics was maintained sufficient to keep the single nephron glomerular filtration rate constant, the pharmacologic inhibition of proximal reabsorption was detected.

On balance it would appear that the in vitro studies are generally in agreement with the results obtained by micropuncture methods, namely, that thiazides and furosemide may inhibit proximal tubule fluid absorption. The mechanism of inhibition and the significance in the context of clinical use of these agents has not been elucidated. It is generally accepted that depletion of the extracellular fluid volume sets in motion secondary physiologic events which increase proximal tubule absorption. Any diuretic effect, whatever its mechanism, is evidently overridden by the forces which promote accelerated proximal tubule reabsorption in the face of extracellular volume depletion.

B. Loop of Henle

In the proximal tubule the mechanism of salt and water transport and the relevant effects of diuretics are poorly understood; however, in the past three years exciting and definitive chronicles have been written about Henle's loop. The provocative discovery that chloride and not sodium is actively transported across the tubule along the length of the thick ascending limb of the loop of Henle was simultaneously reported by two independent groups of investigators (Rocha and Kokko, 1973; Burg and Green, 1973a). The observation was made that sodium chloride was absorbed in this segment while the lumen electrical potential was positive in relation to the bath. Additional evidence in support of this thesis came from the demonstration that the removal of chloride from the bath and perfusate (substituted with sulfate) reduced the potential nearly to zero, whereas the removal of sodium (substituted with choline) increased the positive intraluminal potential. Although the presence of a small amount of "active" sodium transport was not totally excluded in these studies, it was concluded that the bulk of sodium transport along this segment was passive (Burg and Green, 1973a; Rocha and Kokko, 1973).

At the time of this discovery many renal physiologists had come to regard chloride as a "mendicant" ion. This view was based primarily on micropuncture data obtained in the proximal and distal tubules of rats and dogs where electronegativity of the lumen prevailed. Not that evidence to the contrary did not exist, for Rector and Clapp (1962) had suggested a number of years ago that the distal tubule of the rat actively reabsorbed chloride. Moreover, Schwartz and Wallace (1951) and Axelrod and Pitts (1952) had called attention to the disproportionately large amounts of chloride which appeared in the urine following administration of mercurial diuretics. It was proposed that the mercurials primarily inhibited chloride transport in the kidney. But in the intervening decades, sodium was king. The "chloruretic action" of mercurials was hostilely banished from the clinical lexicon. However, in light of recent studies (Burg and Green, 1973b) chloruresis is an "in" word among nephrophiles.

In addition to the organomercurial mersalyl, two other potent "loop diuretics"—furosemide and ethacrynic acid—have been examined recently by Burg and his associates (Burg et al., 1973; Burg and Green, 1973c). These studies were carried out on segments dissected from the cortical portion of the thick ascending limb of Henle's loop. A perfusion arrangement was used which enabled the investigators to examine the effects of the diuretics from both the luminal and peritubular side of the membrane (Figure 1).

As shown in Figure 5, furosemide, when placed in the lumen in very low concentration ($10^{-6} M$), decreased the positive transtubule potential toward zero. Net chloride transport simultaneously decreased. Both effects were greater when a higher concentration of furosemide ($10^{-5} M$) was used in the lumen. In contrast, a higher concentration of the drug in the bath ($10^{-4} M$) elicited a small inhibitory effect (Figure 6). The onset of action with furosemide in the lumen ($10^{-5} M$) occurred within seconds and was rapidly reversed upon removal of the

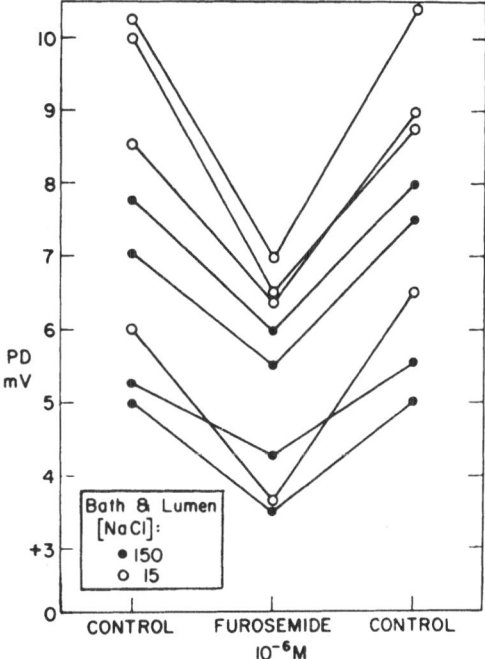

Figure 5. Effect of furosemide in the lumen on transtubule potential across perfused thick ascending limbs of Henle's loop. The depression of transtubule potential occurred within seconds of the addition of furosemide to the lumen. A slightly higher concentration of furosemide (10^{-5} M) in the lumen reduced the luminal potential nearly to zero. (From Burg *et al.*, 1973.)

drug from the perfusate (Burg *et al.*, 1973). These findings are consistent with the rapid onset of action of this drug when administered clinically.

The initial studies with ethacrynic acid in the cortical ascending limb were perplexing (Burg and Green, 1973c). At a concentration of 10^{-4} M in the lumen, ethacrynic acid had no effect. Beyer and associates (1965), however, had found

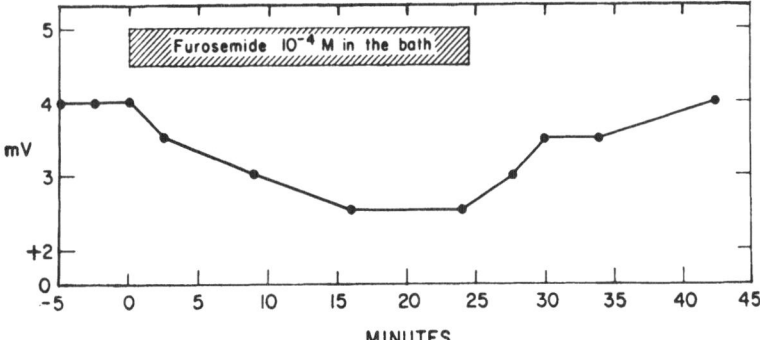

Figure 6. Effect of furosemide in the bath on transtubule potential across a perfused thick ascending limb of Henle's loop. The effect was slower in onset and of lesser magnitude than that elicited with a lesser concentration of furosemide in the lumen. (From Burg *et al.*, 1973.)

that the major excretory product in the urine was an ethacrynic–cysteine complex. Following their lead, a decrease in the electrical potential was observed when a mixture of ethacrynic and cysteine was placed in the lumen (Figure 7). More importantly, the depolarization occurred within seconds after placing a low concentration of the mixture (3×10^{-6} M) in the lumen. As with furosemide, the effects were rapidly reversed when the ethacrynic–cysteine complex was removed from the perfusate. It is noteworthy that, although ethacrynic acid inhibits sulfhydryl-catalyzed reactions *in vitro* (Schultz *et al.*, 1962), the ethacrynic–cysteine mixture is less effective in this regard (reviewed by Burg, 1974). Thus, it appears that the diuretic effect of ethacrynic acid can be dissociated from its inhibitory effect on sulfhydryl-catalyzed reactions *in vitro*.

A relatively low concentration of mersalyl in the lumen (10^{-5} M) also caused the transtubule potential to decrease (Burg and Green, 1973b). The effect with mersalyl was slower than with the nonmercurial diuretics: 5–10 min rather than seconds. After removal of the mersalyl, the potential difference returned to control values within 10–20 min. The slower onset of action *in vitro* is consonant with the slower onset of action of mersalyl observed clinically. The nonmercurial drugs (ethacrynic–cysteine and furosemide, 10^{-5} M) also caused a greater decrease in potential difference (hence chloride transport) than did mersalyl at the same concentration in the perfusate (10^{-5} M). This difference is consistent with the clinical observation that furosemide and ethacrynic acid are more potent diuretics than mercurials.

p-Chloromercuribenzoate (PCMB) is a nondiuretic mercurial agent that *in vitro* possesses a sulfhydryl reactivity similar to mersalyl (reviewed by Burg, 1974). PCMB reverses the diuretic effect of mersalyl *in vivo* (Miller and Farah,

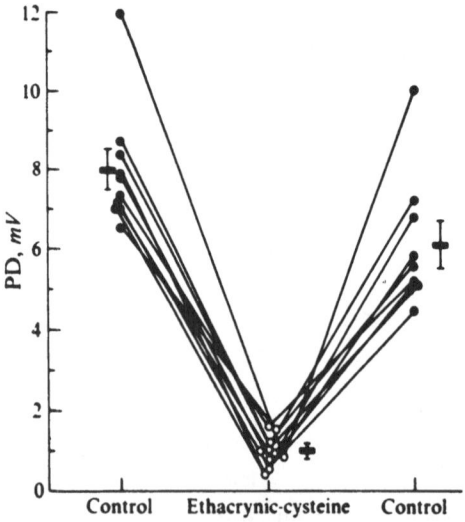

Figure 7. Effect of ethacrynic–cysteine (10^{-5} M) in the lumen of perfused thick ascending limbs of Henle's loop. The decrease in transtubule potential occurred within seconds and reached a steady-state level within 3–10 min after the drug mixture was added to the perfusate. (From Burg and Green, 1973c.)

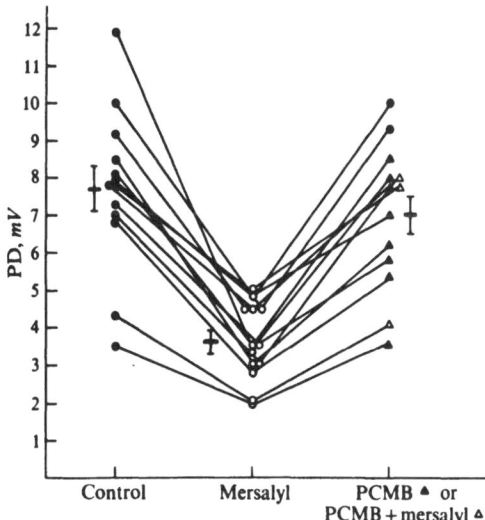

Figure 8. Effect of mersalyl (3×10^{-5} M) in the lumen of perfused thick ascending limbs of Henle's loop. The decrease in transtubule potential occurred within seconds and was reversed within seconds of the addition of p-chloromercuribenzoate (PCMB, 3×10^{-5} M) to the perfusate. PCMB when added to the perfusate alone had no depressive effect on lumen potential. (From Burg and Green, 1973b.)

1962). PCMB in the perfusate immediately reversed the effect of mersalyl (Figure 8), an observation which strengthens the claim that the mercurial action *in vitro* reliably reflects the mode of action *in vivo*.

Since it had been proposed (Weiner *et al.,* 1962) that the "free" mercuric ion was the effective moiety of the organomercurial diuretics *in situ,* mercuric chloride was added to the lumen in other studies. At a low concentration (3×10^{-6} M) mercuric chloride reduced the transtubule potential, but this effect took longer than had been noted with mersalyl. Moreover, the electrical potential was irreversibly decreased by mercuric chloride. In view of these findings it is doubtful that free mercuric ion is the active principle in the diuretic action of mersalyl.

Depression of the potential difference and net solute transport also occurred when each of the diuretics was added to the bath. The time course of these inhibitory effects, however, was more gradual than that obtained with the addition of these agents to the perfusate. Higher concentrations of the drugs were needed to elicit an inhibitory effect (furosemide and mersalyl, 10^{-4} M, ethacrynic acid 10^{-3} M). Moreover, the depressive effects on potential difference and net solute absorption often persisted after the drugs were removed from the bath. Since mersalyl and ethacrynic acid inhibit numerous sulfhydryl-catalyzed reactions *in vitro* (reviewed by Cafruny, 1968; Schultz *et al.,* 1962), it is reasonable to conclude that the irreversible depression of potential difference obtained with these agents represents a nonspecific "toxic" effect and is unrelated to the mechanism of diuretic action *in vivo*.

This last contention is supported by an additional observation (reviewed by Burg, 1974). A buffered saline solution was used in the bath for most of the studies. When serum was used in the bath, the transtubule potential (and net chloride transport) was unaffected by the addition of ethacrynic acid (10^{-4} M) or mersalyl (10^{-4} M) to the bath. The presence of the serum proteins prevented the previously obtained irreversible depression of the transtubule potential. It is generally accepted that mersalyl and ethacrynic acid are significantly protein bound *in vivo*. It is likely then that the "toxic" effects noted *in vitro* are prevented *in vivo* by the binding of the drugs to plasma proteins (reviewed by Burg, 1974).

On the basis of the *in vitro* microperfusion studies, a relatively new view has emerged regarding the mechanism of diuretic action *in vivo*. Furosemide, ethacrynic acid, and mersalyl are diuretics by virtue of their effect to inhibit active chloride transport in the ascending limb of Henle's loop. They elicit their specific inhibitory effects from the luminal side of the tubular membrane, possibly by interacting reversibly with a component of the plasma membrane. Each agent is effective at a luminal concentration that would have little effect on electrolyte transport of other organ systems. Moreover the "effective" concentration of the free drug in urine is relatively high by virtue of the fact that all of these agents are significantly bound to serum proteins.

The phenomenon of protein binding is interesting in another respect. Drugs which are tightly bound to serum proteins are not filtered to a significant extent by the glomerulus. Consequently their entrance to the sensitive receptors on the urinary surface would be severely compromised were filtration the only mode of access. Furosemide (Deetjen, 1966), mersalyl (Campbell, 1960), and ethacrynic acid (Beyer *et al.*, 1965) are secreted into the urine by the organic acid transport mechanism of the proximal tubule, probably in a manner similar to that of *p*-aminohippurate (PAH) (Tune *et al.*, 1969; Grantham *et al.*, 1972). An important clue to the mode of action of furosemide was observed several years ago. Hook and Williamson (1965a) demonstrated that probenecid blocked a furosemide-induced natriuresis in dogs. More than likely probenecid blocked secretion of furosemide into the urine in the proximal tubule and thereby diminished the amount of drug reaching the lumen surface of the ascending limb. Alternatively, probenecid may compete with furosemide at the site of action in the loop of Henle, an opposing view that has not been evaluated by direct study. Nevertheless it is clear that the achievement of very high urinary concentrations of diuretics may be enhanced owing to tubular secretion. Such a mode of action for the potent diuretic substances makes very good sense in the final analysis. Active ion transport is ubiquitous in the body, therefore a means for selectively concentrating drug at the pertinent site in the nephron enhances the clinical usefulness.

Before leaving the loop of Henle, one further point deserves comment. Burg and Green (1973a) and Rocha and Kokko (1973) observed that low concentrations of ouabain (3×10^{-6}–10^{-5} M) reversibly inhibited the transtubule potential and net chloride transport (Figure 9). This finding is difficult to reconcile in the context of the accepted action of the glycoside to interfere with sodium and potassium transport, specifically, because chloride is the ion actively transported in the loop. More than likely, the ouabain effect is a secondary effect of the

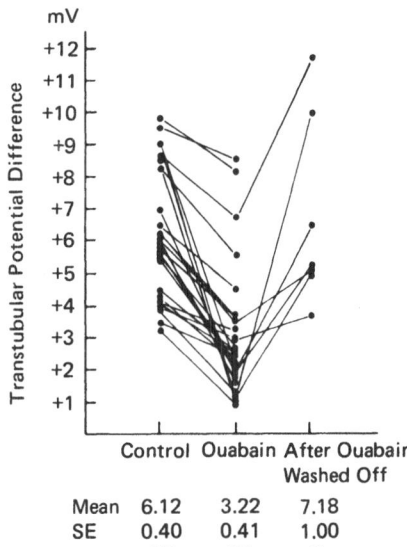

Figure 9. Effect of ouabain ($10^{-5}\,M$) in the bath on transtubule potential of perfused medullary thick ascending limbs of Henle's loop. The effect occurred within a few minutes and was rapidly reversed with removal of ouabain from the bathing fluid. (From Rocha and Kokko, 1973.)

	Control	Ouabain	After Ouabain Washed Off
Mean	6.12	3.22	7.18
SE	0.40	0.41	1.00
n	25	25	8

drug's interference with the cell volume regulatory functions of the sodium–potassium exchange mechanism on the peritubular side of the cell. Viewed in this context, ouabain's effect on chloride transport does not reflect specific interaction with the anion transport mechanism. Rather, as occurs with PAH secretion (Burg and Orloff, 1962; Grantham *et al.*, 1972), the ouabain effect is probably a reflection of inhibition of homocellular transport.

C. Cortical Collecting Tubule

Significant information about the nature of diuretic action in the distal nephron (i.e., beyond the loop of Henle) has also been derived from studies of *in vitro* microperfused tubules. Stoner and associates (1974) recently examined the effects of amiloride on isolated perfused cortical collecting tubules. A perfusion arrangement was used that allowed the investigators to examine the effects of amiloride from both the luminal and peritubular side of the membrane. When placed in the lumen in relatively low concentration ($10^{-5}\,M$), amiloride reversed the transtubule potential from -38.5 mV to 5 mV. This change occurred within a few seconds and was immediately reversible when the amiloride was removed. The net transtubular efflux of sodium and net influx of potassium were almost completely inhibited. These observations are compatible with the natriuretic and antikaliuretic effect of the drug *in vivo*. Amiloride had no effect when added to the bath at a 10-fold higher concentration ($10^{-4}\,M$). Thus, *in vitro* this agent exerts its effects from the luminal side of the membrane. The action of amiloride appeared to be relatively specific for the cortical collecting tubule since it had no effect on isolated perfused thick ascending limbs of Henle (Stoner *et al.*, 1974). Amiloride is a weak organic acid and is excreted in the urine as an intact molecule (Baer *et al.*, 1967). It is possible that this drug, like the more potent "loop" diuretics, is secreted into the urine at the level of the proximal tubule. However, there are no studies available that bear on this issue.

To this point, we have considered diuretics in regard to their primary effects on solute transport. One must also consider the impact of pharmacologic agents on the passive flow of water. Conceivably, a diuretic could have an important inhibitory effect on the hydroosmotic action of antidiuretic hormone (ADH). Important in this regard, Abramow (1974) found a striking effect of ethacrynic acid on the ADH-mediated osmotic water transport in isolated collecting tubules. As illustrated in Figure 10, ethacrynic acid (10^{-5} M) rapidly depressed the hydroosmotic effect of ADH when added to the bathing medium. The inhibitory effect of low concentrations of ethacrynic acid (10^{-5} M), however, was overcome by a high level of ADH in the bath (2 mU/ml). Moreover, ethacrynic acid alone in the bath in relatively high concentration (10^{-4} M) did not affect baseline water permeability. It was concluded that ethacrynic acid interfered with ADH-mediated water movement in the collecting tubule.

Grantham and Burg (1966) and Grantham and Orloff (1968) had previously observed that theophylline or 3',5'-cyclic AMP in the bath elicited increases in osmotic water absorption similar to ADH. On the basis of those observations, it was proposed that ADH stimulated membrane adenyl cyclase to increase the intracellular concentration of cyclic AMP (Grantham and Burg, 1966). To clarify the mechanism of ethacrynic acid–ADH antagonism *in vitro,* Abramow tested the effects of ethacrynic acid on the hydroosmotic effect of dibutyryl adenosine-3',5'-monophosphate and theophylline. Ethacrynic acid did not interfere with the

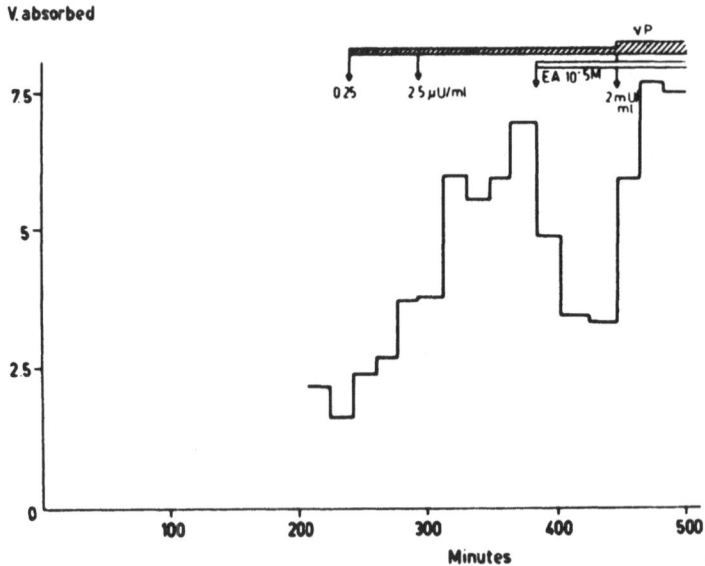

Figure 10. Effect of ethacrynic acid (EA, 10^{-5} M) on the permeability response of isolated cortical collecting tubules to vasopressin (VP, 2.5 μU/ml in the bath). Volume absorption in microliter/cm²/osmol/min. Note that the inhibitory effect of ethacrynic acid on vasopressin-mediated water flow was overcome by high concentrations of vasopressin in the bath. (From Abramow, 1974.)

effect of either agent. Consequently, Abramow (1974) concluded that the antagonistic effect of ethacrynic acid on ADH-mediated water flow occurred at the hormone receptor on the peritubular membrane.

IV. CONCLUSION

From the foregoing account it seems reasonable to predict that the method for studying isolated perfused nephrons will be an important tool for the future study of diuretic action. With improved techniques it should even be possible to study solute and water transport in the distal tubule and papillary collecting duct with some fidelity. Moreover, the explicit mechanisms of diuretic action may be susceptible to solution by this approach. At this early stage, a very important understanding of diuretic action has evolved from these studies. Clearly, the potent loop agents have their principle effect on the urinary side of the epithelial cell. Upon reflection, this mode of action seems infinitely wise, for the cell volume more than likely decreases in consequence of a decrease in solute flow into the cytoplasm. Were these agents to impair solute extrusion on the peritubular side of the cells, intracellular volume would probably increase remarkably as solute and water continued to enter across the urinary surface. Cell swelling in the kidney is not a wholesome activity because of the potential adverse effects on hydrodynamic flow through the narrow tubules and capillaries. Thus, a luminal site of action would seem less likely to predispose to nephrotoxic injury in the course of intense diuresis.

ACKNOWLEDGMENTS

We wish to thank Jan Good and Alice Dworzack for their excellent clerical assistance in the preparation of this manuscript.

REFERENCES

Abramow, M. 1974. Effects of ethacrynic acid on the isolated collecting tubule. *J. Clin. Invest.*, 53:796–804.

Adramow, M. and Dratwa, M. 1974. Effect of vasopressin on the isolated human collecting duct. *Nature, 250:*492–493.

Axelrod, D. R. and Pitts, R. F. 1952. The relationship of plasma pH and anion pattern to mercurial diuresis. *J. Clin. Invest., 31:*171–178.

Baer, F. E. and K. H. Beyer. 1966. Renal pharmacology. *Annu. Rev. Pharmacol., 6:*261–292.

Baer, F. E., Jones, C. B., Spitzer, S. A., and Russo, H. F. 1967. The potassium-sparing and natriuretic activity of *n*-amidino-3,5-diamino-6-chlorophrazine-carboxamide hydrochloride dihydrate (amiloride hydrochloride). *J. Pharmacol. Exp. Ther., 157:*472–485.

Bennett, C. M., Brenner, B. M., and Berliner, R. W. 1968. Micropuncture study of nephron function in the rhesus monkey. *J. Clin. Invest., 47:*203–216.

Bentley, P. J. 1968. Amiloride: A potent inhibitor of sodium transport across the toad bladder. *J. Physiol., 195:*317–330.

Beyer, K. H., Baer, J. E., Michaelson, J. K., and Russo, H. F. 1965. Renotropic characteristics of ethacrynic acid: A phenoxyacetic saluretic–diuretic agent. *J. Pharmacol. Exp. Ther., 147:*1–22.

Brenner, B. M., Falchuk, K. H., Keimowitz, R. I., and Berliner, R. W. 1969a. The relationship between peritubular capillary protein concentration and fluid reabsorption by the renal proximal tubule. *J. Clin. Invest., 48:*1519–1531.

Brenner, B. M., Keimowitz, R. I., Wright, F. S., and Berliner, R. W. 1969b. An inhibitory effect of furosemide on sodium reabsorption by the proximal tubule of the rat nephron. *J. Clin. Invest., 48:*290–300.

Burg, M. B. 1974. The mechanism of action of diuretics in renal tubules. In: *Recent Advances in Renal Physiology and Pharmacology,* pp. 99–109. Ed. by Fanelli, G. M. and Wesson, S. G. University Park Press, Baltimore.

Burg, M. B. and Green, N. 1973a. Function of the thick ascending limb of Henle's loop. *Am. J. Physiol., 224:*659–668.

Burg, M. B. and Green, N. 1973b. Effect of mersalyl on the thick ascending limb of Henle's loop. *Kidney Int., 4:*245–251.

Burg, M. B. and Green, N. 1973c. Effect of ethacrynic acid on the thick ascending limb of Henle's loop. *Kidney Int., 4:*301–308.

Burg, M. B. and Orloff, J. 1962. Effect of strophanthidin on electrolyte content and PAH accumulation of rabbit kidney slices. *Am. J. Physiol., 202:*565–571.

Burg, M. B. and Orloff, J. 1968. Control of fluid absorption in the renal proximal tubule. *J. Clin. Invest., 47:*2016–2024.

Burg, M. B. and Orloff, J. 1970. Electrical potential difference across proximal convoluted tubules. *Am. J. Physiol., 219:*1714–1716.

Burg, M. B. and Weller, P. F. 1969. Iodopyracet transport by isolated perfused flounder proximal renal tubules. *Am. J. Physiol., 217:*1053–1056.

Burg, M. B., Grantham, J., Abramow, M., and Orloff, J. 1966. Preparation and study of fragments of single rabbit nephrons. *Am. J. Physiol., 210:*1293–1298.

Burg, M. B., Helman, S., Grantham, J., and Orloff, J. 1970. Effect of vasopressin on the permeability of isolated rabbit cortical collecting tubules to urea, acetamide, and thiourea. In: *Urea and the Kidney,* pp. 193–199. Ed. by Schmidt-Nielsen, B. Excerpta Medica Foundation, Amsterdam.

Burg, M. B., Stoner, L., Cardinal, J., and Green, N. 1973. Furosemide effect on isolated perfused tubules. *Am. J. Physiol., 225:*119–124.

Burke, T. J., Robinson, R. R., and Clapp, J. R. 1972. Determinants of the effect of furosemide on the proximal tubule. *Kidney Int., 1:*12–18.

Cafruny, E. J. 1968. The site and mechanism of action of mercurial diuretics. *Pharmacol. Rev., 20:*89–116.

Campbell, D. E. S. 1960. Modification by bromcresol green or probenecid of the excretion and diuretic effect of three mercurial diuretics, diurgin, chlormerodrin and mercumatilin. *Acta Pharmacol. Toxicol., 17:*213–232.

Cardinal, J., Lutz, M. D., Burg, M. B., and Orloff, J. 1975. Lack of relationship of potential difference to fluid absorption in the proximal renal tubule. *Kidney Int., 7:*94–102.

Chonko, A. M., Osgood, R. W., Ferris, T. F., and Stein, J. H. 1974. Measurement of nephron filtration rate (V_0) and proximal tubular sodium transport in the rabbit kidney. *Clin. Res., 22:*623A.

Clapp, J. R. and Robinson, R. R. 1968. Distal sites of action of diuretic drugs in the dog nephron. *Am. J. Physiol., 215:*228–235.

Clapp, J. R., Nottebohm, G. A., and Robinson, R. R. 1971. Proximal site of action of ethacrynic acid: Importance of filtration rate. *Am. J. Physiol., 220:*1355–1377.

Dantzler, W. H. 1974. PAH transport by snake proximal renal tubules: Differences from urate transport. *Am. J. Physiol., 226:*634–641.

Deetjen, P. 1966. Micropuncture studies on site and mode of diuretic action of furosemide. *Ann. N.Y. Acad. Sci., 139:*408–415.

DiBona, D. R., Civan, M. M., and Leaf, A. 1969. The cellular specificity of the effect of vasopressin on toad urinary bladder. *J. Membr. Biol., 1:*79–91.

Dirks, J. H. and Seely, J. F. 1970. Effect of saline infusions and furosemide on the dog distal nephron. *Am. J. Physiol., 219:*114–121.

Dirks, J. H., Cirksena, W. J., and Berliner, R. W. 1966. Micropuncture study of the effect of various diuretics on sodium reabsorption by the proximal tubules of the dog. *J. Clin. Invest., 45:*1875–1885.

Duarte, C. G., Chomety, F., and Giebisch, G. 1971. Effect of amiloride, ouabain, and furosemide on distal tubular function in the rat. *Am. J. Physiol., 221:*632–640.

Duggan, D. E. and Noll, R. M. 1972. Effects of ethacrynic acid upon membrane ATPase of dog kidney *in vivo* and *in vitro. Proc. Soc. Exp. Biol. Med., 139:*762–767.

Evanson, R. L., Lockhart, E. A., and Dirks, J. H. 1972. Effect of mercurial diuretics on tubular sodium and potassium transport in the dog. *Am. J. Physiol., 222:*282–289.

Ferguson, D. R. 1966. Effects of frusemide on sodium and water transport by the isolated toad bladder. *Br. J. Pharmacol. Chemother., 27:*528–531.

Goldberg, M., McCurdy, D. K., Foltz, E. L., and Bluemle, L. W., Jr. 1964. Effects of ethacrynic acid (a new saluretic agent) on renal diluting and concentrating mechanisms: Evidence for site of action in the loop of Henle. *J. Clin. Invest., 43:*201–216.

Goldberg, M., Beck, L. H., Puschett, J. B., and Schubert, J. J. 1973. Sites of action of benzothiadiazines, frusemide and ethacrynic acid. In: *Modern Diuretic Therapy in the Treatment of Cardiovascular and Renal Disease,* pp. 135–143. Ed. by Lant, A. F. and Wilson, G. M. Excerpta Medica Foundation, Amsterdam.

Gottschalk, C. W. 1961. Micropuncture studies of tubular function in the mammalian kidney. *The Physiologist, 4:*35–55.

Gottschalk, C. W. and Mylle, M. 1959. Micropuncture study of the mammalian urinary concentrating mechanism: Evidence for the countercurrent hypothesis. *Am. J. Physiol., 196:*927–936.

Grantham, J. 1973. Sodium transport in isolated renal tubules. In: *Modern Diuretic Therapy in the Treatment of Cardiovascular and Renal Disease,* pp. 220–228. Ed. by Lant, E. F., and Wilson, G. M. Excerpta Medica Foundation, Amsterdam.

Grantham, J. and Burg, M. B. 1966. Effect of vasopressin and cyclic AMP on permeability of isolated collecting tubules. *Am. J. Physiol., 211:*255–259.

Grantham, J. and Burg, M. B. and Orloff, J. 1970. The nature of transtubular Na and K transport is isolated rabbit renal collecting tubules, *J. Clin. Invest., 49:*1815–1826.

Grantham, J. and Orloff, J. 1968. Effect of prostaglandin E₁ on the permeability response of the isolated collecting tubule to vasopressin, adenosine 3′,5′-monophosphate, and theophylline. *J. Clin. Invest., 47:*1154–1161.

Grantham, J., Burg, M. B., and Orloff, J. 1970. The nature of transtubular Na and K transport in isolated rabbit renal collecting tubules. *J. Clin. Invest., 49:*1815–1826.

Grantham, J., Qualizza, P. B., and Welling, L. W. 1972. Influence of serum proteins on net fluid reabsorption of isolated proximal tubules. *Kidney Int., 2:*66–75.

Grantham, J., Qualizza, P. B., and Irwin, R. L. 1974. Net fluid secretion in proximal straight renal tubules *in vitro:* Role of PAH. *Am. J. Physiol., 226:*191–197.

Green, R., Windhager, E. E., and Giebisch, G. 1974. Protein oncotic pressure effects on proximal tubular fluid movement in the rat. *Am. J. Physiol., 226:*265–276.

Hamburger, R. J., Lawson, N. L., and Dennis, V. W. 1974. Effects of cyclic adenosine nucleotides on fluid absorption by different segments of proximal tubule. *Am. J. Physiol., 227:*396–401.

Hargitay, B. and Kuhn, W. 1951. Das Multiplikationsprinzip als Grundlage der Harnkonzentrierung in der Niere. *Z. Elektrochem., 55:* 539–558.

Hays, R. M. and Leaf, A. 1962. Studies on the movement of water through the isolated toad bladder and its modification by vasopressin. *J. Gen. Physiol., 45:*905–919.

Helman, S. I., Grantham, J. J., and Burg, M. B. 1971. Effect of vasopressin on electrical resistance of renal cortical collecting tubules. *Am. J. Physiol., 220:*1825–1832.

Holzgreve, H. 1969. The pattern of inhibition of proximal tubular reabsorption by diuretics. In: *Renal Transport and Diuretics,* pp. 229–234. Ed. by Thurau, K. and Jahrmarker, H. Springer-Verlag, Berlin.

Hook, J. B. and Williamson, H. E. 1965a. Influence of probenecid and alterations in acid–base balance of the saluretic activity of furosemide. *J. Pharmacol. Exp. Ther., 149:*404–408.

Hook, J. B. and Williamson, H. E. 1965b. Lack of correlation between natriuretic activity and inhibition of renal Na–K-activated ATPase. *Proc. Soc. Exp. Biol. Med., 120:*358–360.

Imai, M. and Kokko, J. P. 1972. Effect of peritubular protein concentration on reabsorption of sodium and water in isolated perfused proximal tubules. *J. Clin. Invest., 51:*314–325.

Imai, M. and Kokko, J. P. 1974. Transtubular oncotic pressure gradients and net fluid transport in isolated proximal tubules. *Kidney Int., 6:*138–156.

Knox, F. G., Wright, F. S., Howards, S. S., and Berliner, R. W. 1969. Effect of furosemide on sodium reabsorption by proximal tubule of the dog. *Am. J. Physiol., 217:*192–198.

Koefoed-Johnsen, F. and Ussing, H. H. 1953. The contributions of diffusion and flow to the passage of D_2O through living membranes. *Acta Physiol. Scand., 28:*60–76.

Kokko, J. P. 1970. Sodium chloride and water transport in the descending limb of Henle. *J. Clin. Invest., 49:*1838–1846.

Kokko, J. P. 1972a. Qualitative and quantitative importance of the constituents used in microperfusion experiments. *Yale J. Biol. Med., 45:*332–338.

Kokko, J. P. 1972b. Urea transport in the proximal tubule and the descending limb of Henle. *J. Clin. Invest., 51:*1999–2008.

Kokko, J. P. 1973. Proximal tubule potential difference. *J. Clin. Invest., 52:*1362–1367.

Kokko, J. P. and Rector, F. C. 1971. Flow dependence of transtubular potential difference in isolated perfused segments of rabbit proximal convoluted tubule. *J. Clin. Invest., 50:*2745–2750.

Kokko, J. P., Burg, M. B., and Orloff, J. 1971. Characteristics of NaCl and water transport in the renal proximal tubule. *J. Clin. Invest., 50:*69–76.

Lewy, J. E. and Windhager, E. E. 1968. Peritubular control of proximal tubular fluid reabsorption in the rat kidney. *Am. J. Physiol., 214:*943–954.

Lutz, M. C., Cardinal, J., and Burg, M. B. 1973. Electrical resistance of renal proximal tubule perfused in vitro. *Am. J. Physiol., 225:*729–734.

Miller, T. B. and Farah, A. E. 1962. Inhibition of mercurial diuresis by nondiuretic mercurials. *J. Pharmacol. Exp. Ther., 135:*102–111.

Morgan, T., Todokoro, M., Martin, D., and Berliner, R. W. 1970. Effect of furosemide on Na^+ and K^+ transport studied by microperfusion of the rat nephron. *Am. J. Physiol., 218:*292–297.

Radtke, H. W., Rumrich, G., Kinne-Saffran, E., and Ullrich, K. J. 1972. Dual action of acetazolamide and furosemide on proximal volume absorption in the rat kidney. *Kidney Int., 1:*100–105.

Rector, F. C., Jr. and Clapp, J. R. 1962. Evidence for active chloride reabsorption in the distal renal tubule of the rat. *J. Clin. Invest., 41:*101–107.

Rector, F. C., Jr., Brunner, F. P., Sellman, J. C., and Seldin, D. W. 1966. Pitfalls in the use of micropuncture for the localization of diuretic action. *Ann. N.Y. Acad. Sci., 139:*400–407.

Richards, A. N. and Schmidt, C. F. 1924. A description of the glomerular circulation in the frog's kidney and observations concerning the action of adrenalin and various other substances upon it. *Am. J. Physiol., 71:*178–208.

Rocha, A. S. and Kokko, J. P. 1973. Sodium chloride and water transport in the medullary thick ascending limb of Henle. *J. Clin. Invest., 52:*612–623.

Rocha, A. S. and Kokko, J. P. 1974. Permeability of medullary nephron segments to urea and water: Effect of vasopressin. *Kidney Int. 6:*379–387.

Schafer, J. A. and Andreoli, T. E. 1972. The effect of antidiuretic hormone on solute flows in mammalian collecting tubules. *J. Clin. Invest., 51:*1279–1286.

Schmidt, U. and Dubach, U. C. 1970. The behaviour of Na^+K^+-activated adenosine triphosphatase in various structures of the rat nephron after furosemide application. *Nephron, 7:*447–458.

Schultz, E. M., Cragoe, E. J., Jr., Bicking, J. B., Bolhofer, W. A., and Sprague, J. M. 1962. α,β-Unsaturated ketone derivatives of aryloxyacetic acids, a new class of diuretics. *J. Med. Pharm. Chem., 5:*660–662.

Schwartz, W. B. and Wallace, W. M. 1951. Electrolyte equilibrium during mercurial diuresis. *J. Clin. Invest., 30:*1089–1104.

Seely, J. F. and Dirks, J. H. 1969. Micropuncture study of hypertonic mannitol diuresis in the proximal and distal tubule of the dog kidney. *J. Clin. Invest., 48:*2330–2340.

Seldin, D. W. and Rector, F. C., Jr. 1973. Evaluation of clearance methods for localization of site of action of diuretics. In: *Modern Diuretic Therapy in the Treatment of Cardiovascular and Renal Disease,* pp. 97–111. Ed. by Lant, A. F. and Wilson, G. M. Excerpta Medica Foundation, Amsterdam.

Stoner, L. C., Burg, M. B., and Orloff, J. 1974. Ion transport in cortical collecting tubule; Effect of amiloride. *Am. J. Physiol., 227:*453–459.

Suki, W., Rector, F. C., Jr., and Seldin, D. W. 1965. The site of action of furosemide and other sulfonamide diuretics in the dog. *J. Clin. Invest., 44:*1458–1469.

Sullivan, L. P., Tucker, J. M., and Scherbenske, M. J. 1971. Effect of furosemide on sodium transport and metabolism in toad bladder. *Am. J. Physiol., 220:*1316–1324.

Tune, B. M. and Burg, M. B. 1971. Glucose transport by proximal renal tubules. *Am. J. Physiol, 221:*580–585.

Tune, B. M., Burg, M. B., and Patlak, C. S. 1969. Characteristics of p-aminohippurate transport in proximal renal tubules. *Am. J. Physiol., 217:*1957–1063.

Vogl, A. 1950. The discovery of the organic mercurial diuretics. *Am. Heart J., 39:*881–883.

Wearn, J. T. and Richards, A. N. 1924. Observations on the composition of glomerular urine, with particular reference to the problem of reabsorption in the renal tubules. *Am. J. Physiol., 71:*209–227.

Weiner, I. M., Levy, R. I., and Mudge, G. H. 1962. Studies on mercurial diuresis: Renal excretion, acid stability and structure–activity relationships of organic mercurials. *J. Pharmacol. Exp. Ther., 138:*96–112.

Welling, L. W. and Grantham, J. J. 1972. Physical properties of isolated perfused renal tubules and tubular basement membranes. *J. Clin. Invest., 51:*1063–1075.

Wirz, H., Hargitay, B., and Kuhn, W. 1951. Lokalisation des Konzentrierungsprozesses in der Niere durch direkte Kryoskopic. *Heb. Physiol. Pharmacol. Acta., 9:*196–207.

Chapter **3**

Study of Renal Action of Diuretics by Micropuncture Techniques

Franklyn G. Knox and Gary R. Marchand

Department of Physiology and Biophysics
Mayo Clinic, Rochester, Minnesota 55901

I. INTRODUCTION

The collection of tubule fluid from discrete segments of the nephron with micropuncture techniques has significantly advanced the fundamental knowledge of renal physiology. Proof of the hypothesis that urine production begins with the formation of a protein-free ultrafiltrate of plasma awaited development of techniques for the collection and analysis of fluid from Bowman's space. In 1929, A. N. Richards (1929) used the micropuncture technique to confirm this hypothesis in amphibia. Recently, micropuncture techniques have been applied to the direct investigation of the effect of diuretics on single nephron function. The methods can be used to localize the tubule site of action, and the observed changes in tubule fluid reabsorptive rates and electrolyte concentrations can be used to infer mechanisms of action. The methodologies presented herein are considered in the context of their applicability to the study of renal pharmacology. A more detailed monograph of micropuncture techniques together with concepts of nephron function has been provided by Windhager (1968).

The choice of an animal species for micropuncture depends on two major factors: the nephron segment under investigation and whether the diuretic response is species dependent. For example it has been demonstrated that the diuretic response to ethacrynic acid is attenuated in rats. The animal of choice for the puncture of Bowman's space is the Munich–Wistar rat since this species has glomeruli readily identifiable on the surface of the kidney.[1] The squirrel

---

[1] Discovered in the laboratory of Dr. Klaus Thurau, Physiological Institute, Munich, Germany.

monkey is also suitable for this purpose; however, the expense of this model limits widespread application. Micropuncture of the proximal tubule is readily accomplished in both rats and dogs. In this case the advantage of dogs lies in the increased capability to measure total renal function with comparison to the wealth of clearance data available for the dog. In addition the effect of the drug may be restricted to the kidney by arterial administration. Although distal micropuncture can be accomplished in the dog, the rat is the model of choice since distal tubules are more readily identified and punctured in the rat. Finally, papillary structures, including the collecting duct, are accessible for micropuncture in young rats and hamsters which have papillae that extend into the renal pelvis.

Consideration should be given to study of the diuretic under conditions of sodium retention thereby mimicking the clinical use of the drugs. For example, the effects of spironolactone are best studied in models of hyperaldosteronism since the competitive antagonists of aldosterone are most effective in the presence of high circulating levels of aldosterone. Although a chronic model of sodium retention has been developed in the rat (Stumpe et al., 1973), the dog has been studied more intensively and the dog model is technically less difficult (Davis and Howell, 1953; Davis et al., 1964).

II. PREPARATION FOR MICROPUNCTURE

A. Anesthesia

The investigation of renal function by the micropuncture technique requires that the animal be anesthetized throughout the duration of the experiment. The effect of anesthesia upon tubular function as determined in micropuncture experiments is largely unknown. In addition, different anesthetics may have differing effects upon renal function. Elmer et al. (1972) compared the renal function of rats anesthetized with the thiobarbiturate, inactin, or the oxybarbiturate, sodium amytal. Proximal fluid reabsorption, as estimated by the transit time of lissamine green, was significantly depressed in the inactin-anesthetized rat. The authors suggested that the anesthetic employed may account for the observed differences in TF/P inulin from different laboratories. These specific effects of anesthetics can be controlled by making measurements before and after administration of the diuretic in the same anesthetized animal. This approach lends itself well to determining the acute effects of the diuretic but has obvious limitations in determining the chronic effects of diuretics, a clinically relevant issue.

B. Surgical Preparation

To facilitate surgical preparation, food is usually withheld approximately 12–18 hr prior to micropuncture. This necessary maneuver dictates that animals are studied in a state of sodium deprivation. Therefore the possibility that the postprandial excretions of electrolytes may be very important in diuretic effects is difficult to evaluate with micropuncture techniques.

In addition to the standard placement of catheters, the kidney must be thoroughly dissected free from surrounding attachments. Particular care must be exercised to avoid obstruction of the ureter and renal vein by bands of connective tissue. Such obstruction will lead to a tense, poorly functioning kidney. The kidney is then placed in a holder to isolate it from abdominal and respiratory motion. At this point care must be exercised to avoid stretching the renal artery. A compromised arterial inflow can be recognized by palpation of a soft kidney and patchy distribution of blood flow. In the study of diuretics, the choice of ureteral catheter size is an important consideration. The outflow resistance of PE10 catheters has been calculated by Cortell *et al.* (1972) to be 20 times greater than that of PE50 catheters. The authors observed that as the urine flow rate was increased during furosemide or mannitol diuresis, the rate of increase of both proximal and distal intratubular pressure was greater when PE10 catheters were used. Thus at high urine flow rates the smaller catheter would be expected to produce a functional obstruction.

C. Identification of Tubule Segments for Micropuncture

The majority of tubules visible on the surface of the kidney are convolutions of the proximal tubule. Figure 1 shows the latest accessible convolution of a proximal tubule which has been injected with latex. Subsequently, this tubule was dissected free and is shown in Figure 2. The point shown by the arrow corresponds to the point of this proximal tubule which appears on the surface of the kidney (see Figure 1). Typically in the dog or rat only about 60% of the proximal convoluted tubule is accessible to micropuncture. However, in primates 80% of the proximal convoluted tubule is on the surface of the kidney (Bennett *et al.,* 1968).

Nephron segments, that is, late proximal and distal tubule segments, are easily identified by the observation of the transit time of dyes through the nephron. Since Steinhausen (1963) first used lissamine green dye in renal micropuncture studies, the dye has been used widely. The distinctive appearance of the dye within the tubules allows identification of tubule segments along the nephron and also permits estimation of the transit time of tubule fluid through these segments. In the rat, for example, dye appears in the late proximal, early distal, and late distal tubule approximately 10, 20, and 35 sec, respectively, after the initial appearance in the renal microvasculature. The selective micropuncture of late proximal tubules is important for the detection of changes in reabsorption as subsequently discussed. Furthermore, the physiologic characteristics of the early and late distal tubules are markedly different, and therefore it is important to identify these distinct segments of the distal nephron. Samples collected from the early distal tubule may be representative of function in the thick ascending limb of Henle's loop as well as the distal convoluted tubule, while samples from the late distal tubule may be representative of changes in the early collecting system as well as the distal convoluted tubule.

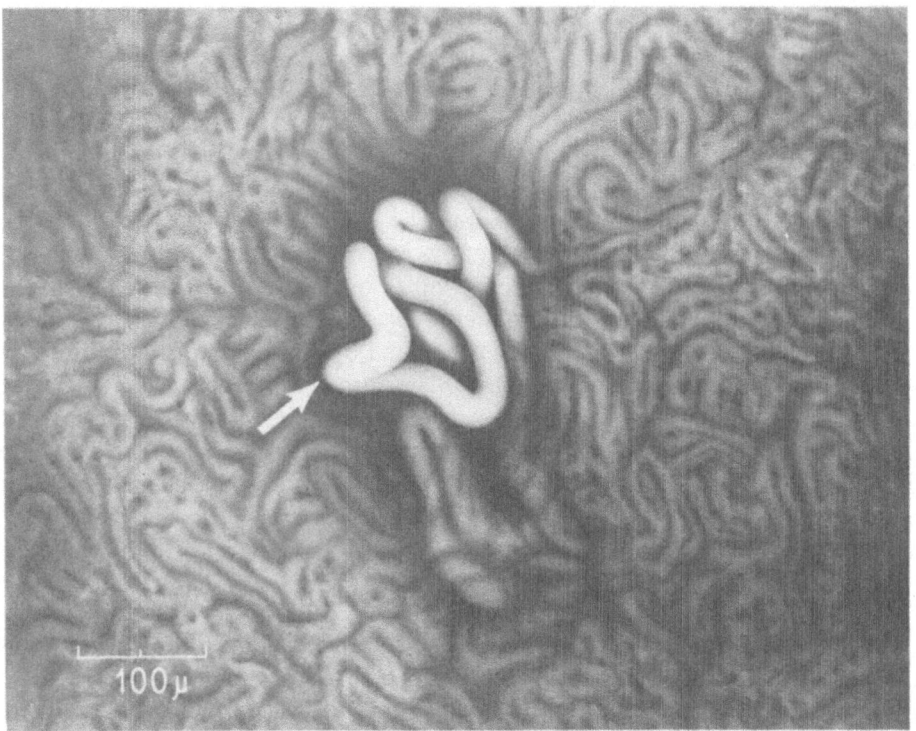

Figure 1. Photomicrograph of the latest accessible surface convolution (arrow) of a proximal tubule of a dog kidney. The tubule has been injected with latex. The photograph has been retouched for clarity of presentation.

A prerequisite to the use of a dye as an aid in the investigation of tubular sodium reabsorption is that the dye itself should not influence sodium reabsorption. However, several studies have indicated that lissamine green may directly inhibit sodium transport. Dörge and Nagel (1969) and Christensen and Frederiksen (1972) have demonstrated a decrease in the short-circuit current across the frog skin produced by lissamine green, while in the rat, Roch-Ramel and Jotterand (1970) and Heller (1971) have demonstrated natriuretic effects of lissamine green in doses comparable to those used in micropuncture studies. We have examined the effect of lissamine green dye on sodium reabsorption by the proximal tubule and urinary sodium excretion in dogs (Lynch *et al.*, 1973). Multiple injections (0.2 ml each) of dye caused no detectable changes in fractional reabsorption by the proximal tubule, single nephron filtration rate, or glomerular filtration rate. Neither was sodium excretion significantly different from that in the contralateral noninjected kidney. Infusion of dye (0.2 ml/min) into the micropuncture kidney was associated with a small but significant unilateral natriuresis. The data indicated that lissamine green dye can be natriuretic; however, doses used to identify late proximal tubule segments had no effect on sodium excretion, fractional reabsorption by the proximal tubule, or single nephron filtration rate.

Given this potential for a natriuretic effect of the dye, the preferred experimental design is to perform mapping of the kidney surface one hour before micropuncture studies are commenced. In this manner the effect of the dye is dissipated prior to diuretic administration, and no further dye injections are given during the course of subsequent experimental testing. This consideration is especially important for the study of diuretics in which the natriuretic response is small.

Other dyes, such as FDC green dye, have been used for location of nephron segments. In our experience these dyes have been somewhat more difficult to visualize than lissamine green, and since the precaution of making all green injections and mapping one hour before commencement of micropuncture is adequate for control of possible natriuretic effects of the dye, lissamine green remains the localizing agent of choice.

An alternative method for localizing late proximal tubule segments is the injection of a microdroplet of stained castor oil into a tubule segment. If the droplet repeatedly reappears in later tubule segments, the puncture site is considered an early tubule segment and samples are not collected. However, if the droplet disappears within 2–3 sec and does not reappear on the surface, the puncture site is considered to be in the late proximal tubule segment. This method can be used more readily in the dog kidney since the chances of puncturing the distal tubule are considerably more remote than in the rat kidney.

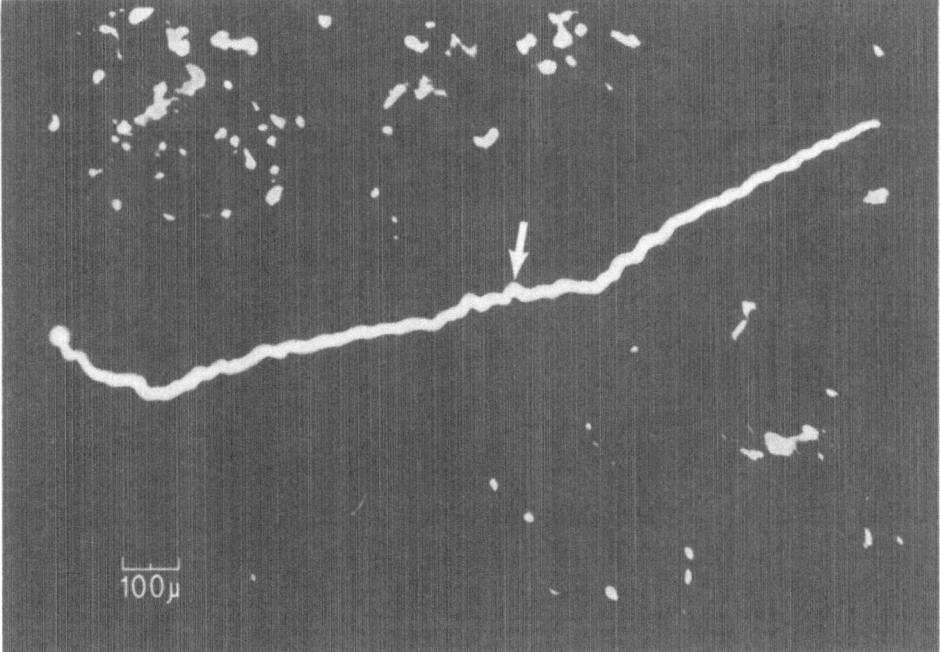

Figure 2. Photomicrograph of the entire proximal convoluted tubule presented in Figure 1. The arrow indicates the point along this nephron segment which corresponds to the latest accessible surface convolution.

In the rat, where distal nephron segments are more numerous on the kidney surface, the lissamine green injection method is preferable to the oil droplet method.

III. MICROPUNCTURE METHODOLOGIES

In the study of the natriuretic effects of diuretics, the first factor to be considered in the intrarenal regulation of sodium reabsorption is the filtered load. The filtered load of sodium is in turn primarily governed by the glomerular filtration rate. The glomerular filtration rate may be decreased by the disease state necessitating the use of the diuretic or may be secondarily decreased by the diuretic under study. In addition to determination of the single nephron filtered load, micropuncture techniques can be utilized to examine the effects of diuretics on the driving forces governing filtration. Diuretics may increase intratubule pressure or may alter arteriolar resistances which in turn will effect the net filtration pressure.

A. Micropuncture of Bowman's Space

Historically, the evidence that the glomerular filtrate was an ultrafiltrate of plasma was provided by A. N. Richards (1929) from his determination of the composition of fluid collected from Bowman's space of amphibia. Until recently, micropuncture of the adult mammalian glomerulus was impossible since the glomeruli are located below the surface of the kidney. The discovery of a mutant strain of Wistar rats, the so-called Munich–Wistar rat, has enabled investigators to study the composition and the dynamics of formation of glomerular filtrate. As expected, the TF/P inulin was equal to unity throughout a large range of plasma concentrations. In addition, the TF/P sodium was also approximately one (Harris *et al.*, 1974).

Micropuncture of Bowman's space permits physiological evaluation of drug-related alterations in glomerular capillary permeability and/or solute ultrafilterability. The constancy of these factors is assumed in the absence of direct determination, i.e., collection from Bowman's space, and is fundamental to interpretation of fluid and electrolyte reabsorption in the remaining nephron.

B. Measurement of Forces for Glomerular Filtration

To investigate the mechanism by which an agent affects single nephron glomerular filtration rate (SNGFR), the forces for filtration can be directly assessed by micropuncture of glomerular structures in mammalian species with glomeruli on the surface of the kidney. Thus the primary determinants of glomerular filtration, including glomerular capillary pressure (Brenner *et al.*, 1971a) and the pressure in Bowman's space, can be directly measured. Oncotic pressure can be estimated from the protein concentration of afferent and efferent arteriolar plasma. Application of a servo-nulling device (Wiederhielm *et al.*,

1964) for the measurement of hydrostatic pressures in superficial renal cortical structures was first reported by Falchuk and Berliner (1971). The apparatus consists of an electrical Wheatstone bridge, one arm of which is a micropuncture pipet filled with hypertonic sodium chloride. The oncotic pressures are calculated from measurements of protein concentrations. The mean glomerular capillary protein concentration is calculated from measurements of systemic protein concentration, which reflect afferent arteriolar protein concentration, and measurements of efferent arteriolar protein concentration obtained by direct micropuncture. The mean glomerular capillary protein concentration is then calculated based on an exponential increase of protein concentration along the length of the glomerular capillary subsequent to the formation of protein-free ultrafiltrate.

Since glomeruli are not accessible for micropuncture in the dog, estimates of glomerular capillary pressure can be obtained by the stop-flow method which involves injecting a long column of castor oil and measuring the resultant intratubular pressure proximal to the blockade. The pressure measured is equal to the net ultrafiltration pressure, i.e., glomerular capillary hydrostatic pressure minus the glomerular capillary oncotic pressure. Since ultrafiltration is abolished by the presence of the oil block, glomerular capillary oncotic pressure is assumed to equal systemic oncotic pressure. Therefore, glomerular capillary pressure (P_G) is calculated as the sum of stop-flow pressure (SFP) and systemic oncotic pressure (π_G).

$$P_G = SFP + \pi_G$$

Similar values for glomerular capillary hydrostatic pressure have been obtained by both direct micropuncture and stop-flow methods in the same rat (Blantz *et al.*, 1972).

C. Measurement of Single Nephron Filtration Rate

1. Determination

The principle for the measurement of single nephron filtration rate is similar to that for determination of filtration rate for the kidney as a whole. The corresponding formulas are:

$$GFR \text{ (ml/min)} = \dot{V} \text{ (ml/min)} \times (U/P)_{\text{in}}$$

and

$$SNGFR \text{ (nl/min)} = \dot{V}_{TF} \text{ (nl/min)} \times (TF/P)_{\text{in}}$$

where *GFR* and *SNGFR* are the filtration rates for the kidney and single nephron, respectively. The flow rate of tubule fluid, $\dot{V}_{TF}$, is obtained by a timed quantitative collection of the tubule fluid at the point of micropuncture. The concentration of inulin is then determined in tubule fluid and divided by that in plasma (TF/P) to provide an index of volume reabsorption to the point of micropuncture.

The quantitative collection of tubule fluid is accomplished by the injection of an oil block into the tubule with subsequent aspiration of tubule fluid at a rate sufficient to maintain the block in a constant position. Several laboratories have evaluated this technique in detail.

2. Analysis of Error

The first consideration is the placement of the pipet. Davidman *et al.* (1971) have shown that measurement of single nephron filtration rate was not influenced by changes in tip size or by the direction of the pipet within the tubule. The major hazard in placement of the pipet is formation of a fistula between underlying convolutions of a proximal tubule. To detect possible fistula formation, Andreucci *et al.* (1971) used a second pipet to inject lissamine green during the collection of tubular fluid. The appearance of dye in adjacent loops was noted in 10% of all punctures. Without the injection of lissamine green, the detection of fistula formation was not possible. This error should be suspected when excessively high values for single nephron filtration rate are obtained due to artifactually elevated $\dot{V}_{TF}$.

The next major consideration is the placement of an adequate oil block, since contamination of collected tubular fluid with fluid from a more distal part of the nephron, i.e., distal to the oil block, could significantly increase the estimation of single nephron GFR. Although it appears that such retrograde contamination is not a significant problem during hydropenia, several laboratories have suggested that it is a potential source of error during conditions of elevated tubular pressures.

Rector *et al.* (1966a) reported that very high TF/P inulin ratios (10–100) which were obtained during elevated ureteral pressure were associated with the use of a relatively short oil block. Subsequently Brenner *et al.* (1969) examined the effect of furosemide, an agent which has been shown to increase intratubular pressure, on fractional reabsorption by the proximal tubule. When oil blocks of conventional length (2–3 tubule diameters) were used for collection of proximal tubular fluid, TF/P inulins were either unchanged or increased during the administration of furosemide. In contrast, when longer oil blocks were used, fractional reabsorption was depressed during furosemide. Thus it was concluded that significant retrograde contamination occurred during the elevated intratubular pressure produced by furosemide administration.

The next step in the determination of single nephron filtration rate is to initiate collection by application of suction to the micropuncture pipet. It has been suggested that changes in intratubular pressure produced during collection of filtrate may be transmitted to the glomerulus and thereby spuriously affect single nephron GFR (Schnermann *et al.*, 1969). Brenner and Daugharty (1972) investigated this possibility by measuring upstream intratubular pressures during the application of either controlled or excessive suction or during spontaneous collection of fluid (see Figure 3). Although the application of excessive suction reduced proximal intratubular pressure, there was no significant effect on single nephron filtration rate. Simultaneous recording of intratubular hydrostatic pressure indicated that while pressure dropped significantly at the collection site, the

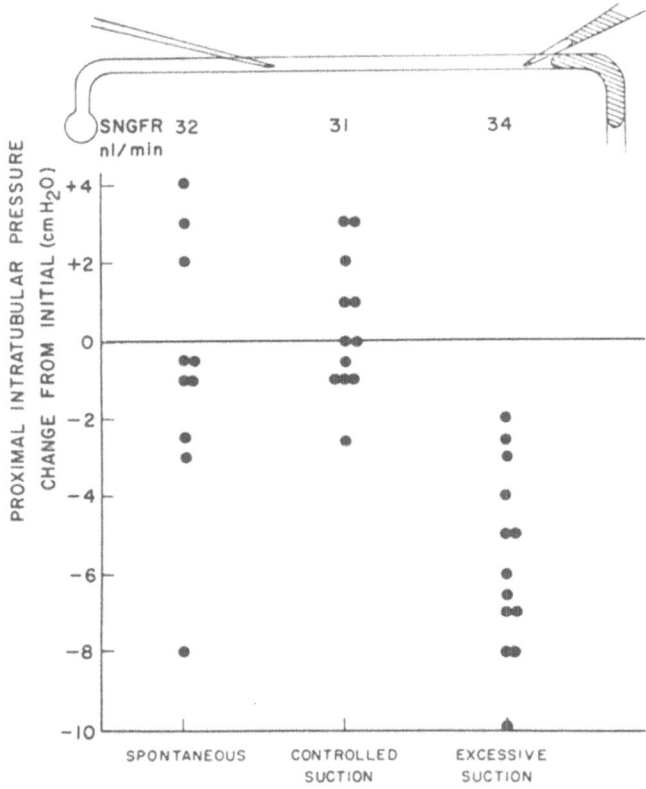

Figure 3. Effects of variations on fluid sampling techniques on proximal intratubular pressures. Values for SNGFR obtained for each technique are also shown. (From Brenner and Daugharty, 1972, by permission.)

pressure within the first convolution emerging from Bowman's space did not change. They concluded that the proximal tubule has the characteristics of a nonlinear (Starling) resistor. Since the glomerulus is located below the surface of the kidney, a sufficient length of tubule is usually interposed between the collection site and the glomerulus so that suction will not alter effective filtration pressure.

Similar to the results found by Brenner and his colleagues, Davidman *et al.* (1971) found that intentional reductions in intratubule pressure were not reflected by measurable changes in single nephron filtration rate. Furthermore, they found that standard collection techniques do not significantly alter intratubule pressure.

Langer *et al.* (1968) reported that castor oil produces a more effective blockade of the tubule than mineral oil and therefore reduces the possibility of retrograde contamination. In addition castor oil does not affect the morphology of the tubular epithelial cells whereas mineral oil does.

Errors also arise from the collection of samples from the distal side of the oil block. This occurs when the oil block is between the collection pipet and the glomerulus and fluid is collected in a retrograde manner from more distal nephron convolutions. This problem arises during high intratubule pressures and can be avoided by observing the downstream displacement of the oil block following injection.

Timing of the collection period is begun upon introduction of the oil block, thereby accounting for filtrate formed before initiating sample collection. In addition, the transient changes in nephron filtration rate induced by the injection of the oil block are minimized when collection times are extended to 2 min (Andreucci *et al.*, 1971).

To avoid a decrease in intratubular pressure, Gertz *et al.* (1969) applied a counterpressure to the collection pipet. This technique resulted in comparatively low filtration rates. When Schnermann *et al.* (1971) used this technique they noted that intratubular pressure during collection was greater than free-flow pressure in the same nephron. These observations suggest that there is transmission of increased intratubular pressure to the glomerulus. The consequent reduction of effective filtration pressure may explain the relatively low single nephron glomerular filtration rates observed by Gertz.

A potential pitfall in the determination of single nephron filtration rate from the distal tubule is leakage from the micropuncture site. This phenomenon has been documented by Bartoli and Earley (1973) as a major cause for underestimation of single nephron filtration rate collected from distal nephrons.

3. Macula Densa Feedback Hypothesis

Thurau and Schnermann (1965) and Schnermann *et al.* (1970) have proposed a feedback system for the regulation of SNGFR. They suggest that the release of angiotensin by the macula densa cells is a function of the fluid delivered to the macula densa. The angiotensin produced by the macula densa cells is assumed to modulate glomerular arteriolar resistance and therefore glomerular hydrostatic pressure. Insertion of the oil block interrupts the flow of fluid to the macula densa. Thus when an oil block is inserted into a proximal nephron, this block ceases the normal orthograde flow of fluid to the macula densa and could activate a feedback mechanism so that the measured single nephron filtration rate would not be representative of the filtration rate of that nephron in the absence of an oil block. Navar *et al.* (1974) have reported studies in dogs consistent with a macula densa feedback for the regulation of single nephron filtration rate. In these studies collections from proximal nephrons, in the absence of flow to the macula densa, resulted in higher single nephron filtration rates than collections from distal nephrons, that is, in the presence of flow to the macula densa.

Similar studies have been performed in the rat in which samples from distal tubules could be more easily obtained and compared with samples from proximal tubules (Knox *et al.*, 1974; Maddox *et al.*, 1974). Collections were made both in the presence and absence of flow to the macula densa, and the autoregulatory capability of single nephrons was tested. No significant difference in single nephron filtration rate or in autoregulatory capability was detected between collections in the presence of flow to the macula densa as compared with collections in the absence of flow to the macula densa. Similar studies in dogs (Knox *et al.*, 1974) also showed good autoregulation of single nephron filtration rate in the absence of flow to the macula densa. Thus it was concluded that autoregulation of single nephron filtration rate is unaltered by interruption of tubule fluid flow to the macula densa, and therefore the micropuncture method is reliable for the measurement of single nephron filtration rate.

Studies with interruption of flow to the macula densa do not evaluate the possible effects of increases in tubule flow rates above physiologic levels. Microperfusion studies by Schnermann *et al.* (1973) and Lohfert *et al.* (1971) indicate that increases in perfusion rate result in decreases in glomerular capillary pressure. Thus they suggest that during elevations of distal sodium delivery, filtration may be modulated by afferent arteriolar constriction. These findings could have considerable importance in the investigation of diuretics since inhibition of fluid reabsorption proximal to the macula densa would result in increases in fluid flow above physiologic levels. In addition, Wright and Schnermann (1974) have shown that this feedback mechanism can be interfered with by the diuretics themselves. They perfused the loop of Henle at different rates and measured the filtration rate of the same nephron. Increases in loop perfusion, from physiologic rates of 10 nl/min to rates well above the physiologic range of 40 nl/min, decreased single nephron filtration rate from 30 to 19 nl/min. The single nephron filtration rate response to increased perfusion rate was

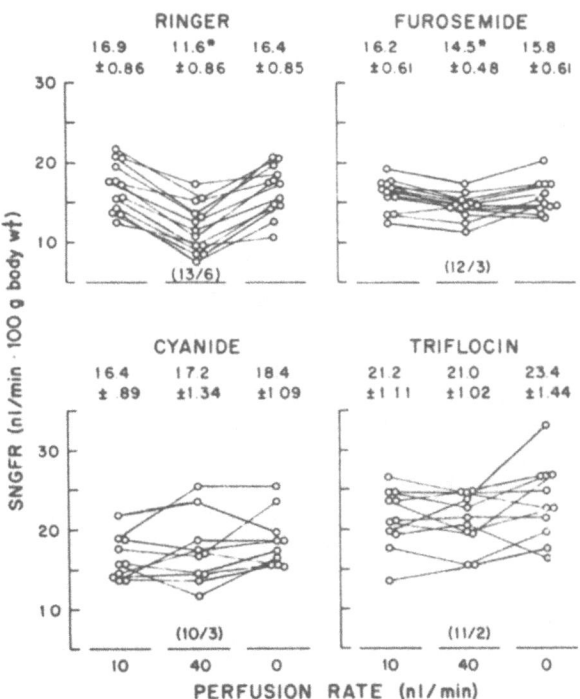

Figure 4. Effects of loop perfusion rate and transport inhibitors on SNGFR. (From Wright and Schnermann, 1974, by permission.)

reduced by furosemide, triflocin, and cyanide (see Figure 4). Thus diuretics that are assumed to inhibit sodium chloride transport by macula densa cells interfered with the feedback mechanism. For example, following the administration of furosemide, delivery of tubule fluid to the macula densa would be markedly elevated. The effect of an elevation in tubule fluid flow rate would be predicted to decrease single nephron filtration rate if it were not for the direct effect of the diuretic on transport by the macula densa cells. This inhibitory effect of furosemide on transport by the macula densa cells inhibits the feedback mechanism so that the net result is little change in single nephron filtration rate when flow to the macula densa is interrupted by the placement of an oil block. These considerations dictate careful evaluation of both the effect of increased delivery of fluid to the macula densa and the direct effects of the drug on the macula densa when interpreting the possible role of a feedback mechanism in the determination of single nephron filtration rate.

D. Proximal Tubule Micropuncture

1. Determination of Absolute Reabsorption: Comparison of Free-Flow and Split-Drop Methods

The effects of diuretics on the absolute reabsorption of fluid can be evaluated with two independent methods: the free-flow and the split-drop (Gertz, 1963) methods. Measurement of absolute reabsorption of isotonic fluid (C) from the proximal tubule with the free-flow method is performed as follows: The volume of tubule fluid collected (V_c) is subtracted from the single nephron filtration rate (V_0) and thereby gives the absolute volume of tubule fluid reabsorbed. The volume of tubule fluid reabsorbed is then divided by the length of tubule from the glomerulus to the point of micropuncture (L). Thus the absolute reabsorptive rate (C) is expressed in nl/sec/mm of tubule length and is calculated as

$$C = \frac{V_0 - V_c}{L} = \frac{V_c[(TF/P)_{in} - 1]}{L}$$

Since the single nephron filtration rate is the keystone for this measurement, the precautions listed earlier are crucial for the accurate determination of absolute reabsorptive rate.

To obtain an accurate estimate of TF inulin, samples should be collected from as near the end of the proximal tubule as possible for the following reasons. The combined sampling and analytic error in the estimation of TF/P inulin is approximately $\pm 10\%$ S.D. The effect of a 10% error in the calculation of fractional reabsorption by the proximal tubule has been calculated by Rector *et al.* (1966b) and is shown in Figure 5. It is clear that the 10% error results in a greater variation in the calculated percent reabsorption when the inulin ratios are low than when the inulin ratios are high. It is evident that if samples were obtained from the early proximal tubule, the inherent error can conceal significant changes in percent reabsorption. In addition, a small inhibitory effect

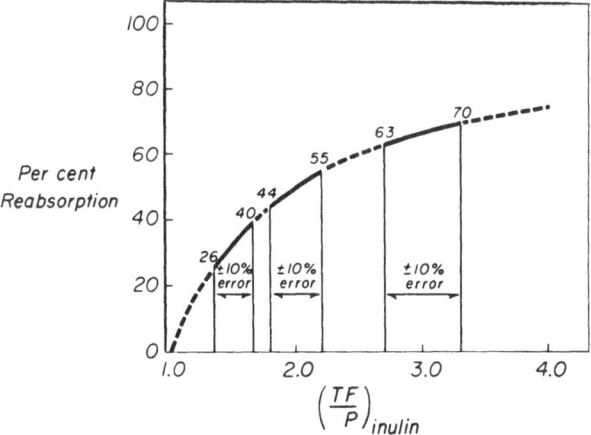

Figure 5. The effect of combined sampling and analytic error of ±10% in the measurement of tubular fluid inulin on the calculated per cent reabsorption of glomerular filtrate. The error in percent reabsorption is greatly magnified at lower inulin TF/P ratios. (From Rector *et al.*, 1966a, by permission.)

of the diuretic may be trivial when examined over a short segment of tubule but may have a significant cumulative effect when extended over the entire accessible portion of the tubule.

Absolute reabsorptive rate for the proximal tubule as obtained by the split-drop technique of Gertz is as follows: A large drop of stained castor oil is injected into a surface convolution of the proximal tubule through one barrel of a double-barreled pipet. The castor oil drop is then split with a drop of saline solution injected through the other barrel of the pipet. As the saline drop is reabsorbed by the tubule epithelium, the castor oil columns approach one another. The rate of shrinkage of the saline drop is measured with sequence photography or with videotape (Figure 6) (Lynch *et al.*, 1972). The time for

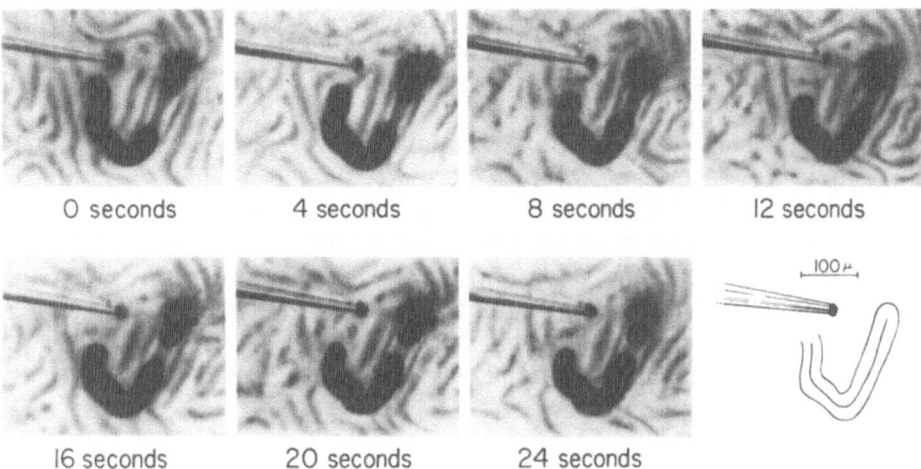

Figure 6. Sequential photomicrographs of a shrinking drop in a proximal tubule of a normal hydropenic dog.

reabsorption of one-half of the volume of the saline drop is determined from the sequential measurements of the volume of the saline drop as a function of time. From this measurement of $t_{1/2}$ and the tubule radius (r), absolute reabsorptive rate can be calculated and expressed again in nl/sec/mm:

$$C = \left(\frac{0.693\ \pi r^2}{t_{1/2}}\right) 10^{-3}$$

Several sources of error in the measurement of reabsorptive capacity using the split drop have been identified. The underlying assumption of the technique is that the rate of shrinking of the drop is a function of the reabsorptive activity of the epithelia to which it is exposed and is proportional to some index of the remaining volume of the drop. Nakajima et al. (1970) and Gyory (1971) have demonstrated that the rate of shrinking of the drop is proportional to the volume of an assumed plane-ended cylinder between the meniscal bases of the drop. Use of another index of volume, such as the actual volume of the drop, results in a changing relationship between the volume and exposed surface area as the drop progressively shrinks. Although the resultant $t_{1/2}$ is independent of initial drop length, a minimum of 50 μm was suggested. The authors concluded that even with the calculation of $t_{1/2}$ based on a drop length between meniscal bases, the technique is subject to limitations of several variables which are difficult to control. The variables included the viscosity of the oil used, the relative lengths of the proximal and distal oil columns, and the consequent differences in fractional resistance to movement, as well as the effect of different oils upon epithelial function. In addition the authors investigated the effect of pressure gradients across the proximal oil column by comparing the $t_{1/2}$ of two simultaneous shrinking drops in the same tubule, the proximal drop subjected to filtration pressure and the distal drop isolated from it. They observed a biphasic shrinking rate for the more distal drop in several nephrons. During the initial phase, the $t_{1/2}$ of the distal drop was longer than the $t_{1/2}$ of the proximal drop. Coincident with complete reabsorption of the proximal drop, the $t_{1/2}$ of the distal drop decreased and became equal to the $t_{1/2}$ observed for the proximal drop. These observations suggest that the reabsorption of the drop may be influenced by filtration pressure.

Indeed, Grandchamp and Boulpaep (1972) have reported that hydrostatic pressure within a shrinking drop is decreased in the absence of continued filtration. Under this circumstance they observed hydrostatic pressure within the drop to be comparable to intratubular free-flow hydrostatic pressure. On the other hand, pressure within the drop was equal to stop-flow pressure if filtration was allowed to continue. Furthermore, they observed that the reabsorptive rate increased when the intraluminal pressure was elevated. These data support the conclusion that variations in intratubular pressure influence the reabsorptive half-time of the shrinking drop.

Gyory (1971) reported that reabsorption was not independent of tubular radius. Based upon the correlation between $t_{1/2}$ and tubule radius, he concluded that reabsorptive capacity per unit surface area was constant and therefore both $t_{1/2}$ and radius must be measured precisely. Thus, another potential source of error is the measurement of the radius of the split drop. Significant variations in tubule diameter can be obtained depending upon whether measurements of the castor oil column, which may distend the tubule, or measurements of the saline drop, which are more difficult to visualize, are used in the calculation. This discrepancy is illustrated in Figure 7 where the radius of the tubule measured with the split drop, and taken as the radius of the castor oil column, was 30% larger than the radius in free flow taken as the radius of a lissamine green column (Wright *et al.*, 1969). Both sets of measurements were obtained from the same kidneys.

A comparison of the absolute rates of sodium reabsorption per unit length (C) was determined for the proximal tubule of the dog using both free-flow and shrinking-drop methodology (Wright *et al.*,1969). The value for absolute reabsorption calculated from the free-flow method was approximately 50% higher than the split-drop method, even though all measurements were made in the same kidneys.

The fact that examination of the possible sources of the discrepancy and the limitations of both the free-flow and split-drop methodologies did not reveal a clear explanation for the 50% difference in absolute reabsorptive rate suggests two possibilities. First, the two methodologies are theoretically sound, but several of the known variables may be in systemic error. Second, a primary variable, such as filtration rate, may play a major role in the free-flow determination of reabsorptive rate but not in the split-drop determination. This latter interpretation is supported by studies which compared the estimation of reabsorption by the two methods following a reduction in GFR. Constriction of the aorta failed to affect reabsorption of the split drop but significantly reduced

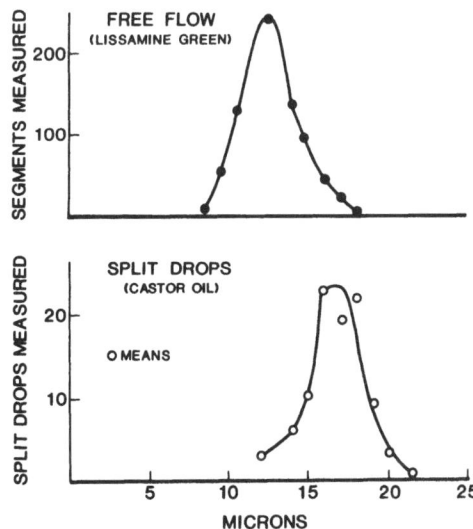

Figure 7. Comparison of the frequency distribution of tubular diameter measured during free-flow or shrinking-drop methodology.

the reabsorptive rate determined during free flow (Knox *et al.*, 1969). Thus, if a diuretic depresses GFR, it is not possible to assess effects on proximal reabsorption during free flow without quantitation of the effect of decreased GFR per se. These studies suggest that whereas free-flow micropuncture is materially affected by changes in filtration rate, the split-drop methodology is not. On the other hand, if a drug molecule must enter the nephron (whether by filtration or secretion) in order to reach its site of action, the split-drop method potentially limits this access.

Additional comparisons between the two methods have been made before and after infusion of hyperoncotic albumin solution (Wright *et al.*, 1969). Although the data obtained using the two different methods gave different values for reabsorptive rate, both methods showed parallel reductions in absolute rates of sodium reabsorption by the proximal tubule following infusion of hyperoncotic albumin solution. Thus these studies indicate that both free-flow and split-drop micropuncture methodologies can be used to evaluate diuretics.

2. Recollection Technique and Analysis of Error

The recollection technique as developed by Dirks *et al.* (1966) is the strongest experimental design for the application of micropuncture methods to the study of diuretics. The principle is to make collections from the same point in the same tubule before and after administration of a diuretic. Thus variations from animal to animal, from kidney to kidney, and from nephron to nephron are well controlled. Samples are collected from single nephrons, and then the point of micropuncture is recorded by making a map of the surface of the kidney and by the injection of a small amount of dye into the interstitium close to the micropuncture point. In mapping the nephron segments on the surface of the kidney, it is helpful to also indicate the direction of tubule fluid flow. As many as 10 nephrons can be punctured for subsequent recollection following the administration of the diuretic under study. Care must be taken to avoid multiple punctures of the same nephron for the initial collections. This can be avoided by assuming that each nephron encompasses a radius of about 10 tubule diameters (see Figure 1).

Mandin *et al.* (1971) reported that when single nephron filtration rates were measured during hydropenia and then after acute volume expansion, repunctured tubules had increases in measured filtration rate of 38% more than the filtration rate for the kidney as a whole. On the other hand, when new tubules were punctured during volume expansion, the single nephron filtration rate and whole kidney filtration rate changed proportionally. They concluded that disproportionate increases in single nephron filtration rate after volume expansion are due to an artifact unique to the recollection methodology. However, studies by Schneider *et al.* (1972) did not confirm an artifact unique to the recollection micropuncture methodology. In these studies similar values were obtained after saline infusion from recollected tubules and previously unpunctured tubules (Figure 8). Although no definitive explanation for the difference between the results of Schneider *et al.* (1972) and those of Mandin *et al.* (1971) was apparent,

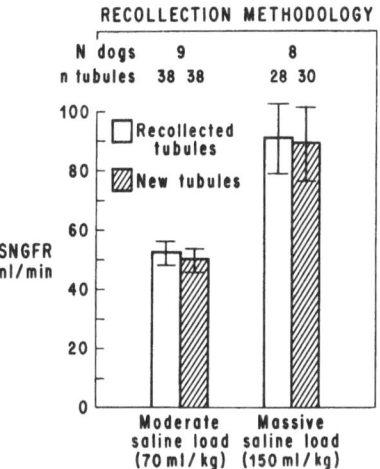

Figure 8. Comparison of SNGFR from new tubules or recollected tubules during maneuvers expected to enhance possible artifactual differences.

several features of the collection methodology in saline-loaded animals should be emphasized. Micropuncture collections during saline diuresis are considerably more difficult to control than during hydropenia because of the high intratubular pressures and tubule fluid flow rates associated with the diuresis. High intratubular pressures could produce, for example, retrograde flow of tubule fluid around an inadequate oil block and result in calculated single nephron filtration rates which are aberrantly high. In the study by Schneider *et al.* (1972), retrograde collection of tubule fluid was avoided by the use of a distal block of castor oil which was approximately 6–8 tubule diameters in length. This procedure has been shown to prevent retrograde flow of tubule fluid under other conditions of high intratubular pressure. Brenner *et al.* (1971b) and Davidman *et al.* (1971) have also evaluated the recollection micropuncture technique following infusion of Ringer's solution in the rat. No difference between collections from new tubules and recollected tubules was found. Thus the recollection micropuncture technique, with the distinct inherent advantage that samples are taken from the same point in the same tubule before and after experimental intervention, is probably the strongest experimental design.

Dirks *et al.* (1966) investigated the effects of several diuretics on proximal tubular reabsorption utilizing the recollection micropuncture technique. The agents investigated included hydrochlorothiazide, ethacrynic acid, furosemide, and acetazolamide. Based on the absence of changes in fractional reabsorption, the authors concluded that there was no evidence for a depression of proximal tubular reabsorption with any of the agents except acetazolamide. Subsequently, evidence has accumulated in the literature which suggests that when changes in glomerular filtration rate produced by these drugs are taken into consideration, a depression of proximal reabsorption can be demonstrated (Brenner *et al.*, 1968; Puschett *et al.*, 1971). Using the recollection technique, Clapp *et al.* (1971) noted that ethacrynic acid reduced the fractional reabsorption of fluid in the proximal tubule when filtration rate remained constant. However, if filtration rate was moderately reduced, fractional reabsorption was unchanged; if filtration rate fell markedly, fractional reabsorption was increased. The authors concluded that unpredictable variations in filtration rate may have obscured the depression of proximal reabsorption. Similarly, Fernandez and Puschett (1973) reported that chlorothiazide inhibited proximal reabsorption in those animals in which glomerular filtration rate decreased by less than 25%. However, fractional fluid reabsorption was unaltered if glomerular filtration decreased by greater than 26%. Knox et al. (1969) reported that the administration of furosemide produced a decrease in nephron filtration rate of 36% and no change in fractional reabsorption by the proximal tubule. As mentioned earlier, they reported that decreased GFR in the absence of a diuretic was associated with an increase in fractional reabsorption. Thus, it was concluded that the decrease in GFR obscured an inhibition of fractional reabsorption by the proximal tubule.

3. Role of Proximal Delivery on Resultant Natriuresis

Berliner et al. (1966) have pointed out that a diuretic which depresses only proximal reabsorption of salt and water would be only moderately effective in causing salt excretion since a considerable part of that which escaped proximal reabsorption would be reabsorbed distally. Secondly and, in their view, more important, the effects of a diuretic will vary markedly with the state of hydration of the animals. In studies with ethacrynic acid, in which urine volume was not replaced with a saline infusion, there was a tendency for urine flow to fall in response to this fluid loss. In these studies, fractional reabsorption by the proximal tubule was markedly increased. In additional experiments, in which the losses of extracellular fluid were prevented by infusions of isotonic saline, the increases in reabsorption by the proximal tubule were avoided. Similarly, Weiner et al. (1971) reported that salt and water depletion produced by furosemide increased proximal reabsorption determined by the split-drop method in rats. Thus in studies of the primary affects of diuretics, the volume state of the animal should be kept constant by replacement of urinary losses. On the other hand, Knox (1970) has demonstrated that during furosemide diuresis either plasma volume expansion with albumin or extracellular volume expansion with saline produced a further increase in the fractional excretion of sodium. Thus an increase in the proximal delivery of fluid may enhance the natriuretic activity of the diuretic.

E. Distal Nephron Micropuncture

The availability of distal tubules on the surface of the mammalian kidney is considerably less than that of proximal tubules. A map of the surface must be prepared using lissamine green dye for identification of the distal convolution. In addition several technical problems must be recognized when attempting distal micropuncture. Usually only a short segment is visible on the surface which limits the length of oil block which can be visualized. Although hydrostatic pressure and volume flow of fluid are low during hydropenia, they are much greater during conditions of diuresis. Thus, maintaining control of the oil block during diuresis is difficult, and the potential to collect fluid distal to the micropuncture site is greater. Furthermore, Kramp *et al.* (1970) reported that the osmolality of distal tubular fluid from the rat was artifactually lowered when collection was accelerated. Finally, since the distal convoluted tubule appears to be functionally heterogeneous, that portion on the surface which is available to micropuncture probably varies between nephrons.

1. Structural–Functional Correlations

Recent evidence suggests that the distal convoluted tubule may consist of three functionally different segments. Based on electrophysiological measurements, Wright (1974) has reported the possibility that the very early distal tubule may have functional characteristics similar to the thick ascending limb of Henle's loop. Woodhall and Tisher (1973) have demonstrated that the distal tubule accessible for·micropuncture consists of at least two physiologically distinct epithelial structures. They found that tubular fluid which enters the early distal tubule remains hypotonic until it enters the initial collecting tubule and only at that point is vasopressin-induced osmotic equilibration possible. Furthermore, they indicate that differences in availability of distal convoluted tubules, as opposed to collecting tubules, exist between various strains of rats. Gross *et al.* (1974) have reported the identification of a distal convoluted tubule segment which is distinct from the thick ascending limb of Henle's loop and from the cortical collecting tubule. The physiologic characteristics of the distal convoluted tubule differ those of the cortical collecting tubule in that the cortical collecting tubule requires either exogenous or endogenous mineralocorticoids to maintain a maximal negative potential difference while the potential difference in the distal convoluted tubule was independent of mineralocorticoid effect.

These observations suggest that three physiologically distinct distal segments are potentially available for micropuncture on the surface of the rat kidney. The earliest segment is the terminal portion of the ascending limb of Henle's loop, a middle segment is the distal convoluted tubule, and a terminal segment is the initial collecting tubule (see Figure 9). Interpretations of data therefore must include consideration of these various epithelial cell types. For this reason Woodhall and Tisher (1973) emphasize that both structural and functional techniques should be employed in such studies.

Tisher and Clapp (1972) have described a method for the histological identification of the tubule at the site of micropuncture. Following the collection of tubular fluid, the nephron is perfused *in vivo* with a fixative suitable for tissue preservation for both light and electron microscopy. Finally, the site of micropuncture is marked by the intraluminal injection of latex. Thus the relationship between structure and function within an identified segment of an individual nephron may be determined.

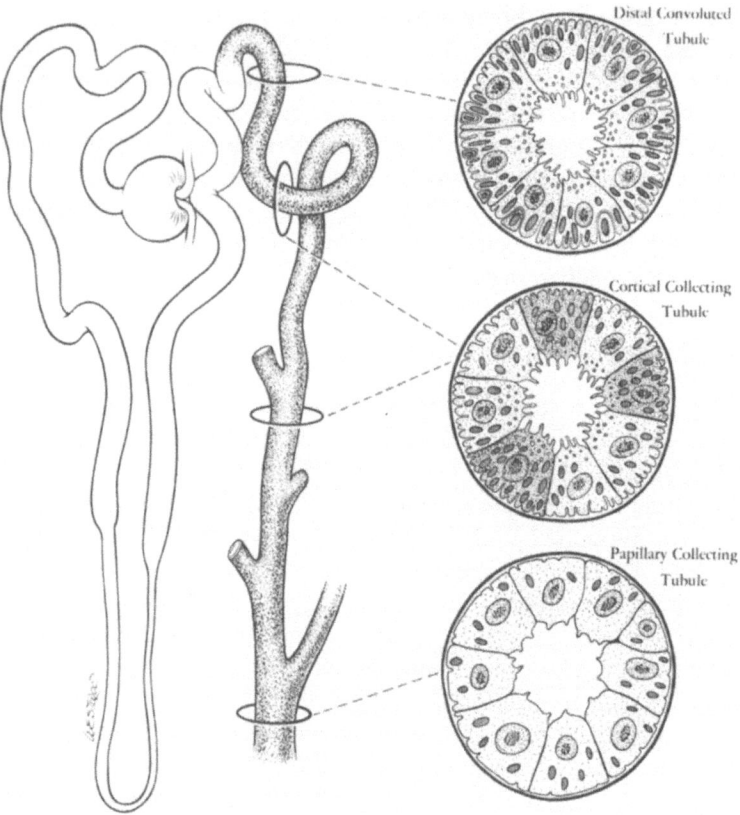

Figure 9. Illustration of the morphologically and physiologically dissimilar segments of the distal nephron and collecting duct. The thick ascending limb of Henle's loop is represented by the unshaded segment adjacent to distal convoluted tubule.

2. Evaluation of Reabsorption in the Loop of Henle

Although the thick ascending limb of loop of Henle is relatively inaccessible to direct micropuncture, the technique has been utilized to indirectly evaluate the effect of diuretics on this nephron segment. For example, free-flow micropuncture studies clearly indicated that loop diuretics inhibit NaCl reabsorption at some site between the late proximal tubule and early distal tubule, most likely the ascending limb of Henle's loop. Clapp and Robinson (1968) demonstrated that furosemide increased the distal TF/P osmolal ratio in dogs. Dirks and Seely (1970) observed that the administration of furosemide to saline-expanded dogs resulted in a reduction in the distal TF/P inulin ratio and abolished the distal sodium gradient. The technique used in these experiments was unable to discriminate the ionic species actively transported and primarily inhibited by the drug. Subsequent studies with the isolated perfused tubule technique, which is the preparation of choice for the direct assessment of loop diuretics, clarified the specific transport mechanism inhibited by the drug. The loop diuretics, ethacrynic acid and furosemide, inhibit chloride transport and consequently sodium reabsorption in the thick ascending limb of Henle's loop (Burg and Green, 1973; Burg *et al.*, 1973).

3. Analysis of Error

Rector *et al.* (1966b) have analyzed pitfalls in the use of distal micropuncture for the localization of diuretic action. They point out that alterations in distal tubule reabsorption cannot be established with certainty by sampling tubule fluid at a single site in the distal tubule because small alterations in reabsorption proximal to this point may produce big changes in the volume of fluid entering the distal convolution and thus obscure any distal effects of the diuretic.

Kunau *et al.* (1975) have avoided this problem in studying the effect of chlorothiazide by micropuncture of both early and late segments of the distal nephron and by increasing delivery from the proximal tubule in control animals. For the latter purpose, a group of rats was studied with benzolamide, a carbonic anhydrase inhibitor. Fractional sodium and chloride delivery from the proximal tubule was similarly increased both with chlorothiazide and with benzolamide. However, benzolamide had no effect on chloride reabsorption in the distal convoluted tubule. In contrast chlorothiazide markedly inhibited distal tubule chloride reabsorption, increasing the fraction of filtered chloride present in the late distal tubule from 1.2 to 6.2%. Thus these studies amply demonstrate the application of distal tubule micropuncture to the study of diuretics.

Duarte *et al.* (1971) have investigated the effect of amiloride, ouabain, and furosemide on distal tubular function in the rat. In these studies the collection site was localized and expressed as a percent of the distal tubule. Amiloride had little if any effect upon the distal TF/P sodium ratio. Ouabain increased late distal TF/P sodium ratios but had no apparent effect upon early distal samples. Furosemide administration resulted in TF/P sodium ratios approaching unity along the entire length of distal tubule which was punctured.

F. Collecting Duct Micropuncture

Stein and Reineck (1974) have recently reviewed the functions of the collecting duct in the regulation of sodium reabsorption. From the available evidence it is clear that the collecting duct is capable of active sodium transport and further that this nephron segment can reabsorb physiologically significant quantities of sodium. Indeed, although the absolute quantities of fluid and ions reabsorbed are relatively small, the collecting duct epithelium is the nephron site where the steepest transepithelial concentration gradients are established. Since the collecting duct is the site of final regulation of sodium excretion, the potential effects of diuretics on this nephron segment are of great importance.

1. Determination of Collecting-Duct Function

Evaluation of collecting-duct function by comparison of the delivery of fluid from the late distal tubule with the final urinary excretion rate has limitations.

First, differences between late distal tubules and final urine may not be entirely due to reabsorption by the collecting duct but rather to a mixture of tubule fluid originating from superficial and deep nephrons. The second major problem is that the structures beyond the late distal tubule consist of the cortical collecting tubule and the papillary collecting duct. The functional properties of these two tubular segments may not be similar. Since the cortical collecting tubule is largely inaccessible to micropuncture, the isolated perfused tubule is the technique of choice for the study of diuretics in this segment. On the other hand, direct micropuncture of the papillary collecting duct is possible and offers distinct advantages over the indirect approach described.

Micropuncture of the papilla requires the choice of an animal species in which the papilla can be exposed. The golden hamster is widely used for this reason since the papilla protrudes approximately 2 mm into the renal pelvis (Windhager, 1964). Young rats have also been used, and in this case the papilla is exposed for about 1 mm in length (Diezi et al., 1973; Sakai et al., 1965).

To assess papillary collecting-duct function, micropuncture is performed as far proximally as possible toward the base of the papilla. Subsequently, a sample is obtained from the tip of the papilla by axial introduction of the pipet into the opening of the collecting duct. The distance between the two collection sites is then measured and the data are presented in terms of reabsorptive capacity per mm of papillary collecting duct.

2. Analysis of Error

It is important to recognize that the concentrating ability of the exposed papilla is less than that of the unexposed kidney (Gertz et al., 1966; Schmidt-Nielsen, 1969). This loss of concentrating ability is probably due to a loss of urea from the papilla. The subsequent decrease in concentrating ability lowers inulin concentration ratios in papillary collecting ducts of the exposed papilla.

In the study of diuretic action on the collecting duct it is important to consider the characteristics of the collecting duct in the presence of increased tubule load. Studies by Diezi et al. (1973) show that the reabsorptive rate for sodium increases significantly both in fractional as well as absolute terms when the load entering the papillary collecting ducts is increased. The absolute rate of sodium reabsorption approaches a plateau as sodium load is markedly increased. This observation may be the consequence of the extracellular fluid volume expansion inhibiting sodium transport by the collecting duct in these experiments or may represent an inherent limitation in the absolute capacity for sodium reabsorption. Since most diuretics markedly augment the delivery of sodium to the collecting system, this feature must be carefully controlled when evaluating the effects of diuretics on the papillary collecting system.

Finally, it must be noted that the terminal papillary collecting duct represents the fusion of several major collecting systems. The possible heterogeneity of contributions from these collecting systems must be recognized when comparisons between the base and tip of the papilla are drawn.

ACKNOWLEDGMENTS

The authors wish to thank Dr. Cobern E. Ott, Dr. Jean-Louis Cuche, and Dr. Jose A. Diaz-Buxo for their suggestions in the preparation of the manuscript, and Ms. Carma Jean Fink for her secretarial assistance.

REFERENCES

Andreucci, V. E., Herrera-Acosta, J., Rector, F. C., Jr., and Seldin, D. W. 1971. Measurement of single-nephron glomerular filtration rate by micropuncture: Analysis of error. *Am. J. Physiol., 221:*1551.

Bartoli, E. and Earley, L. E. 1973. Measurements of nephron filtration rate in the rat with and without occlusion of the proximal tubule. *Kidney Int., 3:*372.

Bennett, C. M., Brenner, B. M., and Berliner, R. W. 1968. Micropuncture study of nephron function in the rhesus monkey. *J. Clin. Invest., 47:*203.

Berliner, R. W., Dirks, J. H., and Cirksena, W. J. 1966. Action of diuretics in dogs studied by micropuncture. *Ann. N.Y. Acad. Sci., 139:*424.

Blantz, R. C., Israelit, A. H., Rector, F. C., Jr., and Seldin, D. W. 1972. Relation of distal tubular NaCl delivery and glomerular hydrostatic pressure. *Kidney Int., 2:*22.

Brenner, B. M., and Daugharty, T. M. 1972. The measurement of glomerular filtration rate in single nephrons of the rat kidney. *Yale J. Biol. Med., 45:*200.

Brenner, B. M., Bennett, C. M., and Berliner, R. W. 1968. The relationship between glomerular filtration rate and sodium reabsorption by the proximal tubule of the rat nephron. *J. Clin. Invest., 47:*1358.

Brenner, B. M., Keimowitz, R. I., Wright, F. S., and Berliner, R. W. 1969. An inhibition effect of furosemide on sodium reabsorption by the proximal tubule of the rat nephron. *J. Clin. Invest., 48:*290.

Brenner, B. M., Troy, J. L., and Daugharty, T. M. 1971a. The dynamics of glomerular ultrafiltration in the rat. *J. Clin. Invest., 50:*1776.

Brenner, B. M., Daugharty, T. M., Ueki, I. F., and Troy, J. L. 1971b. Quantitative assessment of proximal tubule function in single nephrons of the rat kidney. *Am. J. Physiol., 220:*2058.

Burg, M. and Green, N. 1973. Effect of ethacrynic acid on the thick ascending limb of Henle's loop. *Kidney Int., 4:*301.

Burg, M., Stoner, L., Cardinal, J., and Green, N. 1973. Furosemide effect on isolated perfused tubules. *Am. J. Physiol., 225:*119.

Christensen, P. and Frederiksen, O. 1972. The effect of lissamine green on gall bladder fluid absorption and frog skin sodium transport in vitro. *Arch. Ges. Physiol., 331:*160.

Clapp, J. R. and Robinson, R. R. 1968. Distal sites of action of diuretic drugs in the dog nephron. *Am. J. Physiol., 255:*228.

Clapp, J. R., Nottebohm, G. A., and Robinson, R. R. 1971. Proximal site of action of ethacrynic acid: importance of filtration rate. *Am. J. Physiol., 220:*1355.

Cortell, S., Davidman, M., Gennari, F. J., and Schwartz, W. B. 1972. Catheter size as a determinant of outflow resistance and intrarenal pressure. *Am. J. Physiol., 223:*910.

Davidman, M., Lalone, R. C., Alexander, E. A., and Levinsky, N. G. 1971. Some micropuncture techniques in the rat. *Am. J. Physiol., 221:*1110.

Davis, J. O. and Howell, D. S. 1953. Mechanisms of fluid and electrolyte retention in experimental preparations in dogs. II. With thoracic inferior vena cava constriction. *Circ. Res. 1:*171.

Davis, J. O., Urquhart, J., Higgins, J. T., Rubin, E. C., and Hartroft, P. M. 1964. Hypersecretion of aldosterone in dogs with chronic aortic-caval fistula and high output heart failure. *Circ. Res., 14:*471.

Diezi, J., Michoud, P., Aceves, J., and Giebisch, G. 1973. Micropuncture study of electrolyte transport across papillary collecting duct of the rat. *Am. J. Physiol., 224:*623.

Dirks, J. H. and Seely, J. F. 1970. Effect of saline infusions and furosemide on the dog distal nephron. *Am. J. Physiol., 219:*114.

Dirks, J. H., Cirksena, W. J., and Berliner, R. W. 1966. Micropuncture study of the effects of various diuretics on sodium reabsorption by the proximal tubules of the dog. *J. Clin. Invest., 45:* 1875.

Dörge, A. and Nagel, W. 1969. Die Wirkung von Lissamingrün auf den Natriumtransport an der isolierten Bauchhaut von *Rana temporaria. Arch. Ges. Physiol., 313:*11.

Duarte, C. G., Chomety, C., and Giebisch, G. 1971. Effect of amiloride, ouabain, and furosemide on distal tubular function in the rat. *Am. J. Physiol., 221:*632.

Elmer, M., Eskildsen, P. C., Kristensen, L. O., and Leyssac, P. P. 1972. A comparison of renal function in rats anesthetized with inactin and sodium amytal. *Acta Physiol. Scand., 86:*41.

Falchuk, K. H. and Berliner, R. W. 1971. Hydrostatic pressures in peritubular capillaries and tubules in the rat kidney. *Am. J. Physiol., 220:*1422.

Fernandez, P. C. and Puschett, J. B. 1973. Proximal tubular actions of metolazone and chlorothiazide. *Am. J. Physiol., 225:*954.

Gertz, K. H. 1963. Transtubuläre Natriumchloridflüsse und Permeabilität für Nichtelektrolyte in proximalen und distalen Konvolute der Rattinniere. *Arch. Ges. Physiol., 276:*336.

Gertz, K. H., Schmidt-Nielsen, B., and Pagel, H. D. 1966. Exchange of water, urea and salt between the mammalian renal papilla and the surrounding urine. *Fed. Proc., 25:*327.

Gertz, K. H., Braun-Schubert, G., and Brandis, M. 1969. Zur Method der Messung der Filtrationstrate einzelner nahe der Nierenoberflache gelegener Glomeruli. *Pflugers Arch., 310:*109.

Grandchamp, A. and Boulpaep, E. L. 1972. Effect of intraluminal pressure on proximal tubular sodium reabsorption. A shrinking drop micropuncture study. *Yale J. Biol. Med., 45:*275.

Gross, J. B., Imai, M., and Kokko, J. P. 1974. Functional comparison of the distal convoluted tubule and the cortical collecting tubule. *Am. Soc. Nephol., 7:*34.

Gyory, A. Z. 1971. Re-examination of the split oil droplet method as applied to kidney tubules. *Pflugers Arch., 324:*328.

Harris, C. A., Baer, P. G., Chirito, E., and Dirks, J. H. 1974. Composition of mammalian glomerular filtrate. *Am. J. Physiol., 227:*972.

Heller, J. 1971. The influence of lissamine green on tubular reabsorption of electrolytes and water in rats. *Arch. Ges. Physiol., 323:*27.

Knox, F. G. 1970. Effect of increased proximal delivery on furosemide natriuresis. *Am. J. Physiol., 218:*819.

Knox, F. G., Wright, F. S., Howards, S. S., and Berliner, R. W. 1969. Effect of furosemide on sodium reabsorption by proximal tubule of the dog. *Am. J. Physiol., 217:*192.

Knox, F. G., Ott, C. E., Cuche, J. L., Gasser, J., and Haas, J. 1974. Autoregulation of single nephron filtration rate in the presence and the absence of flow to the macula densa. *Circ. Res., 34:*836.

Kramp, R. A., Collindres, R. E., and Gottschalk, C. W. 1970. Effect of collection technic on the osmolality of distal tubular fluid of the rat. *Am. Soc. Nephol., 4:*44.

Kunau, R. T., Weller, D. R., and Webb, H. L. 1975. Clarification of the site of action of chlorothiazide in the rat nephron. *J. Clin. Invest., 56:*401.

Langer, K. H., Thoenes, W., and Wiederholt, M. 1968. Licht-und elektronenmikroskopische Untersuchungen am proximalen Tubuluskonvolut der Rattenniere nach intraluminaler Ölinjektion. *Arch. Ges. Physiol., 302:*149.

Lohfert, H., Lichtenstein, I., Butz, M., and Hierholzer, K. 1971. Continuous measurement of renal intratubular pressures with a combined pressure transducer microperfusion system. *Pflugers Arch., 327:*191.

Lynch, R. E., Schneider, E. G., Willis, L. R., and Knox, F. G. 1972. Absence of mineralocorticoid-dependent sodium reabsorption in dog proximal tubule. *Am. J. Physiol., 223:*40.

Lynch, R. E., Schneider, E. G., Strandhoy, J. W., Willis, L. R., and Knox, F. G. 1973. Effect of lissamine green dye on renal sodium reabsorption in the dog. *J. Appl. Physiol., 35:*169.

Maddox, D. A., Troy, J. L., and Brenner, B. M. 1974. Autoregulation of filtration rate in the absence of macula densa-glomerulus feedback. *Am. J. Physiol., 227:*123.

Mandin, H., Israelit, A. H., Rector, F. C., Jr., and Seldin, D. W. 1971. Effect of saline infusions on intrarenal distribution of glomerular filtrate and proximal reabsorption in the dog. *J. Clin. Invest., 50:*514.

Nakajima, K., Clapp, J. R., and Robinson, R. R. 1970. Limitations of the shrinking-drop micropuncture technique. *Am. J. Physiol., 219:*345.

Navar, L. G., Burke, T. J., Robinson, R. R., and Clapp, J. R. 1974. Distal tubular feedback on the autoregulation of single nephron glomerular filtration rate. *J. Clin. Invest., 53:*516.

Puschett, J. B., Goldstein, S., Godshall, S., Staum, B. B., and Goldberg, M. 1971. Effects of filtration rate and plasma sodium concentration on proximal sodium transport. *Am. J. Physiol., 221:*788.

Rector, F. C., Jr., Brunner, F. P., and Seldin, D. W. 1966a. Mechanism of glomerular tubular balance. I. Effect of aortic constriction and elevated ureteropelvic pressure on glomerular filtration rate, fractional reabsorption, transit time and tubule size in proximal tubule of the rat. *J. Clin. Invest., 45:*590.

Rector, F. C., Jr., Brunner, F. P., Sellman, J. C., and Seldin, D. W. 1966b. Pitfalls in the use of micropuncture for the localization of diuretic action. *Ann. N.Y. Acad. Sci., 139:*400.

Richards, A. 1929. Methods and results of direct investigations of the function of the kidney. *Beaumont Foundation Lectures,* Williams and Wilkins, Baltimore.

Roch-Ramel, F. and Jotterand, N. 1970. Natriuretic effect of lissamine green. *Experientia 26:*683.

Sakai, F., Jamison, R. L., and Berliner, R. W. 1965. A method for exposing the rat renal medulla in vivo; micropuncture of the collecting duct. *Am. J. Physiol., 209:*663.

Schmidt-Nielsen, B. 1969. Comparative physiology of urea excretion. In: *Progress in Nephrology,* pp. 1–12. Ed. by Peters, G. and Roch-Ramel, F. Springer, Berlin.

Schneider, E. G., Lynch, R. E., Willis, L. R., and Knox, F. G. 1972. Single-nephron filtration rate in the dog. *Am. J. Physiol., 222:*667.

Schnermann, J., Horster, M., and Levine, D. Z. 1969. The influence of sampling techniques on the micropuncture determination of GFR and reabsorptive characteristics of single rat proximal tubules. *Pflugers Arch., 309:*48.

Schnermann, J., Wright, F. S., Davis, J. M., Stackelberg, W. V., and Grill, G. 1970. Regulation of superficial nephron filtration rate by tubulo-glomerular feedback. *Pflugers Arch., 318:*147.

Schnermann, J., Davis, J. M., Wunderlich, P., Levine, D. Z., and Horster, M. 1971. Technical problems in the micropuncture determination of nephron filtration rate and their functional implications. *Pflugers Arch., 329:*307.

Schnermann, J., Persson, E. G., and Agerup, B. 1973. Tubuloglomerular feedback. Nonlinear relation between glomerular hydrostatic pressure and loop of Henle perfusion rate. *J. Clin. Invest., 52:*862.

Stein, J. H. and Reineck, H. J. 1974. The role of the collecting duct in the regulation of excretion of sodium and other electrolytes. *Kidney Int., 6:*1.

Steinhausen, M. 1963. Ein Methode zur Differenzierung proximaler und distaler Tubuli der Nierenrinde von Ratten *in vivo* und ihre Anwendung zur Bestimmung tubularer Stromungsgeschwindigkeiten. *Arch. Ges. Physiol., 277:*23.

Stumpe, K. O., Sölle, H., Klein, H., and Krück, F. 1973. Mechanism of sodium and water retention in rats with experimental heart failure. *Kidney Int., 4:*309.

Thurau, K. and Schnermann, J. 1965. Die Natriumkonzentration an den Macula Densa-Zellen als regulierender Faktor für das Glomerulumfiltrat (Mikropunktionsversuche). *Klin. Wochenschr., 43:*410.

Tisher, C. C. and Clapp, J. R. 1972. Intraluminal latex injection: An aid to the histological identification of renal tubules. *Kidney Int., 2:*54.

Weiner, M. W., Weinman, E. J., Kashgarian, M., and Hayslett, J. P. 1971. Accelerated reabsorption in the proximal tubule produced by volume depletion. *J. Clin. Invest., 50:*1379.

Wiederhielm, C. A., Woodbury, J. W., Kirk, S., and Rushmer, R. F. 1964. Pulsatile pressures in the microcirculation of frog's mesentary. *Am. J. Physiol., 207:*173.

Windhager, E. E. 1964. Electrophysiological study of renal papilla of golden hamsters. *Am. J. Physiol., 206:*694.

Windhager, E. E. 1968. *Micropuncture Techniques and Nephron Function.* Butterworth and Co., Cambridge, England.

Woodhall, P. B. and Tisher, C. C. 1973. Response of the distal tubule and cortical collecting duct to vasopressin in the rat. *J. Clin. Invest., 52:*3095.

Wright, F. S. 1974. Relation of electrical potential difference to potassium secretion by the distal renal tubule. *Proc. 25th Int. Cong. Physiol. Sci.,* New Delhi, India.

Wright, F. S. and Schnermann, J. 1974. Inteference with feedback control of glomerular filtration rate by furosemide, triflocin, and cyanide. *J. Clin. Invest., 53:*1695.

Wright, F. S., Howards, S. S., Knox, F. G., and Berliner, R. W. 1969. Measurement of sodium reabsorption by proximal tubule of the dog. *Am. J. Physiol., 217:*199.

Chapter **4**

The Use of Clearance Methods for the Determination of Sites of Action of Diuretics in the Kidney

Garabed Eknoyan

Department of Medicine, Baylor College of Medicine
and Veterans Administration Hospital
Houston, Texas

Manuel Martinez-Maldonado

Departments of Medicine and Physiology
University of Puerto Rico School of Medicine
and Veterans Administration Center
San Juan, Puerto Rico

and

Wadi N. Suki

Department of Medicine, Baylor College of Medicine
and The Methodist Hospital
Houston, Texas

I. INTRODUCTION

Clearance studies, although at best indirect and inferential methods for the study of renal function, have been instrumental in providing an impressive body of information as to the parts of the nephron where diuretics exert their action. Indeed, well after the advent of the more direct and specific micropuncture and isolated tubule techniques, they continue to provide considerable information relative to the renal effects of diuretics and of other pharmacologic agents. This is in part due to the ease and technical facility with which clearance studies can be done, the general availability of the tools necessary to perform clearance measurements, and the reliability and reproducibility of the data obtained from clearance studies. These data, however, must be interpreted cautiously in the framework, and with full appreciation, of the normal function of the various segments of the nephron.

It was the early attempts to relate the rate of urea excretion to the blood urea as a clinical measure of renal function that led to the development of the clearance concept (Smith, 1943). Because of its back-diffusion, the excretion of urea at low urine flow rates is complex and led Ambard and Weill (1912) to the use of a clearance equation that contained two square-root radicals. The actual clearance formula was first suggested by Addis (1917). Van Slyke, working with McLean, Austin and Stillman (Smith, 1943) and later with Möller and McIntosh (Möller *et al.*, 1929), first used the term "clearance" and showed that the excretion efficiency of the kidney could be expressed simply as the "volume of blood cleared of urea by one minute's excretion." They called this the "maximum blood urea clearance." However, the breakthrough in the establishment of clearance methodology was the recognition by Rehberg (1926a,b) that a substance which is freely filtered and neither reabsorbed nor secreted can be used to estimate the glomerular filtration rate. The subsequent work of Homer Smith (1943, 1951) led to the development of the more sophisticated and reliable methods which he so elegantly used to develop the facts and theory on which much of modern renal physiology is based.

As a rule, clearance measurements are limited to plasma except in the rare circumstance where an excreted substance (such as PAH) is transported by the blood cells as well as by plasma. The plasma clearance of any substance is that volume of plasma which has been "cleared" of a particular substance per unit time or that volume of plasma required to supply the amount of the substance appearing in the urine during any unit time period. The standard clearance formula, UV/P, refers therefore to the minimum volume of plasma that could supply the amount of the substance excreted in the urine if the plasma were completely "cleared" of that substance. The figures derived from such calculations provide no direct information about the mechanism of excretion so far as the role of glomerular filtration, tubular reabsorption, or tubular secretion. Consequently, most functional implications of clearance studies are derived from comparing the magnitude of the renal clearance of a substance to that of a substance such as inulin which can be used as an accurate index of glomerular filtration rate. Inulin is an inert fructose polymer with a molecular weight of 5200 and is freely filterable at the glomerulus; it is neither reabsorbed nor secreted by the tubules (Smith, 1951, 1956). It has been used more extensively in clearance studies than any of the other indices of GFR, such as vitamin B_{12}, chelating compounds, or contrast media (Levinsky and Levy, 1973).

As stated earlier, it is the facility with which clearance studies can be performed in the intact animal which led to their widespread use in renal physiology in general and in the study of the sites of action in the kidney of a number of agents, including diuretics. Using clearance techniques, the site of action of a diuretic may be localized to the proximal tubule, to the ascending limb of the loop of Henle, or to the distal tubule and collecting duct. This is, however, based on a number of assumptions which, although qualitatively correct, do not always provide precise quantitative information. We will first briefly review the normal pattern of transport throughout the nephron and then indicate the limitations and pitfalls of the use of each to localize the tubular sites of action of diuretics.

II. THE PROXIMAL TUBULE

Localization of proximal tubular action is based on the assumption that if more of a proximally reabsorbed substance is excreted into the urine than is normally delivered out of the proximal tubule, then the diuretic administered must have inhibited proximal reabsorption. Such a conclusion may be derived from the magnitude of natriuresis produced by the diuretic agent. This is commonly expressed as the fraction of filtered sodium excreted in the urine and calculated from the formula C_{Na}/GFR where C_{Na} *is the clearance of sodium,* $U_{Na}V/P_{Na}$, and *GFR* the glomerular filtration rate or $U_{In}V/P_{In}$. This value is usually expressed as a percent of the *GFR*. Since 50–60% of the glomerular filtrate is reabsorbed in the proximal tubule, and as much as 30–40% of filtered sodium might be reabsorbed more distally, an excretion of 50% or greater of the filtered load of sodium must be observed to infer a proximal site of action (Seldin *et al.,* 1966). Therefore, information on fractional excretion is not useful unless a massive diuresis is produced. However, knowledge of the fate of sodium beyond the proximal tubule and control of the experimental conditions does permit a better utilization of this information. Thus, the bulk of the sodium delivered out of the proximal tubule is reabsorbed in the ascending limb of the loop of Henle to generate solute-free water, and in the distal nephron, where it provides the driving force for potassium and hydrogen secretion (Seldin *et al.,* 1966). By conducting the experiment during water diuresis, the sodium chloride reabsorbed in the loop may be approximated by the measurement of free-water clearance (C_{H_2O}) and the sodium reabsorbed in the distal nephron estimated from potassium excretion (Suki *et al.,* 1965; Seldin *et al.,* 1966; Eknoyan *et al.,* 1967). Thus, delivery out of the proximal tubule may be estimated as the sum of fractional excretion of Na, K, and C_{H_2O} according to the formula:

$$\text{Fractional distal delivery of Na} = \left[\left(\frac{U_{Na+K} V}{P_{Na}} + C_{H_2O} \right) \div GFR \right] \times 100$$

A proximal tubular site of action may also be inferred from changes in the ionic composition of the urine relative to substances principally absorbed in the proximal tubule. This type of information, however, can be interpreted only in terms of nephron sites of action when the reabsorption of an ion has been localized to specific nephron segments by the more direct micropuncture studies. It should be noted in this regard that an ion species rejected proximally, because of the action of a diuretic, may be reabsorbed at a more distal site where the diuretic under consideration may not exert an effect. The characteristics of an ideal proximal marker are shown in Table I. Unfortunately, none of the substances handled in the proximal tubule (glucose, bicarbonate, phosphate, urate, calcium, and magnesium) fulfills all these criteria.

In some species, urate perhaps comes closest to fulfilling these criteria. In man, reduced uric acid clearance and hyperuricemia have been shown to develop when extracellular volume is reduced by salt restriction and chlorothiazide administration (Suki et al., 1967; Steele and Oppenheimer, 1969). In the rat, microinjection and free-flow microperfusion studies have shown that urate is reabsorbed in the proximal but not in the distal tubule (Kramp et al., 1971; Weinman et al., 1975). Bidirectional urate transport in the proximal tubule has, however, been shown (Mudge et al., 1968; Greger et al., 1971). The demonstration of reduced urate excretion by pyrazinoate in man and primates, however, would indicate the presence of a secretory site (Mudge et al., 1968; Skeith and Healey, 1968; Gutman et al., 1969; Fanelli and Bohn, 1970) which may be located anywhere along the tubule. This constitutes a limitation to the use of urate as a marker of proximal reabsorption.

Parallel changes in the renal excretion of sodium, phosphate (Suki et al., 1969), calcium (Walser, 1961; Blythe et al., 1968), and magnesium (Massry et al., 1967) have been demonstrated under a variety of conditions, including following the administration of diuretics (Eknoyan et al., 1970). None of these ions, however, fulfill the criteria listed in Table I. Changes in the plasma level of all three are known to occur, and all three are subject to the influence of a number of hormones, principally that of parathyroid hormone (Eknoyan et al., 1970). Both calcium and magnesium are protein bound, and their use would require measurements of ultrafilterable plasma levels. Micropuncture studies have shown that the ratio of tubular fluid-to-plasma concentration of calcium is close to unity at the end of the accessible portion of the proximal tubule (Lassiter et al., 1963). Magnesium, on the other hand, attains ratios greater than unity (Le Grimellec, 1975), and in some studies its tubular fluid-to-plasma ratio has been shown to be the same as that of inulin, indicating the absence of proximal absorption (Brunette et al., 1969). Both calcium and magnesium are reabsorbed to a considerable extent in the loop of Henle (Lassiter et al., 1963; Brunette et al., 1969; Le Grimellec, 1975). Therefore, neither ion is a suitable marker of proximal reabsorption.

Based on the earlier suggestions that most of the reabsorption of the

Table I. Characteristics of Ideal Proximal Marker

Should have steady plasma level
Should not be protein bound
TF/P ratio should be 1 throughout proximal tubule
Should not be reabsorbed beyond proximal tubule
Should not be secreted

inorganic phosphate filtered is completed by the end of the proximal tubule (Strickler *et al.*, 1964; Agus *et al.*, 1971), phosphate has been suggested as a proximal marker. These results, however, have been challenged and evidence for distal phosphate reabsorption presented (Amiel *et al.*, 1970; Knox *et al.*, 1973; Wen, 1974b; Le Grimellec, 1975). Thus, the suggestion that PO_4 may be the ideal proximal marker is no longer tenable.

Glucose is almost completely reabsorbed in the proximal tubule (Frohnert *et al.*, 1970). The capacity for glucose absorption at this site is considerably in excess of the absorptive activity at prevailing blood glucose levels. It would therefore require considerable depression of reabsorption to develop significant glucosuria in the presence of normal filtered loads of glucose. This can be overcome, however, if the animals are glucose loaded and the studies performed at blood glucose levels above tubular maximum.

Bicarbonate is also reabsorbed primarily (85–90%) in the proximal tubule, the remainder being reabsorbed in the distal tubule (Gottschalk *et al.*, 1960). Volume expansion, which is well known to inhibit proximal sodium reabsorption, has also been shown to depress proximal tubular bicarbonate reabsorption (Kurtzman, 1970). The considerable amounts of HCO_3^- (10–15%) reabsorbed distally would limit the value of changes in HCO_3^- excretion as an index of proximal effect. As with glucose, however, bicarbonate loading should overcome this limitation.

III. THE LOOP OF HENLE

Perhaps the most successful application of clearance techniques to the study of the site of action of diuretics in the kidney has been an analysis of their effect on urine concentration and dilution. It is now well established that the principal process mediating the concentration and dilution of the urine is the absorption of chloride and sodium and generation of hypotonic tubular fluid in the water-impermeable thick ascending limb of the loop of Henle. The clearance of solute-free water (C_{H_2O}) and the reabsorption of solute-free water ($T^{C_{H_2O}}$) reflect principally on the ability of the ascending limb to reabsorb solute, and the measurement of these parameters permits the localization of an effect of a diuretic agent to this segment of the nephron (Suki *et al.*, 1965; Seldin *et al.*, 1966; Eknoyan *et al.*, 1967).

Studies of solute-free water clearance and reabsorption are done under conditions of maximal urine dilution or concentration. To calculate these values the final urine is considered to consist of two moieties:

1. The volume of urine containing the solutes at an osmolal concentration equal to that of plasma (P_{osm}) and defined as the osmolar clearance, which is calculated by the standard clearance formula of

$$V\left(\frac{U_{osm}}{P_{osm}}\right) = C_{osm}$$

2. The volume of solute-free water added to or removed from the C_{osm} to

produce the final urine volume or, in other words, the volume of solute-free water added to or abstracted from the urine to achieve the final urine concentration (U_{osm}) elaborated under the specific experimental conditions. This volume is by definition the difference between urine volume (V) and osmolar clearance (C_{osm}) and is referred to as free-water clearance (C_{H_2O}). It is calculated by the formula: $C_{H_2O} = V - C_{osm}$.

During maximal hydration, antidiuretic hormone is suppressed, the final urine is dilute, V is greater than C_{osm}, and C_{H_2O} is positive. During antidiuresis and in the presence of antidiuretic hormone the final urine is concentrated; V, therefore, is less than C_{osm} and the value of C_{H_2O} is negative. The term free-water reabsorption ($T^{C_{H_2O}}$) was introduced to obviate the use of negative C_{H_2O} values and is calculated by the formula: $T^{C_{H_2O}} = C_{osm} - V$.

IV. THE DISTAL TUBULE

A distal tubular site of action may be inferred from the changes in the excretion of potassium and hydrogen which are secreted, often linked with changes in sodium, at this segment of the nephron (Suki *et al.*, 1965; Seldin *et al.*, 1966; Malnic *et al.*, 1966; Malnic and Giebisch, 1972). The secretory system of both ions, however, operates far below capacity. An inhibition of their secretion may not be reflected in changes in their rates of excretion if the delivery of sodium to this site were increased, because of a more proximal effect of the diuretic, thereby increasing their excretion. The problem associated with the use of potassium as a distal marker may be circumvented by studying potassium-adapted animals infused with potassium chloride and potassium ferrocyanide so as to elicit maximum potassium secretion. Under this circumstance a drop in potassium excretion would clearly localize the site of action of the diuretic under consideration to the site of potassium secretion (Berliner *et al.*, 1950; Suki *et al.*, 1965).

The problem associated with hydrogen secretion is more difficult to overcome since any increase in distal HCO_3^- delivery would obscure any effect of the diuretic on distal hydrogen secretion.

V. THE USE OF CLEARANCE OF WATER AND SODIUM FOR THE DETERMINATION OF SITE OF ACTION OF DIURETICS: LIMITATIONS AND PITFALLS

In man and in the experimental animal a well established method for the detection of the site of action of diuretics is the analysis of changes in renal water and electrolyte excretion (Suki *et al.*, 1973a). This section will concentrate mostly on how changes in water, Na, Cl, and K excretion can be interpreted to localize the site of action of diuretics.

There are four principal nephron segments in which diuretics may inhibit tubular reabsorption (Figure 1). The proximal nephron, during clearance studies, may be thought of as the proximal convoluted tubule including the pars recta.

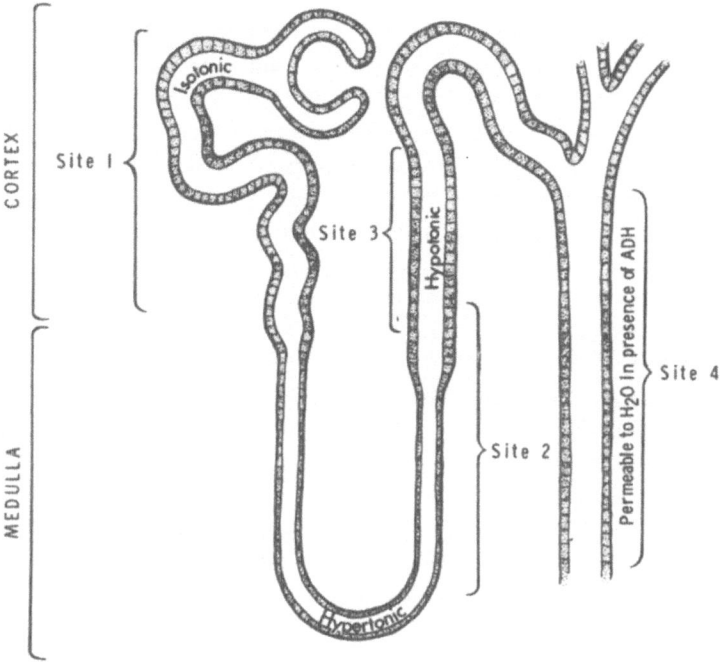

Figure 1. Principal nephron sites in which diuretics may inhibit tubular reabsorption.

Despite controversy as to whether active NaCl transport occurs in the thin ascending limb of the loop of Henle, this segment will be considered as part of the medullary diluting segment and therefore a possible target site for diuretic action (Imai and Kokko, 1974; Jamison, 1974). The medullary portion of the thick ascending limb is also part of the medullary diluting segment. The cortical portion of the ascending limb will be referred to as the cortical diluting segment. Finally, the collecting duct, which contributes to both concentration and dilution of urine, may be affected by diuretic administration.

VI. DIURETIC ACTION IN THE PROXIMAL TUBULE

The most reliable technique presently available which can provide knowledge on the site of action of diuretics is the study of the excretion and reabsorption of solute-free water (C_{H_2O} and $T^{C_{H_2O}}$). Use of the former depends on the fact that during water diuresis (inhibition of antidiuretic hormone secretion) the distal nephron, from the bend of the loop to the end of the collecting duct, is relatively impermeable to water. In addition, because of increased medullary blood flow, solute concentration in the interstitium of the medulla approaches that of plasma and the loss of water from the descending limb is minimized. Thus, the volume reaching the collecting duct will be essentially the same as the volume leaving the proximal tubule. Even in the absence of antidiuretic hormone (ADH), back-diffusion of water from luminal fluid of the collecting ducts does occur consequent to the concentration gradient between the lumen and the medullary interstitium generated by NaCl transport in the ascending limb. Although fluid loss from descending limb and collecting duct is unmeasurable, the generalization can be made that urine flow (V), under conditions of complete ADH suppression, represents the same volume of fluid leaving the proximal tubule per unit time. If all other variables were to remain constant, changes in urine volume may reflect changes in proximal tubular reabsorption (Rector *et al.*, 1964; Seldin *et al.*, 1966; Eknoyan *et al.*, 1967). Theoretically, if a diuretic affected NaCl transport *only* and no further changes in fluid composition were to occur distally, any increment in V would indicate a proximal tubular effect. In reality a number of changes do occur, rendering the use of V as an index of proximal tubular reabsorption cumbersome at best. First is the fact that the *degree* of change in V is crucial. Normally between 50–60% of the filtered water is reabsorbed by the end of the segment of the proximal tubule accessible to micropuncture. Clearly, unless V represented over 50% of the total filtered volume, it could be erroneous to interpret changes as resulting from a proximal effect. A second problem may arise from the fact that, even if no change in distal sodium chloride reabsorption is effected by the diuretic, the increased delivery of substrate may enhance reabsorption in the loop of Henle, increase the medullary gradient, and lead to loss of water from descending limb and collecting duct. Under the appropriate circumstances this might result in no change in V despite a considerable proximal effect (Martinez-Maldonado *et al.*, 1974). Third, a diuretic may inhibit reabsorption of solute in the ascending limb. If this occurs throughout the length of the ascending limb, the medullary solute concentration will drop, preventing loss of water from descending limb and collecting duct, leading to a rise in V in the absence of a proximal effect of the diuretic. Finally, should a diuretic act only in the cortical diluting segment of the ascending limb, V may also rise as a consequence of the delivery into the collecting duct of fluid with a higher osmolality and curtailment of back-diffusion of free water.

Another index of proximal tubular reabsorption could be the fractional excretion of sodium, particularly if corrected for distal potassium secretion $\{[U_{Na+K} V/(P_{Na} \times GFR)] \times 100\}$. Here again, as in the case of V, the value of this parameter would have to exceed 50%. Problems with the use of fractional distal sodium delivery may be further compounded by the possibility that some of the sodium chloride not reabsorbed proximally may be reclaimed in the loop such that sodium excretion may not exceed 50% of the filtered load. A possible way to circumvent this problem can be had during water diuresis inasmuch as the increased reabsorption of sodium distally will be reflected in an increase in free-water clearance. It is possible, therefore, to calculate the sum of $\{[U_{Na+K} V/(P_{Na} \times GFR)] \times 100\} + [(C_{H_2O}/GFR) \times 100]$ which, when in excess of 50%, indicates a proximal effect of the diuretic. In fact, this approach has permitted the correct inference that furosemide exerts an inhibitory effect on proximal tubular reabsorption (Seldin *et al.*, 1966), an observation subsequently confirmed by micropuncture (Rector *et al.*, 1967; Knox *et al.*, 1969; Brenner *et al.*, 1969). This analysis, nevertheless, is not without obstacles and pitfalls. If the proximal effect is modest, it may be missed even during the most careful performance of the clearance study. Furthermore, painstaking attention must be paid to maintaining the experimental subject "in balance." Diuretic-induced fluid losses may lead to contraction of extracellular fluid volume which in turn will enhance proximal tubular reabsorption and reduce distal delivery. This will nullify the action of the diuretic and hamper the interpretation of the clearances. On the other hand, overzealous attempts to replenish the urinary losses may overexpend extracellular fluid (ECF) volume and also complicate the inferential analysis. Since C_{H_2O} and V depend on absolute suppression of ADH for their maximal expression, release of the hormone because of deterioration of the subject or by volume contraction (Czaczkes et al., 1964; Czaczkes and Kleeman, 1964) will alter distal tubular water reabsorption and obscure understanding of the changes. In view of the hazards of altering the clearance of sodium, C_{H_2O}, and V by changes in ECF volume, the importance of obtaining steady-state control collections during which these parameters are constant before introducing the diuretic cannot be overemphasized.

An important aspect of studies designed to investigate the site of action of diuretics is that they should not be performed on a background of conditions which may in themselves mask the effects one wishes to uncover. Water diuresis should be sustained and infusions of hypotonic glucose or mannitol have been used for this purpose. Glucosuria may follow glucose infusion and may raise V, giving the false impression that a proximal effect occurred (Barton et al., 1972). Mannitol, on the other hand, may interfere with the demonstration of an otherwise modest proximal effect since it may result in inhibition of sodium reabsorption at this site consequent to a limiting concentration gradient being reached (Windhager et al., 1959; Windhager and Giebisch, 1961). Furthermore, it will obligate water distally and increase the generation of C_{H_2O} (Seely and Dirks, 1969).

VII. DIURETIC ACTION IN THE ASCENDING LIMB OF HENLE'S LOOP

Free-water generation and free-water reabsorption are rough indices of distal electrolyte reabsorption. The former is not dependent on the responsiveness of the collecting duct to ADH since water diuresis eliminates this variable. Determination of free-water reabsorption in conjunction with C_{H_2O} is of value since it permits separation of the functional state of the medullary diluting segment from that of the cortical diluting segment (Suki et al., 1965; Seldin et al., 1966).

Both of these parameters, C_{H_2O} and $T^{C_{H_2O}}$, depend on the rate of delivery of NaCl to the ascending limb. Thus, marked reductions in GFR will reduce C_{H_2O} and $T^{C_{H_2O}}$ by reducing the rate of delivery of NaCl to distal sites (Berliner and Davidson, 1957; Levinsky et al., 1959). Similarly, enhanced proximal reabsorption, as in extracellular fluid volume contraction, will also curtail $T^{C_{H_2O}}$ and C_{H_2O}. On the other hand, C_{H_2O} and $T^{C_{H_2O}}$ may be enhanced under conditions of

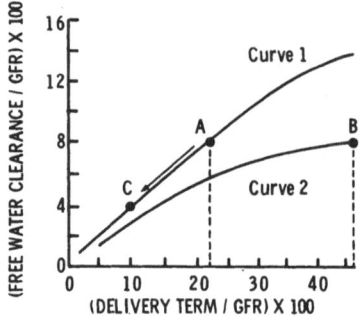

Figure 2. Reference to absolute values of $(C_{H_2O}/GFR) \times 100$ would be inappropriate for an inferential analysis of the functional state of the loop of Henle. As may be seen in curves 1 and 2, C_{H_2O} is identical at points A and B, yet a greater fraction of the distal delivery is being reabsorbed in the case of A than in the case of B, indicating abnormal function in the latter. The amount of C_{H_2O} has been halved at point C but the fraction of distal fluid reabsorbed remains constant, indicating that it is delivery which has been altered (either reduced filtered load or increased proximal reabsorption) rather than loop function.

increased distal delivery. Factors acting directly on the loop will reduce C_{H_2O} and $T^{C_{H_2O}}$. In the case of $T^{C_{H_2O}}$ it appears clear that the rate of osmolar clearance (C_{osm}) is an adequate term to assess grossly the NaCl reaching the diluting site, particularly since this is usually accomplished by the infusion of hypertonic saline in the presence of maximal doses of ADH. However, the term that best describes distal delivery during water diuresis is not as clear. The importance of the issue can be appreciated from the realization that an absolute value for C_{H_2O}, in and of itself, may not provide the necessary information (Figure 2). Reference must always be made to the level of delivery at which that particular C_{H_2O} value is attained. The appropriateness of the delivery term is crucial when assessing whether the loop of Henle is directly inhibited or not. By expressing C_{H_2O} as a fraction of the distal delivery term, one can more precisely determine loop function. To be sure, whichever delivery term is utilized, its range during control and experimental conditions must be comparable.

To determine changes in loop reabsorption, reductions in C_{H_2O} *alone* are not reliable (Figure 2). An alternative is to express C_{H_2O} as a fraction of V, (C_{Na} + C_{H_2O}) or of (C_{Cl} + C_{H_2O}). Correcting these values to a standard GFR helps eliminate variations due to fluctuations in GFR[1].

Changes in C_{H_2O}/V are fraught with the same problems which affect the use of C_{H_2O} or V alone. A rise in V and C_{H_2O} simply due to a decrease in back-diffusion will decrease this ratio without necessarily indicating an effect on loop function. An increase in back-diffusion of fluid will have the converse effect (Martinez-Maldonado *et al.*, 1974). It is evident, then, that complete inhibition of ADH secretion must be continuously present during C_{H_2O} measurements.

Measurement of $T^{C_{H_2O}}$ and medullary tissue concentration is of value in this regard. In animal studies, reductions in $T^{C_{H_2O}}$ (in reference to C_{osm}) and medullary

---

[1] All further reference to these parameters is to the values corrected by GFR. For the sake of clarity the GFR term will be left out.

solute (Na, K, Cl) concentration will indicate that the reduction in C_{H_2O}/V (or $C_{H_2O}/C_{H_2O} + C_{Na}$ or $C_{H_2O}/C_{H_2O} + C_{Cl}$) observed during water diuresis is the result of inhibition of the medullary diluting segment. On the other hand, should $T^{C_{H_2O}}$ remain normal, an effect in the cortical diluting segment could be inferred (Suki *et al.*, 1965).

The use of V as a delivery term is not suitable during osmotic (glucose, mannitol, urea) diuresis since it overestimates NaCl delivery (Barton *et al.*, 1972; Martinez-Maldonado, 1975). In this circumstance $C_{H_2O} + C_{Na}$ is a better estimate. When the osmotic agent is a nonabsorbable anion such as HCO_3^-, C_{Na} must be replaced by C_{Cl} (Rosin *et al.*, 1970). Increased delivery of $NaHCO_3$ to the loop, either by administration of acetazolamide or hypotonic $NaHCO_3$, imposes a limit on the formation of C_{H_2O} when either V or $C_{H_2O} + C_{Na}$ is used as the delivery term. In fact, the similarity between $NaHCO_3$ and mannitol suggests that the former behaves as a nonreabsorbable solute in the loop. To circumvent this, Rosin and his collaborators (1970) suggested the use of the term $C_{Cl} + C_{H_2O}$ as the delivery term. When plotted in such a way, C_{H_2O} was identical to that obtained during hypotonic saline diuresis. It should be pointed out that when hypotonic saline is utilized for the determination of C_{H_2O}, no major difference is apparent between V, $C_{H_2O} + C_{Na}$, or $C_{H_2O} + C_{Cl}$ as delivery terms.

Reference has been made to the analysis of data used to determine whether a diuretic exerts an effect on the medullary or cortical diluting segments. In general, diminished $T^{C_{H_2O}}$ and C_{H_2O}, particularly if medullary tissue solute concentration is also reduced, indicates inhibition of *both* segments. A diminished C_{H_2O} with a normal $T^{C_{H_2O}}$ and normal medullary solute concentration indicates inhibition of the cortical diluting segment only. Theoretically, it is conceivable that a diuretic may have an exclusive site of action in the medullary diluting segment, but the sodium chloride which escapes reabsorption is reabsorbed distally. Should the cortical diluting segment have the necessary reabsorptive capacity, the fluid emerging into the early distal convolution might be just as dilute as normal and C_{H_2O} would also be normal. Yet, medullary solute concentration would be reduced.

VIII. DIURETIC ACTION IN DISTAL TUBULE AND COLLECTING DUCT

Little sodium and water reabsorption takes place in the distal tubule (Clapp and Robinson, 1966), and it is impossible to analyze changes in its function from C_{H_2O} and $T^{C_{H_2O}}$ studies. On the other hand, the collecting duct reabsorbs sodium actively (Windhager and Giebisch, 1961; Windhager 1964), and its permeability, under basal conditions or in response to ADH, determines the amount of water reabsorbed. Sodium reabsorption during water diuresis will further dilute the urine and increase C_{H_2O}, while during hydropenia it will enhance water back-diffusion ($T^{C_{H_2O}}$). A diuretic having an exclusive site of action on sodium reabsorption in the collecting duct will reduce C_{H_2O} without affecting V during water diuresis and will reduce $T^{C_{H_2O}}$ and raise C_{osm} during hydropenia. A diuretic which exclusively inhibits the effect of ADH on water permeability at this site will reduce $T^{C_{H_2O}}$ at any level of C_{osm}, but C_{H_2O} will be normal, as will all the delivery terms. If the diuretic enhances basal permeability of the collecting duct, it will reduce C_{H_2O} and all the delivery terms by augmenting back-diffusion. However, it will not alter $T^{C_{H_2O}}$ or C_{osm} because of the equilibrium which exists between tubular fluid and interstitium except at very high rates of urine flow.

IX. THE USE OF CLEARANCE OF SOLUTES OTHER THAN SODIUM FOR THE DETERMINATION OF SITE OF ACTION OF DIURETICS: LIMITATIONS AND PITFALLS

The search for markers of reabsorption in the various segments of the nephron has led to the consideration of the various components of the tubular fluid contributed by the glomerular filtrate. Parallel changes between the renal excretion of sodium and another electrolyte were first observed for calcium. Walser (1961) observed that saline infusion increased calcium almost in exact proportion to the increase in sodium excretion so that the ratio of the clearance of ionized calcium to that of sodium was almost unity. Subsequently, a number of investigators have demonstrated a covariance with sodium absorption of the absorptive processes of a number of electrolytes and nonelectrolytes present in tubular fluid including calcium (Blythe *et al.*, 1968), magnesium (Massry *et al.*, 1967), phosphate (Suki *et al.*, 1969), bicarbonate (Kurtzman, 1970), uric acid (Suki *et al.*, 1967, and glucose (Kurtzman *et al.*, 1972). Since these ions and nonionic compounds are absorbed at different sites in the nephron, changes in their renal handling following the administration of diuretic agents have been utilized to glean information on the site(s) in the nephron where these agents exert their effects. Because of the complexities of the renal handling of these substances and the several regulatory and counterregulatory influences on their respective absorptive processes, extreme caution must be exercised in designing the experiments and interpreting the data. The utilization of the clearance of these components of tubular fluid for the purpose of localizing the sites of action of diuretics will be discussed separately for each substance against a background of what is known of its normal renal handling.

A. Calcium

At the normal blood pH of 7.4, 35% of the calcium in serum is bound to proteins; the remaining 65% is free (53% ionized and 12% complexed). The free calcium is filtered at the glomerulus (ultrafilterable calcium, UF_{Ca}), but only 2% of this is excreted daily. Thus, a very efficient system exists for reabsorbing calcium from the glomerular filtrate (Epstein, 1968). Most of the filtered calcium (50%) is reabsorbed in the proximal convoluted tubule in a proportion almost similar to that in plasma ultrafiltrate, resulting in a TF/UF_{Ca} of 1.0–1.2 (Lassiter *et al.*, 1963; Duarte and Watson, 1967; Le Grimellec *et al.*, 1973; Le Grimellec,

1975). Another large fraction (40%) is reabsorbed between the end of the accessible portion of the proximal tubule and the early distal tubule, most likely in the ascending limb of the loop of Henle. The reabsorption of calcium at this latter site must be quite avid since the TF/UF_{Ca} in the early distal tubule is only 0.35 (Le Grimellec et al., 1973). The remaining 8% of the filtered calcium must be reabsorbed in the distal convoluted tubule and the collecting duct.

It is apparent from the foregoing that, independent of where diuretic agents were to inhibit transport, an increase in calcium excretion might be expected to result. This, however, is not the case, and the information obtained from studies on the effects of diuretics on calcium excretion has been both interesting and challenging with respect to interpretation. Early after thiazides were introduced, it was observed that their acute administration resulted in very small increases in calcium excretion (Lamberg and Kuhlbäck, 1959). It was subsequently shown that calcium excretion actually fell following prolonged administration (Higgins et al., 1964). The mechanism of this observation was obscure until it was suggested that shrinkage of extracellular fluid (ECF) volume induced by the diuretic caused enhanced absorption of calcium proximal to the site of action of the diuretic, probably in the proximal convoluted tubule or the loop of Henle (Suki et al., 1967). A corollary to this hypothesis is that the absorption of calcium is dissociated from that of sodium at the site of action of these drugs, a suggestion supported by recent micropuncture studies (Edwards et al., 1973). The concept that ECF volume shrinkage mediates the hypocalciuric effect of thiazide diuretics has been challenged, however, since their action resembles that of parathyroid hormone and is not observed in hypoparathyroid patients (Parfitt, 1972, Brickman et al., 1972). Furthermore, large doses of chlorothiazide over a long period of time are associated with parathyroid hyperplasia in the dog (Pickleman et al., 1969). Although parathyroidectomized rats do exhibit hypocalciuria after thiazides (Suki et al., 1973b), this issue is far from settled. Nevertheless, it can be concluded that during any experiment on renal handling of calcium, especially when diuretics are being tested, sodium and water losses must be carefully replaced (Eknoyan et al., 1970). If, despite these measures, calcium excretion fails to rise concomitant with the rise in sodium, it is safe to assume that the diuretic in question exerts its effect on the cortical diluting segment (where the absorption of sodium and of calcium appears to be dissociated) unless the agent is an inhibitor of carbonic anhydrase (vide infra).

Unlike the thiazides, both furosemide and ethacrynic acid produce proportionate changes in sodium and in calcium clearance (Eknoyan et al., 1970). It has been assumed that this effect is the result of inhibition of electrolyte absorption in the medullary segment of the ascending limb of Henle's loop. Whether an inhibitory effect on the proximal tubule may have also played a role cannot be ascertained, but it can be stated with certainty that unless the loop of Henle is also inhibited, inhibition of proximal reabsorptive function cannot result in hypercalciuria. Thus, acetazolamide inhibits the reabsorption of calcium in addition to that of sodium, bicarbonate, and water in the proximal tubule. However, while urine sodium and bicarbonate excretion rises, calcium excretion does not increase (Beck and Goldberg, 1973). Therefore, failure of a diuretic to increase calcium excretion, particularly if the agent under consideration is an inhibitor of carbonic anhydrase, may occur despite significant inhibition of proximal reabsorption.

B. Magnesium

Approximately 70% of the serum magnesium is not bound to protein and is filtered in the glomerulus. The fate of the filtered magnesium varies with the animal species being studied. Thus, in the dog, magnesium is reabsorbed in the proximal tubule in the same proportion as its concentration in the filtrate, and about 40% of the filtered load is reabsorbed at this site (Brunette et al., 1969; Wen et al., 1970). In the rat, however, magnesium reabsorption lags behind that of sodium. TF/UF_{Mg} at the end of the rat proximal convoluted tubule is 1.6–1.8 or even greater (Le Grimellec, 1975) and only between 27–31% of the filtered load is reabsorbed at this site (Brunette et al., 1974). No magnesium is lost in the descending limb, but about half of the filtered load is reabsorbed in the ascending limb: 50% in the dog (Wen et al., 1970) and 55–60% in the rat (Brunette et al., 1974). Some 5% of the filtered load is reabsorbed in the early, but not the late, distal tubule in the rat (Brunette et al., 1974). No reabsorption is evident distal to this site. No convincing evidence exists for magnesium secretion in the absence of hypermagnesemia.

It is apparent from the foregoing that any diuretic which exerts an effect in the proximal tubule, loop of Henle, or early distal tubule might be expected to increase magnesium excretion. This indeed appears to be the case since all the diuretics so far examined, including the thiazide diuretics, have been reported to increase magnesium excretion (Eknoyan et al., 1970). Clearly, magnesium is of poor discriminatory value for the purposes of localization of diuretic action.

C. Phosphate

Phosphate is largely ultrafilterable (97%) in the normal state, and the filtered load in the intact animal is reabsorbed predominantly in the proximal tubule (Strickler et al., 1964) so that the fraction delivered out of this segment closely approximates that excreted in the urine. In the proximal tubule phosphate is reabsorbed more briskly than sodium so that TF/P is approximately 0.7 (Agus et al., 1971).

This primarily proximal reabsorption of phosphate renders it an almost ideal candidate for serving as a marker for proximal tubular events. Phosphate, however, is influenced by a number of factors which may develop in the course of experimental studies. It has been shown that renal phosphate reabsorption varies with the state of ECF volume (Suki et al., 1969). Thus, shrinkage of ECF volume in the course of an experiment with diuretics may curtail or abolish the phosphaturia induced by the agent. Constant and careful replacement of urinary sodium and water losses, therefore, is mandatory in experiments of this type.

Furthermore, changes in parathyroid hormone will profoundly alter proximal tubular phosphate and sodium reabsorption. Stimulation of parathyroid hormone raises TF/P phosphate and reduces TF/P inulin, thereby markedly increasing distal delivery of sodium, water, and phosphate and enhancing phosphate excretion (Agus *et al.*, 1973). A similar situation may result in the course of experiments with diuretics. For example, the administration of furosemide increases calcium excretion and lowers the serum calcium. If sodium and water losses are replaced without calcium, the serum calcium will be diluted further and parathyroid hormone may be stimulated. It is important, therefore, to always replace calcium losses in addition to the losses of water and other electrolytes. In an effort to remedy this problem and circumvent the development of secondary hypoparathyroidism, experiments have been performed in thyroparathyroidectomized (TPTX) dogs (Eknoyan *et al.*, 1970). In these experiments all the diuretics examined lowered phosphate reabsorption and increased its excretion. This was construed as evidence that virtually all the diuretics exert an effect in the proximal tubule. These observations, however, are subject to an alternate explanation. In the hypoparathyroid state phosphate delivery out of the proximal tubule is considerably in excess of urinary phosphate excretion (Wen, 1974b). Consequently, a site for phosphate reabsorption that is normally suppressed by PTH is unraveled. This site is in greatest likelihood located in the loop of Henle (Brunette *et al.*, 1973). An increase in phosphate excretion in TPTX animals, therefore, may not represent an action of the diuretic in the proximal tubule but rather in the loop of Henle.

It may be concluded that in intact animals studies utilizing changes in phosphate excretion to localize actions of diuretics in the proximal tubule may be possible provided that the losses of sodium, water and calcium are carefully replaced. Studies on TPTX animals are more difficult to interpret.

D. Hydrogen Ion Secretion–Bicarbonate Reabsorption

Hydrogen ion appears to be secreted throughout the nephron (Rector *et al.*, 1965). Bicarbonate reabsorption, therefore, also takes place throughout the nephron, since even in the distal convoluted tubule the minimum achieved pH of 6.4 is not sufficient to render the tubular fluid bicarbonate-free (Malnic *et al.*, 1972). Qualitatively, however, most of the bicarbonate filtered is reabsorbed in the proximal tubule (Bennett *et al.*, 1960; Malnic *et al.*, 1972). The protonation of buffers, on the other hand, and the acidification of the final urine occurs in the distal convoluted tubule and the collecting duct. In the collecting duct, because of the unfavorable surface/volume relationship, the CO_2 resulting from the titration of the residual bicarbonate and the formation of carbonic acid is trapped in the urine, thereby raising its P_{CO_2} (Uhlich *et al.*, 1968).

The characteristics of the hydrogen ion secretion process outlined above may be utilized for the purpose of localizing the sites of action of diuretic agents provided the right conditions are met. A major increase in bicarbonate excretion in the normally hydrated animal may be construed as evidence for an action on the proximal tubule. On the other hand, an agent may inhibit proximal absorption of bicarbonate without bicarbonaturia resulting, if the degree of proximal inhibition is modest and the distal hydrogen ion secretion is intact.

Moderate increases in the load of bicarbonate to the distal nephron can be effectively reabsorbed. Under circumstances such as these, an effect on bicarbonate absorption can be more easily discerned during bicarbonate loading, although in this latter experimental condition a modest inhibition of bicarbonate absorption cannot be safely used to assign a site of action in the proximal tubule. More importantly, the reabsorption of bicarbonate is subject to major variations if extracellular volume is altered. Reabsorption may be reduced by the bicarbonate infusion itself, by the use of hypertonic solutions of sodium bicarbonate for the purpose of raising the serum bicarbonate concentration, and by the excessive replacement of urinary losses (Kurtzman, 1970). This relationship of HCO_3^- absorption to changes in fluid volume requires that experiments be carefully planned and conducted.

The acidification process in the distal tubule and collecting duct may also be used to localize action in this segment of the nephron. Salt deprivation, treatment with mineralocorticoids, and infusion of a nonreabsorbable anion such as sulfate provide maximum stimulus for urinary acidification and the protonation of urinary buffers (Schwartz *et al.*, 1955). Under these conditions, a rise in the urine pH and a reduction in the excretion of titratable acid are indications for a site of action in the distal nephron.

An increase in urine Pco_2 has been adduced as evidence for inhibition of bicarbonate absorption proximal to the collecting duct and the consequent increase in the delivery of bicarbonate to this site (Latner and Burnard, 1950). While this is valid, it must be cautioned that in addition to the delivery of bicarbonate to the collecting duct, the urine Pco_2 is also increased by the augmented delivery of phosphate to this site and decreased by increased urine flow rate and by inhibition of hydrogen ion secretion in this segment (Portwood *et al.*, 1959; Halperin *et al.*, 1974). These factors must all be taken into account and strictly controlled if this approach were to be undertaken to localize drug action.

E. Glucose

Glucose is freely filtered in the glomerulus and rapidly reabsorbed in the early portion of the proximal convoluted tubules so that 98% of the filtered load is reabsorbed by the end of this segment. No further glucose is reabsorbed in the loop of Henle or distal convoluted tubule, but only 0.1% of the filtered glucose is excreted in the final urine suggesting that some 2% is reabsorbed in the collecting duct (Frohnert *et al.*, 1970). The capacity of the distal absorptive site, however, must be considerable since proximal and tubular glucose absorption may be depressed considerably without an apparent glucosuria (Wen, 1974a). Consequently, for an agent to induce glucosuria at prevailing normal blood sugar levels, it would have to also exert a distal effect in addition to a proximal effect. Changes in glucose excretion at normal blood levels, therefore, are not suitable for pharmacological localization purposes. To circumvent this limitation, experiments may be performed during glucose loading. Glucose administration, however, may enhance proximal tubular reabsorption (Schloeder and Stinebaugh, 1970; Suki *et al.*, 1974) and blunt drug-induced diuresis (Levin *et al.*, 1969). In larger doses glucose may also induce an osmotic diuresis and thereby translocate absorption from one segment of the nephron to another. In conclusion, studies of renal glucose handling are not suitable for the localization of the site of action of diuretics.

F. Uric Acid

The renal handling of uric acid has been extensively investigated, and several excellent reviews on the excretion of uric acid in animals (Weiner and Fanelli, 1975), nonhuman primates (Fanelli and Beyer, 1975), and in man (Steele and Rieselbach, 1975) have been published. Most of the information collected to date is derived from studies employing various inhibitors of uric acid absorption and/or secretion. These agents, however, may have multiple effects or may exert different effects in different species. Thus, conclusions drawn from such studies are open to criticism and subject to different interpretations (Holmes *et al.*, 1972). The shortcomings of these studies notwithstanding, it is generally accepted that uric acid is to a large extent filtered and subsequently reabsorbed and secreted. The exact order of the latter two events and the site(s) in the nephron where they may take place remains a subject of considerable debate. It is likely that both processes take place to varying extents in the proximal tubule. If this were true, studies of the renal handling of uric acid would be expected to be of poor value in localizing the sites in the nephron where diuretics exert their effects.

Most diuretics available for use in man have been shown to raise the serum uric acid (Kelley, 1975). This has been attributed by Suki *et al.* (1967) to enhancement of tubular absorption of uric acid as a consequence of the shrinkage of extracellular fluid volume and enhancement of proximal tubular absorption. This suggestion has been supported by further studies in man (Steele, 1969; Steele and Oppenheimer, 1969) and in the rat (Weinman and Eknoyan, 1975; Weinman *et al.*, 1975). Other effects of diuretics such as hyperlacticacidemia (Schirmeister *et al.*, 1969), change in uric acid distribution between body fluid compartments (Zweifler and Thompson, 1965), and increased uric acid production (Ayvazian and Ayvazian, 1961) may contribute to the hyperuricemia and further complicate the interpretation of this observation.

REFERENCES

Addis, T. 1917. Ratio between the urea content of the urine and of the blood after the administration of large quantities of urea. *J. Urol.*, 1:263.

Agus, Z. S., Puschett, J. B., Senesky, D., and Goldberg, M. 1971. Mode of action of parathyroid hormone and cyclic adenosine 3′,5′-monophosphate on renal tubular phosphate reabsorption in the dog. *J. Clin. Invest.*, 50:617.

Agus, Z. S., Gardner, L. B., Beck, L. H., and Goldberg, M. 1973. Effects of parathyroid hormone on renal tubular reabsorption of calcium, sodium, and phosphate. *Am. J. Physiol.*, 224:1143.

Ambard, L. and Weill, A. 1912. Les lois numeriques de la sécrétion rénales de l'urée et du chlorine de sodium. *J. Physiol. Pathol. Gen., 14:*753.

Amiel, C., Kuntziger, H., and Richet, G. 1970. Micropuncture study of handling of phosphate by proximal and distal nephron in normal and parathyroidectomized rat. Evidence for distal absorption. *Pfluegers Arch., 317:*93.

Ayvazian, J. H. and Ayvazian, L. F. 1961. A study of the hyperuricemia induced by hydrochloro-thiazide and acetazolamide separately and in combination. *J. Clin. Invest., 40:*1961.

Barton, L. J., Lackner, L. H., Rector, F. C., Jr., and Seldin, D. W. 1972. The effect of volume expansion on sodium reabsorption in the diluting segment of the dog kidney. *Kidney Int., 1:*19.

Beck, L. H. and Goldberg, M. 1973. Effects of acetazolamide and parathyroidectomy on renal transport of sodium, calcium, and phosphate. *Am. J. Physiol., 224:*1136.

Bennett, C. M., Brenner, B. M., and Berliner, R. W. 1960. Micropuncture study of nephron function in the rhesus monkey. *J. Clin. Invest., 47:*203.

Berliner, R. W. and Davidson, D. G. 1957. Production of hypertonic urine in the absence of pituitary antidiuretic hormone. *J. Clin. Invest., 36:*1416.

Berliner, R. W., Kennedy, T. J., and Hilton, J. G. 1950. Renal mechanisms for excretion of potassium. *Am. J. Physiol., 162:*348.

Blythe, W. B., Gitelman, H. J., and Welt, L. G. 1968. Effect of expansion of the extracellular space on the rate of urinary excretion of calcium. *Am. J. Physiol., 214:*52.

Brenner, B. M., Keimowitz, R. I., Wright, F. S., and Berliner, R. W. 1969. An inhibitory effect of furosemide on sodium reabsorption by the proximal tubule of the rat nephron. *J. Clin. Invest., 48:*290.

Brickman, A. S., Massry, S. G., and Coburn, J. W. 1972. Changes in serum and urinary calcium during treatment with hydrochlorothiazide: Studies on mechanisms. *J. Clin. Invest., 51:*945.

Brunette, M., Wen, S.-F., Evanson, R. L., and Dirks, J. H. 1969. Micropuncture study of magnesium reabsorption in the proximal tubule of the dog. *Am. J. Physiol., 216:*1510.

Brunette, M. G., Taleb, L., and Carriere, S. 1973. Effect of parathyroid hormone on phosphate reabsorption along the nephron of the rat. *Am. J. Physiol., 225:*1076.

Brunette, M. G., Vigneault, N., and Carriere, S. 1974. Micropuncture study of magnesium transport along the nephron in the young rat. *Am. J. Physiol., 227:*891.

Clapp, J. R. and Robinson, R. R. 1966. Osmolality of distal tubular fluid in the dog. *J. Clin. Invest., 45:*1847.

Czaczkes, J. W. and Kleeman, C. R. 1964. The effect of various states of hydration and the plasma concentration on the turnover of antidiuretic hormone in mammals. *J. Clin. Invest., 43:*1649.

Czaczkes, J. W., Kleeman, C. R., and Koening, M. 1964. Physiologic studies of antidiuretic hormone by its direct measurement in human plasma. *J. Clin. Invest., 43:*1625.

Duarte, C. G. and Watson, J. F. 1967. Calcium reabsorption in proximal tubule of the dog nephron. *Am. J. Physiol., 212:*1355.

Edwards, B. R., Baer, P. G., Sutton, R. A. L., and Dirks, J. H. 1973. Micropuncture study of diuretic effects on sodium and calcium reabsorption in the dog nephron. *J. Clin. Invest., 52:*2418.

Eknoyan, G., Suki, W. N., Rector, F. C., Jr., and Seldin, D. W. 1967. Functional characteristics of the diluting segment of the dog nephron and the effect of extracellular volume expansion on its reabsorptive capacity. *J. Clin. Invest., 46:*1178.

Eknoyan, G., Suki, W. N., and Martinez-Maldonado, M. 1970. Effect of diuretics on urinary excretion of phosphate, calcium, and magnesium in thyroparathyroidectomized dogs. *J. Lab. Clin. Med., 76:*257.

Epstein, F. H. 1968. Calcium and the kidney. *Am. J. Med., 45:*700.

Fanelli, G. M., Jr. and Beyer, K. H., Jr. 1975. Uric acid in nonhuman primates with special references to its renal transport. *Annu. Rev. Pharmacol., 14:*355.

Fanelli, G. M., Jr. and Bohn, D. L. 1970. Functional characteristics of renal urate transport in the *Cebus* monkey. *Am. J. Physiol., 218:*627.

Frohnert, P. P., Höhmann, B., Zwiebel, R., and Baumann, K. 1970. Free flow micropuncture studies of glucose transport in the rat nephron. *Pfluegers Arch., 315:*66.

Gottschalk, C. W., Lassiter, W. E., and Mylle, M. 1960. Localization of urine acidification in the mammalian kidney. *Am. J. Physiol., 198:*581.

Greger, R., Lang, F., and Deetjen, P. 1971. Handling of uric acid by the rat kidney. I. Microanalysis of uric acid in proximal tubular fluid. *Pfluegers Arch. Eur. J. Phys., 324:*279.

Gutman, A. B., Yü, T. F., and Berger, L. 1969. Renal function in gout. III. Estimation of tubular secretion and reabsorption of uric acid by use of pyrazinamide. *Am. J. Med., 47:*575.

Halperin, M. L., Goldstein, M. B., Haig, A., Johnson, M. D., and Stinebaugh, B. J. 1974. Studies on the pathogenesis of Type I (distal) renal tubular acidosis as revealed by the urinary P_{CO_2} tension. *J. Clin. Invest., 53:*669.

Higgins, B. A., Nassim, J. R., Collins, J., and Hilb, A. 1964. The effect of bendrofuazide on urine calcium excretion. *Clin. Sci., 27:*457.

Holmes, E. W., Kelley, W. N., and Wyngaarden, J. B. 1972. The kidney and uric acid excretion in man. *Kidney Int., 2:*115.

Imai, M. and Kokko, J. P. 1974. Sodium chloride, urea, and water transport in the thin ascending limb of Henle. *J. Clin. Invest., 53:*393.

Jamison, R. L. 1974. Recent advances in the physiology of Henle's loop and the collecting tubule system. *Circ. Res., 34:*191.

Kelley, W. N. 1975. Effects of drugs on uric acid in man. *Annu. Rev. Pharmacol., 15:*327.

Knox, F. G., Wright, F. S., Howards, S. S., and Berliner, R. W. 1969. Effect of furosemide on sodium reabsorption by proximal tubule of the dog. *Am. J. Physiol., 217:*192.

Knox, F. G., Schneider, F. G., Willis, L. R., Strandhoy, J. W., and Coburn, E. O. 1973. Site and control of phosphate reabsorption by the kidney. *Kidney Int., 3:*347.

Kramp, R. A., Lassiter, W. E., and Gottschalk, C. W. 1971. Urate-2-^{14}C transport in the rat nephron. *J. Clin. Invest., 50:*35.

Kurtzman, N. A. 1970. Regulation of renal bicarbonate reabsorption by extracellular volume. *J. Clin. Invest., 49:*586.

Kurtzman, N. A., White, M. G., Rogers, P. W., and Flynn, J. J., III. 1972. Relationship of sodium reabsorption and glomerular filtration rate to renal glucose reabsorption. *J. Clin. Invest., 51:*127.

Lamberg, B. A. and Kuhlbäck, B. 1959. Effect of chlorothiazide and hydrochlorothiazide on the excretion of calcium in urine. *Scand. J. Clin. Lab. Invest., 11:*351.

Lassiter, W. E., Gottschalk, C. W., and Mylle, M. 1963. Micropuncture study of renal tubular reabsorption of calcium in normal rodents. *Am. J. Physiol., 204:*771.

Latner, A. L. and Burnard, E. D. 1950. Idiopathic hyperchloraemic renal acidosis of infants. *Q. J. Med., 19:*285.

Le Grimellec, C. 1975. Micropuncture study along the proximal convoluted tubule. Electrolyte reabsorption in first convolutions, *Pfluegers Arch., 354:*133.

Le Grimellec, C., Roinel, N., and Morel, F. 1973. Simultaneous Mg, Ca, P, K, Na and Cl analysis in rat tubular fluid. I. During perfusion of either inulin or ferrocyanide. *Pfluegers Arch., 340:*181.

Levin, N. W., Mandelbaum, J., and Colwell, J. A. 1969. Effect of glucose on furosemide-induced electrolyte excretion. *J. Lab. Clin. Med., 74:*980.

Levinsky, N. G. and Levy, M. 1973. Clearance techniques. In: *Handbook of Physiology*, Section 8, Renal Physiology, pp. 103–117. Ed. by Orloff, J. and Berliner, R. W. American Physiological Society, Bethesda, Maryland.

Levinsky, N. G., Davidson, D. G., and Berliner, R. W. 1959. Effects of reduced glomerular filtration on urine concentration in the presence of antidiuretic hormone. *J. Clin. Invest., 38:*730.

Malnic, G. and Giebisch, G. 1972. Mechanism of renal hydrogen ion secretion. *Kidney Int., 1:*280.

Malnic, G., Klose, R. M., and Giebisch, G. 1966. Microperfusion study of distal tubular potassium and sodium transfer in rat kidney. *Am. J. Physiol., 211:*548.

Malnic, G., de Mello Aires, M., and Giebisch, G. 1972. Micropuncture study of renal tubular hydrogen ion transport in the rat. *Am. J. Physiol., 222:*147.

Martinez-Maldonado, M. 1975. Renal diluting capacity (C_{H_2O}) in the rat: Comparison of infusion of saline with mannitol (M), glucose (G) and urea (U) solutions. *Clin. Res., 23:*369A.

Martinez-Maldonado, M., Eknoyan, G., and Suki, W. N. 1974. Influence of volume expansion on renal diluting capacity in the rat. *Clin. Sci. Molec. Med., 46:*331.

Massry, S. G., Coburn, J. W., Chapman, L. W., and Kleeman, C. R. 1967. Effect of NaCl infusion on urinary Ca^{++} and Mg^{++} during reduction in their filtered loads. *Am. J. Physiol., 213:*1218.

Möller, E., McIntosh, J. F., and Van Slyke, D. D. 1929. Studies of urea excretion. *J. Clin. Invest., 6:*427.

Mudge, G. H., Cucchi, G., Platts, M., O'Connell, J. M. B., and Berndt, W. O. 1968. Renal excretion of uric acid in the dog. *Am. J. Physiol., 215:*404.

Parfitt, A. M. 1972. The interactions of thiazide diuretics with parathyroid hormone and vitamin D. Studies in patients with hypoparathyroidism. *J. Clin. Invest., 51:*1879.

Pickleman, J. R., Straus, F. H., II, Forland, M., and Paloyan, E. 1969. Thiazide-induced parathyroid stimulation. *Metabolism, 18:*867.

Portwood, R. M., Seldin, D. W., Rector, F. C., Jr., and Cade, R. 1959. The relation of urinary CO_2 tension to bicarbonate excretion. *J. Clin. Invest., 38:*770.

Rector, F. C., Jr., Van Giesen, G., Kiil, F., and Seldin, D. W. 1964. Influence of expansion of extracellular volume on tubular reabsorption of sodium independent of changes in glomerular filtration rate and aldosterone activity. *J. Clin. Invest., 43:*341.

Rector, F. C., Jr., Carter, N. W., and Seldin, D. W. 1965. The mechanism of bicarbonate reabsorption in the proximal and distal tubules of the kidney. *J. Clin. Invest., 44:*278.

Rector, F. C., Jr., Sellman, J. C., Martinez-Maldonado, M., and Seldin, D. W. 1967. The mechanism of suppression of proximal tubular reabsorption by saline infusions. *J. Clin. Invest., 46:*47.

Rehberg, P. B. 1926a. Studies on kidney function. The rate of filtration and reabsorption in the human kidney. *Biochem. J., 20:*447.

Rehberg, P. B. 1926b. Studies on kidney function. II. The excretion of urea and chlorine analyzed according to a modified filtration reabsorption theory. *Biochem. J., 20:*461.

Rosin, J. M., Katz, M. A., Rector, F. C., Jr., and Seldin, D. W. 1970. Acetazolamide in studying sodium reabsorption in diluting segment. *Am. J. Physiol., 219:*1731.

Schirmeister, J., Man, N. K., and Hallauer, W. 1969. Study on renal and extrarenal factors involved in the hyperuricemia induced by furosemide. In: *Progress in Nephrology,* pp. 59–63. Ed. by Peters, G. and Roch-Ramel, F. Springer-Verlag, New York.

Schloeder, F. X. and Stinebaugh, B. J. 1970. Renal tubular sites of natriuresis of fasting and glucose-induced sodium conservation. *Metabolism, 19:*1119.

Schwartz, W. B., Jenson, R. L., and Relman, A. S. 1955. Acidification of the urine and increased ammonium excretion without change in acid–base equilibrium: Sodium reabsorption as a stimulus to the acidifying process. *J. Clin. Invest., 34:*673.

Seely, J. F. and Dirks, J. H. 1969. Micropuncture study of hypertonic mannitol diuresis in the proximal and distal tubule of the dog kidney. *J. Clin. Invest., 48:*2330.

Seldin, D. W., Eknoyan, G., Suki, W. N., and Rector, F. C., Jr. 1966. Localization of diuretic action from the pattern of water and electrolyte excretion. *Ann. N.Y. Acad. Sci., 139:*328.

Skeith, M. D. and Healey, L. A. 1968. Urate clearance in *Cebus* monkeys. *Am. J. Physiol., 214:*582.

Smith, H. W. 1943. *Lectures on the Kidney,* pp. 74–77. University Extension Div., University of Kansas, Lawrence, Kansas.

Smith, H. W. 1951. *The Kidney—Structure and Function in Health and Disease,* pp. 39–80. Oxford University Press, New York.

Smith, H. W. 1956. *Principles of Renal Physiology.* Oxford University Press, New York.

Steele, T. H. 1969. Evidence for altered renal urate reabsorption during changes in volume of the extracellular fluid. *J. Lab. Clin. Med., 74:*288.

Steele, T. H. and Oppenheimer, S. 1969. Factors affecting urate excretion following diuretic administration in man. *Am. J. Med., 47:*564.

Steele, T. H. and Rieselbach, R. E. 1975. Renal urate excretion in normal man. *Nephron, 14:*21.

Strickler, J. C., Thompson, D. D., Klose, R. M., and Giebisch, G. 1964. Micropuncture study of inorganic phosphate excretion in the rat. *J. Clin. Invest., 43:*1596.

Suki, W. N., Rector, F. C., Jr., and Seldin, D. W. 1965. The site of action of furosemide and other sulfonamide diuretics in the dog. *J. Clin. Invest., 44:*1458.

Suki, W. N., Hull, A. R., Rector, F. C., Jr., and Seldin, D. W. 1967. Mechanism of the effect of thiazide diuretics on calcium and uric acid. *J. Clin. Invest., 46:*1121.

Suki, W. N., Martinez-Maldonado, M., Rouse, D., and Terry, A. 1969. Effect of expansion of extracellular fluid volume on renal phosphate handling. *J. Clin. Invest., 48:*1888.

Suki, W. N., Eknoyan, G., and Martinez-Maldonado, M. 1973a. Tubular sites and mechanisms of diuretic action, *Annu. Rev. Pharmacol., 13:*91.

Suki, W. N., Eknoyan, G., Samaan, N., Dichoso, C., Johnson, P. G., and Martinez-Maldonado, M. 1973b. Idiopathic hypercalciuria: Its diagnosis, pathogenesis and treatment. In: *Cornell Seminars in Nephrology,* pp. 229–246. Ed. by Baker, E. L. John Wiley & Sons, New York.

Suki, W. N., Hebert, C. S., Stinebaugh, B. J., Martinez-Maldonado, M., and Eknoyan, G. 1974. Effects of glucose on bicarbonate reabsorption in the dog kidney. *J. Clin. Invest., 54:*1.

Uhlich, E., Baldamus, C. A., and Ullrich, K. J. 1968. Verhalten von CO_2-Druck und Bicarbonat in Gegenstromsgetem des Nierenwerks, *Pfluegers Arch. Eur. J. Physiol., 303:*31.

Walser, M. 1961. Calcium clearance as a function of sodium clearance in the dog. *Am. J. Physiol., 200:*1099.

Weiner, I. M. and Fanelli, G. M., Jr. 1975. Renal urate excretion in animal models. *Nephron, 14:*33.

Weinman, E. J. and Eknoyan, G. 1975. Chronic effects of chloróthiazide on reabsorption by the proximal tubule of the rat. *Clin. Sci. Molec. Med., 49:*107.

Weinman, E. J., Eknoyan, G., and Suki, W. N. 1975. The influence of the extracellular fluid volume on the tubular reabsorption of uric acid. *J. Clin. Invest., 55:*283.

Wen, S. F. 1974a. Significance of distal glucose transport in regulating glucose excretion. *Clin. Res., 22:*550A.

Wen, S. F. 1974b. Micropuncture studies of phosphate transport in the proximal tubule of the dog. The relationship to sodium reabsorption. *J. Clin. Invest., 53:*143.

Wen, S. F., Evanson, R. L., and Dirks, J. H. 1970. Micropuncture study of renal magnesium transport in proximal and distal tubule of the dog. *Am. J. Physiol., 219:*570.

Windhager, E. E. 1964. Electrophysiological study of the renal papilla of golden hamsters. *Am. J. Physiol., 206:*694.

Windhager, E. E. and Giebisch, G. 1961. Micropuncture study of renal tubular transfer of sodium chloride in the rat. *Am. J. Physiol., 200:*581.

Windhager, E. E., Whittembury, G., Oken, D. E., Schatzman, H. J., and Solomon, A. K. 1959. Single proximal tubules of the *Necturus* kidney. III. Dependence of H_2O movement on NaCl concentration. *Am. J. Physiol., 197:*313.

Zweifler, A. J. and Thompson, G. R. 1965. Correction of thiazide hyperuricemia by potassium chloride and ammonium chloride. *Arthritis Rheum., 8:*1134.

Chapter **5**

Effects of Diuretics on Renal Transport of Potassium

Gerhard Giebisch

Department of Physiology
Yale University School of Medicine
New Haven, Connecticut 06510

I. INTRODUCTION

This chapter is an assessment of the effects of the more important diuretics on the renal transport processes governing the excretion of potassium ions. Our knowledge of the effects of diuretics on the tubular potassium transport system has advanced with new insights into the physiology of potassium transport. These advances, concerned with mapping of potassium transport along the nephron and with the cellular mechanism of renal tubular potassium transport, have been based largely on work carried out at the single nephron level. The following study attempts to evaluate the action of diuretics within the framework of these newly acquired concepts.

II. THE PHYSIOLOGY OF POTASSIUM EXCRETION

A. Tubular Sites of Potassium Reabsorption and Secretion—Clearance and Stop-Flow Experiments

Maintenance of a normal potassium balance requires a urinary excretion rate of not more than 10–20% of the filtered load of potassium. However, this amount can be dramatically reduced to less than 1% by dietary potassium deprivation. These observations demonstrate the kidney's ability to reabsorb potassium. Under several experimental and pathological conditions, it can clearly be shown that the amount of potassium may also exceed that delivered to the tubules by glomerular filtration. Hence, it is necessary to include a tubular secretory mechanism in the overall renal tubular operation regulating renal potassium excretion.

Concerning the relative importance of reabsorptive and secretory processes in setting the rate of urinary potassium excretion, a variety of techniques including the use of clearance, stop-flow, and micropuncture techniques have clearly shown that secretory and reabsorptive mechanisms in some distal portions of the nephron are not only the major sources of urinary potassium but also the principal sites of tubular regulation of potassium excretion. The arguments leading to these conclusions have been reviewed (Berliner, 1961; Brenner and Berliner, 1973; Schultze, 1973; Wright, 1974; Giebisch, 1971, 1974a) and are, briefly, the following.

1. After receiving diuretics in successively larger doses, experimental animals lose enough sodium and fluid to reduce glomerular filtration rate (GFR) significantly, and the delivery of potassium to the tubules may fall by as much as 30–40% of its original value (Berliner, 1961; Berliner and Kennedy, 1948). Despite this significant reduction in the filtered load of potassium, the rate of urinary potassium excretion may remain remarkably constant. Berliner and his associates argued that it would be difficult to reconcile these results solely within a filtration–reabsorption theory of renal potassium excretion. In particular, they pointed out that changes in reabsorption which might take place in proportion to the rate of glomerular filtration would have resulted in excretion of a constant fraction of the filtered potassium load but not in excretion of a constant *absolute* amount of potassium. Accordingly, the appearance in the urine of such a fixed amount of potassium as its filtered load fell was thought more likely to represent secretion of potassium into the urine at a constant rate. Berliner and his associates also postulated that most of the filtered potassium had to be reabsorbed by the tubular epithelium at nephron sites upstream of those involved in the secretory process (Berliner, 1961).

Subsequently, this theory received further support by experiments carried out in dogs in which the filtered potassium load was reduced by clamping one renal artery while the urine was being collected separately from the two kidneys (Davidson *et al.*, 1958). Provided sodium excretion was maintained at elevated levels, the filtered load of potassium could be reduced by arterial compression by some 30% without leading to differences in potassium excretion between the two kidneys. Again, these results showed absence of a tight relationship between filtered load and urinary excretion rates of potassium. It was concluded that secretion of potassium occurs normally at distal nephron sites after the tubular fluid had been rendered free of potassium by extensive reabsorption during passage along more proximal regions of the nephron.

2. Further information on the mode of tubular potassium transport was gained in experiments in which potassium excretion was stimulated by potassium loading and an anion species, such as ferrocyanide, that is neither reabsorbed nor secreted, but is used to suppress urinary chloride excretion (Berliner, 1961; Berliner *et al.*, 1950). This results in excretion of a urine rich in

potassium but poor in anions other than ferrocyanide. The important finding was that the minimum amount of potassium secreted, i.e., that excreted in excess of the filtered moiety, was significantly greater than the total amount of all urinary anions other than ferrocyanide. Since the latter is excreted solely by glomerular filtration, it follows that potassium ions could not have been secreted with an anion but must have been exchanged during the secretory process for some filtered cation. In view of their abundance in the urine sodium ions were assumed to be the most likely ion species. Thus, cation exchange across a distal tubular segment of low anion permeability, rather than tubular secretion with an anion, emerged as the operation thought to account for potassium secretion.

3. The view that potassium secretion is dependent on tubular exchange for sodium was further supported by a number of observations indicating that urinary potassium excretion was indeed sensitive to the amount of sodium excreted into the urine. If the absolute rate of sodium excretion was considered representative of the sodium load reaching the distal tubular site of potassium secretion, several findings were consistent with the idea that sodium delivery might become rate limiting for potassium secretion. Relevant observations show that reduction of sodium excretion by dietary sodium restriction prevents the powerful kaliuretic effect of adrenal mineralocorticoids (Davis and Howell, 1953; Howell and Davis, 1954; Relman and Schwartz, 1952; Seldin et al., 1956). Davidson et al. (1958) have also made relevant observations in dogs in which glomerular filtration rate of one kidney had been acutely reduced by some 30–40%. As pointed out before this maneuver is ineffective in reducing urinary potassium excretion provided special precautions are taken—such as administration of mercurial diuretics, diamox, or sodium sulfate—to maintain sodium excretion at relatively high levels. In sharp contrast sodium excretion drops precipitously when filtration rate is acutely depressed and such precautions are not taken (Davidson et al., 1958; Thompson and Pitts, 1952). A dramatic fall in urinary potassium excretion occurred with the decrease in urinary sodium output. The implication was that the fall in the amount of sodium available for distal exchange with potassium had become rate limiting and was responsible for the depression in renal potassium excretion.

The dependence of potassium secretion upon sodium delivery to some distal nephron sites had received further support by results from stop-flow experiments (Sullivan et al., 1960; Malvin et al., 1958; Pitts et al., 1958; Vander, 1961; Sullivan, 1961; Walker et al., 1961). These experiments provided evidence not only that the secretory site was distal to that of potassium reabsorption but also demonstrated the sensitivity of potassium secretion to the luminal sodium concentration. Normally, but particularly when potassium excretion is stimulated, the "potassium peak" in stop-flow experiments is contained within the very first urinary samples which are collected after release of the ureteral clamp. Samples collected prior to the potassium peak contain little potassium and sodium, thus showing that potassium reabsorption precedes secretion. Importantly though, if the stop-flow technique was modified so as to allow sodium-poor tubular fluid to proceed to the site where potassium secretion takes place [by briefly interrupting ureteral occlusion (Walter et al., 1961)], the tubular accumulation of potassium was dramatically reduced. This suppression of potassium secretion is reversible since readmission of sodium-rich proximal fluid to distal nephron sites leads to the prompt reappearance of high potassium concentrations in stop-flow samples. It is clear that the luminal sodium concentration exerts a strong regulatory effect upon distal tubular potassium transport: When potassium transport is stimulated, the presence of sodium assured maximum potassium secretion. Absence or reduction of sodium in the lumen, on the other hand, suppresses potassium secretion and frequently even induces net potassium reabsorption.

The influence of the luminal sodium supply on renal potassium excretion has also been evaluated in the doubly perfused amphibian kidney (Vogel and Tervooren, 1964). This preparation is stable over a period of several hours and allows selective and extensive ion substitutions in either the aortic perfusion fluid supplying the glomerular filtrate or the portal perfusion fluid which feeds into the peritubular capillary network surrounding the tubules. When the potassium concentration in the double-perfused frog kidney was kept at normal concentrations in the peritubular perfusion fluid in which sodium had been replaced by mannitol or raffinose, the effects of changes in the luminal sodium concentrations could be studied. It could be demonstrated that potassium excretion into the urine was critically dependent on the sodium concentration of the fluid supplying the glomerular filtrate. Thus, whereas the potassium excretion remains low in the absence of sodium, it is significantly stimulated as the luminal sodium concentration is elevated. Again, this demonstrates the sodium sensitivity of the excretory process of potassium.

Two points should be stressed with respect to the dependence of potassium excretion upon the urinary sodium supply. First, the situation is complicated by observations that prior chronic sodium deprivation does not depress but may actually even enhance the kidney's ability to excrete an exogenous potassium load (Anderson and Laragh, 1958; Wright et al., 1971; Peterson, 1975). From the above discussion one might have expected a blunted kaliuretic response to potassium loading in sodium-deficient animals. Thus, low sodium excretion does not always compromise the excretory potential for potassium. The enhanced secretory response of low-sodium animals to potassium loading will be further discussed in Section III-B. A second point concerns the site within the nephron where low sodium concentrations exert their effect upon potassium transport. An important finding of micropuncture studies in non-potassium-loaded animals on a low-sodium regime was that reduction of urinary potassium excretion was shown to be due largely to stimulation of potassium reabsorption along the collecting duct (Malnic et al., 1966b). Thus, the tubular sodium effect extends clearly beyond a depression of secretion alone. This necessitates some reevaluation of the nature of the effects of sodium on tubular potassium secretion.

4. Several lines of evidence obtained in renal clearance experiments also point to an important relationship between the acid–base balance of the organism and the rate of renal potassium excretion (Berliner, 1961; Brenner and Berliner, 1973; Giebisch, 1971; Berliner et al., 1951, 1954; Malnic et al., 1971; Rector, 1973). In general, alkalosis induces enhanced potassium loss whereas acute

acidosis reduces potassium excretion. Results from stop-flow experiments (Sullivan *et al.*, 1960; Pitts *et al.*, 1958) have clearly shown that it is the distal nephron which responds to acid–base stimuli and which modulates the rate of potassium secretion. Nevertheless, it should be noted that the initial response of the tubule to acid–base disturbances may differ sharply from that which obtains during the prolonged imposition of alkalosis or acidosis (Malnic *et al.*, 1971; Gennari and Cohen, 1975).

B. Importance of the Distal Tubule, the Cortical Collecting Tubule, and the Collecting Duct in Regulating Potassium Excretion—Micropuncture and Microperfusion Data

A large body of evidence has become available from micropuncture studies in the amphibian (Wiederholt *et al.*, 1971), rodent (Wright *et al.*, 1971; Malnic *et al.*, 1964, 1966b, 1971; Peterson, 1975; Lechène *et al.*, 1969; DeRouffignac *et al.*, 1969; Watson *et al.*, 1964; Duarte *et al.*, 1971), canine (Bennett *et al.*, 1967; Evanson *et al.*, 1972; Dirks and Seely, 1970) and monkey kidney (Bennett *et al.*, 1968) that the distal convoluted tubule is the main site of regulating urinary potassium excretion. The distal tubule responds to metabolic stimulation either by secretion or reabsorption of potassium ions. In contrast, changes of proximal tubular potassium handling or modification of potassium transport along Henle's loop, with some notable exceptions, are not important in the regulation of potassium excretion.

Figures 1–3 provide information on the mode of renal tubular potassium handling in three experimental conditions ranging from control experiments (Figure 1) to studies during maximal potassium conservation (Figure 2) and including a situation of maximal stimulation of urinary potassium excretion (Figure 3) (Malnic *et al.*, 1964).

Figure 1 summarizes data on concentration differences and fractional excretion rates in a control group of rats excreting an amount of potassium equivalent to some 17% of the filtered potassium load. The general pattern of tubular potassium handling is a small reduction of proximal tubular potassium concentrations below plasma levels, a significant fall of early distal tubular fluid/ plasma TF/P concentration ratios, followed by a progressive increase of these ratios as a function of distal tubular length, and a final further increase of potassium concentrations with the passage of tubular fluid through the collecting tubule and collecting duct system.

When the changes in tubular potassium concentrations are corrected for reabsorptive water movement, it can be seen that some 70% of the filtered potassium load has been reabsorbed by the time the tubular fluid has reached the end of the proximal convoluted tubule. At the earliest distal tubular puncture site some 95% of the filtered potassium has been reabsorbed. Net movement of potassium along the distal convoluted tubule can be deduced from the positive slope of the regression line correlating potassium/inulin TF/P ratios to distal tubular length. Calculations using mean early distal and final urinary excretory data lead to the conclusion that as much as 70% of the potassium in the final

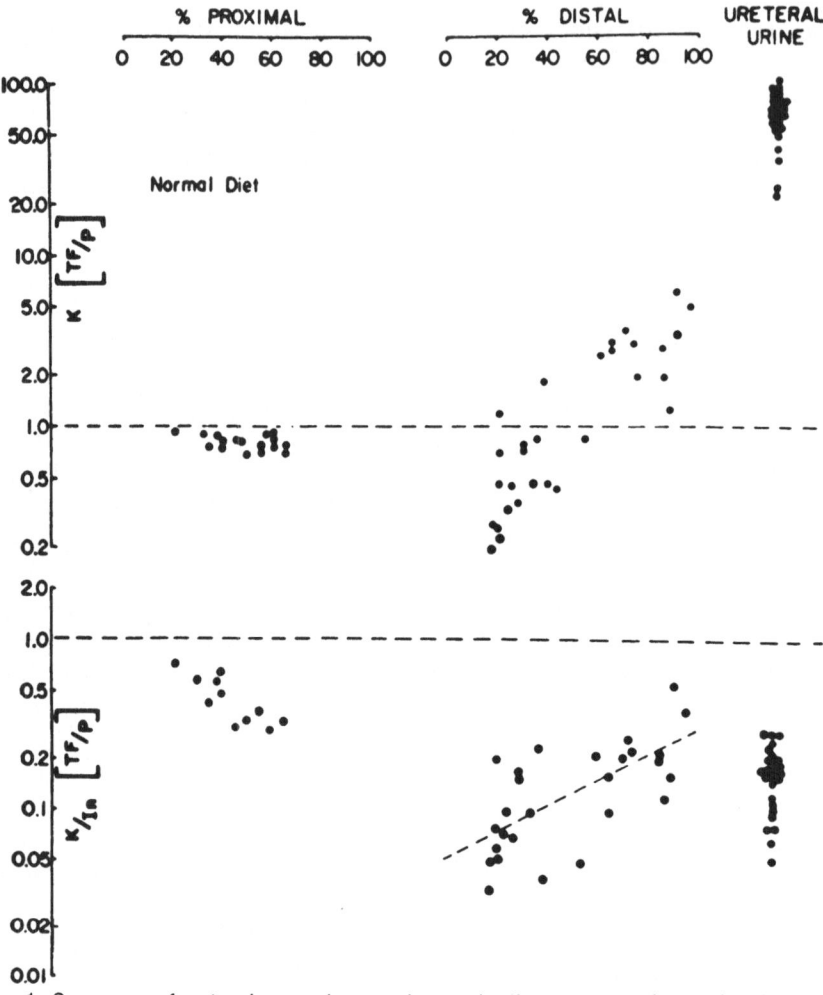

Figure 1. Summary of potassium and potassium-to-inulin concentration ratios from rats on control diet. Upper panel: tubule fluid/plasma concentration ratios along the nephron. Lower panel: potassium/inulin tubular fluid/plasma concentration ratios. Values represent the fraction of filtered potassium remaining within the lumen. Urinary values are also included. (From Malnic *et al.*, 1964.)

urine may derive from distal tubular secretion. This value may underestimate the true secretory contribution since the earliest distal tubular puncture sites are about 20% distal tubular length and more extensive net reabsorption of potassium may have obtained at the very beginning of this tubular segment. Such a transport pattern along the earliest part of the distal tubule could clearly accentuate the contribution of distal tubular potassium secretion to the amount of potassium in the final urine.

Comparison of late distal fractional excretion rates with values of the final ureteral urine indicates absence of net movement or net reabsorption along the collecting duct epithelium. A similar transport pattern emerges from micropuncture experiments on single papillary collecting ducts in the rat (Diezi *et al.*,

1973). In animals on a normal potassium and sodium intake, net secretion is absent, but a small, although variable, degree of potassium reabsorption has been observed along the most terminal nephron segment. Hilger *et al.* (1958) came to similar conclusions based on experiments using microcatheter exploration of collecting ducts in the golden hamster.

Comparison of these data from animals on a control diet with the results of experiments in "low"-K or "high"-K animals demonstrate a number of important similarities and differences (see Figures 2 and 3).

Proximal transport patterns with respect to transepithelial concentration differences were not markedly different in animals on a normal potassium intake from those on either a high- or low-potassium regime, despite the fact that the mean fractional excretion rates of potassium were as low as 3% in low-K animals and as high as 150% in high-K animals.

Similarly, despite these dramatic differences in urinary excretion rates, early distal tubular potassium TF/P ratios are not different in the three groups of animals.

Due to strong osmotic diuresis in the group of high-K animals, a somewhat larger fraction of potassium is present at the early distal tubular level in these animals. Diminished reabsorption of potassium at tubular sites preceding the distal tubule thus can potentially contribute to the moiety of potassium in the final urine.

Along the distal convoluted tubule the increase in potassium concentration ratios varies sharply in animals on a low or high potassium intake. Potassium concentration ratios in low-K animals rise only moderately, and inspection of the lower section of Figure 2 indicates that this increase can be accounted for fully by the rate of distal tubular water reabsorption. Thus, net potassium secretion has been completely suppressed in these animals. The regression line of distal tubular potassium/inulin TF/P ratios shows a negative slope which, however, is not statistically different from zero. Nevertheless, in other studies in which dietary potassium deprivation was maintained over longer periods of time, we have observed a reversal of the direction of net transport, i.e., net reabsorption of potassium along the distal convoluted tubule in low-potassium states (Duarte *et al.*, 1971).

Whereas distal tubule potassium secretion is abolished by pretreatment with a low-potassium diet, secretion is strongly stimulated by a regime in which administration of a high-K diet and infusion of a carbonic anhydrase inhibitor and an exogenous potassium load maximally stimulate excretion rates to values approaching twice the amount filtered. As can be seen from inspection of Figure 3, potassium TF/P ratios rise steeply along the distal tubule. Significant net addition of potassium occurs and potassium/inulin TF/P ratios above unity can be observed by the time tubular fluid reaches the middle of the distal tubule. Again, a large fraction—some 85% at least—of the urinary potassium moiety may have entered the lumen by secretion. We and others have observed that it is at the distal tubular level that changes in acid–base balance (Malnic *et al.*, 1971), diuretics (Duarte *et al.*, 1971; Dirks and Seely, 1970; Evanson *et al.*, 1972; Bennett *et al.*, 1967, 1968) and adrenal steroids (Hierholzer *et al.*, 1965;

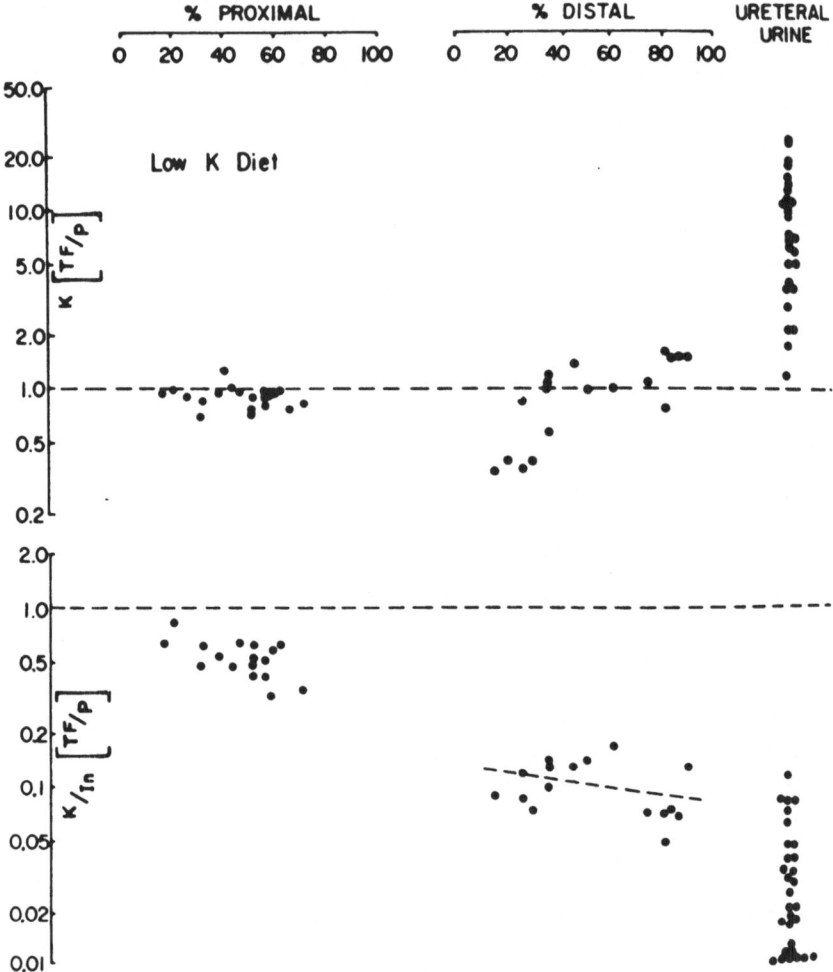

Figure 2. Summary of potassium and potassium-to-inulin concentration ratios as function of nephron length in animals kept on a low potassium diet for several weeks prior to the experiment. (From Malnic *et al.*, 1964.)

Hierholzer and Lange, 1974), as well as changes in dietary potassium intake (Wright *et al.*, 1971; Malnic *et al.*, 1971), affect the rate of potassium excretion by varying the amount of potassium being secreted along the distal tubule.

In contrast to the distal tubule, the loop of Henle is not significantly involved in the regulation of urinary potassium excretion. Micropuncture data obtained in loops of the exposed rodent kidney show that the potassium concentration increases towards the hairpin turn (Brenner and Berliner, 1973; Jamison *et al.*, 1967; Jamison, 1970) and that there is a close relationship between the potassium concentration in loop fluid and the medullary interstitial osmotic pressure (DeRouffignac and Morel, 1969). The transport pattern of potassium in the loop of Henle is consistent with some recycling across loops so that potassium loss occurs from the ascending limb (low early distal potassium/

inulin TF/P ratios) whereas net addition may take place along the descending limb of Henle's loop (potassium concentrations along the descending limb increase at a rate exceeding that of inulin). Some potassium added to the loop may also be derived as a result of reabsorption from the collecting ducts. However, the very similar and effective reduction of early distal tubular potassium concentrations by potassium reabsorption along the ascending limb of Henle's loop and the early distal tubule, irrespective of final urinary excretory patterns of potassium, makes it virtually certain that the events governing potassium recycling in the loop of Henle are not important in the regulation of potassium balance.

Comparison of fractional excretion rates at the late distal tubular level with

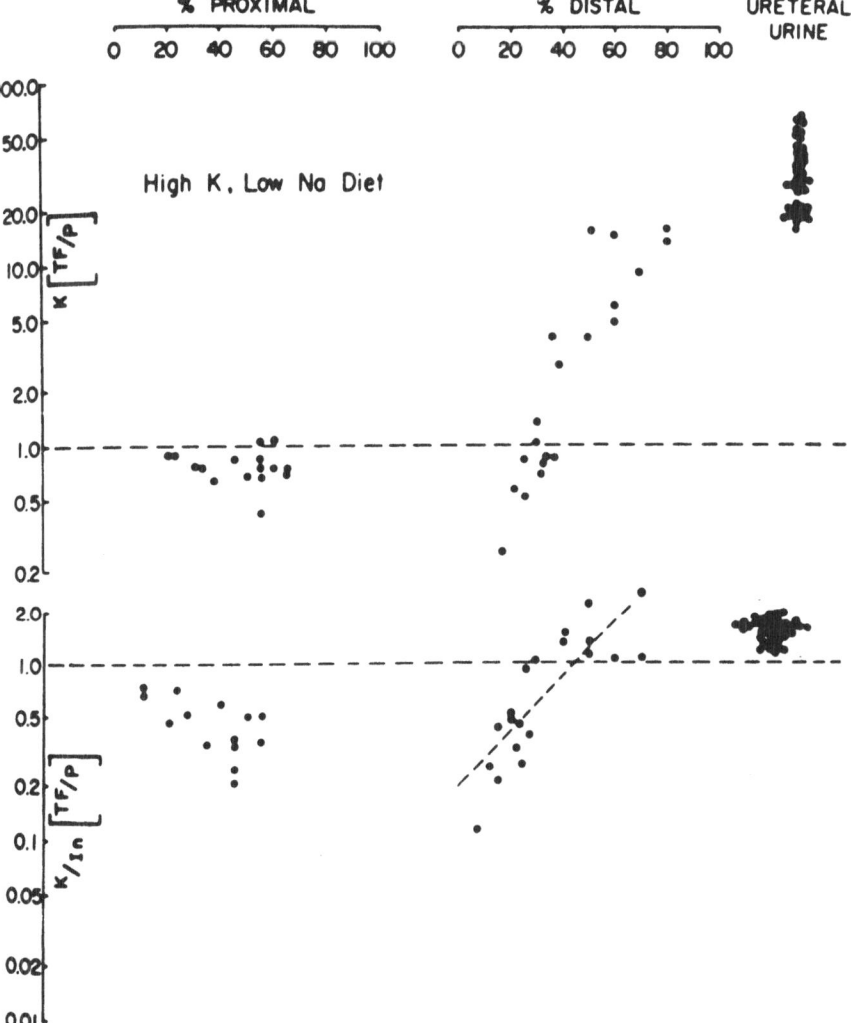

Figure 3. Summary of potassium and potassium-to-inulin concentration ratios in animals in which urinary potassium excretion had been maximally stimulated. (From Malnic et al., 1964.)

those in the final urine demonstrates an additional role of the collecting duct epithelium in the control of urinary potassium excretion. In general, only a modest and quite variable secretory contribution of this tubular segment can be shown even in strongly kaliuretic rats (Malnic et al., 1964, 1966b). This conclusion is confirmed by puncture of individual papillary collecting ducts (Diezi et al., 1973, Jamison, 1970) and by microcatheter studies in potassium-loaded golden hamsters (Hierholzer, 1961).

Recently, evidence has become available that the collecting ducts may, however, under special conditions contribute incisively to urinary potassium excretion. Thus, in low-sodium states (pretreatment of rats with a low-sodium diet and infusion of sodium-free solutions) animals respond to an exogenous load of potassium with accelerated excretion of potassium. This stimulation of potassium secretion takes place at levels beyond the distal convoluted tubule, i.e., the collecting tubules and collecting ducts (Wright et al., 1971; Peterson, 1975). Also, in rats in which total renal mass had been reduced by contralateral nephrectomy and additional surgical removal of renal tissue, the stimulation of renal potassium secretion after a potassium load (Schultz et al., 1971) is largely the result of augmented secretion along the collecting duct epithelium (Bank and Aynedjian, 1973; Finkelstein and Hayslett, 1974).

Recent studies in vitro have confirmed the role of the collecting duct epithelium in the process of potassium secretion. Experiments performed on single, isolated collecting ducts in vitro showed the ability of these tubular segments to secrete potassium ions against steep concentration gradients (Grantham et al., 1970; Burg and Grantham, 1971). Secretion of potassium could be shown to be sensitive to the luminal sodium concentration and to be critically dependent on luminal contact time. Secretion of potassium along these isolated collecting tubules could be inhibited by amiloride (Burg and Stoner, 1974) and acidification of the luminal perfusion fluid (Boudry et al., 1976).

The ability to effect net reabsorption of potassium is more evident at the level of the collecting duct epithelium than along the distal tubule. Two conditions in particular are characterized by extensive net reabsorption of potassium ions from the lumen. First, pretreatment of rats with a low-potassium diet stimulates potassium reabsorption both along the distal convoluted tubule but more so along the collecting ducts. This conclusion is based on the comparison of late distal with final urinary excretion rates of potassium (Malnic et al., 1964) as well as on the direct observation in micropuncture experiments on papillary collecting ducts: Fractional excretion rates of potassium fall significantly along individual papillary collecting ducts toward the papillary tip (Diezi et al., 1973). Secondly, practically identical results obtain in low-sodium animals in which the administration of sodium-free infusion fluids and pretreatment with a low-sodium diet lower urinary potassium excretion (Peterson, 1975; Malnic et al., 1966b). These low excretion rates of potassium are due to reabsorption of this ion along the terminal collecting duct system. Again, this conclusion is based both on the comparison of late distal with urinary excretion data (Peterson, 1975; Malnic et al., 1966b) as well as on micropuncture data of single collecting ducts (Diezi et al., 1973).

It is clear from these considerations that the distal tubule and the collecting tubule and collecting duct jointly participate in the regulation of urinary potassium excretion. Both systems may be activated to secrete potassium, but in those species studied the distal tubular epithelium is more frequently involved in the secretory response. In contrast, the collecting duct epithelium reabsorbs potassium frequently; particularly in low-potassium and low-sodium states this part of the nephron contributes effectively to the conservation of potassium ions.

C. Electrophysiology of the Distal Tubule and Collecting Duct

The distal nephron is divided into several functionally and morphologically distinct parts (Wright, 1974; Burg and Stoner, 1974). These differences include changes of the electrical potential differences along the distal tubular epithelium and the cortical collecting ducts. Figure 4 schematically summarizes some of these features and some transport patterns of the distal nephron.

The thick ascending limb of Henle's loop or the cortical portion of the thick ascending limb of Henle's loop (I) is characterized by a lumen-positive electrical potential difference thought to be generated by active chloride reabsorption (Burg and Green, 1973a–c; Rocha and Kokko, 1973). Whether or not sodium and potassium reabsorption are solely driven by the transepithelial electrical potential difference is not certain. In particular, details of the reabsorptive mechanism of potassium transport at the level of the ascending limb of Henle's loop are unknown. Yet this nephron segment's functional activity is important in that it very effectively lowers the luminal potassium concentration and thus obligatorily reduces the potassium content of early distal tubular fluid to very low levels.

The distal tubule proper, i.e., that part accessible to puncture from the kidney surface, is made up of an early (II) segment, morphologically similar to the thick ascending limb of Henle's loop, and the late distal convoluted tubule (III), sharing some morphological features such as the presence of dark, intercalated cells, with the epithelium of the cortical collecting tubule. The early

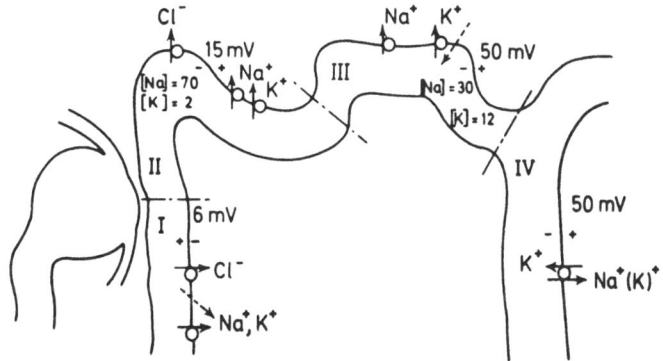

Figure 4. Subdivisions of the distal nephron including electrical potential differences and some transport parameters. (From Wright, 1974.)

distal tubule (II) is a tubular segment with an electrical potential difference intermediate between that of the thick ascending limb of Henle's loop and the strongly negative electrical potential difference across the late distal tubule (Wright, 1971a,b). The early distal tubule is the site of active chloride, potassium and sodium reabsorption (Wright, 1974; Burg and Green, 1973a; Giebisch and Windhager, 1973). The late distal tubule (III) has an electrical potential difference of about -50 mV, lumen negative (Giebisch et al., 1966; Malnic and Giebisch, 1972a; Wright, 1971a). It is the main tubular site of potassium secretion. Potassium reabsorption also, but only rarely, occurs at this nephron site. The late distal tubule is also characterized by active sodium and chloride pumps effecting net reabsorption of these ions against sizable electrochemical potential gradients (Malnic et al., 1966a; Malnic and Giebisch, 1972a; Khuri et al., 1975). The cortical collecting tubule (IV) extends from the junction of several distal tubules to the outer medulla and in the rat is unbranched. Its electrical polarization is similar to that of the late distal tubule. The cortical collecting tubule is a site of active potassium secretion and active sodium reabsorption (Burg and Stoner, 1974; Grantham et al., 1970), a process probably linked directly by a carrier mechanism. Not shown is the papillary collecting duct which extends into the medullary region, contains multiple branchings, and has a thicker epithelium than the cortical collecting tubule. It should be noted in passing that all segments of the distal nephron are able to secrete hydrogen ions (Rector, 1973; Malnic, 1974; Malnic and Giebisch, 1972b).

In addition to the magnitude of the transepithelial potential difference, several additional electrical properties of the distal tubular epithelium are relevant with respect to its function as the main site of potassium secretion. Thus, the peritubular membrane potential of distal tubule cells is strongly negative by some -70 mV (Malnic and Giebisch, 1972a; Sullivan, 1968; Wiederholt and Giebisch, 1974). Although the problem has not been systematically studied, it appears likely that the peritubular cell potential of early and late distal tubule cells is not different. Accordingly, the transepithelial potential differences between the early and late distal tubule are due to differences of the electrical polarization of the luminal cell membrane such that the absolute magnitude of the luminal potential difference declines during transition from the early to the late distal tubule. The underlying mechanism of the progressively increasing depolarization of the luminal cell boundary has not as yet been elucidated.

The magnitude of the transepithelial potential difference across the epithelium of the distal tubule (Malnic and Giebisch, 1972a; Giebisch et al., 1966; Wiederholt and Giebisch, 1974), as well as across that of the cortical collecting tubule (Grantham et al., 1970), is sensitive to the luminal sodium concentration. Reduction of the luminal sodium concentrations lowers the transepithelial potential difference at both nephron sites. In the Amphiuma kidney, changes in the luminal sodium concentration manifest themselves largely by electrical potential changes across the peritubular, not luminal, cell membrane (Wiederholt and Giebisch, 1974). Thus, the cell negativity rises with an elevation of the luminal sodium concentration. The most likely explanation for the above is that with the increase in luminal sodium content, cell sodium concentration rises. This leads to activation of a sodium–potassium exchange pump in the peritubular cell membrane and, assuming a coupling ratio of Na:K in excess of unity, to hyperpolarization of the peritubular cell boundary. Thus, by activation of a peritubular electrogenic sodium pump, the potential difference across the peritubular cell membrane is partly under control of the distal tubular sodium concentration. The precise mechanism of the generation of the electrical potential difference across the cortical collecting duct is unknown except for its strong dependence on active sodium transport (Grantham *et al.*, 1970).

Two additional electrophysiological properties of distal tubular and collecting tubule cells deserve mention. Several studies using electrophysiological methods have shown that the peritubular cell membrane of distal tubule cells has a high potassium permeability (Sullivan, 1968; Wiederholt and Giebisch, 1974). This view is based on the observation that stepwise increase in the peritubular potassium concentration progressively depolarizes the peritubular cell membrane. The effect is best explained by a reduction of the transmembrane concentration difference of potassium and the associated lowering of the diffusion gradient of this ion. Whether a similarly high potassium permeability also characterizes the peritubular membrane of collecting tubule or collecting duct cells is not known at present, but it appears to be a likely possibility.

It can also be shown that the luminal membranes of distal tubule cells have an inherently high potassium permeability: The luminal potential difference can be effectively reduced by increasing the luminal potassium concentration (Giebisch *et al.*, 1966; Malnic and Giebisch, 1972a; Wiederholt and Giebisch, 1974). This extensive leakiness to potassium ions accounts for the relatively high transepithelial potassium conductance of this tubular segment (Malnic and Giebisch, 1972a). In contrast, the potassium permeability of the collecting duct epithelium is much lower, a functional behavior essential for restricting the loss of potassium from the collecting duct lumen after its secretion into the distal tubule (Burg and Stoner, 1974). The low potassium permeability of the collecting duct epithelium is thus instrumental in generating the high urinary potassium concentrations which develop as a consequence of (1) distal tubular secretion, (2) abstraction of fluid along the collecting tubule, and (3) variable secretion of potassium along the collecting tubule and collecting ducts. In contrast, the relatively high potassium permeability of the distal tubule proper explains the dependence of distal tubular potassium secretion upon the transtubular electrical potential difference.

D. Cellular Models of Potassium Transport

Figures 5 and 6 summarize cell models of potassium transport which have emerged from studies of the electrochemical potential gradients across the luminal and peritubular cell membranes (Berliner, 1961; Wright, 1974, Giebisch, 1971; Giebisch and Windhager, 1973; Giebisch and Malnic, 1973).

Figure 5 schematically represents two mechanisms for potassium secretion and reabsorption. From the available information it is likely that the cell model

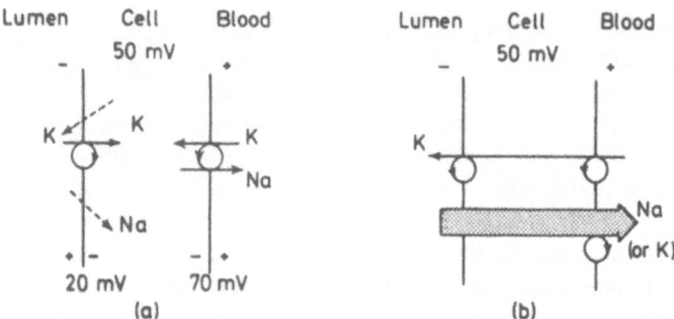

Figure 5. Schematic representation of possible mechanisms of distal tubular and collecting tubule handling of potassium. The main differences between models (a) and (b) are the higher permeabilities to Na and K across the luminal cell membrane and the presence of an active reabsorptive potassium pump within the luminal membrane of (a). Model (b) is distinguished by presence of an active secretory K pump at the luminal cell membrane. At the peritubular site, active potassium uptake is a feature of both cell models. (From Wright, 1974.)

shown in Figure 5a is preferentially applicable to the distal tubule, whereas that in Figure 5b incorporates a number of features more likely to be found within cells of the isolated cortical collecting tubule (Wright, 1974).

The main features of the distal tubular cell model include an active Na–K exchange pump which extrudes sodium from the cell, in exchange for potassium, across the peritubular cell membrane. The tubule cell is electrically negative and has a low sodium concentration with respect to the peritubular sodium concentration; accordingly, sodium ions must be extruded against a sizable electrochemical potential gradient. The situation is less clearcut with respect to the presumed active nature of potassium accumulation within tubule cells. Khuri and his associates have recently measured the potassium activity by means of special potassium-sensitive microelectrodes and observed distal tubular cell activities of only 40–50 mEq/liter (Khuri *et al.*, 1972a,b). This value lowers the effective transmembrane potassium activity gradient across the peritubular cell membrane considerably. The electrical potential difference across the peritubular membrane may thus become large enough to transfer potassium, passively, into the cell (Khuri *et al.*, 1972a).

Following this line of argument, one could envisage that the peritubular potential difference is generated directly by an electrogenic sodium pump (Khuri *et al.*, 1972a). If sodium and potassium movement were tightly coupled and were to occur by a neutral carrier-exchange mechanism at a ratio of 1:1, the pump would then not contribute *directly* to the electrical potential difference. Rather, the pump would generate a high potassium concentration within the tubule cell and thereby establish a steep concentration difference across the peritubular cell membrane. Since the latter membrane has a high potassium permeability, a potassium diffusion potential would be generated, its magnitude critically depending on the transmembrane potassium concentration difference. In contrast, if the movement of sodium and potassium were completely uncoupled, active pump-driven sodium extrusion per se would generate the transmembrane electrical potential difference (cell negative) and thereby provide the driving force for passive potassium translocation into the cell.

Whatever the precise mechanism of peritubular potassium transfer may be, it is likely that both mechanisms are present. Available evidence indicates that the stimulation of peritubular sodium extrusion may directly hyperpolarize renal tubule cells (Whittembury, 1971; Proverbio and Whittembury, 1975; Giebisch, 1974b; Takokoro and Boulpaep, 1972), including those of the distal tubule (Wiederholt and Giebisch, 1974). These findings support the presence of an element of electrogenic sodium extrusion. On the other hand, it can also be demonstrated, by kinetic studies of potassium transfer across the peritubular cell membrane of distal tubule cells, that significant changes of the rate of peritubular potassium uptake may occur in the absence of changes in the peritubular electrical potential difference (deMello-Aires et al., 1973). This view would support the presence of electrically neutral stimulation of peritubular potassium uptake and the operation of Na–K exchange at a ratio close to unity.

Hence, it is most reasonable to envision an active exchange mechanism of sodium and potassium within the peritubular cell membrane in which a variable coupling ratio permits pumping in an electrically neutral or an electrogenic mode. Peritubular potassium uptake has recently been shown to play a major role in the control of transepithelial potassium transport.

Less is known about the peritubular Na–K transport system at the level of the cortical collecting tubule, but some indirect evidence suggests that exchange of Na and K may involve an electrogenic active transport mechanism that contributes directly to cell polarization (Grantham et al., 1970).

Further inspection of Figures 5a and 5b indicates that the two cell models differ with respect to the transport properties of the luminal cell membrane. Thus, the luminal cell membrane of distal tubule cells has a fairly high potassium permeability which would probably permit potassium ions to diffuse passively and sufficiently fast from cell to lumen at a rate controlled by the magnitude of the transmembrane electrochemical potential difference. In contrast, an active transport step from cell to lumen, in addition to one actively transferring potassium from blood to cell, is an integral part of the model in Figure 5b which represents the mode of potassium transfer at the level of cortical collecting ducts (Wright, 1974; Grantham et al., 1970). The key argument in support of this additional active-transport step is the unlikely high magnitude of cellular potassium activities which would be necessary to achieve passive movement of this ion across the luminal membrane of collecting tubule cells (Wright, 1974; Grantham et al., 1970).

Another difference between the luminal cell membrane of distal and collecting tubule cells concerns the presence of an active reabsorptive potassium pump in the luminal cell membrane opposing the potassium leak from cell to lumen (Malnic et al., 1966a). The presence of such a mechanism is firmly established at the distal tubular level by: (1) the observation that the mammalian distal tubule may actively reabsorb potassium from lumen to peritubular fluid in states of potassium deprivation (Duarte et al., 1971) [it normally does so in some aquatic amphibia (Wiederholt *et al.*, 1971]; (2) the comparison of steady-state and free-flow transepithelial concentration differences of potassium ions with the magnitude of the normal electrical potential difference (Malnic *et al.*, 1964, 1966a,b, 1971, Wright *et al.*, 1971). It can be shown that luminal potassium concentrations are consistently below the level predicted from electrochemical equilibrium. This finding suggests the presence of an active transport mechanism opposing potassium diffusion across the luminal cell membrane. From considerations of the electrochemical potential difference it is certain that such a reabsorptive potassium pump is located within the luminal cell membrane (Brenner and Berliner, 1973; Giebisch, 1971). (3) Finally, treatment with ouabain increases, both in rats (Duarte *et al.*, 1971; Strieder *et al.*, 1974) and in *Amphiuma* (Wiederholt *et al.*, 1971), the luminal potassium concentration, a finding that suggests inhibition of a reabsorptive potassium pump by this cardiac steroid.

Whereas the presence of active potassium reabsorption has thus been firmly established at the level of the distal tubule, it is not known whether such a mechanism is also present at the level of the cortical *collecting tubule. In vitro,* isolated segments of the cortical collecting tubule are characterized by net potassium secretion and not reabsorption, but these tubules had, prior to their isolation, not been specifically stimulated to reabsorb potassium (Grantham *et al.*, 1970; Burg and Grantham, 1971; Burg and Stoner, 1974). Accordingly, the existence of potassium reabsorption in these cortical collecting tubules has not been established. In contrast, micropuncture experiments clearly indicate that active potassium reabsorption can be induced across the terminal papillary *collecting duct* epithelium by either potassium or sodium restriction (Diezi *et al.*, 1973).

Figure 6 presents a somewhat more detailed distal tubular transport scheme which incorporates additional transport aspects, particularly those that have emerged from studies using radioactive tracers (Wiederholt *et al.*, 1971; de-Mello-Aires *et al.*, 1973). In a compartmental analysis of distal tubular potassium transport it can be shown that with stimulation of potassium secretion (by metabolic alkalosis, diamox, or potassium loading) the cellular transport pool of potassium (S_2) increases. Conversely, potassium depletion lowers the cellular potassium pool. These changes in the cellular potassium content are due exclusively to alterations in potassium uptake across the peritubular cell border. The view that the potassium content of distal tubule cells varies with the secretory rate has been confirmed by measurements with potassium-sensitive microelectrodes (Khuri *et al.*, 1972a) and by measurements of transepithelial electrical potential differences across the peritubular cell membrane (Wright, 1971b, 1974). Since the peritubular cell potential difference is, at least in part, generated by a potassium diffusion potential, changes in the transmembrane potential may be assumed to reflect parallel alterations—qualitatively at least—in intracellular potassium concentrations. An important conclusion from these studies is that many stimuli known to affect transepithelial potassium secretion do so by acting to modulate peritubular potassium uptake. Changes in cell pH and the peritubular potassium concentration are relevant examples.

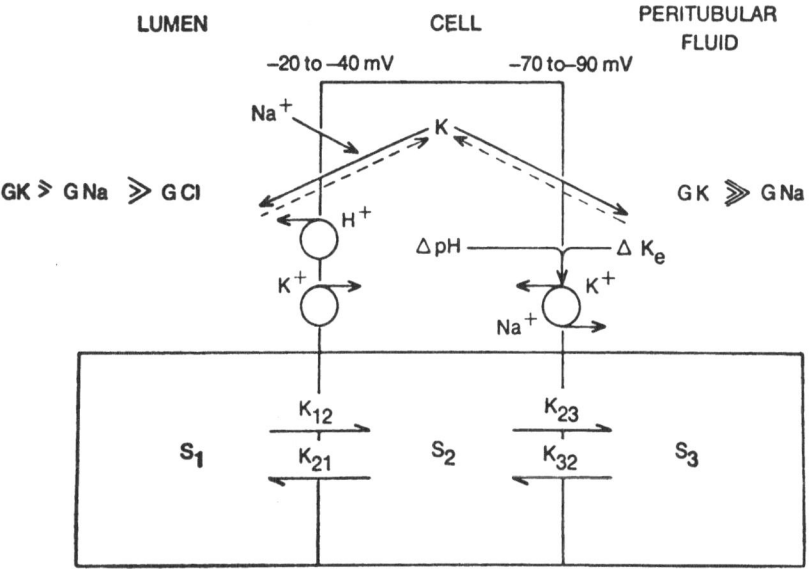

Figure 6. Some properties of a single distal tubule cell including presentation of a three-compartment system consisting of the tubular lumen, the cell compartment and the peritubular fluid compartment. S_1, S_2, and S_3 denote amount of solute (K) in individual compartments, and k values define unidirectional solute (K) movement across the luminal and peritubular cell membrane, respectively. (From Giebisch and Malnic, 1973.)

Inspection of Figure 6 further shows that the luminal cell membrane is partly depolarized, thus aiding the movement of potassium across this cell boundary. The electrical potential difference here is normally of adequate magnitude to allow potassium ions to cross the luminal cell membrane passively (Giebisch, 1971; Giebisch and Windhager, 1973). It also shows that it actively pumps hydrogen ions into the lumen (Rector, 1973; Malnic, 1974) and that sodium ions enter the cell down an electrochemical potential gradient. It is likely that sodium ions interact with the cell membrane since electrical potential changes after alterations of the luminal sodium concentration manifest themselves predominantly as changes across the peritubular cell membrane (Wiederholt and Giebisch, 1974). This means that sodium ions do not carry current during this translocation process across the membrane. They may interact with an electrically neutral carrier mechanism. As pointed out before, the luminal sodium concentration activating electrogenic sodium extrusion across the peritubular membrane partly controls the cellular negativity. Not shown in Figure 6 is an active chloride pump in the luminal cell membrane. Experiments on distal tubules of the rat have shown both that the luminal chloride permeability is too low (Malnic and Giebisch, 1972a) and the cellular chloride activities too high (Khuri *et al.*, 1975) to allow chloride reabsorption solely by passive reabsorption along an electrochemical potential gradient.

The most important general conclusion relating to the control of distal tubular potassium transport is that, rather than by primary changes in the transport properties of the luminal cell membrane (no change in k_{12} or k_{21}), it is the driving force acting on luminal potassium transfer which is regulated by changes in cellular potassium content and concentration (S_2). This latter variable is controlled by the rate of and by changes in peritubular potassium uptake (Wiederholt et al., 1971; deMello-Aires et al., 1973).

III. FACTORS AFFECTING THE RATE OF DISTAL TUBULE, COLLECTING TUBULE, AND COLLECTING DUCT POTASSIUM TRANSPORT

A. Distal Tubular Flow Rate and Sodium Delivery

A considerable body of evidence indicates that acute reductions of urinary sodium excretion compromise potassium excretion. It has already been pointed out that acute reductions of glomerular filtration rate result not only in a dramatic fall in sodium excretion but simultaneously curtail the renal ability to excrete potassium (Davidson et al., 1958). Further experimental support for the sodium dependence of potassium excretion can be found in stop-flow experiments in which appearance and magnitude of potassium accumulation depends on the luminal sodium concentration (Sullivan, 1961; Vander, 1961; Walker et al., 1961). Finally, it has been shown in microperfusion experiments at the distal tubular (Malnic et al., 1966a) and collecting tubule level (Grantham et al., 1970) that reduction of sodium concentration invariably depresses tubular potassium secretion.

On the other hand, it is also known that delivery of a larger-than-normal load of sodium-containing fluid into the distal nephron is a potent stimulus for potassium secretion. Exploration of this latter phenomenon is of particular importance since it is this mechanism by which many diuretic agents promote urinary potassium loss.

The application of micropuncture methods has made it possible to pinpoint the tubular site at which potassium transport is affected by the availability of sodium ions.

Figure 7 summarizes distal tubular micropuncture data from rats which had been on a low-sodium diet and had received no sodium during the experiment (Malnic et al., 1971). Comparison with control data (see Figure 1) reveals some important differences. (1) Urinary potassium excretion has been dramatically decreased by the low-sodium regime. Compared to the mean control excretion rate of some 17% of the filtered potassium load, only 4% is excreted in the low-sodium animals. (2) Comparison of the potassium concentration ratios along the distal convoluted tubule does not reveal marked differences between the two groups. (3) Fractional potassium secretion along the distal tubule is moderately reduced in low-sodium animals, an effect largely due to reduced distal tubular flow rate. (4) The most striking point, however, is the accentuation of potassium reabsorption beyond the distal tubule in the low-sodium group of animals. Whereas in animals on a normal sodium regime or in animals on a high potassium intake (see Figures 1 and 3) urinary fractional excretion rates of potassium are similar to those at the late distal tubular level, the situation is

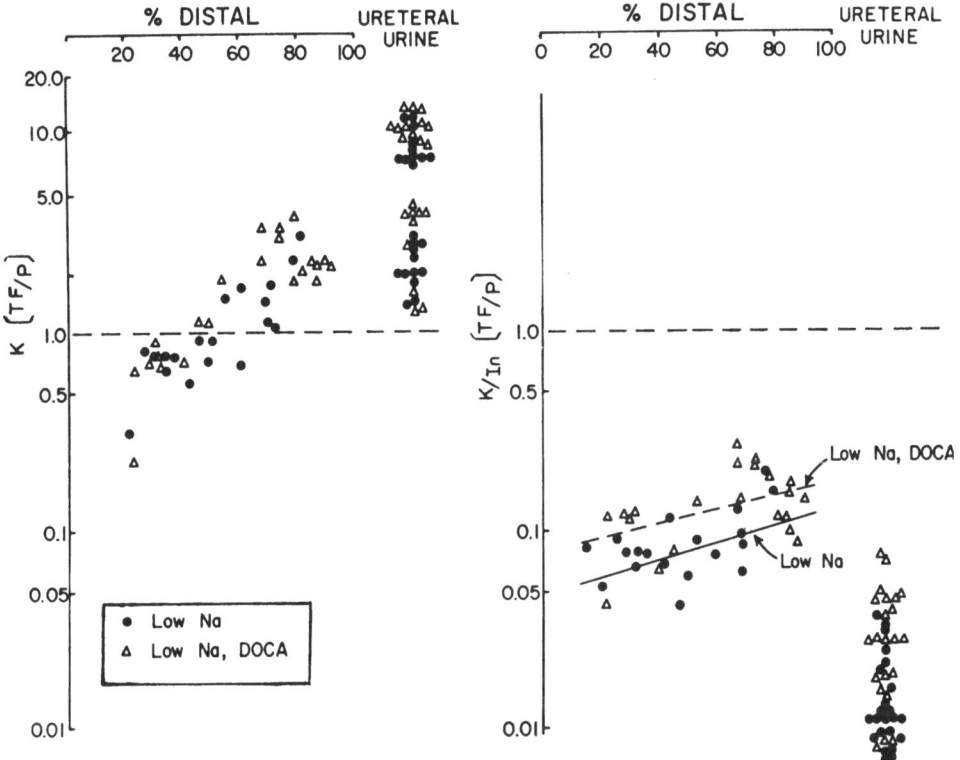

Figure 7. Summary of potassium and potassium-to-inulin concentration ratios from rats kept on a low-sodium diet for several weeks prior to the experiments and receiving sodium-free solutions during the micropuncture study. (From Malnic *et al.*, 1966b)

different in low-sodium animals. Inspection of Figure 7 clearly shows a sharp fall from late distal excretion rates of some 10–15% of the filtered potassium load to only a few percent in the final urine. This fall is due to net reabsorption of potassium along nephron sites beyond the late distal tubule. This conclusion has been fully confirmed by puncture of individual papillary collecting ducts (Diezi *et al.*, 1973). Thus, the collecting duct system emerges as a major site of tubular potassium reabsorption in this state of potassium conservation.

A similar segmental analysis of tubular sodium transport, not shown here, demonstrated that the sodium concentration of distal tubular fluid, the sodium load entering, and the sodium reabsorption along the distal tubule are not limiting factors of distal potassium secretion. (Malnic *et al.*, 1971). These variables remain within the normal range, despite a precipitous fall in urinary sodium output. However, the concentration of sodium fell precipitously along the collecting ducts, a tubular site coinciding with that of extensive potassium reabsorption.

It is proposed that two factors account for the reduction in urinary potassium excretion in conditions in which urinary sodium had been acutely decreased. The first possibility concerns the role of the sharp decline in transepithelial electrical potential difference (lumen negative) which occurs after the fall in luminal sodium concentration. To ensure potassium secretion along the collecting duct system, the delivery of sodium must be sufficient to exceed the amount reabsorbed, thus assuring maintenance of a luminal sodium concentration high enough to keep the electrical potential difference poised toward predominance of secretion. Reduction of this electrical driving force, which normally favors potassium secretion, would leave unopposed active potassium reabsorption and result in the reversal of the direction of net secretion of potassium from secretion to net reabsorption.

The second factor involves the carrier-mediated sodium–potassium exchange mechanism which had been proposed by Grantham *et al.* (1970). A fall of potassium secretion with reduction of sodium delivery to the cortical collecting tubule could also be due to inadequate supply of sodium for carrier-mediated exchange with potassium. This mechanism could account for complete suppression of potassium secretion at best, but it is difficult to envision its participation in the reversal of the direction of potassium transport from secretion to active potassium reabsorption.

The mechanisms of potassium secretion along the distal tubule and the collecting ducts differ significantly with respect to the rate at which luminal steady-state concentrations are achieved. The potassium concentrations in the distal tubule of free-flow samples are identical to those in the steady state during stop-flow conditions (Malnic *et al.*, 1964, 1966a,b), and these transepithelial concentration differences may remain unchanged over a 10-fold increase in distal tubular flow rate (Khuri *et al.*, 1975b). The latter can be increased either by progressive extracellular volume expansion or by increasing flow rate in continuous perfusion experiments through single distal tubules (Morgan and Berliner, 1969). It is obvious that if distal tubular potassium concentrations are independent of flow rate, net secretion of potassium increases with flow rate past the secretory site (Khuri *et al.*, 1975b; Kunau *et al.*, 1974). This relationship does not obtain at the collecting tubule level (Grantham *et al.*, 1970), and it is doubtful whether it occurs along the papillary collecting ducts.

Figure 8 summarizes the effects of increasing distal tubular volume flow rate upon distal potassium secretion (Khuri *et al.*, 1975b). It is apparent that augmenting distal tubular fluid delivery (in this instance induced by saline loading and by progressively larger depression of fluid reabsorption along the proximal tubule) enhances potassium secretion markedly in rats on a normal or high-potassium diet. The magnitude of the stimulatory effect of distal flow rate upon potassium secretion is clearly affected by the state of the potassium secretory system: Similar increments in fluid delivery stimulate potassium secretion more in animals fed a high-potassium diet than in animals with normal potassium intake. Under these two conditions volume flow rate becomes the limiting factor of net potassium secretion. In contrast, increasing fluid delivery to the distal tubule in animals on a low-potassium diet is ineffective in stimulating potassium secretion.

There are many experimental conditions in which the rate of distal tubular potassium secretion is sharply augmented by increasing volume flow rates past

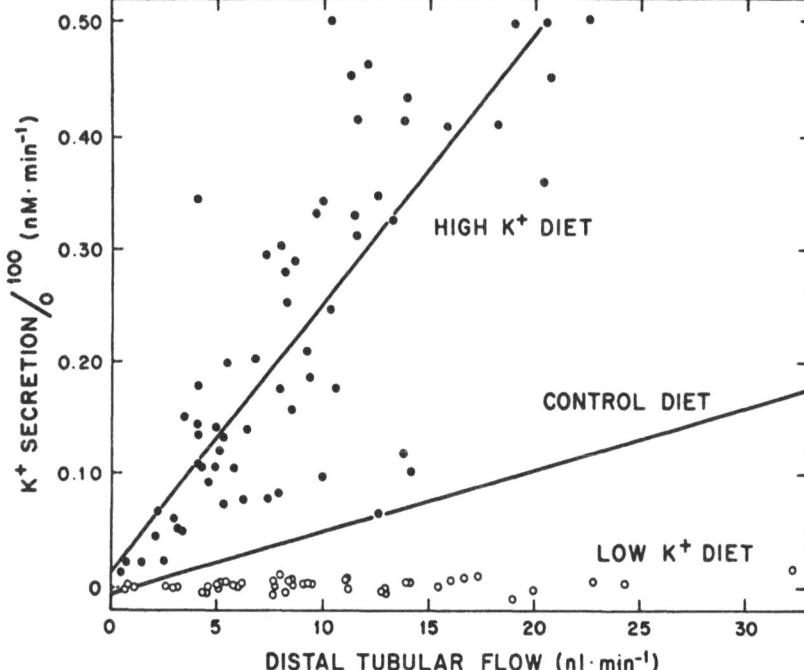

Figure 8. Plot of absolute rates of normalized (0–100%) distal tubular potassium secretion as function of distal tubular volume flow rate. The latter had been varied by loading with saline or saline-urea solutions given at progressively higher rates intravenously. Data are from rats kept on a low, normal and high dietary potassium intake. (From Khuri et al., 1975b.)

the late distal tubule without elevation of the distal tubular potassium concentration. These include: osmotic diuresis induced by mannitol administration (Malnic et al., 1966b; Seely and Dirks, 1969), saline diuresis (Malnic et al., 1966b; Dirks and Seely, 1970; Khuri et al., 1975b), postobstructive diuresis (McDougal and Wright, 1972), diuresis after contralateral nephrectomy (Giebisch et al., 1971), and the kaliuresis after furosemide (Duarte et al., 1971; Dirks and Seely, 1970) and after administration of mercurial diuretics (Evanson et al., 1972).

The possible mechanism by which distal tubular flow rate may enhance potassium secretion has been discussed in some detail elsewhere (Khuri et al., 1975a). Briefly, it is suggested that both the luminal sodium concentration and the peritubular potassium concentration play an important role.

The distal peritubular potassium transfer must sharply increase in order to assure the large enhancement of potassium transfer across the luminal cell membrane necessary to sustain at constant or near constant levels the tubular concentration of potassium despite large increments of distal volume flow rate. One mechanism by which peritubular potassium uptake may increase could be a lowering of the cellular potassium concentration resulting from the washout of potassium ions from distal tubule cells into the lumen. As the cellular potassium concentration declines, the concentration difference against which peritubular potassium uptake occurs is reduced so that potassium uptake increases.[1] However, in potassium-deprived animals the reduction in plasma potassium limits the potential increase in peritubular potassium uptake sharply. Under such conditions, with increasing luminal flow rate the cellular potassium concentration would fall to a much lower level and prevent the increase of potassium egress from tubule to cells with increased flow rate. Thus, whether or not flow rate stimulates potassium secretion would depend critically on the peritubular potassium uptake.

A second factor linking increased distal tubular flow rate to stimulation of distal tubular potassium secretion is the rise of the luminal sodium concentration which occurs uniformly with elevation of tubular flow rates (Khuri *et al.*, 1975a). It can be shown in the amphibian distal tubule that a rise in the luminal sodium concentration increases the transepithelial electrical potential difference (lumen negative) by peritubular hyperpolarization (Wiederholt and Giebisch, 1974). This increase in cell negativity would be expected to stimulate passive peritubular potassium uptake and thus electrically couple sodium to potassium movement.

It is apparent from these considerations that, by affecting flow rate and the luminal sodium concentration, the delivery of sodium ions provides a control mechanism which, in association with peritubular potassium uptake, determines the rate of potassium secretion. The nature of coupling between flow rate, sodium delivery, and electrically mediated potassium secretion at the distal tubular level is characterized by widely varying coupling ratios between the transport rates of sodium and potassium. This exchange ratio may vary by more than an order of magnitude depending both on the state of activity of the sodium reabsorptive and the potassium secretory system. Whereas the electrical driving force depends predominantly on the luminal sodium concentration, the chemical driving force is set by the intracellular potassium concentration which is controlled by the peritubular uptake mechanism.

In addition, potassium secretion may also be stimulated along the cortical collecting ducts by increased sodium delivery: Potassium secretion would be expected to rise as a consequence of the increased luminal negativity and accelerated sodium–potassium exchange.

B. Variations in Dietary Intake of Potassium and Sodium: Potassium Deficiency and Potassium Adaptation

Dietary deprivation of potassium stimulates net reabsorption of potassium along both the distal tubule (Duarte *et al.*, 1971; Malnic *et al.*, 1964) and the collecting ducts (Diezi *et al.*, 1973). Thus, dietary lack of potassium reduces the extent to which the potassium concentration rises along the distal tubule (see

---

[1] Factors that maintain high secretory rates of potassium in the presence of a moderate fall in cellular potassium concentration could be an increase in transepithelial sodium conductance (Malnic and Giebisch, 1972a) facilitating entry of this ion and stimulation of peritubular sodium-potassium exchange. Both events could be triggered by elevation of the luminal sodium concentration which occurs with enhanced distal tubular flow rates (Khuri *et al.*, 1975a).

Figure 2). Similarly, steady-state concentration differences of potassium across the distal tubular epithelium are significantly below those achieved by animals on a normal or elevated potassium intake (Malnic *et al.*, 1966a). Reduction of the dietary intake of potassium also induces net reabsorption of potassium along the papillary collecting duct (Diezi *et al.*, 1973).

It is most likely that the significant reduction of cellular potassium content and of the potassium concentration of distal tubule cells plays a key role in the curtailment of potassium secretion. Several lines of evidence may be cited in support of this thesis. (1) In tracer flux studies on single mammalian distal tubules, peritubular potassium uptake was found to be reduced in potassium-depleted rats, leading to a fall in the cellular transport pool of potassium (DeMello-Aires *et al.*, 1973). (2) Measurements of cellular potassium activities indicated a significant reduction (Khuri *et al.*, 1972a). (3) Electrical potential measurements across the peritubular cell membrane as well as transepithelial potential measurements in potassium-depleted rats indicated a reduction of both parameters (Wright, 1971b, 1974). As indicated above, the fall in the peritubular potential difference is consistent with a parallel reduction in the cellular concentration of potassium.

Thus, there is strong evidence that the potassium content and the potassium concentration of distal tubule cells fall in potassium-deprived animals. As a consequence the secretory influx from cell lumen is expected to drop and leave unopposed the reabsorptive potassium-transport system in the luminal cell membrane. Depending on the extent of the change in cellular potassium concentration, potassium secretion along the distal tubule could be either reduced, suppressed completely, or replaced by net reabsorption. It is tempting to speculate that a similar sequence of events is also responsible for the induction of net potassium reabsorption along the papillary collecting duct.

A chronic high intake of potassium is also known to modify the renal mode of potassium transport. The development of potassium tolerance was well described by Thatcher and Radike (1947) in the late forties and was defined as the ability of animals to survive otherwise lethal acute potassium loads after a period of high dietary potassium intake. Since then several studies have confirmed the notion that increased renal excretion of potassium contributes to the phenomenon of potassium tolerance (Berliner *et al.*, 1950; Wright *et al.*, 1971; Adam and Dawborn, 1972; Peterson, 1975). Accordingly, animals ingesting a potassium-rich diet are characterized by a more rapid and more efficient renal excretory response to exogenous potassium loads. An essentially similar response is that of effective renal excretion of potassium when renal mass has been reduced: A smaller number of nephrons are now exposed to a normal potassium load. After adapting, these nephrons also respond to potassium loading more efficiently (Schon *et al.*, 1974; Schultze *et al.*, 1971).

In studies on single nephrons of potassium-adapted rats it can be shown that potassium secretion is stimulated along the distal tubule (Wright *et al.*, 1971). Despite some uncertainties, it is likely that aldosterone is involved in the development of potassium adaptation; its secretion rate is stimulated in rats maintained on a high potassium intake (Boyd *et al.*, 1971; Boyd and Mulrow,

1972). An interesting relationship also exists between the renal Na–K ATPase system and potassium adaptation. It can be shown that in potassium-adapted kidneys Na–K ATPase levels are significantly elevated (Silva *et al.*, 1973; Schon *et al.*, 1974). Since the latter enzyme system plays a key role in providing energy to many cellular Na–K exchange pumps (Skou, 1965), it is likely that stimulation of the latter transport system within distal tubule cells plays an important role in the renal response to prolonged potassium administration.

Measurements of the rate of cellular uptake of ^{42}K have confirmed directly the enhancement of peritubular potassium uptake and thus underscore the key role of active potassium uptake in the adaptive response (DeMello-Aires *et al.*, 1973). Measurements with potassium-selective microelectrodes also show increased potassium activity in distal tubule cells of potassium-adapted rats (Khuri *et al.*, 1972a), and the increased electrical potential differences across single distal tubule cells of high-K animals are consistent with elevated cell potassium concentrations (Wright, 1971b, 1974). Thus, all the available evidence supports the thesis that changes in the cell content and the cell concentration of potassium of distal tubule cells are fundamentally involved in the adaptive response. Once adaptation is established, the extent to which plasma potassium levels have to rise to produce powerful potassium secretion falls progressively until a dramatic secretory response may take place after a potassium load with only minimal changes in plasma potassium levels. This situation is encountered in herbivorous animals which are normally on a high potassium intake (Rabinowitz and Gunther, 1972; Scott, 1969a,b).

The relationship between renal sodium handling and potassium excretion is complicated by the following observations. Reduction of sodium intake in nonpotassium-challenged rats reduces potassium excretion (Peterson, 1975; Malnic *et al.*, 1966b). However, when such sodium-deprived rats were challenged by either a sodium chloride, sodium and potassium chloride, or by a potassium chloride load, they excreted potassium faster than normal rats (Peterson, 1975). Several studies in a variety of species support this observation (Anderson and Laragh, 1968; Willis *et al.*, 1972; Mohammad *et al.*, 1972, Janata *et al.*, 1970; Sonnenberg, 1971, 1972).

Micropuncture studies show that the low potassium excretion in sodium-depleted unchallenged rats is due to increased potassium reabsorption beyond the distal tubule (Peterson, 1975; Malnic *et al.*, 1966b). However, compared to animals on a normal sodium intake, increased secretion of potassium occurred both along the distal tubule and the collecting ducts upon infusion of sodium and/ or potassium chloride (Peterson, 1975). Importantly, administration of DOCA to rats on a normal sodium diet increased distal potassium secretion to the rates observed in sodium-depleted animals. Thus it is safe to conclude that increased levels of mineralocorticoids contribute to the augmentation of distal tubular potassium secretion in sodium-depleted animals. An analysis of the factors mediating these responses shows that both enhanced delivery of fluid and sodium as well as increased cellular uptake of potassium are important factors in the stimulation of potassium secretion along the distal tubule.

With respect to the relevance of flow modifications along the distal tubule, it can be shown that the delivery of sodium-containing fluid into the distal tubules increased in low-sodium animals after potassium loading above values in animals on a normal sodium intake. Thus, by an unknown mechanism, the low-sodium state sensitizes the proximal tubule and/or the loop of Henle to potassium loading such that the latter now inhibits net sodium and fluid reabsorption more than in animals on a control diet (Peterson, 1975; Brandis et al., 1972). It can also be shown that the administration of sodium chloride, again by an unknown mechanism, directly stimulates cellular potassium uptake (Peterson, 1975). Thus, despite the fact that volume flow rate, sodium delivery, and intratubular sodium concentrations are similar in rats on a control diet given potassium and in rats given both potassium and sodium (as the chloride salts), potassium is secreted twice as fast when both electrolytes are given—at a time when the plasma concentration is significantly lower in those animals receiving sodium with potassium. Apparently, more potassium enters cells during the combined electrolyte infusions. It is reasonable to conclude that as a result of the enhanced cellular entry of potassium achieved by sodium administration, the cellular potassium concentration rose to a higher level and led to stimulation of potassium secretion in those animals receiving potassium *and* sodium.

An unsolved problem at the moment is the elucidation of the factors which specifically activate nephron sites beyond the distal tubule to secrete potassium. It is not clear why animals pretreated with a low-sodium regime respond to potassium loading with enhanced potassium secretion *beyond* the distal tubule, whereas the tubular response to potassium loading in potassium-adapted animals resides within the *distal* tubule proper (Wright et al., 1971; Peterson, 1975).

C. Acid–Base Balance and Potassium Transport

A large body of evidence supports the view that during acute induction of alkalotic conditions renal potassium excretion increases, whereas potassium excretion is reduced in short-term conditions of either respiratory or metabolic acidosis (Berliner, 1961; Rector, 1973; Wright, 1974; Giebisch, 1971; Malnic, 1974; Malnic and Giebisch, 1972b). The site along the nephron where potassium transport is modified during acid–base disturbances has been defined by micropuncture experiments. Thus, potassium secretion increases along the distal convoluted tubule during the infusion of bicarbonate, after administration of carbonic anhydrase inhibitors, and after reduction of arterial pCO_2 by mechanical hyperventilation (Malnic et al., 1964, 1971). In contrast, during acute metabolic or respiratory acidosis potassium secretion along the distal tubule is decreased. (Malnic et al., 1971). In a recent study on isolated, perfused rabbit collecting tubules it was shown that lowering the pH of the perfusion fluid suppressed potassium secretion (Boudry et al., 1976).

It is believed that the changes in potassium secretion after acid–base alterations are primarily due to the effects of cellular pH changes upon peritubular potassium uptake. Several findings may be cited in support of this view: (1) Acid–base-induced changes in potassium secretion are clearly not directly related to changes in plasma potassium concentrations since these are, in general, inversely related. Thus, induction of metabolic or respiratory alkalosis reduced plasma potassium levels, whereas these are elevated in metabolic and respiratory acidosis (Malnic *et al.*, 1971). These observations support previous finding that alkalosis leads to translocation of potassium into cells and acidosis causes a shift of potassium from cells to the extracellular compartment (Pitts, 1953; Malnic *et al.*, 1971). (2) From a comparison of luminal pH values with the distal secretory rate of potassium in a wide variety of acid–base situations it is apparent that changes in distal tubular potassium secretion are not exclusively related to luminal pH (Malnic *et al.*, 1971). Particularly, inducing metabolic or respiratory acidosis may depress distal tubular potassium secretion without lowering tubular pH. Thus, whereas under many experimental conditions luminal pH changes do reflect parallel changes in the extracellular and intracellular fluid compartments, they are not always related to the rate of distal tubular potassium secretion. Thus, at similar distal tubular pH values, elevation of the arterial pCO_2 level or metabolic acidosis both depress potassium secretion. Both maneuvers are known to lower cell pH, and it is thus likely that this cellular pH change, and not luminal pH changes, was responsible for the modification of distal tubular potassium secretion (Malnic *et al.*, 1971). (3) Experimental evidence that the cell potassium content is under the influence of pH changes comes from tracer experiments using ^{42}K. Unidirectional influx of potassium across the peritubular cell membrane is enhanced in metabolic alkalosis (DeMello-Aires *et al.*, 1973) and after diamox (Wiederholt *et al.*, 1971). Potassium activities of distal tubule cells are elevated in metabolic alkalosis and reduced in metabolic acidosis (Khuri *et al.*, 1972a). Thus it appears safe to conclude that cell alkalosis enhances, and acidosis depresses, peritubular potassium uptake. Accordingly, changes in cell potassium are the main factors which control distal tubular potassium concentrations during acid–base disturbances.

Attention should be drawn to the fact that continued acid–base alterations lead to secondary changes in potassium excretion which may differ significantly from those observed in the initial phase of acid–base disturbance. Thus, both chronic metabolic and respiratory acidosis may induce potassium loss rather than potassium retention; the kaliuresis of respiratory alkalosis may last only a short period whereas, in general, during sustained metabolic alkalosis, potassium excretion remains elevated (Malnic *et al.*, 1971; Gennari and Cohen, 1975). Indirect evidence suggests that secondary adjustments of potassium transport are due to changes in sodium delivery and sodium reabsorption along the distal nephron (Gennari and Cohen, 1975). Further direct studies will be necessary however, to evaluate precise nephron sites and the mechanism underlying these long-term adjustments of potassium transport in acid-base disturbances.

D. Mineralocorticoids and Potassium Transport

Mineralocorticoids have important effects on the tubular transport of potassium and sodium (Hierholzer and Lange, 1974). The following are main points of interest (Hierholzer and Lange, 1974). (1) Observations that early distal sodium concentrations are elevated in adrenalectomized rats suggest a defect of sodium reabsorption along Henle's loop. (2) Similarly, distal tubular sodium concentrations are elevated in the adrenalectomized state. (3) The collecting-duct system is another site of action of mineralocorticoids, as evidenced by the observation that steady-state sodium concentrations are elevated in functionally isolated segments of collecting ducts. Normal values are established subsequent to aldosterone treatment (Uhlich *et al.*, 1969). (4) The main site of mineralocorticoid action on potassium transport is at the distal tubular level. Adrenalectomy reduces the ability of this nephron segment to raise the luminal potassium concentration. Hence, distal tubular potassium secretion is reduced.

Two sites of action have been proposed for mineralocorticoids with respect to their stimulatory action on potassium transport. First, using potassium-sensitive microelectrodes, it has been demonstrated that the potassium activity of single distal tubule cells is reduced in adrenalectomized rats. This functional lesion can be restored by aldosterone after a time lag (Wiederholt *et al.*, 1974). These observations are in accord with a stimulatory role of mineralocorticoids on peritubular potassium uptake. In addition, a more rapid effect of aldosterone upon the passive permeability of the luminal membrane of distal tubule cells has also been deduced from electrophysiological measurements. It is suggested that aldosterone also increases the leakiness of the luminal membrane of distal tubule cells to potassium (Wiederholt *et al.*, 1973).

IV. THE EFFECT OF DIURETICS ON POTASSIUM TRANSPORT

A. The Effects of Water and Osmotic Diuresis

Both Mudge *et al.* (1950a,b) and Berliner (1961) have already stressed that intracellular potassium concentration plays a key role in the regulation of potassium excretion. Using clearance methods, Mudge *et al.* (1950a) carried out a number of clearance experiments and showed that changes of cellular hydration per se led to consistent modifications in renal potassium excretion. Thus, administration of hypertonic solutions, inducing contraction of cell water, increased potassium excretion more than the same solutes in isotonic solutions. They also showed that potassium excretion fell to very low levels when the body fluids were diluted during water diuresis. Thus, water diuresis is generally not kaliuretic (Berliner, 1961; Mudge *et al.*, 1950b; Ali *et al.*, 1958; Anslow and Wesson, 1966; Evans *et al.*, 1954; Urbach *et al.*, 1953). The only exception to this view is that of Moehring *et al.* (1972) that hypokalemic plasma levels of rats with hereditary diabetes insipidus can be restored to normal and urinary potassium loss curtailed by the administration of antidiuretic hormone. Conceivably, the protracted elevation of distal tubular flow in the absence of antidiuretic hormone may have offset the tendency for reduced potassium secretion during water diuresis. Factors which might blunt potassium secretion during water diuresis may be dilution of body fluid with concomitant depression of cellular potassium activity and a sharp reduction of distal tubular, collecting tubule, and collecting duct sodium concentrations. These changes have been shown to reduce potassium secretion either via their effect on the electrical potential difference or by directly curtailing carrier-mediated Na–K exchange at the collecting tubule level.

Several studies using both clearance and micropuncture techniques have demonstrated the strongly kaliuretic effect of osmotic diuretics including mannitol (Rabinowitz and Gunther, 1972; Wesson and Anslow, 1948; Malnic et al., 1966b), urea (Rabinowitz and Gunther, 1972; Gonick et al., 1964), and isotonic or hypertonic (Malnic et al., 1966b; Khuri et al., 1976a) sodium chloride administration. Two mechanisms are most prominently involved in the stimulation of potassium excretion by osmotic diuretics. These are the increased fluid delivery and the changes in sodium concentrations along the distal nephron. First, inhibition of sodium and water reabsorption along the proximal tubule (Brenner and Berliner, 1969; Cortney et al., 1965; Landwehr et al., 1967) and Henle's loop (Seely and Dirks, 1969) leads to a large increase in distal tubular flow rate and sodium delivery. In view of the sensitivity of distal tubular potassium secretion to luminal flow rate, it would be expected that the augmentation of distal volume flow should stimulate potassium secretion. Indeed, this factor is the most prominent feature of kaliuresis after osmotic diuresis since the latter never induces an increase in distal tubular potassium concentrations.

It has also been observed that those osmotic diuretics which increase the luminal sodium concentration, such as iso- or hypertonic sodium chloride, sodium sulfate, or sodium bicarbonate solutions, are more potent kaliuretic agents than nonelectrolytes such as urea or mannitol solutions. Administration of the latter results in a much smaller elevation of the sodium concentration along the distal tubule (Khuri et al., 1975a) or even to a marked reduction of the sodium concentration in the final urine (Malnic et al., 1971); sodium chloride, sodium sulfate, or sodium bicarbonate drastically elevate the sodium concentration along the distal nephron.

Representative examples of the effects of loading with nonelectrolyte or sodium-containing osmotic diuretics upon potassium transport are shown in Figures 9 and 10. Despite the fact that fractional excretion rates of water were quite similar in the two experimental situations, it is apparent that the administration of hypertonic sodium chloride is more kaliuretic than that of mannitol. Thus, whereas mannitol loading increased fractional excretion rates of potassium to a mean value of 30% (from control values of some 17%), hypertonic sodium chloride loading resulted in the excretion of almost 50% of the filtered potassium. Both the zero intercept and the slope of the line relating fractional potassium excretion rates to tubular length are different in the two conditions. Thus, a larger fraction of potassium enters the distal tubule during mannitol diuresis. Osmotic diuretics may, in addition to stimulating distal tubular potassium secretion, also contribute to urinary potassium excretion by delivering a larger than normal fraction of the filtered potassium into the distal tubule. It is most reasonable to assume that this increase in early distal potassium delivery is

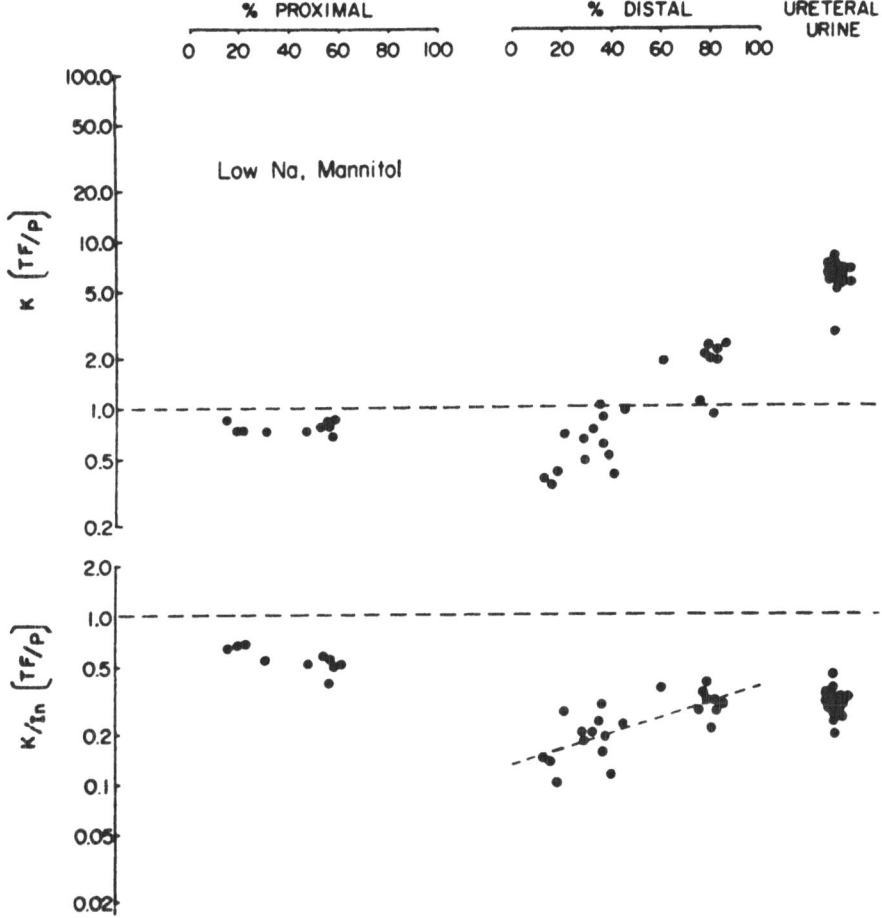

Figure 9. Summary of potassium and potassium-to-inulin concentration ratios from rats on a low-sodium diet receiving 10% mannitol intravenously. (From Malnic *et al.*, 1966b.)

due to diminished potassium reabsorption along the ascending limb of Henle's loop.

The reduced rate of distal tubular potassium secretion in mannitol-loaded animals as compared to sodium chloride-loaded animals coincides with dramatically different sodium concentration patterns along the distal nephron. Whereas the sodium concentration fell along the distal tubule, and more precipitously along the collecting ducts in mannitol-infused animals, a marked increase in distal tubular and final urine sodium concentrations obtains in saline-loaded rats (Malnic *et al.*, 1971; Khuri *et al.*, 1975a). These findings support the notion that the efficiency of osmotic agents in stimulating potassium excretion involves not only the delivery of increased amounts of fluid into the distal tubule but also the ability of such agents to elevate the tubular sodium concentration. Augmentation of the luminal sodium content would be expected to stimulate potassium secretion again by either enhancing the transepithelial and peritubular electrical

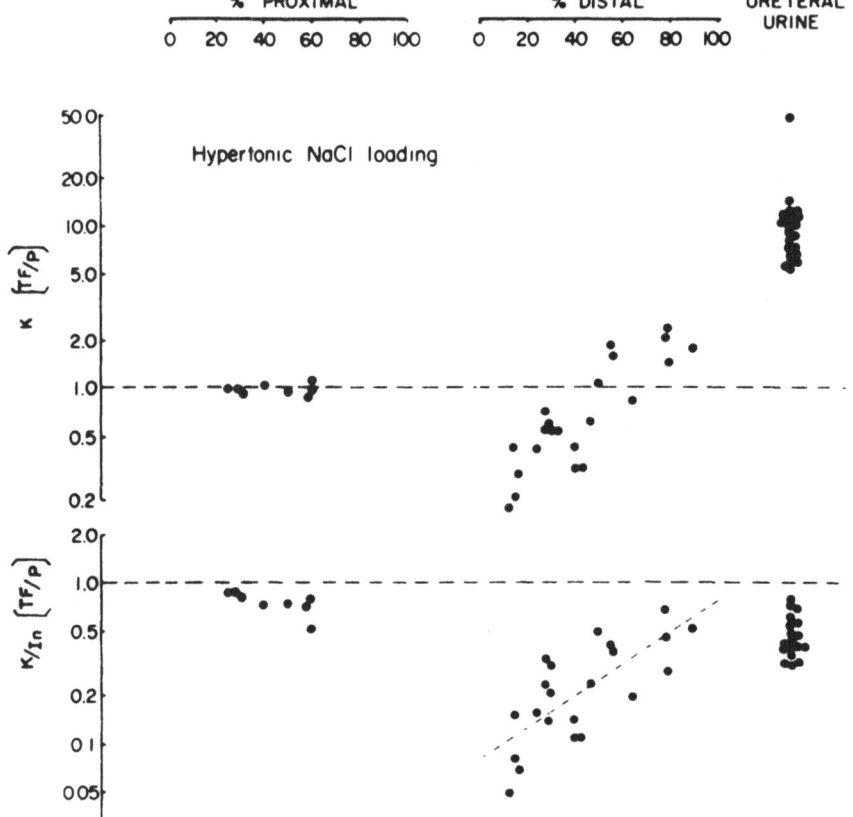

Figure 10. Summary of potassium and potassium-to-inulin concentration ratios from rats during administration of hypertonic sodium chloride. (From Malnic *et al.*, 1966b.)

potential difference or by providing an extra sodium supply to the sodium-sensitive potassium exchange mechanism at the collecting duct level.

B. Diuretics with Primary Action on the Loop of Henle

Several lines of evidence strongly suggest that the effect on potassium secretion of those diuretics having their primary site of action along the loop of Henle is in principal similar to that of an osmotic diuresis with sodium containing fluid. That is to say, they stimulate potassium secretion unspecifically by enhanced fluid and sodium delivery to the distal secretory site of potassium transport.

Experiments on isolated, thick ascending limbs of Henle have clearly established that such diuretics as furosemide (Burg *et al.*, 1973), ethacrynic acid (Burg and Green, 1973c), and mercurials (Burg and Green, 1973a) inhibit fluid reabsorption at this nephron site. With respect to furosemide, this view is also supported by microperfusion experiments of the loop of Henle *in vivo* (Morgan *et al.*, 1970; Morgan, 1974). The *in vitro* perfusion experiments have further indicated that the aforementioned diuretics may, as a common feature, inhibit tubular chloride transport. Micropuncture experiments of early distal tubules have confirmed the inhibitory action of the above-mentioned diuretics and of chlorothiazide at the level of Henle's loop (Duarte *et al.*, 1971; Clapp and Robinson, 1968; Meng, 1967, 1969; Deetjen, 1965, 1966; Deetjen *et al.*, 1969; Malnic *et al.*, 1969). Triflocin has also been shown to depress fluid and sodium transport along Henle's loop (Lockhart *et al.*, 1972; Kauker, 1972).

From clearance experiments it also appears that at least some of these diuretics stimulate potassium transport rather unspecifically (Seldin *et al.*, 1966; Schück and Stribrna, 1968, 1971). A comparable rate of potassium excretion was observed for given increments in urinary sodium excretion, irrespective of the nature of the administered diuretic (furosemide, sulfonamide derivatives) (Seldin *et al.*, 1966).

A representative example of the effects of a diuretic (such as furosemide) with a strong but not exclusive action on Henle's loop is shown in Figures 11 and 12. The following observations are important. (1) Inspection of Figure 11 indicates that administration of this drug dramatically elevates the tubular sodium concentration along the distal tubule. (2) As summarized in the lower section of Figure 11, a much larger than normal fraction of filtered sodium enters the distal tubule. The rate of fractional sodium reabsorption along the distal

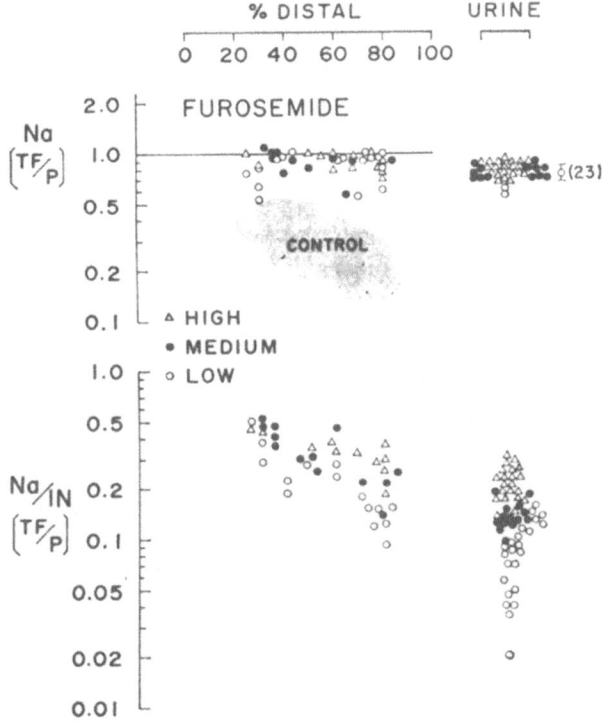

Figure 11. Summary of sodium and sodium-to-inulin concentration ratios from rats infused with three different doses of furosemide. (From Duarte *et al.*, 1971.)

tubule is sharply increased from normal values of less than 10% to peak values approaching 35–40% of the filtered sodium load. This observation is quite consistent with the demonstrated large reserve capacity of the distal tubular epithelium to enhance net reabsorption with increased delivery (Khuri et al., 1975a) and with evidence that furosemide does not act at the distal tubular level (Morgan, 1974; Morgan et al., 1970). (3) Inspection of Figure 12, which summarizes pertinent results of the effects of furosemide on distal tubular potassium transport, shows diminished potassium reabsorption at sites prior to the early distal tubule, as evidenced by the elevation of both early distal tubular fluid/plasma and fractional excretion ratios. (Compare with corresponding values in Figure 1.) (4) In contrast, the progression of tubular/plasma potassium ratios along the remainder of the distal tubule falls into the range of values observed in nondiuretic (see Figure 1) or saline-loaded (see Figure 9) animals, despite the fact that tubular water reabsorption was drastically reduced (urine U/P inulin ratios ranging from a mean value of 10 at the lowest to 3.6 at the highest dose of furosemide). Accordingly, the fraction of potassium which was secreted depended solely on volume flow rate along the distal tubule and not on significant modifications of the transepithelial potassium concentration gradients. Thus, furosemide affects distal tubular potassium transport solely by increasing distal tubular fluid delivery and by elevating the luminal sodium concentration.

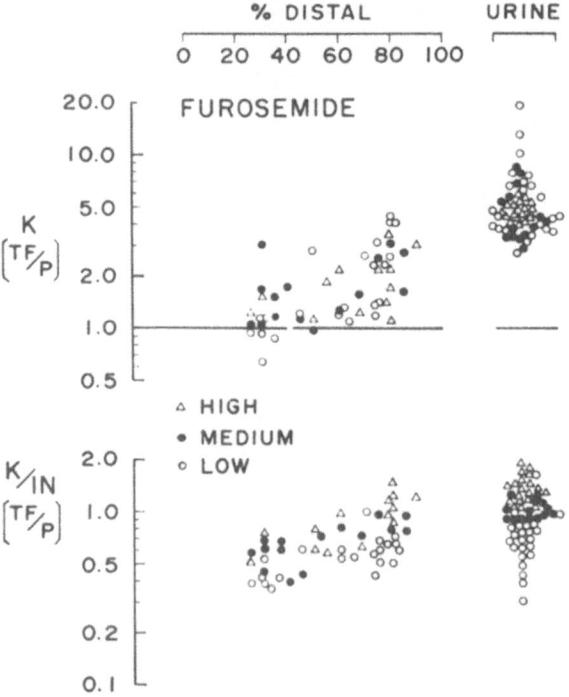

Figure 12. Summary of potassium and potassium-to-inulin concentration ratios from rats infused with three different doses of furosemide. (From Duarte et al., 1971.)

Although direct evidence is less complete, it seems permissible to speculate that with diuretics such as mercurials, ethacrynic acid, chlorothiazide and chlorothiazide derivatives, and triflocin—all of which enhance distal fluid and sodium delivery—a similar mechanism is operative (Goldberg, 1973; Dirks and Seely, 1968). One exception appears to exist: mercurial diuretics inhibit potassium secretion when the latter is stimulated prior to administration of the diuretic compound (Evanson *et al.*, 1972). Some indirect evidence also suggests that ethacrynic acid may inhibit potassium reabsorption along the distal tubule of the dog kidney (Kahn *et al.*, 1971).

C. Diuretics with Direct Action on Distal Tubule and Collecting Tubule Potassium Transport

Three diuretics in particular, ouabain, carbonic anhydrase inhibitors, and mercurial diuretics, can be shown to have a direct effect upon the distal tubular transport of potassium, in addition to their ability to enhance fluid delivery to the distal tubule and thereby nonspecifically stimulate potassium secretion.

Cardiac steroids such as ouabain have well-known diuretic effects and promote urinary loss of sodium and potassium (Cade *et al.*, 1961; Orloff and Burg, 1960; Strieder *et al.*, 1974). In those species in which these compounds inhibit salt and fluid transport at sites proximal to the distal tubule, renal potassium secretion may be unspecifically stimulated by the delivery of larger-than-normal amounts of fluid and sodium to the main tubular site of potassium secretion (see Sections III-A and IV-B). In addition, experiments on the isolated perfused amphibian kidney (Wiederholt *et al.*, 1971) and on rat distal tubules (Duarte *et al.*, 1971) have shown that cardiac steroids are able to promote kaliuresis without an increase of distal fluid and sodium delivery and also to elevate potassium concentrations. Accordingly, these agents stimulate potassium secretion by specifically enhancing luminal potassium concentration in addition to inhibiting sodium and fluid reabsorption along the distal tubule. These findings are best explained by an inhibitory action of cardiac steroids on the active reabsorptive potassium pump in the luminal cell membrane. Suppression of this transport mechanism would leave unopposed the secretory influx of potassium from cell to lumen, favoring the establishment of transepithelial potassium concentration differences approaching those to be expected from the electrical potential difference (Wiederholt *et al.*, 1971).

Figure 13 provides data from a series of distal tubular recollection experiments in which the effects on tubular fluid/plasma concentration ratios of sodium and potassium and respective fractional excretion rates after renal arterial perfusion of ouabain are summarized. It is apparent that a dramatic elevation of tubular sodium and potassium concentration takes place after ouabain administration. Simultaneously, the fractional excretion rates of these ions increase significantly.

While these results are indicative of a more pronounced effect of ouabain on luminal rather than peritubular potassium uptake, attention should be drawn to the fact that significant species differences have been observed in the effects of

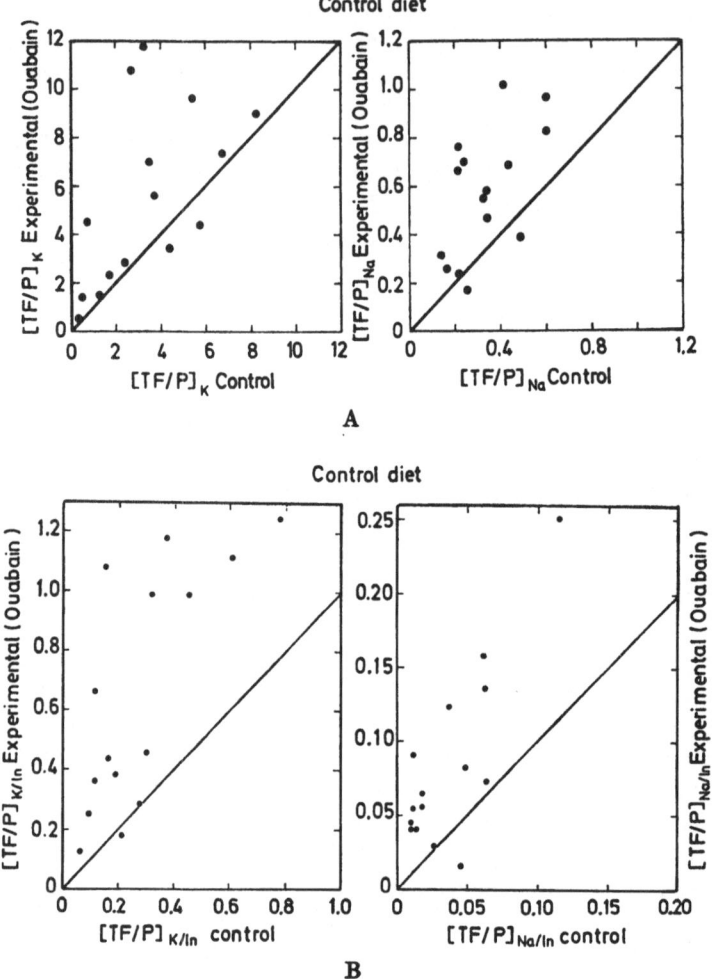

Figure 13. Summary of recollection data of distal tubular potassium and sodium tubular fluid/ plasma concentration ratios and fractional excretion rates before and after receiving ouabain intraarterially. Animals had been on a normal K intake. (From Strieder *et al.*, 1974.)

ouabain. Thus, in the canine (Cade *et al.*, 1961) and avian (Orloff and Burg, 1960) kidney the extent of potassium secretion for a given increment in sodium excretion declines after cardiac glycosides. This indicates an additional and more powerful inhibitory effect on peritubular potassium uptake which is apparently absent in the rat kidney *in vivo*.[2] Potassium excretion rates may still exceed control values of nondiuretic conditions, but this stimulatory effect

[2] We have been unsuccessful in our attempts to demonstrate an inhibitory effect of ouabain upon renal potassium excretion in the rat. In experiments in which renal potassium excretion had been maximally stimulated by the administration of diamox and hypertonic potassium sulfate solution, ouabain, given intraarterially in maximal doses, led to a further increase in renal potassium excretion from preouabain excretion levels of potassium approaching 100% (Fowler, Wiederholt, and Giebisch, unpublished observations).

would be due to enhanced fluid delivery into the distal tubule and not due to a direct effect on tubular potassium concentration. The perfused rat kidney responds to ouabain with reduced potassium excretion when excretion rates had been elevated initially (Bowman *et al.*, 1973).

A similar situation exists with respect to the effect of mercurial diuretics on distal tubular potassium transport in the dog. Confirming earlier conclusions based on clearance experiments (Mudge *et al.*, 1950b; Berliner *et al.*, 1950), Evanson *et al.* (1972) showed that chlormerodrin sharply reduced distal tubular potassium secretion in dogs which had responded to a high dietary intake of potassium with enhanced levels of potassium excretion. The authors concluded that mercurial diuretics most likely blocked peritubular uptake of potassium. Whether mercurials are kaliuretic or not would depend on the relationship between increased delivery of fluid and sodium (loop effect), which tends to enhance potassium secretion, and the inhibitory effect on peritubular potassium uptake (distal tubular effect), which tends to depress potassium secretion.

Finally, part of the kaliuretic action of carbonic anhydrase inhibitors has been shown to take place at the distal tubular level. These compounds increase late distal tubular potassium concentrations in the rat nephron (Malnic *et al.*, 1964) and also increase peritubular potassium uptake in the amphibian distal tubule (Wiederholt *et al.*, 1971). These results are similar to those obtained in animals made alkalotic by infusion of bicarbonate. In both situations it may be assumed that cell pH has been shifted to the alkaline direction (Struyvenberg *et al.*, 1968) as a consequence of which peritubular potassium uptake increased (see Section III-C).

D. Potassium-Sparing Diuretics

From the considerations of the site of action of adrenal mineralocorticoids at the distal tubular level it may be anticipated that the potassium-sparing action of spironolactones, steroid-like compounds known to antagonize the renal effects of mineralocorticoids, also occurs at the distal tubular level (Goldberg, 1973). Although no relevant micropuncture studies are available, such a distal site of action can be deduced from stop-flow experiments (Vander *et al.*, 1960).

Triamterene and amiloride are another group of potassium-sparing diuretics having only mild natriuretic activity (Goldberg, 1973; Baer *et al.*, 1967; Baer, 1973; Guignard and Peters, 1970; Baba *et al.*, 1968). Experiments on single nephrons show that the site of action is the epithelium of the distal tubule (Duarte *et al.*, 1971) and the cortical collecting tubule (Stoner *et al.*, 1974). Similar conclusions have been derived from stop-flow studies (Baer *et al.*, 1967; Ball and Greene, 1963; Nielsen and Lassen, 1963).

Figure 14 illustrates the effects of amiloride on distal tubular potassium transport (Duarte *et al.*, 1971). Data obtained in control, nondiuretic rats are included for comparison. It is apparent that the progressive increase in distal tubular potassium concentration which normally occurs has been dramatically reduced. Under normal conditions the tubular fluid/plasma concentration ratio may reach values as high as 3.0; none of these concentration ratios exceeded

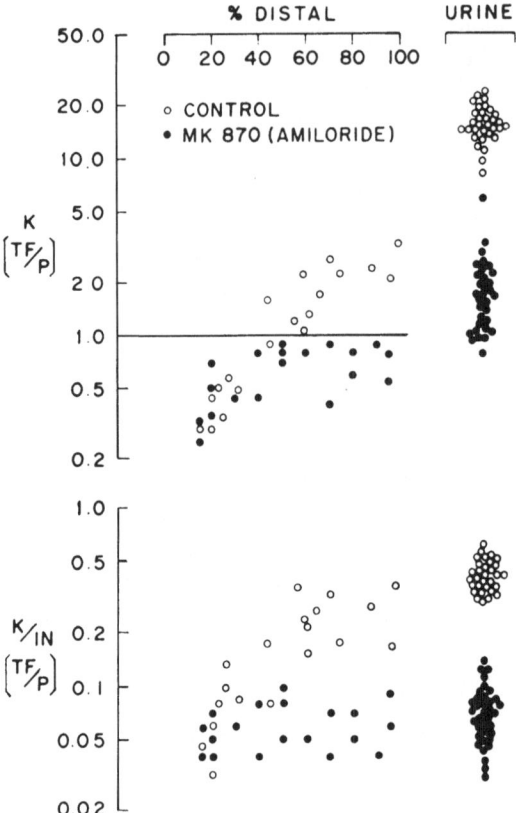

Figure 14. Summary of potassium and potassium-to-inulin concentration ratios from rats on control diet and from amiloride-treated rats. (From Duarte *et al.*, 1971.)

unity after amiloride. Urinary concentration ratios are also sharply lowered. Inspection of the lower part of Figure 14 indicates that potassium secretion was completely suppressed. Importantly, there was a significant rise in the plasma potassium concentration after amiloride administration. It may be concluded that amiloride depresses potassium excretion by sharply blocking its secretion at the distal tubular level. The effect of amiloride on potassium secretion is maintained even when the latter is stimulated (Goldberg, 1973). In sharp contrast to the powerful effect of amiloride on distal tubular potassium secretion, this drug has only a small inhibitory effect on distal tubular sodium transport (Goldberg, 1973; Duarte *et al.*, 1971).

Studies on the effect of amiloride on the cortical collecting tubule *in vitro* show that at this nephron site both potassium and sodium transport are effectively reduced (Stoner *et al.*, 1974). Thus, the very dramatic decrease in potassium transport which is observed at both nephron sites is associated with a proportionately much more effective depression of sodium transport at the level of the cortical collecting tubule than at that of the distal tubule. Also, the electrical effect of amiloride, although qualitatively similar at both nephron sites, is more pronounced at the collecting tubule level. At this site amiloride causes a reversal of the polarity of the potential difference. The positive potential difference, being abolished by diamox, is thought to be due to electrogenic hydrogen ion secretion into the lumen. At the level of the distal tubule, amiloride reduces the electrical negativity but neither abolishes it nor renders the lumen electrically positive (Duarte *et al.*, 1971).

The precise mechanism of action of amiloride at the nephron level is unknown. Evidence is available that amiloride reduces the sodium permeability of the mucosal cell membrane of the toad bladder (Bentley, 1969; Gatzy, 1971; Larsen, 1973; Doerge and Nagel, 1970) and that of the outer membrane of the amphibian frog skin (Biber, 1971). This results in a fall of the transepithelial potential difference. It is tempting to consider that similar changes at the nephron level could mediate the drug effect on potassium transport, the fall in the electrical potential difference reducing passive movement of potassium from peritubular space into the lumen. However, as pointed out before, potassium secretion into the distal tubule is completely suppressed at a time when distal sodium transport is at best moderately reduced and the electrical potential difference is significantly reduced but not abolished. Clearly, more experiments are necessary to evaluate directly whether or not amiloride effects potassium transport independent of its effect on sodium and whether it acts on the luminal or peritubular cell membrane or on both.

An interesting relationship exists between the duration of amiloride administration and its kaliuretic effects (Hohenegger, 1971a,b, 1973; Hohenegger *et al.*, 1971). Thus, during continuous application of amiloride, potassium retention occurs only initially. Subsequently, urinary potassium excretion rises and potassium balance is reestablished. Fecal potassium output also rises during protracted amiloride treatment (Goldman *et al.*, 1971). It can be shown that the "potassium escape" phenomenon is solely related to the state of the body potassium stores prior to and during amiloride administration (Hohenegger, 1973). Thus, when animals are pretreated with a high-potassium diet, potassium escape is accelerated. In contrast, when animals are treated during the period of drug administration with an exchange resin withdrawing potassium at a rate similar to that expected to be retained, no escape phenomenon obtains. It is clear that a strong positive potassium balance is necessary for stimulation of potassium secretion during prolonged amiloride administration. From the available evidence it is most likely that the escape phenomenon is related to the increased potassium content of secretory tubule cells along the distal and collecting tubules.

ACKNOWLEDGMENT

Work in the author's laboratory was supported by grants from the NIH, NSF, and the American Heart Association.

I am grateful to Mrs. M. Sainati and my wife Ilse for assistance in the preparation of this paper.

REFERENCES

Adam, W. R. and Dawborn, J. K. 1972. Potassium tolerance in rats. *Aust. J. Exp. Biol. Med. Sci.,* 50:757–763.

Ali, N. N., Cross, R. B., and Pickford, M. 1958. Electrolyte excretion in diuretic and non-diuretic dogs. *J. Physiol., 141:*177–182.

Anderson, H. M. and Laragh, J. H. 1958. Renal excretion of potassium and normal and sodium depleted dogs. *J. Clin. Invest., 37:*323–331.

Anslow, W. P., Jr. and Wesson, L. G. 1955. Some effects of pressor-antidiuretic and oxytoxic fractions of posterior pituitary extract on sodium, chloride, potassium and ammonium excretion in the dog. *Am. J. Physiol. 1821:*561–566.

Baba, W. J., Lant, A. F., Smith, A. J., Townshend, M., and Wilson, G. W. 1968. Pharmacological effect in animals and normal human subjects of the diuretic amiloride hydrochloride (MK-870). *Clin. Pharmacol. Ther., 9:*318–324.

Baer, J. E. 1973. Potassium-sparing diuretics. In: *Modern Diuretic Therapy in the Treatment of Cardiovascular and Renal Disease,* pp. 148–154. Ed. by Lant, A. F. and Wilson, G. M. Excerpta Medica, Amsterdam.

Baer, J. E., Jones, C. B., Spitzer, S. A., and Russo, H. F. 1967. The potassium-sparing and natriuretic activity of *N*-amidino-3,4-diamino-6-chloropyrazinecarboxamidehydrochloride dihydrate (amiloride hydrochloride). *J. Pharmacol. Exp. Ther., 157:*472–485.

Ball, G. M. and Greene, J. A., Jr. 1963. Localization of site of action of triamterene diuretic. *Proc. Soc. Exp. Biol. Med., 113:*326–328.

Bank, N. and Aynedjian, H. S. 1973. A micropuncture study of potassium excretion by the remnant kidney. *J. Clin. Invest., 52:*1480–1490.

Bennett, C. M., Clapp, J. R. and Berliner, R. W. 1967. Micropuncture study of the proximal and distal tubule in the dog. *Am. J. Physiol., 213:*1254–1262.

Bennett, C. M., Brenner, B. M. and Berliner, R. W. 1968. Micropuncture study of nephron function in the Rhesus monkey. *J. Clin. Invest., 47:*203–216.

Bently, P. J. 1969. Amiloride: A potent inhibitor of sodium transport across the toad bladder. *J. Physiol., 195:*317–331.

Berliner, R. W. 1961. Renal mechanism for potassium excretion. *Harvey Lect. 55:*141–171.

Berliner, R. W., and Kennedy, T. J., Jr. 1948. Renal tubular secretion of potassium in the dog. *Proc. Soc. Exp. Biol. Med., 67:*542–545.

Berliner, R. W., Kennedy, T. J., and Hilton, J. G. 1950. Renal mechanisms for excretion of potassium. *Am. J. Physiol., 162:*348–367.

Berliner, R. W., Kennedy, T. J., Orloff, J. 1951. Relationship between acidification of the urine and potassium metabolism. *Am. J. Med., 11:*274–282.

Berliner, R. W., Kennedy, T. J., and Orloff, J. 1954. Factors affecting the transport of potassium and hydrogen ions by the renal tubule. *Arch. Int. Pharmacodyn. Ther., 97:*299–312.

Biber, T. U. L. 1971. Effect of changes in transepithelial transport on the uptake of sodium across the outer surface of the frog skin. *J. Gen. Physiol., 58:*131–144.

Boudry, J. F., Stoner, L. C., and Burg, M. B. 1976. The effect of lumen pH on potassium transport in renal cortical collecting tubules. *Am. J. Physiol., 230:*239–244.

Bowman, R. H., Dolgin, J., and Carson, R. 1973. Interaction between ouabain and furosemide on Na and K excretion in perfused rat kidney. *Am. J. Physiol., 224:*1200–1205.

Boyd, J. E. and Mulrow, P. J. 1972. Further studies of the influence of potassium upon aldosterone production in the rat. *Endocrinology, 90:*299–301.

Boyd, J. E., Palmore, W. P., and Mulrow, P. J. 1971. Role of potassium in the control of aldosterone secretion in the rat. *Endocrinology, 88:*556–565.

Brandis, M., Keyes, J., and Windhager, E. E. 1972. Potassium-induced inhibition of proximal tubular fluid reabsorption in rats. *Am. J. Physiol., 222:*421–427.

Brenner, B. M. and Berliner, R. W. 1969. Relationship between extracellular volume and fluid reabsorption by the rat kidney. *Am. J. Physiol., 217:*6–12.

Brenner, B. M. and Berliner, R. W. 1973. Transport of Potassium, In: *Handbook of Physiology,*

Section 8: Renal Physiology, pp. 497–520. Ed. by Orloff, J. and Berliner, R. W. American Physiological Society, Washington, D.C.

Burg, M. B. and Grantham, J. J. 1971. Ion movements in renal tubules. In: *Membranes and Ion Transport*, Vol. 3. pp. 49–78. Ed. by Bittar, E. E. Wiley-Interscience, New York.

Burg, M. and Green, N. 1973a. Effect of mersalyl on the thick ascending limb of Henle's loop. *Kidney Int., 4:*245–251.

Burg, M. B. and Green, N. 1973b. Function of the thick ascending limb of Henle's loop *Am. J. Physiol., 224:*659–668.

Burg, M. and Green, N. 1973c. Effect of ethacrynic acid on the thick ascending limb of Henle's loop. *Kidney Int., 4:*301–308.

Burg, M. and Stoner, L. 1974. Sodium transport in the distal nephron. *Fed. Proc., 33:*31–36.

Burg, M., Stoner, L., Cardinal, J., and Green, N. 1973. Furosemide effect on isolated perfused tubules. *Am. J. Physiol., 225:*119–124.

Cade, J. R., Shalhoub, R. J., Canessa-Fisher, M., and Pitts, R. F. 1961. Effect of strophanthidin on the renal tubules of dogs. *Am. J. Physiol., 200:*373–379.

Clapp, J. R. and Robinson, R. R. 1968. Distal sites of action of diuretic drugs in the dog nephron. *Am. J. Physiol., 215:*228–235.

Cortney, M. A., Mylle, M., Lassiter, W. E., and Gottschalk, C. W. 1965. Renal tubular transport of water, solute and PAH in rats loaded with isotonic saline. *Am. J. Physiol., 209:*1199–1205.

Davidson, D. G., Levinsky, N. G., and Berliner, R. W. 1958. Maintenance of potassium excretion despite reduction of glomerular filtration during sodium diuresis. *J. Clin. Invest., 37:*548–555.

Davis, J. O. and Howell, D. S. 1953. Mechanisms of fluid and electrolyte retention in experimental preparation in dogs. II. With inferior vena cava constriction. *Circ. Res., 1:*171–178.

DeMello-Aires, M., Giebisch, G., Malnic, G., and Curran, P. F. 1973. Kinetics of potassium transport across single distal tubules of rat kidney. *J. Physiol. (London), 232:*47–70.

DeRouffignac, C. and Morel, F. 1969. Micropuncture study of water, electrolytes, and urea movements along the loops of Henle in Psammomys. *J. Clin. Invest., 48:*474–486.

DeRouffignac, C., Lechène, C., Guinnebault, M., and Morel, F. 1969. Etude par microponction de l'élaboration de l'urine. III. Chez le mérion non diuretique et en diurese par le mannitol, *Nephron, 6:*643–666.

Deetjen, P. 1965. Mikropunktionsuntersuchungen zur Wirkung von Furosemid. *Pfluegers Arch. Ges. Physiol., 284:*184–191.

Deetjen, P. 1966. Micropuncture studies on site and mode of diuretic action on furosemide. *Ann. N.Y. Acad. Sci., 39:*408–412.

Deetjen, P., Buntig, W. E., Hardt, K. and Rohde, R. 1969. Direct effect of ethacrynic acid in the rat: A micropuncture study concerning the relationship of site and mode of diuretic action. In: *Progress in Nephrology*, pp. 255–261. Ed. by Peters, G. and Roch-Ramel, F. Springer, Berlin.

Diezi, J., Michoud, P., Aceves, J., and Giebisch, G. 1973. Micropuncture study of electrolyte transport across papillary collecting duct of the rat. *Am. J. Physiol., 224:*623–634.

Dirks, H. J. and Seely, J. F. 1968. Micropuncture and diuretics. *Annu. Rev. Pharmacol., 9:*73–84.

Dirks, J. H. and Seely, J. F. 1970. Effect of saline infusions and furosemide on the dog distal nephron. *Am. J. Physiol., 219:*114–121.

Doerge, A. and Nagel, W. 1970. Effect of amiloride on sodium transport in frog skin. II. Sodium transport pool and unidirectional fluxes. *Pfluegers Arch., 321:*91–101.

Duarte, C. G., Chométy, F., and Giebisch, G. 1971. Effect of amiloride, ouabain, and furosemide on distal tubular function in the rat. *Am. J. Physiol., 221:*632–639.

Evans, M. B., Hughes Jones, N. C., Milne, M. D., and Steiner, S. 1954. Electrolyte excretion during experimental potassium depletion in man. *Clin. Sci., 13:*305–316.

Evanson, R. L., Lockhart, E. A., and Dirks, J. H. 1972. Effect of mercurial diuretics on tubular sodium and potassium transport in the dog. *Am. J. Physiol., 222:*282–289.

Finkelstein, F. O. and Hayslett, J. P. 1974. Role of medullary structures in the functional adaptation of renal insufficiency. *Kidney Int., 6:*419–425.

Gatzy, J. T. 1971. The effect of K-sparing diuretics on ion transport across the excised toad bladder. *J. Pharmacol. Exp. Ther., 176:*580–584.

Gennari, F. J. and Cohen, J. J. 1976. The role of the kidney in potassium homeostasis: Lessons from acid–base disturbances. *Kidney Int., 8:1–5.*

Giebisch, G. 1971. Renal potassium excretion. In: *The Kidney, Morphology, Biochemistry, Physiology*, Vol. 3, pp. 329–382. Ed. by Rouiller, Ch. and Muller, A. Academic Press, New York and London.

Giebisch, G. 1974a. Some recent developments in renal electrolyte transport. In: *Recent Advances in Renal Physiology and Pharmacology*, pp. 125–148. Ed. by Wesson, L. and Fanelli, G. M. University Park Press, Baltimore.

Giebisch, G. 1974b. The effects of drugs on the electrophysiological properties of kidney tubules. In: *Drugs and Transport Processes*, pp. 3–22. Ed. by Callingham, E. University Park Press, Baltimore.

Giebisch, G. and Windhager, E. E. 1973. Electrolyte transport across renal tubular membranes. In: *Handbook of Physiology*, Section 8, Renal Physiology, pp. 315–376. Ed. by Orloff, J. and Berliner, R. W. American Physiological Society, Washington, D.C.

Giebisch, G., Malnic, G., Klose, R. M. and Windhager, E. E. 1966. Effect of ionic substitutions on distal potential differences in rat kidney. *Am. J. Physiol., 211:560–568.*

Giebisch, G., Boulpaep, E. L., and Whittembury, G. 1971. Electrolyte transport in kidney tubule cells. *Proc. R. Soc. (London), Ser. B., 262:175–196.*

Giebisch, G. and Malnic, G. 1973. Coupled ion movement across the renal tubule. In: *Transport Mechanisms in Epithelia*, pp. 537–552. Ed. by Ussing, H. H. and Thorn, N. A. Alfred Benzon Symposium V, Munksgaard.

Giebisch, G., Diezi, J., Michoud, P., and Grandchamp, A. 1974. The effect of chronic reduction of GFR on tubular sodium and potassium transport in control and contralaterally nephrectomized rats. In: *International Symposium on Renal Handling of Sodium*, pp. 89–94. Ed. by Wirz, H. and Spinelli, F. S. Karger, Basel.

Goldberg, M. 1973. The renal physiology of diuretics. In: *Handbook of Physiology*, Section 8, Renal Physiology, pp. 1003–1032. Ed. by Orloff, J. and Berliner, R. W. American Physiological Society, Washington, D.C.

Goldman, W. J., Skeggs, H. R., Scott, W., Baer, J. E., and Mattis, P. A. 1971. Effects of the chronic administration of amiloride, hydrochloride (N-amidino-3,5-diamino-6-chlorpyrazinecarboxamide hydrochloride dihydrate) on electrolyte balance in the dog. *J. Pharmacol. Exp. Ther., 179:438–448.*

Gonick, H. C., Coburn, J. W., Rubini, M. E., and Kleeman, C. R. 1964. Effect of urea osmotic diuresis on potassium excretion. *Am. J. Physiol., 206:1118–1122.*

Grantham, J. J., Burg, M. B., and Orloff, J. 1970. The nature of transtubular Na and K transport in isolated rabbit renal collecting tubules. *J. Clin. Invest., 49:1815–1826.*

Guignard, J. P. and Peters, G. 1970. Effects of tramtere and amiloride on urinary acidification and potassium excretion in the rat. *Eur. J. Pharmacol., 10:255–267.*

Hierholzer, K. 1961. Secretion of potassium and acidification in collecting ducts of mammalian kidney. *Am. J. Physiol., 201:318–324.*

Hierholzer, K. and Lange, S. 1974. The effects of adrenal steroids on renal function. In: *MTP International Review of Science, Series I*, Vol. 6, Kidney and Urinary Tract Physiology, pp. 273–334. Ed. by Thurau, K. Butterworth, London.

Hierholzer, K., Wiederholt, M., Holzgreve, H., Giebisch, G., Klose, R. M., and Windhager, E. E. 1965. Micropuncture study of renal transtubular concentration gradients and sodium and potassium in adrenalectomized rats. *Arch. Ges. Physiol., 285:193–210.*

Hilger, H. H., Klümper, J. D., and Ullrich, K. J. 1958. Wasserrückresorption und Ionentransport die Sammelrohrzellen der Säugetierniere. *Pfluegers Arch., 267:218–237.*

Hohenegger, M. 1971a. Potassium-escape phenomenon in rats during continuous application of amiloride. 1. Influence of different daily potassium intake. *Pharmacology, 5:301–306.*

Hohenegger, M. 1971b. Potassium-escape phenomenon in rats during continuous application of amiloride. II. Influence of pretreatment with diets of different potassium content and of adrenalectomy. *Pharmacology, 6:300–307.*

Hoheneger, M. 1973. Potassium-escape phenomenon in rats during continuous application of amiloride. IV. Etiology of the escape phenomenon. *Pharmacology, 9:27–34.*

Hohenegger, M., Marktl, W., and Selzer, H. 1971. Potassium-escape phenomenon in rats during continuous application of amiloride. III. Influence of acid and alkali loading. *Pharmacology, 6:*308–316.

Howell, D. S. and Davis, J. O. 1954. Relationship of sodium retention to potassium excretion by the kidney during the administration of desoxycorticosterone acetate to dogs. *Am. J. Physiol., 179:*359–363.

Jaenike, J. R. and Berliner, R. W. 1960. A study of distal tubular functions by a modified stop-flow technique. *J. Clin. Invest., 39:*481–490.

Jamison, R. L. 1970. Micropuncture study of superficial and juxtamedullary nephrons in the rat. *Am. J. Physiol., 218:*46–55.

Jamison, R. L., Bennet, C. M., and Berliner, R. W. 1967. Countercurrent multiplication by the thin loops of Henle. *Am. J. Physiol., 212:*357–366.

Janata, V., Kuhn, E., Schueck, O., Stribrna, J., Turek, J., and Brodan, V. 1970. Metabolic and functional study of the kidney of rats fed on a low sodium diet. *Physiol. Bohemoslov., 19:*209–218.

Kahn, M. and Bohrer, N. K. 1967. Effect of potassium-induced diuresis on renal concentration and dilution. *Am. J. Physiol., 212:*1365–1375.

Kahn, T., Goldstein, M. H., Alfago, E., and Levitt, M. F. 1971. K transport and its relation to Na transport in the distal tubule of the hydrated dog. *Am. J. Physiol., 221:*1456–1463.

Kauker, M. L. 1972. Micropuncture study of the effect of triflocin on tubular reabsorption in rats. *J. Pharmacol. Exp. Ther., 185:*472–480.

Khuri, R. N., Agulian, S. K. and Kalloghlian, A. 1972a. Intracellular potassium in cells of distal tubule. *Pfluegers Arch., 335:*297–307.

Khuri, R. N., Hajjar, J. J., and Agulian, S. K. 1972b. Measurement of intracellular potassium with liquid ion-exchange microelectrodes. *J. Appl. Physiol., 321:*419–425.

Khuri, R. N., Agulian, S. K., and Bogharian, K. 1975. Electrochemical potential of chloride in distal renal tubule of the rat. *Am. J. Physiol., 227:*1354–1355.

Khuri, R. N., Wiederholt, M., Strieder, N., and Giebisch, G. 1975a. The effects of graded solute diuresis on renal tubular sodium transport in the rat. *Am. J. Physiol., 228:*1262–1268.

Khuri, R. N., Wiederholt, M., Strieder, N., and Giebisch, G. 1975b. The effects of flow rate and potassium intake on distal tubular potassium transfer. *Am. J. Physiol., 228:*1249–1261.

Kunau, R. T., Jr., Webb, H. L., and Borman, S. C. 1974. Characteristics of the relationship between the flow rate of tubular fluid and potassium transport in the distal tubule of the rat. *J. Clin. Invest., 54:*1488–1495.

Landwehr, D. M., Klose, R. M., and Giebisch, G. 1967. Renal tubular sodium and water reabsorption in the isotonic sodium chloride loaded rat. *Am. J. Physiol., 212:*1327–1333.

Larsen, E. H. 1973. Effect of amiloride, cyanide and ouabain on the active transport pathway in toad skin. In: *Transport Mechanisms in Epithelia*, pp. 131–143. Ed. by Ussing, H. H. and Thorn, N. A. A. Benzon Symposium V, Munksgaard, Copenhagen, Academic Press, New York.

Lechène, C., Morel, F., Guinnebault, M., and DeRouffignac, C. 1969. Etude par microponction de l'élaboration de l'urine. I. Chez le rat dans différents états de diurèse. *Nephron, 6:*457–477.

Lockhart, E. A., Dirks, J. H., and Cerriere, S. 1972. Effects of troflocin on renal tubular reabsorption and blood flow distribution. *Am. J. Physiol., 223:*89–96.

Malnic, G. 1974. Tubular handling of H. In: *MTP International Review of Science, Series I*, Vol. 6, Kidney and Urinary Tract Physiology, pp. 79–106. Ed. by Thurau, K. Butterworth, London.

Malnic, G. and Giebisch, G. 1972a. Some electrical properties of distal tubular epithelium in the rat. *Am. J. Physiol., 223:*797–808.

Malnic, G. and Giebisch, G. 1972b. Mechanism of renal hydrogen ion secretion. *Kidney Int., 1:*280–296.

Malnic, G., Klose, R. M., and Giebisch, G. 1964. Micropuncture study of renal potassium excretion in the rat. *Am. J. Physiol., 206:*647–686.

Malnic, G., Klose, R. M., and Giebisch, G. 1966a. Microperfusion study of distal tubular potassium and sodium transfer in rat kidney. *Am. J. Physiol., 211:*548–559.

Malnic, G., Klose, R. M., and Giebisch, G. 1966b. Micropuncture study of distal tubular potassium and sodium transport in rat nephron. *Am. J. Physiol., 211:*529–547.

Malnic, G., Enokibara, H., deMello-Aires, M., and Vieira, F. L. 1969. Effect of furosemide and NaCl loading on chloride excretion in single nephrons of rat kidney. *Pfluegers Arch., 309:*21–37.

Malnic, G., deMello-Aires, M., and Giebisch, G. 1971. Potassium transport across renal distal tubules during acid-base disturbances. *Am. J. Physiol., 211:*1192–1208.

Malvin, R. L., Wilde, W. S., and Sullivan, L. P. 1958. Localization of nephron transport by stop-flow analysis. *Am. J. Physiol., 194:*135–142.

McDougal, W. S. and Wright, F. S. 1972. Defect in proximal and distal sodium transport in post-obstructive diuresis. *Kidney Int., 2:*304–317.

Meng, K. 1967. Mikropunktionsuntersuchungen über die saluretische Wirkung von Hydrochloro-thiazid, Acetazolamid und Furosemid. *Naunyn-Schmiedeberg's Arch. Pharmakol. Exp. Pathol., 257:*355–363.

Meng, K. 1969. Mikropunktionsuntersuchungen über die Wirkung von Diuretica in der Henleschen Schleife. *Klin. Wochenschr., 47:*668–672.

Moehring, J., Schoemig, A., Brekuer, H., and Moehring, B. 1972. ADH induced potassium retention in rats with genetic diabetes insipidus. *Life Sci., 11:*64.

Mohammad, G., DiScala, V. A., and Stein, R. M. 1972. Effects of salt depletion on tubular Na, H_2O and K transfer in dog. *5th Int. Congr. Nephrol. Abstracts,* p. 89, Karger, Basel.

Morgan, T. O. 1974. Intrarenal action of diuretics. In: *Drugs and the Kidney,* Vol. 9, pp. 13–20. Ed. by Edwards, K. D. G. Karger, Basel.

Morgan, T. O. and Berliner, R. W. 1969. A study by continuous microperfusion of water and electrolyte movements in the loop of Henle and distal tubule of the rat. *Nephron, 6:*388–405.

Morgan, T., Tadakoro, M., Martin, D., and Berliner, R. W. 1970. Effect of furosemide on Na^+K^+ transport studied by microperfusion of the rat nephron. *Am. J. Physiol., 218:*292–297.

Mudge, G. H., Foulks, J., and Gilman, A. 1948. The renal excretion of potassium. *Proc. Soc. Exp. Biol. Med., 67:*545–547.

Mudge, G. H., Foulks, J., and Gilman, G. 1950a. Renal secretion of potassium in the dog during cellular dehydration. *Am. J. Physiol., 161:*159–166.

Mudge, G. H., Ames, A., Foulks, J., and Gilman, A. 1950b. Effects of drugs on renal secretion of potassium in the dog. *Am. J. Physiol., 161:*151–158.

Nielsen, O. R. and Lassen, J. B. 1963. Triamterene activity investigated by the stop-flow technique and in vitro studies on carbonic anhydrase. *Acta Pharmacol. Toxicol., 20:*351–356.

Orloff, J. and Burg, M. 1960. Effect of strophanthidin on electrolyte excretion in the chicken. *Am. J. Physiol., 199:*39–54.

Peterson, L. M. N. 1975. The effect of sodium intake on renal potassium excretion. Thesis, Yale University School of Medicine.

Pitts, R. F. 1953. Mechanisms for stabilizing the alkaline reserves of the body. *Harvey Lect., 48:*172–209.

Pitts, R. F., Gurd, R. S., Kessler, R. H., and Hierholzer, K. 1958. Localization of acidification of urine, potassium and ammonia secretion and phosphate reabsorption in the nephron of the dog. *Am. J. Physiol., 194:*125–134.

Proverbio, F. and Whittembury, G. 1976. Cell electrical potentials during enhanced sodium extrusion in guinea pig kidney cortex slices. *J. Physiol., 250:*559–578.

Rabinowitz, L. and Gunther, R. A. 1972. Excretion of sodium and potassium in sheep during osmotic diuresis. *Am. J. Physiol., 222:*810–812.

Rector, F. C., Jr. 1973. Acidification of the urine. In: *Handbook of Physiology,* Section 8, Renal Physiology, pp. 431–454. Ed. by Orloff, J. and Berliner, R. W. American Physiological Society, Washington, D.C.

Relman, A. S. and Schwartz, W. B. 1952. Effect of DOCA on electrolyte balance in normal man and its relationship to sodium chloride intake. *Yale J. Biol. Med., 24:*540–558.

Rocha, A. S. and Kokko, J. P. 1973. Sodium chloride and water transport in the medullary thick ascending limb of Henle. Evidence for active chloride transport. *J. Clin. Invest., 52:*612–623.

Schon, D. A., Silva, P., and Hayslett, J. P. 1974. Mechanism of Potassium excretion in renal insufficiency. *Am. J. Physiol., 227:*1323–1330.

Schück, O. and Stribrna, J. 1968. Distal potassium secretion in man. *Lancet, 21:*972–974.

Schück, O. and Stribrna, J. 1971. Localization of the action of diuretics on renal tubular potassium transport in man. *Physiol. Bohemoslov., 20:*297–305.

Schultze, R. G. 1973. Recent advances in the physiology and pathophysiology of potassium excretion. *Arch. Intern. Med., 113:*885–897.

Schultze, R. G., Taggart, D. D., Shapiro, H., Pennell, J. P., Caglar, S., and Bricker, N. 1971. On the adaptation in potassium excretion associated with nephron reduction in the dog. *J. Clin. Invest., 50:*1061–1068.

Scott, D. 1969a. The effects of variations in water or potassium intake on the renal excretion of potassium in sheep. *Q. J. Exp. Physiol., 54:*16–24.

Scott, D. 1969b. The effect of intravenous infusion of KCl or HCl on the renal excretion of potassium in the sheep. *Q. J. Exp. Physiol., 54:*25–35.

Seely, J. F. and Dirks, J. H. 1969. Micropuncture study of hypertonic mannitol diuresis in the proximal and distal tubule of the dog kidney. *J. Clin. Invest., 48:*2330–2340.

Seldin, D. W., Welt, L. G., and Cort, J. 1956. The role of sodium salts and adrenal steroids in the production of hypokalemic alkalosis. *Yale J. Biol. Med., 29:*229–274.

Seldin, D. W., Eknoyan, G., Suki, W. H., and Rector, F. C. 1966. Localization of diuretic action from the pattern of water and electrolyte excretion. *Ann. N.Y. Acad. Sci., 139:*328.

Silva, P., Hayslett, J. P., and Epstein, F. H. 1973. Chronic K^+ adaptation. Role of Na^+-K-ATPase. *J. Clin. Invest., 52:*2665–2671.

Skou, J. C. 1965. Enzymatic basis for active transport of Na^+ and K^+ across cell membrane. *Physiol. Rev., 45:*596–617.

Sonnenberg, H. 1971. The renal response to blood volume expansion in the rat: Proximal tubular function and urinary excretion. *Can. J. Physiol. Pharmacol., 49:*525–533.

Sonnenberg, H. 1972. Renal response to blood volume expansion: Distal tubular function and urinary excretion. *Am. J. Physiol., 223:*916–924.

Stoner, L. C., Burg, M. B., and Orloff, J. 1974. Ion transport in cortical collecting tubule; effect of amiloride. *Am. J. Physiol., 227:* 453–459.

Strieder, N., Khuri, R. N., Wiederholt, M., and Giebisch, G. 1974b. Studies on the renal action of ouabain in the rat. Effects in the non-diuretic state. *Pfluegers Arch., 349:*91–107.

Struyvenberg, A., Morrison, R. B., and Relman, A. S. 1968. Acid–base behavior of separated canine renal tubules. *Am. J. Physiol., 214:*1155–1162.

Sullivan, L. P. 1961. Effect of sodium and impermeant anions on renal K transport during stopped flow. *Am. J. Physiol., 201:*774–780.

Sullivan, L. P., Wilde, W. S., and Malvin, R. L. 1960. Renal transport sites for K, H, and NH_3. *Am. J. Physiol., 198:*244–254.

Sullivan, W. J. 1968. Electrical potential differences across distal renal tubules of *Amphiuma. Am. J. Physiol., 214:*1096–1103.

Takokoro, M. and Boulpaep, E. L. 1972. Electrophoretic method of ion injection in single kidney cells. *Yale J. Biol. Med., 45:*432–435.

Thatcher, J. S. and Radike, A. W. 1947. Tolerance to potassium intoxication in the albino rat. *Am. J. Physiol., 151:*138–146.

Thompson, D. D. and Pitts, R. F. 1952. Effects of alterations of renal arterial pressure on sodium and water excretion. *Am. J. Physiol., 168:*490–499.

Uhlich, E., Baldamus, C. A., and Ullrich, K. J. 1969. The effect of aldosterone on sodium transport in the collecting ducts of the mammalian kidney. *Pfluegers Arch., 308:*111–121.

Urbach, J. R., Phelps, M. D., Steiger, W. S., and Bellet, S. 1953. Effect of water diuresis on renal excretion of certain urinary solutes in normal man. *J. Appl. Physiol., 6:*243–251.

Vander, A. J. 1961. Potassium secretion and reabsorption in distal nephron. *Am. J. Physiol., 201:*505–510.

Vander, A. J., Wilder, W. S., and Malvin, R. L. 1960. Stop-flow analysis of aldosterone and steroidal antagonist, SC 8109, on renal tubular transport kinetics. *Proc. Soc. Exp. Biol. Med., 103:*525–527.

Vogel, G. and Tervooren, U. 1964. Der Einfluss von Na auf K and Ca Transporte der isolierten perfundierten Amphibienniere. *Pfluegers Arch., 281:*354–364.

Walker, W. G., Cooke, C. R., Payne, J. W., Baker, C. R. F., and Andrew, D. J. 1961. Mechanism of renal potassium secretion studied by a modified stop-flow technique. *Am. J. Physiol., 200:*1133–1138.

Watson, J. F., Clapp, J. R., and Berliner, R. W. 1964. Micropuncture study of potassium concentration in proximal tubule of dog, rat and *Necturus. J. Clin. Invest., 43:*595–605.

Wesson, L. G. and Anslow, W. P., Jr. 1948. Excretion of sodium and water during osmotic diuresis in the dog. *Am. J. Physiol., 153:*465–474.

Whittembury, G. 1971. Relationship between sodium extrusion and electrical potentials in kidney cells. In: *Electrophysiology of Epithelial Cells.* Ed. by Giebisch, G. pp. 153–178. F. K. Schattauer Verlag, Stuttgart and New York.

Wiederholt, M. and Giebisch, G. 1974. Some electrophysiological properties of the distal tubule of *Amphiuma* kidney. *Fed. Proc., 33:*387.

Wiederholt, M., Sullivan, W. J., Giebisch, G., Solomon, A. K., and Curran, P. F. 1971. Transport of potassium and sodium across single distal tubules of *Amphiuma. J. Gen. Physiol., 57:*495–529.

Wiederholt, M., Schoormans, W., Fischer, F., and Behn, C. 1973. Mechanism of action of aldosterone on potassium transfer in the rat kidney. *Pfluegers Arch., 345:*157–178.

Wiederholt, M., Agulian, S., and Khuri, R. N. 1974. Intracellular potassium in the distal tubule of the adrenalectomized and aldosterone treated rat. *Pfluegers Arch., 347:*117–123.

Willis, L. R., Schneider, E. G., Lynch, R. W., and Knox, F. G. 1972. Effect of chronic alteration of sodium balance on reabsorption by proximal tubule of the dog. *Am. J. Physiol., 223:*34–39.

Wright, F. S. 1971a. Increasing magnitude of electrical potential along the renal distal tubule. *Am. J. Physiol., 220:*624–638.

Wright, F. S. 1971b. Alterations in electrical potential and ionic conductance of renal distal tubule cells in potassium adaptation. In: *Proc. Int. Union Physiol. Sci. IX.* p. 609.

Wright, F. S. 1974. Potassium transport by the renal tubule. in *MTP International Review of Science, Series I,* Vol. 6. Kidney and Urinary Tract Physiology, pp. 79–106. Ed. by Thurau, K. Butterworth, London.

Wright, F. S., Strieder, N., Fowler, N. B., and Giebisch, G. 1971. Potassium secretion by the distal tubule after potassium adaptation. *Am. J. Physiol., 221:*437–448.

III

Metabolism

Chapter **6**

The Effect of Diuretics on Kidney Intermediary Metabolism

Saulo Klahr

Renal Division
Department of Medicine
Washington University School of Medicine
St. Louis, Missouri

I. INTRODUCTION

Diuretic agents could conceivably affect tubular sodium reabsorption in a variety of ways: (1) by redistributing intrarenal blood flow or by changing peritubular capillary blood pressure and oncotic pressure; (2) by altering tubular membrane permeability; (3) by directly inhibiting enzymes or hypothetic carrier molecules involved in the translocation of sodium or chloride across cell membranes; or (4) by inhibiting cellular metabolism or the supply of energy available for ion transport (Heidenreich, 1969).

Recent evidence suggesting an effect of diuretics on chloride transport or membrane permeability has been obtained in studies utilizing the isolated perfused thick ascending limb of Henle's loop from rabbit kidney. This structure lies deep within the renal medulla and hence is not accessible to direct analysis (micropuncture) *in vivo*. Microperfusion studies *in vitro* indicate that this segment is water impermeable and that the intraluminal potential is positive, suggesting active chloride reabsorption (Burg and Green, 1973a; Rocha and Kokko, 1973). In this preparation, both furosemide and ethacrynic acid, when added to the luminal side, produced a rapid inhibition of transtubular potential difference (Burg and Green, 1973b; Burg et al., 1973). When the diuretics were removed the potential difference returned rapidly to control levels, suggesting that no irreversible metabolic alteration had occurred. The fact that their effects occurred quite rapidly after addition to the lumen but not after addition to the bath or peritubular site also suggests that intracellular accumulation may not be necessary for their effect. Similar results obtained with mercurial diuretics suggest that these compounds may also work by inhibiting chloride transport or through changes in membrane permeability (Burg and Green, 1973c). In addition, both furosemide and ethacrynic acid have been shown to affect cation permeability in model phospholipid membranes (Singer, 1974). Phosphatidylcholine vesicles have been shown to acquire a negative surface charge in the presence of furosemide or ethacrynic acid. In addition, these vesicles displayed a higher efflux rate for ^{22}Na and ^{86}Rb when exposed to these two diuretics. The increased permeability of cations seemed to be related to the creation of a negative surface charge. While in these vesicles ethacrynic acid also facilitated hydrogen transport, this property was not shared by furosemide.

Although the evidence reviewed above indicates that potent diuretics such as ethacrynic acid, furosemide, and mercurials may exert their major effect through alterations in membrane permeability, an effect of these substances on renal metabolism and a possible relationship of any metabolic alterations to their diuretic effect merits consideration. Before discussing the effects of diuretics on renal intermediary metabolism and the possible relation of such effects to the increased salt and water excretion produced by these agents, it seems appropriate to review first some general principles of normal renal metabolism in order to provide the reader with an adequate background for the discussion that follows.

II. RENAL METABOLISM

A major aim in metabolic studies of the kidney is to elucidate the biochemical pathways by which energy from metabolism is used in renal function. Since the major source of energy in mammals is the aerobic oxidation of substrates, the rate of oxygen uptake by the kidney should provide a gross estimate of total energy production by this organ. However, in addition to aerobic oxidative reactions, other mechanisms such as glycolysis and anaerobic oxidative decarboxylations have been shown to provide significant quantities of energy for renal function (Cohen and Barac-Nieto, 1973). The consumption of oxygen by the kidney *in vivo*, per unit weight, is one of the highest in the organism. Although the weight of the kidney is approximately 0.5% of total body weight, it accounts for approximately 10% of the total oxygen consumption by the body under basal conditions. In addition, the mammalian kidney demonstrates a considerable substrate specificity in that it selectively utilizes certain substrates from arterial blood. The uptake of substrates by the kidney is not always related to their concentrations in blood. For example, there is very little net uptake of glucose across the kidney despite a blood concentration of glucose of approximately 5 mM. In contrast, the kidney takes up considerable amounts of lactate and glutamine despite the fact that under most circumstances the concentrations of lactate and glutamine in blood are of the order of 1 and 0.5 mM, respectively (Pitts, 1972). While total oxygen consumption by the kidney may provide a measurement of total renal energy production and requirements, the rate of substrate uptake and the metabolic pathways by which a particular substrate is utilized may yield information about the mechanisms by which cellular metabolism and cellular functions are coupled.

A. Relation of Renal Oxygen Consumption to Sodium Reabsorption

Sodium reabsorption is quantitatively, by far, the most important transport function of the renal tubules. It seems well established that sodium reabsorption in the kidney is an active process, which requires the bulk of the oxygen consumed by the kidney (see Figure 1).

Ussing *et al.* (1960) first discussed in detail why utilization of oxygen by the intact mammalian kidney might parallel net sodium reabsorption. Studies by Thaysen *et al.* (1960), Lassen *et al.* (1961), and Kramer and Deetjen (1960) demonstrated that total renal oxygen consumption in anesthetized dogs could be subdivided into two components, oxygen consumption of the nonfiltering kidney, termed basal oxygen consumption and equal to approximately 0.1 mmol oxygen/min per 100 g of kidney, and suprabasal oxygen consumption directly proportional to filtration rate and hence to net reabsorption of sodium. It has been estimated by several investigators (Thaysen *et al.*, 1960; Deetjen and Kramer, 1961; Thurau, 1961; Knox *et al.*, 1966) that approximately 28–32 sodium equivalents are reabsorbed per mole of suprabasal oxygen consumed by the normal kidney. It also has been shown that the sodium–oxygen ratio is

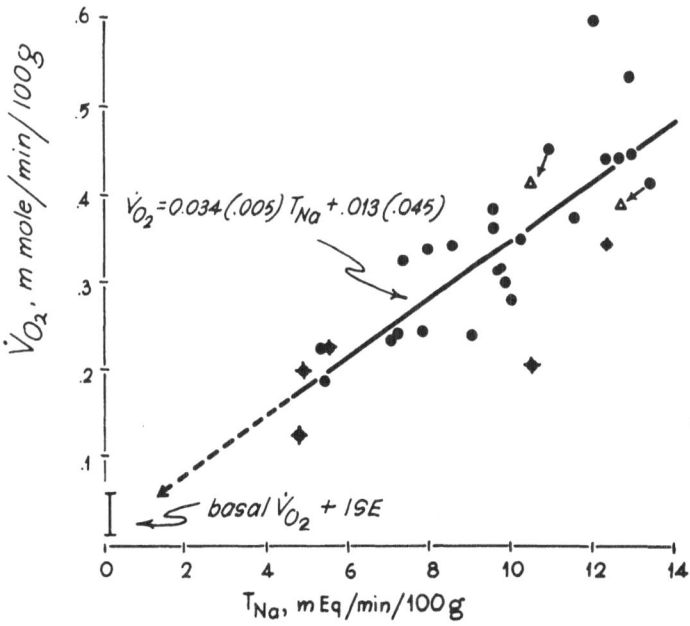

Figure 1. Relationship between oxygen consumption ($\dot{V}_{O_2}$) and sodium transport (T_{Na}) during water diuresis (●) plus elevated ureteral pressure (◑) and following Pitressin infusion (△). (Reproduced by permission from Knox *et al.*, 1966.)

remarkably constant under a wide variety of experimental conditions. A quantitative relationship between increments in oxygen consumption and increments in sodium transport rate was first demonstrated by Ussing and Zerahn (1951) in the frog skin. In this preparation oxygen uptake rate (above a basal oxygen uptake) was proportional to the rate of net sodium transport. Sodium uptake in the frog skin was determined in the absence of sodium in the medium bathing the "pond side" of the skin and was found to amount to approximately 80% of the total oxygen consumption. The assumption was made that none of this oxygen utilization was related to sodium transport. This approach of subtracting a basal value of oxygen uptake from total oxygen consumption has also been used in the study of other tissues that transport solutes transepithelially, the assumption being that basal energy production is not available for other cellular work. Zerahn (1956) calculated that in the frog skin 4–5 equivalents of sodium were transported per equivalent of oxygen utilized. Assuming that 6 moles of ATP are produced per mole of oxygen (ATP/O_2 = 6 or P/O = 3), approximately 3 equivalents of sodium are transported per mole of ATP formed in the frog skin. In the kidney, one mole of oxygen is required for every 28–32 equivalents of sodium reabsorbed. This, as mentioned before, is a remarkably constant figure, derived by several groups of investigators in different preparations and in different animals. If we assume a P/O ratio of 3, that is if 3 ATPs are generated for every atom of oxygen consumed, then 6 ATPs would be produced for every molecule of oxygen. If 30 mEq of sodium are transported per 6 mM of ATP, then 5 mEq of sodium are transported by the kidney for every mM of ATP produced by oxidative metabolism. The kidney thus appears to be a remarkably efficient organ when compared with other organs that transport sodium such as the toad bladder, the frog skin, muscle, and human red cells. In these tissues, using the same kind of calculations, only 3 sodiums are transported per high-energy phosphate bond utilized.

B. Renal Substrate Uptake and Utilization

The metabolism of the medulla and papilla of the kidney has been described as largely anaerobic and glycolytic, whereas that of the cortex has been ascribed to the aerobic oxidation of glucose, lactate, pyruvate, citrate, and the free fatty acid, palmitate (Metcoff and Yoshida, 1971). Most of the studies in the older literature related to substrates used by the kidney were biochemically oriented and were performed on slices or homogenates. However, recent experiments by Pitts and his co-workers (Pitts, 1974) in the *in vivo* functioning kidney of the dog have provided new and significant information regarding the major renal metabolic fuels. Differences were found in the relative rates of oxidation of glutamine and lactate under different conditions of acid–base balance, namely, metabolic alkalosis and metabolic acidosis. While glutamine uptake accounted for about 40% of the total CO_2 produced by the kidney in metabolic acidosis, it only accounted for about 15% in metabolic alkalosis. On the other hand, lactate accounted for only 22.5% of the total renal CO_2 production in metabolic acidosis and it provided about 47.5% of the renal CO_2 in metabolic alkalosis. Conse-

Table I. Percentages of Total Renal CO_2 Derived
from Various Metabolites[a]

Substrate	Acidosis, %	Alkalosis, %
Glutamine	40.0	14.5
Lactate	22.4	47.4
Palmitate	8.4	6.8
Stearate	7.0	3.3
Oleate	6.3	6.2
Citrate	10.8	13.8
Glucose	19.8	26.2
Total	114.7	118.2

[a] Reproduced with permission from Pitts (1974).

quently, about 60–65% of the total CO_2 produced by the kidney was derived from glutamine and lactate, and the greater oxidation of one or the other was dependent on the acid–base status of the animal. The remainder of the CO_2 produced by the kidney is provided by fatty acids (palmitate, stearate, and oleate), approximately 10–15% is derived from citrate, and approximately 20–25% is derived from glucose. In essence, glutamine and lactate appear to be the major substrates of oxidative metabolism in the kidney (see Table I).

C. Relation of Substrate Uptake to Sodium Reabsorption

Attempts to determine which metabolites are oxidized by the kidney to support the high rate of active ion transport have yielded conflicting results. A quantitative comparison of net substrate uptake with oxygen consumption suggested that if completely oxidized, the net renal uptake of free fatty acids and lactate could account for 59 and 35%, respectively, of the simultaneous renal oxygen consumption. This calculation implies that the lactate and fatty acids taken up are oxidized and provide the energy required for renal sodium transport. However, attempts to relate net sodium reabsorption to renal uptake of free fatty acids and lactate have produced contradictory results. Barac-Nieto and Cohen (1968) reported a significant correlation between sodium transport and net renal free fatty acid uptake, but Dies *et al.* (1970b) found no such correlation. Instead Dies *et al.* observed a correlation between net lactate uptake and net sodium reabsorption. In neither of these studies was oxidation of the substrate measured.

More recent evidence indicates that free fatty acids may not be completely oxidized in the kidney (Barac-Nieto and Cohen, 1971). In addition, Chinard *et al.*, (1962) have shown in experiments using the indicator dilution technique that *in vivo* renal lactate metabolism is complex. Similar to the metabolism of free fatty acids, only a portion of the lactate taken up by the dog kidney is oxidized. There was also evidence in this study that lactate is simultaneously produced and utilized by the kidney. Nevertheless, these data indicate that renal lactate oxidation may account for as much as 50% of renal production of CO_2. It is apparent that substrate oxidation rather than net substrate uptake should be measured when examining the metabolic sources of the energy used by the kidney. Recently Brand *et al.* (1974) have attempted to determine whether or not lactate oxidation provides energy for sodium transport in dog kidney. Renal lactate oxidation was measured at normal and reduced rates of sodium reabsorption. Oxidation of uniformly labeled [^{14}C]lactate to CO_2 was calculated from the renal production of $^{14}CO_2$ divided by the renal arterial lactate specific activity. Net renal lactate utilization, CO_2 production, and net sodium reabsorption were measured. After control observations ureteral pressure was elevated bilaterally, and after approximately 50 min of equilibration the metabolic and functional measurements were repeated. During increased ureteral pressure, there was approximately a 50% decrease in glomerular filtration rate, net transport of sodium, and renal production of CO_2, with no significant change in lactate uptake or lactate oxidation. Lactate oxidation accounted for approximately 27% of mean renal CO_2 production in control periods and approximately 50% during increased ureteral pressure. These data suggest that either lactate oxidation is not supplying energy for active sodium transport or is coupled to a moiety of sodium transport which is unaffected by the increased ureteral pressure.

Trimble and Bowman (1973), in studies using the isolated perfused kidney of the rat, showed that sodium reabsorption was highest with glucose in the perfusate, intermediate with palmitate, and lowest with no exogenous substrate present. To evaluate the possible role of endogenous lipid as an energy source for electrolyte transport, they employed α-bromopalmitate, a compound known to inhibit mitochondrial oxidation of long-chain fatty acids. They found that a portion of the energy necessary for sodium transport may be derived from endogenous fatty acid oxidation, since α-bromopalmitate produced significant decreases in sodium reabsorption both in the presence and absence of glucose. When palmitate was the only exogenous substrate, reabsorption of sodium was greater than that observed with no exogenous substrate present but less than that seen with glucose present. Ross *et al.* (1973) have also demonstrated in the isolated perfused rat kidney that glomerular filtration rate and sodium reabsorption are greater when glucose is used as the substrate. Glucose increased the percent of sodium reabsorption from 77 to 98% of the filtered load and lowered the ratio of sodium to potassium in the urine from 6 to 1.2. The major effect of glucose on kidney function could not be obtained with oleate, butyrate, or with acetoacetate. They concluded from their results that glucose rather than long- or short-chain fatty acids was the preferred substrate from which energy for sodium reabsorption is derived.

D. Studies of Renal Metabolism *in Vitro*

A large body of evidence regarding metabolic pathways in the kidney has been obtained from *in vitro* studies utilizing preparations such as kidney slices, isolated tubular suspensions, and kidney homogenates. Caution must be exercised when interpreting such data with regard to functions which can only be performed in a normal manner by the intact kidney *in vivo*. The *in vitro* studies, however, have served as background information for appropriate experimentation in the *in vivo* situation and can only be related to a function of the intact kidney to the extent to which that particular function remains undisturbed. With these reservations in mind some of the relevant *in vitro* data in the area of renal metabolism will be briefly reviewed.

It has been known for a number of years that the metabolism of the renal cortex differs significantly from that of the renal medulla (Gyorgy *et al.*, 1928; Dickens and Weil-Malherbe, 1936). Studies conducted in the rat reveal that the rate of oxygen consumption by slices of renal cortex were three to four times higher than from slices of inner medulla. On the other hand, the medulla was abundantly capable of glycolysis; by contrast, the cortex had a more limited glycolytic activity (Gyorgy *et al.*, 1928). Similar observations have also been obtained in the guinea pig (Dickens and Weil-Malherbe, 1936). Studies of dog kidney slices, incubated in a medium with an osmolality of 300 mOsm, revealed that oxygen consumption by the cortex was 6–7 times higher than that for the medulla per unit of dry weight (Kean *et al.*, 1961). Osmolality had a profound effect on the metabolism of cortex and medulla. Increasing osmolality of the bathing medium inhibited oxygen consumption of both cortex and inner medulla. In contrast, glycolysis in the inner medulla was not inhibited until levels of 1100–1300 mOsm were achieved, whereas in the cortex it was inhibited with only moderate increases in osmolality. Kean *et al.* (1962), in studies in the dog kidney, found 15 times more mitochondrial material in cortex than in inner medulla. Oxygen consumption was inhibited more readily in medullary mitochondrial suspensions than in those from the cortex when osmolality was increased by adding sodium chloride.

With glucose as substrate, the cortex increased CO_2 production in a linear fashion with progressive increases in oxygen tension (Lee and Peter, 1969). Outer medulla did so, too, but to a lesser extent. Outer papilla increased only modestly and papillary tips not at all. In contrast, net lactate production was low in cortex at either low or high oxygen tensions. Outer medulla was capable of shifting from high to low lactate production as medium Po_2 was increased. Lactate production has been shown to remain high at all oxygen tensions in outer papilla and papillary tips. Reduction of Po_2 markedly reduced ATP content in cortical slices, not as dramatically in outer medulla, and not at all in outer papilla and papillary tips. These data suggest that the cortex is entirely oxidative, but capable of utilizing glucose to produce ATP. The medulla appears able to shift from anaerobic to aerobic glycolysis with changing Po_2's. The outer papilla, to a large extent, and the papillary tip, entirely, appear obligatorily dependent upon anaerobic glycolysis (Lee *et al.*, 1962; Lee and Peter, 1969). Abodeely and Lee (1971), comparing palmitate to glucose utilization by slices of rabbit outer renal medulla, found glucose to be the preferential exogenous fuel of respiration in this portion of the kidney. Increasing sodium concentrations increased the rate of substrate oxidation. Ouabain abolished the sodium-induced acceleration of oxygen consumption and of glucose and palmitate oxidation.

These results suggest that glucose may be the preferential fuel of respiration for the production of energy presumably applied to sodium reabsorption in the thick ascending limb.

Bernanke and Epstein (1965) found significant oxygen consumption and large amounts of lactate production in inner medullary slices from hydropenic dogs exposed to 100% oxygen. Lactate production did not increase upon exposure to 5% oxygen, but it rose 50% in 100% nitrogen. Oxygen consumption was greater with succinate as substrate than with glucose. Although ATP content was not measured, calculated theoretical ATP available from oxidative metabolism was in all experimental conditions significantly greater than that available from anaerobic glycolysis.

Weidemann and Krebs (1969) and Krebs *et al.* (1966) using cortex slices from rat kidney found that fatty acids were the prime substrate but that ketone bodies could be utilized by the renal cortex. In contrast, their data provide evidence that lactate can serve as fuel in renal cortex *in vitro* only if its concentration is high and when ketone bodies and fatty acids are absent. Otherwise, lactate was converted preferentially to glucose and not oxidized. In the absence of added substrate they noted a low respiratory quotient, low rates of ammonia production, and minimal concentrations of glycogen, all leading to the conclusion that triglyceride probably provided endogenous oxidative substrate for the renal cortical slices in their experiments.

The overall scheme of *in vitro* experiments suggests that in the mammalian kidney marked differences exist in the metabolism of the cortex, outer medulla, inner medulla, and papilla. The renal cortex is almost completely dependent on oxidative metabolism. The preferential substrates used seem to include fatty acids, glucose, and lactate. In contrast the medulla seems to depend largely upon glucose as substrate source for energy production, although it is also capable of utilizing other substrates. The outer medulla seems capable of shifting from aerobic to anaerobic glycolysis with decreases in the availability of oxygen. The inner medulla and papilla depend heavily upon anaerobic glycolysis, although aerobic glycolysis may be possible under certain conditions.

E. Relation of Renal Metabolism to Salt and Water Reabsorption

Solute transport across epithelia including the renal tubules involves both active and passive components. The term "active transport" can be defined in a number of ways; the one used most often is that this type of transport proceeds against an electrochemical gradient and depends on the integrity of the energy-producing systems of the cell. In terms of thermodynamics, the transport may be called active if it is observed under conditions where all physical and chemical forces are zero. Active transport of a substance can be coupled either directly to the cell metabolism via ATP or other energy-rich substrates, resulting in a so-called primary active transport, or it can be coupled to the flux of another substance whose transport in this case is directly dependent on the cellular metabolism. These so-called cotransports can either be a symport when both substances move in the same direction or an antiport if the directions are opposite. In the proximal tubule cotransport of sodium and *d*-glucose (Schurek *et al.*, 1970) and sodium and amino acids has been considered, and a dependence of sodium absorption on proton transport has been suggested (Steinmetz, 1974).

The metabolic pathways supporting the active transport process in the tubule have interested many investigators. The presence of ATPases which are activated by the solute species transported has been considered evidence in support of a direct coupling between transport and cellular metabolism. In the case of sodium transport the sodium–potassium activated, ouabain-sensitive ATPase, Na–K ATPase, seems to be the link between cellular metabolism and transport. Chapter 7 in this book is devoted to the effects of diuretics on Na–K ATPase.

Metabolic inhibitors with a known mode of action on energy production have been used to investigate whether ATP or other energy-rich intermediates are the immediate energy source for primary active transport processes. Metabolic inhibitors have also been used to study the effect of inhibition of certain metabolic pathways on salt and water reabsorption by different nephron segments. It has been shown that cyanide, an inhibitor of the electron transport chain and hence of oxidative phosphorylation, inhibits salt and water reabsorption in the kidney (Strickler and Kessler, 1963; Weinstein *et al.*, 1969; Martinez-Maldonado *et al.*, 1969; Herms and Malvin, 1963). This inhibitor also has been shown to reduce the concentrating and diluting capacity of the kidney (Weinstein *et al.*, 1969; Martinez-Maldonado *et al.*, 1969, 1970), suggesting that it may affect ion transport in the loop of Henle. Cyanide has also been shown to reduce oxygen consumption (Fujimoto *et al.*, 1964) and the levels of renal ATP (Kessler *et al.*, 1968; Kessler, 1969). Iodoacetamide, a potent inhibitor of glycolysis, has been shown to produce natriuresis (Strickler and Kessler, 1963; Weinstein and Klose, 1969) and reduce the ability of the dog kidney to concentrate and dilute the urine (Martinez-Maldonado, 1969, 1970). Combinations of these two inhibitors, cyanide and iodoacetamide, produce greater natriuresis than when either inhibitor is administered alone (Martinez-Maldonado *et al.*, 1970). Studies utilizing micropuncture techniques have shown inhibition of sodium reabsorption by cyanide in the proximal tubule of *Necturus* (Maunsbach, 1964) and in the proximal tubule of the rat (Windhager and Giebisch, 1961). Maunsbach (1964) also found inhibition of sodium reabsorption in the proximal tubule of *Necturus* with iodoacetate, an inhibitor of anaerobic glycolysis. Schatzman *et al.* (1958) found inhibition of water reabsorption with dinitrophenol and with ouabain when these compounds were added to the fluid used to perfuse the proximal tubule of *Necturus*. Weinstein and Klose (1969) demonstrated by free-flow micropuncture techniques in the rat that the renal intraarterial infusion of either cyanide or iodoacetamide decreased fractional sodium reabsorption in surface tubules to a value approximately 50% of the control. Compensation of fluid reabsorption occurred in the loop of Henle, and reabsorption along surface distal convoluted tubules was not significantly different from the values obtained prior to the infusion of the inhibitor. The increment in sodium excretion in the final urine was modest. In contrast, iodoacetamide had no measurable effect on proximal tubular reabsorption. It produced profound inhibition of distal nephron reabsorption resulting in large natriuresis and increased pressure in distal segments. These data are consistent with some of the *in vitro* experiments, suggesting that the cortex and hence the proximal tubule depend obligatorily upon oxidative metabolism and the medulla and thus the loop of Henle and distal tubule require glycolysis to sustain sodium reabsorption. Additional experiments by Weinstein (1970), using the split-drop technique, revealed that cyanide more than doubled, whereas 2-deoxyglucose and dinitrophenol had no effect on the reabsorptive half-time of isotonic saline perfusate. The addition of deoxyglucose to cyanide in the isotonic sodium perfusate did not produce a greater inhibitory effect than that observed with cyanide alone. The observation that dinitrophenol had no effect on isotonic saline reabsorption in the experiments by Weinstein is different from the observations of Chertok *et al.* (1966) and Fernandez *et al.* (1969). Gyory and Kinne (1971) studied the effects of a series of metabolic inhibitors on fluid reabsorption in the proximal tubule using the split-drop technique. They found that cyanide and CCCP (carbonylcyanide-*m*-chlorophenylhydrazone) inhibited isotonic absorption completely but only when applied via peritubular blood capillary perfusion. On the other hand, oligomycin and antimycin inhibited isotonic transport by 80% when applied intratubularly in conjunction with 0.5% albumin. Thus, inhibition of ATP synthesis, either by inhibition of cytochrome oxidase (cyanide) or by uncoupling the electron flow from phosphorylation (CCCP), abolished transepithelial solute transport. Neither of these substances has an effect on the Na–K ATPase present in isolated plasma membranes. Under conditions where cell metabolism is inhibited but the transport system is not directly affected, it should be possible to stimulate sodium transport if energy is supplied to the cells. For this purpose phosphoenolpyruvate (PEP), which can lead to the synthesis of ATP via the pyruvate kinase reaction, can be used. In tubules perfused with cyanide demonstrating a 75% inhibition of sodium reabsorption, addition of PEP has been shown to partially restore the transport capacity of the tubule. The effect of PEP on sodium transport was also tested when oligomycin or antimycin A were used to suppress intracellular energy production. Only in the presence of 10^{-5} M antimycin A does PEP lead to a partial restoration of isotonic transport. At higher concentrations of antimycin or when oligomycin was present, addition of PEP did not restore fluid reabsorption. At 10^{-5} M antimycin, Na–K ATPase is inhibited by 55%; at higher concentrations of antimycin A and all concentrations of oligomycin the enzyme is inhibited nearly completely. Therefore, inhibition of isotonic absorption by oligomycin and high concentrations of antimycin A can be explained by an action of the inhibitors both on the mitochondria and the transport system for sodium, whereas in the presence of 10^{-5} M antimycin the action on the mitochondria predominates. These results further support the view that Na–K ATPase is involved in some critical step of transepithelial sodium transport. On the basis of experiments carried out in the isolated perfused kidney of the rat, Ross *et al.* (1973) suggested that in the absence of added substrate the energy for sodium reabsorption by the perfused kidney is presumably provided by endogenous substrate. The addition of substrates to the perfusion medium affected the percentage of the filtered sodium which was reabsorbed, as would be expected if oxidation of the fuel provided extra energy required for the active transport of sodium. In addition, there were significant effects on the GFR of adding substrates to the perfusion medium; the nature of this increase is not clear at present. Ross *et al.* also calculated the contribution of a series of fuels tested (glucose, butyrate, and oleate) to GFR and sodium reabsorption. Their data on the effects of substrates on sodium reabsorption are summarized in Table II. These results obtained in the *in vitro* perfused kidney of the rat are in marked contrast to the relative contribution of glucose and fatty acids to the fuel of respiration in kidney cortical slices (Weidemann and Krebs, 1969). The apparent discrepancy between substrate utilization of cortical slices and the perfused organ may simply reflect the extra metabolic requirements to support the high rate of sodium transport in the perfused kidney. However, the preferential role of glucose in supporting sodium reabsorption in this model is striking.

Besarab *et al.* (1974) demonstrated that maximal inhibition of Na–K ATPase by ouabain in the isolated perfused rat kidney decreased sodium reabsorption by about 50% of the filtered load so that about half the sodium continued to be reabsorbed, a process that seemed to depend on metabolic energy, since it was eliminated when inhibitors of the electron-transport chain (cyanide) or glycolysis (iodoacetamide) were used or when glucose was removed during anoxic perfusion. The addition of furosemide did not further depress reabsorption of filtrate when added after ouabain in a single experiment. In kidneys perfused with bovine albumin plus Ringer's bicarbonate, the addition of 25 mM ouabain to completely inhibit Na–K ATPase decreased fractional reabsorption of sodium from 95% to 54% of the filtered load. Subsequent addition of 1 mM acetazolamide reduced sodium reabsorption even further to 34%. Ouabain alone reduced sodium reabsorption to 30% in kidneys perfused without bicarbonate. Restoration of bicarbonate in the medium to 25 mEq/liter was accompanied by a rise in fractional reabsorption to 53%; the further addition of acetazolamide produced a drop back to about 35%. Ethacrynic acid, ethacrynic–cysteine, or 2 mM furosemide decreased fractional reabsorption only slightly when given after ouabain. Perfusing the kidney at 11°C instead of 37°C

Table II. Contribution of Endogenous and Exogenous Substrates to Sodium Reabsorption in Perfused Rat Kidney[a]

Substrate added	GFR, ml/min	Na reabsorbed, %	Total Na reabsorbed, μEq/min per gram wet wt	Total Na reabsorption supported by substrate, %
None	0.29	77.1	32.1	24.7
Fatty acid (butyrate or oleate)	0.62	86.7	77.1	34.7
Glucose (as sole substrate)	0.75	98.2	130.0	75.2

[a] Reproduced by permission from Ross *et al.* (1973).

reduced sodium reabsorption to 10% of the filtered load without further depression being observed when ouabain and acetazolamide were added. Rewarming the kidney to 32°C increased sodium reabsorption to almost 30%. These experiments suggest that there are at least three mechanisms for sodium reabsorption: one pathway dependent on Na–K ATPase that seems to be inhibited by ouabain and partly blocked as well by ethacrynic acid and furosemide; a second, sensitive to acetazolamide and involving bicarbonate reabsorption; and a third residual mechanism sensitive to temperature and contributing approximately one third of sodium reabsorption. The lack of an additive effect of furosemide or ethacrynic acid on sodium reabsorption when ouabain was present at maximal inhibitory concentrations may indicate that these diuretics work through the Na–K ATPase mechanism. However, the results may also be interpreted to suggest that uptake, concentration, and secretion of these diuretics into the tubular lumen was impaired in the presence of ouabain, resulting in no further effect on sodium reabsorption when they were added after the glycoside.

III. EFFECTS OF DIURETICS ON RENAL METABOLISM

When analyzing the effects of diuretic agents on renal metabolism it is important to distinguish between those metabolic effects which presumably are secondary to decreased ion reabsorption and those which are primary in nature.

A. The Effects of Diuretics on Renal Oxygen Consumption *in Vivo*

As discussed above, a number of studies have shown a stoichiometric relationship between oxygen consumption and sodium reabsorption by the mammalian kidney under a wide variety of conditions. Certain experimental maneuvers have been reported to alter the ratio between net sodium reabsorbed and oxygen consumed by the kidney. The infusion of mannitol (Kiil *et al.*, 1961; Knox *et al.*, 1966) and that of the carbonic anhydrase inhibitor, dichlorphenamide (Kessler *et al.*, 1964), has been shown to lower the amount of sodium reabsorbed either without a change in or with a proportionally lesser reduction in oxygen consumption. Thus, the ratio of net sodium reabsorbed to oxygen consumed falls during the administration of these two agents. Studies by Thurau (1961) have shown that the decreased sodium reabsorption produced by hydrochlorothiazide results in a fall in oxygen consumption and the ratio of sodium reabsorption to net oxygen consumption remains unchanged. Mercurial diuretics and mercurial compounds without diuretic activity have been shown by Deetjen and Kramer (1961) and Kessler *et al.* (1964) not to affect the ratio between sodium reabsorbed and oxygen consumed. Fulgraff (1969) has reported that furosemide administration may depress tubular sodium reabsorption in dogs to 70% of the filtered load without changing renal oxygen consumption. Administration of ethacrynic acid to anesthetized dogs resulted in a decrease in sodium reabsorption from 96 to 71% of the filtered load whereas oxygen consumption remained constant (Wolf *et al.*, 1969). Mean renal blood flow was increased to 134% of the control levels, but renal arteriovenous difference oxygen was lowered, respectively. Thus, the ratio of sodium transported to oxygen consumed was decreased significantly after injection of ethacrynic acid. The results obtained with furosemide and ethacrynic acid were interpreted to indicate that the inhibition of sodium transport produced by these diuretics occurs not through an effect on metabolism but through an effect on membrane permeability.

In those instances (mannitol or dichlorphenamide administration) where net sodium reabsorption decreased without a proportional change in oxygen consumption, a number of possible explanations must be considered: (1) The quantity of sodium that has been reabsorbed into the peritubular capillaries may back-leak at increasing rates into the tubular lumen. (2) The agent may have increased the energy requirements for active transport of sodium. (3) A component of sodium reabsorption not dependent on metabolism may have been reduced to a greater extent than a second component which is oxygen dependent. For example, if segmental differences in oxygen consumption exist between different portions of the nephron, a marked reduction in sodium reabsorption in a segment of the nephron where sodium reabsorption is predominantly aerobic (proximal tubule) may result in increased sodium reabsorption at the level of the loop and theoretically may lead to decreased oxygen consumption, with no alterations in total sodium transport, and to a shift from aerobic metabolism to glycolytic metabolism if reabsorption in the thick ascending limb is not completely dependent on oxidative phosphorylation. On the other hand, a shift in the proportion of sodium reabsorbed to the proximal tubule where the transfer may be oxygen dependent, at the expense of the loop of Henle, may increase the oxygen cost of sodium reabsorption. An uncoupling of oxidative phosphorylation, a situation in which oxygen consumption will persist, but the formation of high-energy intermediates would be compromised, may also affect the ratios between oxygen consumption and sodium reabsorption.

The effects of mannitol on sodium reabsorption and oxygen consumption have been attributed by Kiil *et al.* (1961) and by Knox *et al.* (1966) to an enhanced back-diffusion of sodium in the proximal tubule. This back-leak from peritubular capillary to lumen would decrease net sodium reabsorption without altering oxygen consumption. The effect of dichlorphenamide, an inhibitor of carbonic anhydrase, on the sodium-to-oxygen ratios is not completely clear. Carbonic anhydrase inhibitors have been shown not to decrease oxygen consumption by slices of kidney cortex, medulla, or cortical mitochondria. The ATP content of cortex and medulla are not reduced *in vivo* despite a natriuresis suggesting that enhanced passive back-diffusion of sodium (perhaps secondary to the intratubular retention of bicarbonate in the tubular lumen) may be a likely mechanism.

Fulgraff (1969) suggested that both ethacrynic acid and furosemide may act at the level of the nephron by changing membrane permeability either by increasing it, thereby enhancing the back-leak of Na, or by decreasing it and thereby increasing the energy cost of transport. However, as we will discuss subsequently, both of these diuretics have extensive metabolic effects. A major effect of these diuretics on portions of the nephron where oxidative phosphorylation is not the major mechanism responsible for sodium reabsorption is also a plausible explanation for the dissociation. If one assumes that most of the oxygen in the kidney is consumed in the proximal tubule and that most of the energy for chloride and sodium reabsorption in the thick ascending limb of Henle is derived via glycolysis, with the effects of ethacrynic acid and furosemide mainly confined to this segment, one may observe decreased sodium reabsorption without a major effect on oxygen consumption even in the absence of a permeability effect. On the other hand, Washington and Holland (1966) have reported that during osmotic diuresis or saline loading urinary Po_2 is reduced. Since both saline and osmotic diuresis result in increased sodium delivery to and enhanced sodium reabsorption in the ascending limb, these authors proposed that the drop in urine Po_2 results from enhanced oxygen consumption for the reabsorptive process. The reduced urine Po_2 is returned to normal by ethacrynic acid which also raised urine Po_2 during hydropenia. Since ethacrynic acid inhibits sodium reabsorption principally in the medullary segments of the ascending limb of Henle's loop, the rise in urine Po_2 was attributed to inhibition of active sodium transport and therefore oxygen consumption at this site.

Different rates of oxygen consumption by different nephron segments complicate the interpretation of the effects of diuretics on the fixed relationship between sodium reabsorption and oxygen consumption. Recent studies have attempted to explore the relationship between proximal and distal sodium reabsorption and the overall rate of oxygen consumption by the kidney. Weinstein and Szyjewicz (1974), using the rat, demonstrated that when net sodium reabsorption was shifted fractionally from the proximal tubule to the loop of Henle as a result of volume expansion with isotonic saline, the net amount of sodium reabsorbed per oxygen consumed by the whole kidney increased. This occurred without a significant change in total renal oxygen consumption. Absolute sodium reabsorption in the proximal tubule remained constant. Single nephron and whole kidney filtration rate increased proportionally. Quantitatively then, the effects of volume expansion in these studies on sodium reabsorption were to increase absolute sodium reabsorption in the distal nephron without changing absolute sodium reabsorption in the proximal tubule. Simultaneously, during volume expansion more net sodium reabsorption occurred for the same amount of oxygen consumed. These data are most consistent with the idea that the distal nephron, primarily the loop of Henle, where absolute reabsorption of filtrate increases during isotonic volume expansion, is less oxygen dependent than the proximal tubule as suggested previously by Weinstein and Klose (1969). On the other hand, Kjekshus et al. (1969) have suggested from studies conducted in dogs subjected to decreases in GFR, during distal blockade with ethacrynic acid and chlorothiazide, that similar stoichiometric relationships between sodium reabsorption and oxygen consumption exist in the proximal and distal parts of the nephron.

It should be pointed out that inferences as to the mechanism of action of diuretics based on changes in Q_{O2}/T_{Na} may not be warranted because, in addition to the possible effects of redistribution of fluid reabsorption between different nephron segments on such ratios, measurements of oxygen consumption have major technical pitfalls. In addition, total renal oxygen consumption is the sum of basal and transport-associated oxygen consumption, each of which may vary independently, and the effect of diuretic agents on basal oxygen consumption is unknown.

B. Effects of Diuretics on the Local Metabolic Rate of the Kidney

The external work performed by the kidney in concentrating various solutes in urine relative to plasma is small. Therefore, practically all energy expended in the kidney is converted to heat. Aukland and his co-workers (1969) have applied the technique of decreases in local heat generation to localize the action of diuretics *in vivo* utilizing the kidney of the dog.

It has been proposed that heat generation may be estimated from the rate of heat accumulation during occlusion of the renal artery by recording the rise of local temperature. The rate of heat accumulation estimated in this way equals the metabolic rate immediately before occlusion if: (1) metabolic heat is removed from the site of measurement exclusively by blood flow and is therefore quantitatively accumulated during circulatory arrest, and (2) the metabolic rate and tissue volume remain unchanged during the first seconds of arterial occlusion. As for the first assumption, heat-clearance measurements suggest that removal of metabolic heat from the renal cortex and outer zone of the medulla is mainly by blood flow (convection) whereas clearance from the inner medulla and papilla is affected mainly by heat diffusion (conduction) towards the cortical medullary border. Since heat diffusion will also continue along established temperature gradients during circulatory arrest, no immediate temperature rise would be expected in the inner medulla, suggesting that measurements would have to be restricted to the cortex and outer medulla. Aukland *et al.* (1969) measured the initial rate of temperature rise during arterial occlusion with fine thermocouples placed in the kidneys of anesthetized dogs for estimation of local metabolic rates. After establishing a steady urine flow, measurements of heat-accumulation rates were started by occluding the renal artery for 5–10 sec with 2–5-min intervals. This control period, lasting 30–60 min, also included measurements of PAH and creatinine clearances. Thereafter the diuretics to be tested were given as a single dose intravenously, and heat-accumulation measurements were continued for the next 30–60 min with two clearance periods of 5–10 min duration. Mersalyl reduced metabolic rates, per unit tissue volume, of the outer medulla to 65% of control without significant reduction in the cortex, suggesting inhibition of sodium transport in the loops of Henle. Chlorothiazide lowered cortical metabolic rate to 76% of control with no change in outer medulla, indicating an action in the convoluted tubules. Ethacrynic acid and furosemide acted mainly on the loops of Henle, as indicated by reductions of outer medullary metabolic rates to 21 and 32% of control values, respectively. Cortical metabolic rate also fell to 78 and 85% of control, suggesting additional effects on cortical nephron segments. Swelling of the kidney during diuresis accounted for a reduction in metabolic rate of about 10% of control. These experiments do not provide any clues as to whether the decrease in metabolic rate per unit tissue was primary or secondary to the effects of the diuretic tested.

C. The Effects of Diuretics on Renal Metabolism of Substrates *in Vivo*

Recent studies (Boineau *et al.*, 1974) have evaluated the effects of furosemide on renal lactate metabolism and CO_2 production *in vivo* in dogs. Dogs were made slightly alkalotic by the administration of sodium bicarbonate prior to study so as to increase the utilization of lactate by the kidney. A constant continuous infusion of tracer amounts of uniformly labeled [^{14}C]lactate was given intravenously. Initial samples of urine, arterial blood, and renal venous blood were collected during control periods and after the administration of 1 mg furosemide per kilogram body weight given intravenously as a bolus. Urine flow was shown to increase threefold, and fractional sodium excretion increased 10 times following administration of furosemide. GFR decreased by about 30%, and renal blood flow remained unchanged. Total renal CO_2 production decreased markedly in the first 10 min after furosemide administration and returned to control rates about 10 min following furosemide administration. There was no effect on the renal extraction of lactate or its conversion to CO_2. The percentage of CO_2 derived from lactate increased immediately following furosemide administration and returned to control levels 10 min after the administration of furosemide. The authors concluded that the decrease in renal CO_2 production suggested a temporary decrease in renal energy production following the administration of furosemide. The observed temporary increase in the percentage of CO_2 contributed from lactate suggested a depression in the renal utilization of substrates other than lactate during furosemide administration. These studies suggest that furosemide does not affect the utilization of lactate by the kidney of the dog *in vivo*. On the other hand, Dies *et al.* (1970a,b) had shown previously that the infusion of furosemide into dogs resulted in a significant decrease in the net renal uptake of lactate and nonesterified fatty acids. In their experiments, furosemide given in large doses decreased sodium reabsorption from 3286 to 1788 μEq/min and increased fractional sodium excretion from 2.6 to 33%. Total renal blood flow remained approximately constant. Arterial lactate increased from 1.29 ± 0.18 to 1.45 ± 0.17 μmol/ml, and arterial nonesterified fatty acids remained constant. Renal utilization of nonesterified fatty acids decreased from 9.10 ± 1.08 to 4.51 ± 1.8 μmol/min, and the renal utilization of lactate diminished from 23.41 ± 3.06 to 12.56 ± 3.52 μmol/min. The depression in renal utilization of nonesterified fatty acids by furosemide may be related in these experiments to a specific competition between the two compounds for a common entrance pathway into renal tubular cells. Probenecid blocks both the diuretic effects of furosemide (Hook and Williamson, 1965) and the renal uptake of nonesterified fatty acids (Dies *et al.*, 1970b). It had been shown previously by Barac-Nieto and Cohen (1968) that the administration of chlorothiazide, another diuretic whose action is blocked by probenecid (Beyer and Baer, 1961), or of probenecid itself almost completely blocked the renal utilization of nonesterified fatty acids, although the natriuresis produced by these drugs was moderate or nil. In the studies of Dies *et al.* furosemide decreased renal utilization of nonesterified fatty acids much less than chlorothiazide or probenecid did in the experiments of Barac-Nieto and Cohen, despite the fact that furosemide lowered transport of sodium much more. From these observations it seems probable that the depression in renal utilization of nonesterified fatty acids produced by furosemide is not related to the ability of this drug to decrease sodium transport.

Regarding the effects of diuretics on substrate uptake, it should be pointed out that furosemide, ethacrynic acid, and chlorothiazide are transported into the cell from the peritubular circulation by the organic acid transport system. Many of the substrates that the kidney utilizes may also be transported by the same pathway. Hence, decreases in substrate uptake during diuretic administration may not be directly related to their natriurctic effect but to the fact that they may block substrate uptake directly at the peritubular site by a competitive type of phenomena. Whether some of the diuretic effects can be ascribed to this decreased substrate uptake is unknown. However, the data demonstrating that inhibition of uptake of nonesterified fatty acids by chlorothiazide is quite marked while the natriuresis is small and the opposite data with furosemide seem to indicate that this mechanism may not be important in the diuretic effect.

D. Effect of Diuretic Agents on Oxygen Consumption by Renal Slices *in Vitro*

Several investigators have evaluated the effect of diuretics on oxygen consumption by renal cortical and medullary slices. Evidence that diuretics may exert their effect by interfering with kidney cell metabolism and mitochondrial oxidative phosphorylation has been advanced. Concentrations of ethacrynic acid ranging between 0.1 and 1 mM have been shown to depress oxygen consumption and decrease intracellular potassium concentrations of kidney slices from rats, rabbit, and dogs (Jones and Landon, 1967; MacKnight, 1969; Landon and Fitzpatrick, 1969; Epstein, 1972; Podevin and Boumendil-Podevin, 1972; De-Jairala *et al.*, 1972). A recent report by Case *et al.* (1973) has shown that ethacrynic acid reduces oxygen consumption in rabbit kidney cortical slices, even when pretreated with sufficient ouabain to inhibit Na–K ATPase or in slices pretreated with amiloride. Ethacrymic acid can also reduce oxygen consumption, without change in tissue electrolytes, in slices incubated in sodium-free medium. It also decreases oxygen consumption in isolated kidney mitochondria. Case *et al.* (1973) also demonstrated that at low doses (0.01 mM) ethacrynic acid inhibited phosphate utilization of mitochondria incubated with succinate in the presence of ADP and a hexokinase trap. At this dosage no significant effect on oxygen consumption was noted and the P/O ratio fell. Higher doses, 0.1 and 1 mM, reduced phosphate utilization progressively so that the P/O ratio fell to zero. Others (Gaudemer and Foucher, 1967; Goldschmidt *et al.*, 1970) have also shown previously that ethacrynic acid has effects on isolated mitochondria. The observations that in slices incubated for 3 hr in choline medium ethacrynic acid reduced oxygen consumption without associated changes in cell electrolytes, plus the finding that the drug reduced utilization of phosphate and oxygen consumption of isolated mitochondria suggests that the metabolic effects of ethacrynic acid are not secondary to depression of ion transport by the drug. Case *et al.* (1973) suggested from their data that ethacrynic acid may inhibit sodium transport by interfering with oxidation and phosphorylation in mitochondria of transporting cells. On the other hand, inhibition of respiration of mitochondria isolated from cortical tissue could not be demonstrated following the *in vivo* administration of 10 mg per kilogram body weight of ethacrynic acid to rabbits (Landon and Fitzpatrick, 1972). However, recently a report has appeared (Sawa *et al.*, 1974) suggesting that ethacrynic acid administration to the rat may decrease oxygen consumption by mitochondria isolated from cortex, outer medullary region, and liver. Epstein (1972) has shown that ethacrynic acid affects active transport of sugars by rabbit kidney cortical slices *in vitro* and that it also decreases oxygen uptake both in the presence and in the absence of sodium in the bathing medium. A rapid diminution of tissue ATP content occurred during tissue incubation with ethacrynic acid. Gordon (1968) has shown that in tightly coupled mitochondria preparations, isolated from rat liver and kidney, ethacrynic acid inhibits respiration and acts in some respects as an uncoupling agent. It can thus be postulated that the fall in oxygen uptake brought about by ethacrynic acid is secondary to inhibition of mitochondrial ATP production. This suggestion is strengthened by the observation that membrane ATPase-stimulated mitochondrial respiration is inhibited by doses of ethacrynic acid (0.05 mM) which do not inhibit ATPase *in vitro* (Landon and Forte, 1971). It has also been suggested Suki *et al.*, 1973) that medullary mitochondria may be more sensitive to ethacrynic acid than cortical mitochondria.

Among mercurial diuretics, meralluride results in a fall in intracellular potassium and inhibition of tissue respiration of rat kidney slices *in vitro*. These effects have been attributed to inhibition of ATPase activity. On the other hand, the nondiuretic mercurial, *p*-chloromercurybenzoate (PCMB), has been shown not to have an effect on ATPase activity, respiration, or intracellular potassium of the slices. Both meralluride and PCMB increase tissue water in incubated kidney slices. When a mercurial diuretic is injected and slices are obtained, initial concentrations of intracellular potassium remain at normal levels even though Na–K ATPase activity is depressed. If these tissues with inhibited ATPase activity are sliced and incubated, they do lose potassium and show an inhibited respiration similar to slices incubated *in vitro* with a mercurial diuretic (Landon and Fitzpatrick, 1969). It has been stated that mitochondrial respiration is not inhibited by organic mercurials *in vivo* or by organic mercurials *in vitro* in the presence of cytoplasmic protein, and the effects of mercurials on cell metabolism have been explained as secondary to membrane and transport changes. Yoshida *et al.* (1971) have reported that chlormerodrin also inhibits respiration of rat renal cortical and medullary slices. In contrast, neither amiloride or acetazolamide exhibited any influence upon oxygen uptake. Hydrochlorothiazide was only slightly inhibitory. Chlormerodrin was also shown to suppress the rate of oxygen uptake by mitochondria. Grief and Jacobs (1958) have reported that chlormerodrin lowered the P/O ratio in renal mitochondria prepared from normal kidney. When mercury-labeled chlormerodrin was administered 4 hr prior to killing the animal, it failed to lower the P/O ratio in kidney mitochondria. In experiments in which chlormerodrin was administered for 14 days prior to killing the rats, the drug suppressed the rate of oxygen uptake and P/O ratio in renal mitochondria of such animals.

The effects of diuretic administration on isolated rat renal cortical and outer medullary and liver mitochondrial oxygen consumption and swelling have been recently published Sawa *et al.*, 1974). Oxygen consumption was significantly higher in cortical as compared to outer medullary mitochondria. When ethacrynic acid, furosemide, chlorothiazide, acetazolamide, chlormerodrin, and triflocin were injected, it was reported that all diuretics exerted an inhibitory effect on cortical, outer medullary, and liver mitochondrial oxygen consumption. Mercury was found to be the most important inhibitor followed by ethacrynic acid, triflocin, furosemide, chlorothiazide, and finally acetazolamide. The inhibitory effect of equimolar doses of nondiuretic analogs of mercury and triflocin was lower by 28 and 29%, respectively. The effects of diuretics on mitochondrial swelling were also studied utilizing concentrations of diuretics that inhibited oxygen consumption by 50%. At these doses, furosemide, chlorothiazide, and acetazolamide had only a slight effect on liver mitochondria. Ethacrynic acid had the greatest effect followed by mercury. By contrast, mercury had the greatest effect on cortical and outer medullary mitochondrial swelling followed by ethacrynic acid and furosemide, while chlorothiazide and acetazolamide had only a slight effect. These results suggested to the authors that, as in the dog, a difference exists between cortical and outer medullary mitochondria in the rat and that diuretics exert a direct inhibitory effect on renal mitochondrial function which is different from the effect on hepatic mitochondria and is greater than that of the nondiuretic analogs that were examined.

E. Effects of Diuretics on Renal Glycolysis *in Vitro* and *in Vivo*

Suggestive evidence has accumulated, as discussed elsewhere in this chapter, to indicate that the inner medulla and papilla are structures within the kidney that can derive their energy supply from glycolysis. Suggestive evidence is also available to indicate that the outer medulla is capable of aerobic or anaerobic metabolism. Several groups have demonstrated that ethacrynic acid inhibits glycolysis in intact tissues (Jones and Landon, 1967; Gordon and deHartog, 1971) and in the membrane-free cytoplasmic fractions of cells (Klahr *et al.*, 1971a,b; Gordon and deHartog, 1971). The effects of ethacrynic acid on glycolysis have been examined in cytoplasmic membrane-free preparations obtained from the renal cortex and medulla of rabbits and rats in an effort to examine the effects of this agent on glycolysis independent of its action on sodium transport (Klahr *et al.*, 1971a). Lactate production in the absence and presence of ethacrynic acid was studied using fructose-1,6-diphosphate, glucose-6-phosphate, or 3-phosphoglycerate and membrane-free preparations. The effects of furosemide on this process were also studied in a similar manner. Table III depicts the effects of increasing concentrations of ethacrynic acid or furosemide on the formation of lactate from fructose-1,6-diphosphate by membrane-free preparations of rat renal cortex. The inhibition of glycolysis by both compounds was dose dependent. With 0.5 mM ethacrynic acid inhibition of lactate production averaged 31%; with a 1 mM concentration, it averaged 54%; finally, with 10 mM ethacrynic acid inhibition was 79%. Furosemide (1 mM) produced a slight inhibition which was not statistically significant. On the other hand, 5 mM furosemide resulted in a significant decrease in lactate formation in every experiment, and somewhat greater inhibition was observed when 10 mM furosemide was added to the incubation mixture. Similar results were obtained using membrane-free preparations from rat renal medulla and preparations from rabbit cortex or medulla. Preincubation of the membrane-free preparations with ethacrynic acid resulted in a greater inhibition of lactate when the substrate was added. This was not the case with furosemide. It was also shown that dithiothreitol (Cleland's reagent), a sulfhydryl protective agent, partially blocked the effect of ethacrynic acid on glycolysis while it had no effect on the effect of furosemide. Analogs of ethacrynic acid devoid of SH binding ability did not decrease lactate formation from fructose-1,6-diphosphate significantly. Ethacrynic acid did not inhibit lactate formation when 3-phosphoglyceric acid was the substrate used. These results suggest that the effect of ethacrynic acid on the glycolytic pathway is localized between the site of entry of fructose-1,6-diphosphate and the site of formation of 3-phosphoglyceric acid. On the other hand, addition of furosemide to cell-free preparations incubated with 3-phosphoglyceric acid resulted in a significant inhibition of lactate production (Klahr et al., 1973). These results suggest a different site and mode of action on glycolysis of these two diuretic agents. It has been shown by Klahr et al. (1971a) and Gordon and deHartog (1971) that ethacrynic acid inhibits the enzyme,

Table III. Effects of Increasing Concentrations of Ethacrynic Acid and Furosemide on Lactate Formation[a]

	Control	Lactate (μmol/ mg protein·hr) mean ± S.E.
Ethacrynic acid	601 ± 28	
0.5 mM		414 ± 8
1 mM		278 ± 25
10 mM		128 ± 6
Furosemide	513 ± 66	
1 mM		405 ± 72
5 mM		230 ± 56
10 mM		198 ± 21

[a] Membrane-free preparations of renal cortex were used. Fructose-1,6-diphosphate was used as substrate. Reproduced by permission from Klahr et al. (1973).

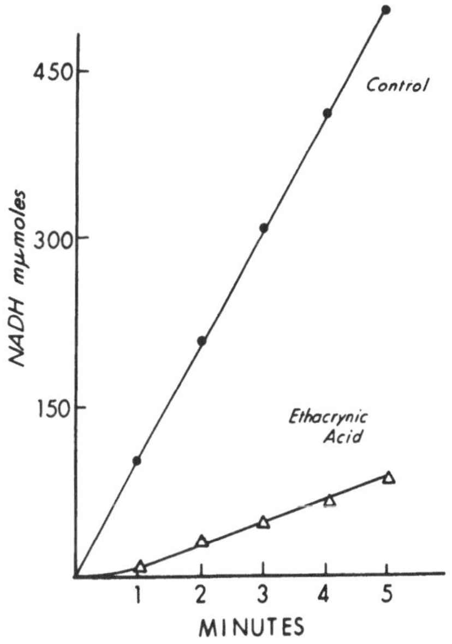

Figure 2. Inhibition of rabbit muscle glyceraldehyde-3-phosphate dehydrogenase by 1 m*M* ethacrynic acid. (Reproduced by permission from Klahr *et al.*, 1971b.)

glyceraldehyde-3-phosphate dehydrogenase, both from rabbit muscle and kidney cortex and medulla (Figure 2). Phosphoglycerate kinase activity is also inhibited but to a much lesser extent. Optimum inhibitory activity is observed when the inhibitor and the enzyme are brought together prior to assay, but preincubation is not essential to demonstrate inhibition. Gordon has presented evidence to suggest that ethacrynic acid inhibits glyceraldehyde-3-phosphate dehydrogenase by competing with or displacing NAD at a sulfhydryl site on the enzyme. Similar results have been obtained in Ehrlich ascites tumor cells (Gordon, 1968).

The preceding observations are of interest in view of the observations by Landon and Fitzpatrick (1969) that addition of membranes to membrane-free cytoplasmic preparations endowed with glycolytic activity resulted in a greater stimulation of the rate of glycolysis. The sole requirement for a maximal stimulation of glycolytic activity by the addition of membranes is the maintenance of ADP at levels of 0.5 m*M* or higher. The membrane stimulation of the glycolytic pathway occurred at the triosephosphate level. It apparently is the result of a specific coupling of two cytoplasmic enzymes in the glycolytic pathway and membranes. The two enzymes in the glycolytic pathway that are involved in such a coupling catalyze the conversion of 3-phosphoglyceraldehyde to 3-phosphoglycerate. In this reaction ATP is formed. This formation of ATP in the cytoplasma is coupled with the utilization of ATP by membrane systems. The reaction can be written as follows:

3-phosphoglyceraldehyde + Pi + NAD $\rightleftharpoons$
   1,3-diphosphoglycerate + NADH (glyceraldehyde phosphate dehydrogenase)

1,3-diphosphoglycerate + ADP $\rightleftharpoons$
                     3-phosphoglycerate + ATP (phosphoglycerate kinase)

         ATP $\rightleftharpoons$ ADP + Pi (membrane ATPase)

In the presence of membranes the equilibrium of the reaction is shifted in the direction of increased glycolysis. When coupled to the membrane, the reaction does not alter the levels of ADP or ATP. A portion of the membrane ATPase activity is inhibited by ouabain, and this ouabain sensitive ATPase system is apparently involved in the coupled transport of sodium and potassium across the plasma membrane. The observed coupling would then link sodium transport and glycolysis. A similar suggestion has been made by Parker and Hoffman (1967) in erythrocytes. An effect of ethacrynic acid at this site may be critical in terms of ATP supply from glycolysis to sodium transport.

Evidence has also accumulated suggesting that furosemide may inhibit glyceraldehyde-3-phosphate dehydrogenase (Klahr et al., 1971b; Yoshida and Metcoff, 1972). Furosemide apparently also inhibits another site in the glycolytic pathway located between pyruvate and lactate formation, presumably by inhibiting lactate dehydrogenase. It is of interest that both the glyceraldehyde-3-phosphate dehydrogenase step and the lactate dehydrogenase step involve the participation of NAD or NADH as cofactors. Therefore, the possibility exists that furosemide may inhibit glycolysis by affecting NAD–NADH concentrations. Indeed, it is of interest that incubation of NADH with furosemide resulted in the rapid disappearance of NADH measured either fluorometrically or spectrophotometrically (Klahr et al., 1973). Furthermore, it has been suggested recently by Zesch et al. (1969) that furosemide leads to a decrease in the renal content of reduced glutathion (GSH). The maximal GSH decrease coincided with the peak sodium excretion, and as the diuretic effect subsided GSH concentrations increased. Zesch et al., therefore, postulated that the reduction of renal GSH may be related to the natriuretic effect of furosemide. They suggested that the decrease in GSH was due to an inhibition in glutathion reductase by furosemide. These observations suggest that furosemide may affect the redox potential of cells.

Klahr et al. (1973) have also shown that injection of ethacrynic acid, into one renal artery in vivo, leads to decreased glycolysis by membrane-free homogenates of that kidney as compared to homogenates obtained from the contralateral noninjected kidney. However, when furosemide was injected intraarterially no effect of the drug on glycolysis, by membrane-free homogenates obtained from that kidney, was observed. On the other hand, Yoshida and Metcoff (1970, 1972) have demonstrated that the intravenous injection of 20 mg furosemide/kg body wt affected the concentrations of glycolytic intermediates in the kidney of the rat. These authors demonstrated a crossover point between triosephosphate and 1,3-diphosphoglyceric acid and therefore suggested that the intravenous injection of furosemide may inhibit glycolysis in the kidney by an effect at the level of glyceraldehyde-3-phosphate dehydrogenase.

Whether or not the inhibition of glycolysis observed in the presence of ethacrynic acid or furosemide plays a role in the natriuresis produced by these compounds is not clear. Recent studies designed to evaluate the effects of furosemide, ethacrynic acid, and iodoacetate administration on renal function and metabolism have been conducted in the perfused rat kidney (Bowman et al., 1973). When rat kidneys were perfused with furosemide and ethacrynic acid, both substances had diuretic and natriuretic activity at concentrations of $10^{-4} M$ and caused net secretion of potassium. There was a fall in glomerular filtration rate with both drugs, and ethacrynic acid caused marked glucose excretion when a moderately high concentration of the drug was employed. Concentrations of both drugs which were diuretically effective did not inhibit overall glycolysis in the perfused kidney (Table IV). Since this glycolytic evaluation did not completely rule out the possibility that glycolysis at localized sites may have been inhibited by the diuretics, sodium transport was also studied in kidneys which were perfused with a low level of iodoacetate. In spite of a demonstrable inhibition of glycolysis by iodoacetate, there was no increased sodium excretion. Bowman *et al.* (1973), therefore, concluded that the diuretic effects of furosemide and ethacrynic acid are not related to inhibition of renal glycolysis. Furthermore, in their studies inhibition of renal glycolysis with iodoacetate did not appear to greatly increase sodium excretion and to modify sodium reabsorption. These latter results are at variance with data obtained by others *in vivo* (Martinez-Maldonado *et al.*, 1970) and in the isolated perfused kidney of the rat (Besarab *et al.*, 1974).

F. Effects of Diuretics on Renal Gluconeogenesis

While gluconeogenesis from a number of substrates has been demonstrated in renal cortical slices incubated *in vitro* (Krebs *et al.*, 1963), no significant differences between arterial and renal venous blood glucose concentrations have been observed. Using normal unanesthetized dogs McCann and Jude (1958) were able to measure an increase in renal venous glucose over arterial concentrations of only 1.9 mg/100 ml. Steiner *et al.* (1968) and Roxe *et al.* (1970) reported even smaller values. On the other hand, data in eviscerated animals

Table IV. Metabolic Intermediates in Kidneys Perfused with Furosemide, Ethacrynic Acid, or Iodoacetate μmol/g dry wt[a]

	Control	Furosemide, 2 mM	Ethacrynic acid, 2 mM	Iodoacetate, 0.05 mM
Glucose-6-P	216 ± 15	238 ± 28	362 ± 18	220 ± 5
Fructose-1,6-diP	49 ± 3.3	43 ± 3	82 ± 4	285 ± 24
Triose-P	80 ± 9.1	118 ± 19	111 ± 41	248 ± 21
3-P-Glycerate	274 ± 39	318 ± 20	317 ± 42	776 ± 61
Phosphoenolpyruvate	58 ± 9.3	nm[b]	nm[b]	173 ± 26
Pyruvate	287 ± 14	196 ± 25	259 ± 34	271 ± 17
Lactate	2974 ± 350	4180 ± 740	4077 ± 621	1966 ± 204
Citrate	2054 ± 93	3135 ± 485	4268 ± 87	1765 ± 65
α-Ketoglutarate	3190 ± 192	2376 ± 239	376 ± 59	1433 ± 63
ATP	8420 ± 542	8190 ± 450	5050 ± 360	7924 ± 16

[a] Kidneys were rapidly frozen after 60 minutes of perfusion. Reproduced by permission from Bowman *et al.* (1973).
[b] nm = not measured.

suggest a large renal net glucose extraction (Reinecke and Hauser, 1948). The fact that there is renal extraction of glucose if [^{14}C]glucose is administered while there is no net extraction of unlabeled glucose across the kidney suggests that glucose may be used and at the same time be produced by the kidney simultaneously from other precursors. Fulgraff and his co-workers (1972) have studied the effects of wide concentration ranges of furosemide, ethacrynic acid, and chlorothiazide on glucose formation by rat kidney cortical slices. They measured the formation of glucose from fructose, pyruvate, lactate, and α-ketoglutarate. Studies were carried out at two pHs, pH 7.25 and 7.49, both with and without substrates. Furosemide stimulated the rate of gluconeogenesis in a concentration-dependent manner when fructose, pyruvate, or lactate were present as substrate. The percent increase in glucose formation was greater at pH 7.49, but the rates achieved with the maximal effective concentrations were about the same at both pH values. The rate of glucose formation was only slightly enhanced when the substrates used were malate and α-ketoglutarate. Ethacrynic acid enhanced the rate of glucose synthesis from fructose, pyruvate, and lactate but had no stimulating effects if malate or α-ketoglutarate were the substrates. The effects of ethacrynic acid were seen at lower concentrations than those required for furosemide, but the maximal rates which could be observed were in the same order of magnitude. On the other hand, chlorothiazide had no effect on gluconeogenesis. While ethacrynic acid increased glucose production from fructose up to a concentration of 10^{-6} M, higher concentrations of ethacrynic acid tended to depress gluconeogenesis.

The findings suggest that furosemide influences enzyme activities at such sites, that the reactions catalyzed by pyruvate carboxylase, phosphoenolpyruvate carboxykinase, and the enzymes proximal to the triosephosphates are accelerated. It is, nevertheless, somewhat unexpected that glucose synthesis from malate and α-ketoglutarate, which share the gluconeogenic pathway with the former substrates from oxaloacetate onwards, is influenced only to a minor degree since malate dehydrogenase is not considered to be a rate-limiting enzyme. The effect of furosemide on gluconeogenesis, however, may relate to the fact that this diuretic may inhibit the oxidation of glucose or its glycolysis and hence glucose formed will not be broken down through the glycolytic pathway or oxidized. In this context, it should be noted that furosemide inhibits glucose oxidation by renal cortex and medulla *in vitro* (Burck and Petruch, 1970) and reduces the activity of hexokinases especially in the medulla (Janata and Schuck, 1971; Janata and Lege, 1972a,b) and glyceraldehyde-3-phosphate dehydrogenase in cortex and medulla noncompetitively with NAD (Yoshida and Metcoff, 1972; Klahr *et al.*, 1973). The other possibility is that the effect of gluconeogenesis induced by furosemide is mediated by changes in the concentrations of certain regulatory substances such as ATP or cyclic AMP. Ethacrynic acid also increased gluconeogenesis, and the effects were similar to those obtained with furosemide when fructose, pyruvate, or lactate were present as substrates. Even concentrations of ethacrynic acid as small as 10^{-7} M stimulated glucose synthesis, and the maximal effective concentrations were lower than those required with furosemide. The percent increase was, however, in the same range with both substances. Similar comments to those used for furosemide can be applied to the possible mechanisms by which ethacrynic acid influences gluconeogenesis. Ethacrynic acid certainly decreases glycolysis and glucose oxidation. These effects may result in increased levels of glucose production from certain substrates if the glucose formed is not reutilized. Friedrichs and Schoner (1973) found only a 10–12% stimulation of renal gluconeogenesis from pyruvate with low concentration of ethacrynic acid or furosemide. Higher concentrations inhibited gluconeogenesis. The relation, if any, between these observations and the diuretic effect of these drugs is completely unclear.

G. Effects of Diuretics on Renal Adenyl Cyclase

Experiments reported recently by Ebel (1974) indicate that 1 mM furosemide and 1 mM ethacrynic acid inhibit adenyl cyclase in homogenates obtained from kidney cortex and inner medulla. On the other hand, amiloride was without any effect. Furosemide partially blocked the increased production of cyclic AMP induced by PTH, and ethacrynic acid had a more profound effect. Ethacrynic acid also blocked the increase in cyclic AMP produced by 0.1 mM isoproterenol. In inner medulla, furosemide partially blocked the effect of ADH on adenyl cyclase and ethacrynic acid had a profound inhibitory effect. Whether inhibition of renal adenyl cyclase by these drugs plays any role in their diuretic effect is unknown. However, increases rather than decreases in cyclic AMP have been shown to interfere with sodium reabsorption (Agus *et al.*, 1971).

H. A Synopsis of the Renal Metabolic Effects of Ethacrynic Acid, Furosemide, Mercurial Diuretics, and Thiazides

1. Ethacrynic Acid
   Main renal site of action: Thick ascending limb of Henle's loop
   Metabolic effects
      In vitro:
         1. Inhibits membrane transport ATPase
         2. Inhibits mitochondrial oxidative phosphorylation
         3. Inhibits glycolysis
         4. Inhibits sulfhydryl-enzyme systems (glyceraldehyde-phosphate dehydrogenase, succinic dehydrogenase, etc.)
         5. Inhibits or stimulates (?) renal gluconeogenesis (contradictory results may be dose related)
      In vivo:
         1. Decreases ratio of Na reabsorbed to oxygen consumed
         2. Inhibition of glycolysis?

2. Furosemide
   Main renal site of action: Thick ascending limb of Henle's loop
   Metabolic effects
      In vitro:
         1. Inhibits membrane transport ATPase

    2. Inhibits glycolysis (at higher concentrations than ethacrynic
acid)
    3. Inhibits respiration of kidney slices—mitochondrial effect?
    4. Inhibits carbonic anhydrase
    5. Decreases fatty acid uptake
    6. Effects on gluconeogenesis?
  In vivo:
    1. Decreases ratio of Na reabsorbed to oxygen consumed
    2. Inhibits carbonic anhydrase

3. Thiazide Diuretics

Main renal site of action: Diluting segment of Henle's loop—distal tubule
Metabolic effects
  In vitro:
    1. Varying degrees of inhibition of carbonic anhydrase
    2. Inhibits mitochondrial O_2 consumption?
    3. Inhibition of succinoxidase activity (high concentrations
       $2 \times 10^{-2} M$ to $2 \times 10^{-3} M$ required)
    4. Inhibition of phosphodiasterase
  In vivo:
    1. Decreases renal O_2 consumption with no change in the ratio of
Na reabsorbed to O_2 consumed
    2. Inhibition of carbonic anhydrase
    3. Decreases renal fatty acid uptake

4. Mercurial Diuretics

Main renal site of action: Thick ascending limb of Henle's loop
Metabolic effects
  In vitro:
    1. Inhibits O_2 uptake of kidney slices
    2. Inhibits membrane stimulation of cytoplasmic glycolysis
    3. Inhibits sulfhydryl-enzyme systems
    4. Inhibits mitochondrial respiration
  In vivo:
    1. No effect on the ratio of Na reabsorbed to O_2 consumed

IV. SUMMARY

    A large number of drugs capable of altering electrolyte reabsorption by the
kidney have been introduced in the last 15 years. In contrast to the relatively
advanced state of our knowledge regarding cellular mechanisms associated with
pharmacological action of drugs in other fields, the cellular reactions responsible
for diuresis remain obscure. In the present chapter we have attempted to present
the evidence for and against a possible action of diuretic agents on salt and water

reabsorption in the kidney tubule through their effects on metabolism. Not all the therapeutic agents used as diuretics have been discussed. This has been done on purpose since drugs such as spironolactones, amiloride, etc., probably work through mechanisms that do not involve primary metabolic alterations. On the other hand, the evidence emerging would suggest that the renal metabolic alterations produced by diuretic agents should be interpreted with caution. Since a tight coupling exists between ion transport and cell metabolism, many of the changes in renal metabolism observed after administration of diuretics could be secondary to alterations in ion transport. Most of the evidence for a primary metabolic effect of diuretics has been obtained with ethacrynic acid in *in vitro* systems. However, even in the case of this diuretic, recent evidence (Burg and Green, 1973b) suggests that this agent may inhibit ion reabsorption through an effect on permeability. Another word of caution regards the fact that most studies on the action of diuretics have concentrated on their potential effects on sodium transport. The recent data published by Burg and his colleagues would suggest that a primary effect of the potent diuretics now in use may be on the reabsorption of chloride. A discussion of this subject is presented elsewhere in this book. A unitarian concept for the action of diuretics may not always be possible, and some diuretics may block ion transport by a variety of mechanisms. At certain concentrations they may just produce an effect on permeability. However, administration of large doses of certain diuretics (ethacrynic acid, furosemide) may lead to metabolic effects that may result in increased diuretic potency of these agents. Obviously, not all the literature on the subject has been covered in this chapter, and some areas have been omitted for the sake of brevity and clarity. We hope to have provided the reader with some insight into the relationships between ion transport and metabolism and how diuretics affect such a relationship.

ACKNOWLEDGMENTS

The original work described in this chapter was supported by U.S.P.H.S. grant AM-09976.

The secretarial assistance of Mrs. Patricia Verplancke and Mrs. Patricia Persons is gratefully appreciated.

REFERENCES

Abodeely, D. A. and Lee, J. B. 1971. Fuel of respiration of outer renal medulla. *Am. J. Physiol.,* 220:1693.

Agus, Z. S., Puschett, J. B., Senesky, D., and Goldberg, M. 1971. Mode of action of parathyroid hormone and cyclic adenosine 3′,5′-monophosphate on renal tubular phosphate reabsorption in the dog. *J. Clin. Invest., 50:*617.

Aukland, K., Johannesen, J., and Kiil, F. 1969. In vivo measurements of local metabolic rate in the dog kidney. Effect of mersalyl, chlorothiazide, ethacrynic acid and furosemide. *Scand. J. Clin. Lab. Invest., 23:*317.

Barac-Nieto, M. and Cohen, J. J. 1968. Nonesterified fatty acid uptake by dog kidney: Effects of probenecid and chlorothiazide. *Am. J. Physiol., 215*:98.

Barac-Nieto, M. and Cohen, J. J. 1971. The metabolic fates of palmitate in the dog kidney in vivo. Evidence for incomplete oxidation. *Nephron, 8*:488.

Bernanke, D. and Epstein, F. H. 1965. Metabolism of the renal medulla. *Am. J. Physiol., 208*:541.

Besarab, A., Silva, P., and Epstein, F. H. 1974. Evidence for multiple sodium pumps in the isolated perfused rat kidney. *J. Clin. Invest., 53*:6a.

Beyer, K. H. and Baer, J. E. 1961. Physiological basis for the action of newer diuretic agents. *Pharmacol. Rev., 13*:517.

Boineau, F., King, V. F., Goldgeier, M., Strauss, W., and Balagura, S. 1974. Effects of furosemide on renal metabolism of lactate. *Kidney Int., 6*:25A.

Bowman, R. H., Dolgin, J., and Coulson, R. 1973. Furosemide, ethacrynic acid and iodoacetate on function and metabolism in perfused rat kidney. *Am. J. Physiol., 224*:416.

Brand, P. H., Cohen, J. J., and Bignall, M. C. 1974. Independence of lactate oxidation from net Na^+ reabsorption in dog kidney in vivo. *Am. J. Physiol., 227*:1255.

Burck, H. C. and Petruch, F. 1970. Atmungsänderung von Nierenschnitten unter Furosemid, *Klin. Wochensch., 48*:376.

Burg, M. and Green, N. 1973a. Function of the thick ascending limb of Henle's loop. *Am. J. Physiol., 224*:659.

Burg, M. and Green, N. 1973b. Effect of ethacrynic acid on the thick ascending limb of Henle's loop. *Kidney Int., 4*:301.

Burg, M. and Green, N. 1973c. Effect of mersalyl on the thick ascending limb of Henle's loop. *Kidney Int., 4*:245.

Burg, M., Stoner, L., Cardinal, J., and Green, N. 1973. Furosemide effect on isolated perfused tubules. *Am. J. Physiol., 225*:119.

Case, D. B., Gunther, S. J., and Cannon, P. J. 1973. Ethacrynate-induced depression of respiration in transport systems and kidney mitochondria. *Am. J. Physiol., 224*:769.

Chertok, R. J., Hulet, W. H., and Epstein, B. 1966. Effects of cyanide, amytol and DNP on renal sodium absorption. *Am. J. Physiol., 219*:978.

Chinard, F. P., Enns, T., and Nolan, M. F. 1962. Indicator dilution studies with diffusable indicators. *Circ. Res., 10*:473.

Cohen, J. J. and Barac-Nieto, M. 1973. Renal metabolism of substrates in relation to renal function. In: *Handbook of Physiology,* Section 8, Renal Physiology, pp. 909–927. Ed. by Orloff, J. and Berliner, R. W. American Physiological Society, Washington, D.C.

Deetjen, P. and Kramer, K. 1961. Die Abhängigkeit des O_2-Verbranchs der Niere von der Na Rukresorption. *Arch. Ges. Physiol., 273*:636.

DeJairala, S. W., Vieyra, A., and MacLaughlin, M. 1972. Influence of ethacrynic acid and ouabain on the oxygen consumption and potassium and sodium content of the kidney external medulla of the dog. *Biochim. Biophys. Acta, 279*:320.

Dickens, F. and Weil-Malherbe, H. 1936. Metabolism of normal and tumour tissue XIV. A note on the metabolism of kidney. *Biochem. J., 30*:659.

Dies, F., Herrera, J., Matos, M., Avelar, E., and Ramos, G. 1970a. Substrate uptake by the dog kidney in vivo. *Am. J. Physiol., 218*:405.

Dies, F., Ramos, G., Avelar, E., and Matos, M. 1970b. Relationship between renal substrate uptake and tubular sodium reabsorption in the dog. *Am. J. Physiol., 218*:411.

Ebel, H. 1974. Effects of diuretics on renal NaK-ATPase and adenyl cyclase. *Arch. Pharmacol., 281*:301.

Epstein, R. W. 1972. The effects of ethacrynic acid on active transport of sugars and ions and on other metabolic processes in rabbit kidney cortex. *Biochem. Biophys. Acta., 274*:128.

Fernandez, J., Capek, K., Heller, J., and Novakova, A. 1969. The effect of uncouplers of oxidative phosphorylation on sodium transport in the proximal renal tubule of the rat. *Experientia, 25*:125.

Friedrichs, D. and Schoner, W. 1973. Stimulation of renal gluconeogenesis by inhibition of the sodium pump. *Biochim. Biophys. Acta, 304*:142.

Fujimoto, M., Nash, F. D., and Kessler, R. H. 1964. Effects of cyanide, Q_{10} and dinitrophenol on renal sodium reabsorption and oxygen consumption. *Am. J. Physiol., 206*:1327.

Fulgraff, G. 1969. Effects of diuretics on the relation between oxygen consumption and sodium transport. In: *Proc. 4th Int. Congr. Nephrol.*, Vol. 2, pp. 119–126. Ed. by Alwall, N., Berglund, F., and Josephson, B. S. Karger, Basel.

Fulgraff, G., Nunemann, H., and Sudhoff, D. 1972. Effects of the diuretics furosemide, ethacrynic acid and chlorothiazide on gluconeogenesis from various substrates in rat kidney cortex slices. *Arch. Pharmacol., 273*:86.

Gaudemer, Y. and Foucher, B. 1967. Influence of sodium ethacrynate on some reactions involved in the mechanism of oxidative phosphorylation. *Biochim. Biophys. Acta, 131*:255.

Goldschmidt, D., Morelis, R., Gaudemer, Y., and Gautheron, D. 1970. The effect of ethacrynate on oxygen uptake and cation transport in rat liver mitochondria. *Bull. Soc. Chem. Biol., 52*:523.

Gordon, E. E. 1968. Site of ethacrynic acid action on Ehrlich ascites tumor cells. *Biochem. Pharmacol., 17*:1237.

Gordon, E. E. and deHartog, M. 1971. Localization and characterization of the inhibitory action of ethacrynic acid on glycolysis. *Biochem. Pharmacol., 20*:2339.

Grief, R. L. and Jacobs, G. S. 1958. Effect of mercurial diuretics upon oxidative phosphorylation in rat kidney mitochondria. *Am. J. Physiol., 192*:599.

Gyorgy, P., Keller, W., and Brehme, T. 1928. Nierenstoffwechsel und Nierenentwicklung. *Biochem. Z., 200*:356.

Gyory, A. Z. and Kinne, R. 1971. Energy sources for transepithelial sodium transport in rat proximal tubules. *Pfluegers Arch., 327*:234.

Heidenreich, O. 1969. Introductory remarks: Problems of the mode of action of diuretics on the cellular and subcellular level. In: *Proc. 4th Int. Congr. Nephrol.*, Vol. 2, pp. 116–118. Ed. by Alwall, N., Berglund, F., and Josephson, B. S. Karger, Basel.

Herms, W. and Malvin, R. L. 1963. Effects of metabolic inhibitors on urine osmolality and electrolyte excretion. *Am. J. Physiol., 204*:1065.

Hook, J. B. and Williamson, H. E. 1965. Influence of probenecid and alterations in acid–base balance on the saluretic activity of furosemide. *J. Pharmacol. Exp. Ther., 149*:404.

Janata, V. and Lege, L. 1972a. Metabolic investigations of the rat kidney after chronic administration of polythiazide, furosemide and ethacrynic acid. *Int. J. Clin. Pharmacol., 62*:125.

Janata, V. and Lege, L. 1972b. Metabolic investigations of the rat kidney after chronic administration of polythiazide, furosemide and ethacrynic acid. *Int. J. Clin. Pharmacol., 63*:214.

Janata, V. and Schuck, O. 1971. Metabolic investigations of the rat kidney after administration of polythiazide, furosemide and ethacrynic acid. I. Changes in carbohydrate metabolism in the cytoplasmic fraction of the renal cortex and medulla. *Int. Klin. Pharmakol. Ther. Toxikol., 4*:196.

Jones, V. D. and Landon, E. J. 1967. The effect of ouabain, meralluride and ethacrynic acid on respiration and glycolysis in kidney slices. *Biochem. Pharmacol., 16*:2163.

Kean, E. L., Adams, F. H., Winters, R. W., and Davies, H. E. 1961. Energy metabolism of the renal medulla. *Biochim. Biophys. Acta, 54*:474.

Kean, E. L., Adams, F. H., Davies, H. C., Winters, R. W., and Davies, R. E. 1962. Oxygen consumption and respiratory pigments of mitochondria of the inner medulla of the dog kidney. *Biochim. Biophys. Acta, 64*:503.

Kessler, R. H. 1969. The effects of glucose and inhibitory compounds on renal nucleotides in vivo. In: *Proc. 4th Int. Congr. Nephrol.*, Vol. 2, pp. 137–143. Ed. by Alwall, N., Berglund, F., and Josephson, B. S. Karger, Basel.

Kessler, R. H., Landwehr, D., Quintanilla, A., Weseley, S. A., Kaufman, W., Arcila, H. and Urbaitis, B. K. 1968. Effects of certain inhibitors on renal sodium reabsorption and ATP specific activity. *Nephron, 5*:474.

Kessler, R. H., Weinstein, S. W., Nash, F. D., and Fujimoto, M. 1964. Effects of chlormerodrin, *p*-chloromercuribenzoate and dichlorphenamide on renal sodium reabsorption and oxygen consumption. *Nephron, 1*:221.

Kiil, F., Aukland, K., and Refsum, H. E. 1961. Renal sodium transport and oxygen consumption. *Am. J. Physiol., 201*:511.

Kjekshus, J., Aukland, K., and Kiil, F. 1969. Oxygen cost of sodium reabsorption in proximal and distal parts of the nephron. *Scand. J. Clin. Lab. Invest., 23*:307.

Klahr, S., Bourgoignie, J., Yates, J., and Bricker, N. 1971a. Ethacrynic acid and furosemide: Metabolic effects independent of cation transport inhibition. In: *Proc. 1st Eur. Biophys. Congr., 3:*409.

Klahr, S., Yates, J., and Bourgoignie, J. 1971b. Inhibition of glycolysis by ethacrynic acid and furosemide. *Am. J. Physiol., 221:*1038.

Klahr, S., Bourgoignie, J., and Yates, J. 1973. Effects of ethacrynic acid and frusemide on renal metabolism. In: *Modern Diuretic Therapy in the Treatment of Cardiovascular and Renal Disease,* pp. 241–252. Ed. by Lant, A. F. and Wilson, G. M. Excerpta Medica, Amsterdam.

Knox, F. G., Fleming, J. S. and Rennie, D. W. 1966. Effects of osmotic diuresis on sodium reabsorption and oxygen consumption of kidney. *Am. J. Physiol., 210:*751.

Kramer, K. and Deetjen, P. 1960. Beziehungen des O_2-Verbranchs der Niere zu Durchblutung und Glomerulusfiltrat. *Arch. Ges. Physiol., 27:*782.

Krebs, H. A., Bennet, D. A. H., De Gasquet, P., Gascoyne, T., and Yoshida, T. 1963. Renal gluconeogenesis: The effect of diet on the gluconeogenic capacity of rat kidney cortex slices. *Biochem. J., 86:*22.

Krebs, H. A., Hems, R., Wiedemann, M. J., and Speake, R. N. 1966. The fate of isotopic carbon in kidney cortex synthesizing glucose from lactate. *Biochem. J., 101:*242.

Landon, E. J. and Fitzpatrick, D. F. 1969. The action of diuretics on respiration and glycolysis in the kidney. In: *Proc. 4th Int. Congr. Nephrol.,* Vol. 2, pp. 127–136. Ed. by Alwall, N., Berglund, F., and Josephson, B. S. Karger, Basel.

Landon, E. J. and Fitzpatrick, D. F. 1972. Ethacrynic-acid and kidney cell metabolism. *Biochem. Pharmacol., 21:*1561.

Landon, E. J. and Forte, L. R. 1971. Cellular mechanisms in renal pharmacology. *Ann. Rev. Pharmacol., 11:*171.

Lassen, N. A., Munck, O., and Thaysen, J. H. 1961. Oxygen consumption and sodium reabsorption in the kidney. *Acta Physiol. Scand., 51:*371.

Lee, J. B. and Peter, H. M. 1969. Effect of oxygen tension on glucose metabolism in rabbit kidney cortex and medulla. *Am. J. Physiol., 217:*1464.

Lee, J. B., Vance, V. K., and Cahill, G. F., Jr. 1962. Metabolism of C^{14} labelled substrates by rabbit kidney cortex and medulla. *Am. J. Physiol., 203:*27.

MacKnight, A. D. C. 1969. Effects of ethacrynic acid on the electrolyte and water contents of rat renal cortical slices. *Biochim. Biophys. Acta, 173:*223.

Martinez-Maldonado, M., Eknoyan, G., and Suki, W. N. 1969. Effects of cyanide on renal concentration and dilution. *Am. J. Physiol., 217:*1363.

Martinez-Maldonado, M., Eknoyan, G., and Suki, W. N. 1970. Importance of aerobic and anaerobic metabolism in renal concentration and dilution. *Am. J. Physiol., 218:*1076.

McCann, W. P. and Jude, J. R. 1958. The synthesis of glucose by the kidney. *Bull. Johns Hopkins Hosp., 103:*77.

Maunsbach, A. B. 1964. Effects of cyanide and iodoacetate on ultrastructure and electrical potential differences in Necturus proximal tubule cells. *Fed. Proc., 23:*545.

Metcoff, J. and Yoshida, T. 1971. Renal function and renal metabolism. *Pediat. Clin. N. Am., 18:*639.

Parker, J. C. and Hoffman, J. F. 1967. The role of membrane phosphoglycerate kinase in the control of glycolytic rate by active cation transport in human red blood cells. *J. Gen. Physiol., 50:*893.

Pitts, R. F. 1972. Metabolic fuels of the kidney. In: *Proc. 5th Int. Congr. Nephrol.,* Vol. 2, pp. 2–15. Ed. by Villarreal, H. S. Karger, Basel.

Pitts, R. F. 1974. Metabolism of the kidney. In: *Physiology of the Kidney and Body Fluids,* pp. 259–269. Year Book Medical Publishers, Chicago.

Podevin, R. A. and Boumendil-Podevin, E. F. 1972. Effects of temperature, medium K^+, ouabain and ethacrynic acid on transport of electrolytes and water by separated renal tubules. *Biochim. Biophys. Acta, 282:*234.

Reinecke, R. M. and Hauser, P. J. 1948. Renal gluconeogenesis in the eviscerated dog. *Am. J. Physiol., 153:*205.

Rocha, A. S. and Kokko, J. P. 1973. Sodium chloride and water transport in medullary thick ascending limb of Henle: Evidence for active chloride transport. *J. Clin. Invest., 52:*612.

Ross, B. D., Epstein, F.H., and Leaf, A. 1973. Sodium reabsorption in the perfused rat kidney. *Am. J. Physiol., 225:*1165.

Roxe, D. M., DiSalvo, J., and Balagura, S. 1970. Renal glucose production in the intact dog. *Am. J. Physiol., 218*:1676.

Sawa, H., Hyde, S., and Eknoyan, G. 1974. Effect of diuretics on isolated rat kidney mitochondria. *Kidney Int., 6*:92A.

Schatzman, H. J., Windhager, E. E., and Solomon, A. K. 1958. Single proximal tubules of *Necturus* kidney. *J. Gen. Physiol., 44*:659.

Schurek, H. J., Lohfert, H., and Hierholzer, K. 1970. Na-Resorption in der isoliert perfundierten Rattenniere (Abhängigkeit von Substrangebot und Na-load). *Arch. Ges. Physiol., 319:*R85.

Singer, M. A. 1974. Effects of furosemide and ethacrynic acid on cation transport across phospholipid bilayer membranes. *Can. J. Physiol. Pharmacol., 52*:930.

Steiner, A. L., Goodman, A. D., and Treble, D. H. 1968. Effect of metabolic acidosis on renal gluconeogenesis in vivo. *Am. J. Physiol., 215*:211.

Steinmetz, P. R. 1974. Cellular mechanisms of urinary acidification. *Physiol. Rev., 54*:890.

Strickler, J. C. and Kessler, R. H. 1963. Effects of certain inhibitors on renal excretion of salt and water. *Am. J. Physiol., 205*:117.

Suki, W. N., Eknoyan, G., and Martinez-Maldonado, M. 1973. Tubular sites and mechanisms of diuretic action. *Annu. Rev. Pharmacol., 13*:91.

Thaysen, J. H., Lassen, N. A., and Munck, O. 1960. Sodium transport and oxygen consumption in the mammalian kidney. *Excerpta Med., 29*:44.

Thurau, K. 1961. Renal Na-reabsorption and O_2 uptake in dogs during hypoxia and hydrochlorothiazide infusion. *Proc. Soc. Exp. Biol. Med., 106*:714.

Trimble, M. E. and Bowman, R. H. 1973. Renal Na^+ and K^+ transport: Effects of glucose, palmitate and α-bromopalmitate. *Am. J. Physiol., 225*:1057.

Ussing, H. H. and Zerahn, K. 1951. Active transport of sodium as the source of electric current in short-circuited isolated frog skin. *Acta Physiol. Scand., 23:*110.

Ussing, H. H., Kruhoffer, P., Thaysen, J. H., and Thorn, N. A. 1960. Alkali metal ions in biology. In: *Handbuch der Experimentellen Pharmakologie*, pp. 260–261. Ed. by Eichler, O. and Farah, A. Springer-Verlag, Berlin.

Washington, J. A., II and Holland, J. M. 1966. Urine oxygen tension: Effects of osmotic and saline diuresis and of ethacrynic acid. *Am. J. Physiol., 210*:243.

Weidemann, M. J. and Krebs, H. A. 1969. The fuel of respiration of rat kidney cortex. *Biochem. J., 112*:149.

Weinstein, S. W. 1970. Proximal tubular energy metabolism, sodium transport and permeability in the rat. *Am. J. Physiol., 219*:978.

Weinstein, S. W. and Klose, R. M. 1969. Micropuncture studies on energy metabolism and sodium transport in the mammalian nephron. *Am. J. Physiol., 217*:498.

Weinstein, S. W. and Szyjewicz, J. 1974. Individual nephron function and renal oxygen consumption in the rat. *Am. J. Physiol., 227*:171.

Weinstein, E., Manitius, A., and Epstein, F. H. 1969. The importance of aerobic metabolism in the renal concentrating process. *J. Clin. Invest., 48*:1855.

Windhager, E. E. and Giebisch, G. 1961. Comparison of short circuit current and net water movement in single perfused proximal tubules of rat kidney. *Nature, 191*:1205.

Wolf, K., Bieg, A., and Fulgraff, G. 1969. On the mode of action of diuretics II. Effects of ethacrynic acid on renal oxygen consumption and tubular sodium reabsorption in dogs. *Eur. J. Pharmacol., 7*:342.

Yoshida, A., Yamada, T., and Koshikawa, S. 1971. Effect of diuretics on energy metabolism. *Biochem. Pharmacol., 20*:1933.

Yoshida, T. and Metcoff, J. 1970. Inhibition of furosemide of glyceraldehyde-3-phosphate dehydrogenase step in rat kidney. *Proc. Am. Soc. Nephrol., 4*:88.

Yoshida, T. and Metcoff, J. 1972. Furosemide inhibits renal glyceraldehyde-3-phosphate dehydrogenase (GA3PDH) and redox potential during natriuresis in the rat. *Fed. Proc., 31*:331.

Zerahn, K. 1956. Oxygen consumption and active sodium transport in the isolated and short-circuited frog skin. *Acta Physiol. Scand., 36*:300.

Zesch, A., Senft, G., and Losert, W. 1969. Biochemical studies on mechanisms of compounds influencing tubular Na^+ transport: II. 6-Aminonicotinamide, furosemide. In: *Progress in Nephrology* pp. 275-280. Ed. by Peters, G. and Roch-Ramel, F. Springer-Verlag, Berlin.

Chapter **7**

Renal ATPase as a Receptor for Drugs Acting on the Kidney

Manuel Martinez-Maldonado

Departments of Medicine and Physiology
University of Puerto Rico School of Medicine
and
Veterans Administration Center
San Juan, Puerto Rico 00936

and

Arnold Schwartz

Department of Cell Biophysics
Baylor College of Medicine
Houston, Texas 77025

I. INTRODUCTION

The search for the biochemical basis of active sodium transport was advanced decisively by the discovery of Na^+–K^+ ATPase by Skou (1957). Subsequent identification of this enzyme system in cell membranes from numerous organs (Skou, 1964, 1965) solidified the contention of its importance in cation transport. Early findings of its presence in kidney (Bonting *et al.*, 1961; Kinsolving *et al.*, 1963) led to considerable investigative activity and partial elucidation of its role in active cation transport in this organ. Of great interest is the possibility that renotropic drugs and hormones may exert at least some of their renal effects through an action on the enzyme system. The purpose of this discussion is to review the evidence for the Na^+–K^+ ATPase as a receptor or "intermediary" in the mechanism of action of drugs and hormones and its relation to the regulation of ion and water transport by the kidney.

II. EVIDENCE FOR ROLE IN SODIUM TRANSPORT

A. Pharmacological Studies

Early indirect evidence was accrued from the effect of cardiac glycosides on renal function (Farber *et al.*, 1951; Hyman *et al.*, 1956, Strickler and Kessler, 1961). These agents were shown by Skou to be specific inhibitors of the sodium plus potassium activated enzyme (Skou, 1957, 1960). The inhibition by cardiac glycosides of Na^+-K^+ ATPase was found to be universal and independent of the cellular origin of the enzyme. In various species the infusion of ouabain, or other active cardiac glycosides, results in an increase in water and electrolyte excretion. A direct tubular effect in dogs and chickens was clearly established by a number of investigators (Wilde and Howard, 1960; Orloff and Burg, 1960; Cade *et al.*, 1961). Evidence to this effect in man has also been obtained (Farber *et al.*, 1951; Hyman *et al.*, 1956). A tubular action has also been demonstrated in rats (Duarte *et al.*, 1971; Strieder *et al.*, 1974), snakes, and other amphibians (Schatzmann *et al.*, 1958; Dantzler, 1974).

More recently simultaneous reports from three different laboratories (Martinez-Maldonado *et al.*, 1969; Hook, 1969; Nelson and Nechay, 1970) demonstrated that in the dog, the natriuresis which follows ouabain or digoxin administration into one renal artery correlates with the degree of inhibition of Na^+-K^+ ATPase isolated from the perfused dog kidney. Furthermore, the *in vitro* binding of radioactive cardiac glycosides to the Na^+-K^+ ATPase isolated from kidneys infused *in vivo* with the drug is reduced proportionally to the degree of inhibition present, suggesting that the enzyme is a pharmacological receptor for the glycosides (Allen *et al.*, 1971).

Measurement of renal metabolic rates by heat accumulation techniques has shown that ouabain reduces metabolism in both cortex and medulla, while leading to a significant natriuresis (Sejersted *et al.*, 1971). Evidence that these events are causally related was obtained in additional studies by demonstrating that ethacrynic acid, which led to a natriuresis comparable to that observed with ouabain, also reduced metabolic rates to the same levels as ouabain (Lie *et al.*, 1974).

Direct evidence for a renal effect of cardiac glycosides in some species comes from studies with isolated tubular segments. In proximal tubules and collecting ducts of rabbits and snakes, ouabain abolishes the normally present transtubular potential gradient (Grantham *et al.*, 1970; Burg and Orloff, 1970; Kokko *et al.*, 1971; Imai and Kokko, 1974). A similar result has been observed in isolated perfused rabbit ascending limb (Rocha and Kokko, 1973; Burg and Green, 1973).

Other pharmacological agents (diuretic agents are discussed later) have also implicated the Na^+-K^+ ATPase system in renal reabsorptive functions. The administration of maleic acid to rats produces an experimental Fanconi syndrome, manifested by proteinuria, glucosuria, and aminoaciduria due to inhibition of proximal tubular function. This is associated with inhibition of Na^+-K^+ ATPase in cortical tissue (Kramer and Gonick, 1973). Furthermore, maleic acid has been shown to inhibit Na^+–K^+ ATPase activity in homogenates prepared from frog skin tissue (Kramer and Burgard, 1974), suggesting (if we can extrapolate to mammalian preparations) that the general disturbance of proximal reabsorption seen in rats may indeed be the result of enzyme inhibition. Whether the observed changes in glucose and amino acid reabsorption in experimental Fanconi syndrome are secondary to alterations in Na^+ transport is not clear. An effect on glucose reabsorption *in vivo* by cardiac glycosides has not been shown conclusively. In the dog, Kupfer and Kosovsky (1965) failed to find increased glucose excretion or any effect on glucose *Tm*. On the other hand, utilizing a "heartless" dog preparation, Czáky and his collaborators (1964) were able to show that ouabain inhibited renal glucose reabsorption. Further studies on this point are clearly needed. *In vitro* data do suggest, however, that ouabain interferes with glucose transport (Gordon, 1965). Studies of cortical or medullary kidney slices of adult female rats showed that net glucose uptake by both cortex and medulla are significantly inhibited by ouabain at concentrations of 10^{-3} and 10^{-5} M, respectively. Metabolism of $[^{14}C]$glucose to $[^{14}C]CO_2$ by cortex and medulla was also depressed by ouabain at concentrations of 10^{-4} M and 10^{-5} M, respectively. Respiration, however, was affected only at the highest concentrations of ouabain used. Lithium and choline, replacing sodium in the medium, abolished the effects of 10^{-4} M ouabain, yet significant inhibition of metabolism of $[^{14}C]$glucose to $[^{14}C]CO_2$ by cortex persisted in the lithium and choline media. Incubation of the tissues in standard medium in a nitrogen atmosphere abolished the effects of ouabain that were observed in an aerobic atmosphere suggesting that Na^+-dependent active glucose transport occurs.

Although data exist from both *in vivo* and *in vitro* experiments, the relationship between overall sodium and amino acid transport and Na^+–K^+ ATPase is beyond the scope of this discussion.

B. Physiological Studies

Important evidence that the enzyme system participates in the regulation of renal electrolyte transport was advanced by Katz and Epstein (1967). Unilateral nephrectomy in rats, which leads to increased filtered load and total reabsorption in the remaining kidney, resulted in a significant increase in the "specific activity" of Na^+–K^+ ATPase isolated from the remaining kidney. This was attributed to an enhancement of Na^+ movement through the "pump." Other membrane-bound enzymes and Mg^{2+} ATPase were not altered, indicating that the increase in activity was specific for Na^+–K^+ ATPase. Furthermore, bilateral adrenalectomy which reduces filtered load and absolute reabsorption prevented the adaptative elevation in enzyme activity. It should be pointed out that $[^3H]$ ouabain binding studies were not performed in these experiments, precluding the conclusion that "pump" sites may have increased along the nephron. The relationship between filtered and reabsorbed load may well be a major determinant of the activity of the enzyme *in vivo*. Nechay and Nelson (1970) found a significant relationship between filtered load and enzyme activity in dogs, suggesting that enzyme activity reflects the level of *total* sodium reabsorptive capacity of the kidney.

Fanestil (1968), on the other hand, examined the relationships among (1) compensatory enlargement, (2) excretory load, (3) excreting renal tissue (kidney tissue which produces urine actually excreted from the animal), and (4) functional renal mass (kidney tissue which produces urine, part of which is excreted and part of which is reabsorbed as a result of surgical manipulation). For this last group rats in which part of a ureter had been excised (unilaterally hydronephrotic and unilaterally nephrectomized rats) were utilized in addition to a control sham-operated group. No change in Mg^{2+} ATPase activity (ouabain insensitive) was detected in any of the groups as compared to control. Animals with only 50% excretory capacity but normal functional renal mass had normal $Na^+–K^+$ ATPase and normal renal weight. In contrast, those animals which had decreased functional mass, the hydronephrotic and nephrectomized groups, developed compensatory renal enlargement and increased $Na^+–K^+$ ATPase activities. It was not possible from these experiments to dissociate compensatory renal enlargement from induction of $Na^+–K^+$ ATPase. Both compensatory renal enlargement and induction of $Na^+–K^+$ ATPase seemed to be related to the mass of functional renal tissue rather than to the mass of excreting renal tissue remaining in the animal. One rationalization of those results is that the apparent induction of $Na^+–K^+$ ATPase is not the result of a shift of the excretory load to a single kidney but rather a shift of metabolic demands to that organ. However, renal function studies were not performed, so a relationship between sodium reabsorption and renal ATPase cannot be ruled out.

Studies of selective postnatal development of $Na^+–K^+$ ATPase in rabbit renal heavy microsomal fraction have also yielded evidence for a physiological role of the enzyme in renal transport (Davis and Dixon, 1971). Total ATPase and $Na^+–K^+$ ATPase increased gradually with age from newborn to adult. Magnesium-dependent ATPase, however, remained essentially unchanged and equivalent to the adult levels at all ages. $Na^+–K^+$ ATPase was essentially absent at birth and at 5 weeks of age approached levels comparable to those of the adult. This observed rise in ATPase was accounted for by the selective increase in the $Na^+–K^+$-activated component. These changes correlate well with the reported maturation of the renal transport mechanisms for amino acids, PAH, and sodium ion during the perinatal period. These observations on the development of the rabbit kidney before 5 weeks of age are comparable to the results obtained in the rat. During normal growth in male rats, 3 weeks to 3 months of age, the rate of increase in kidney weight and GFR are the same and the ratio of GFR to gram kidney weight is constant after 4–5 weeks of age (Potter *et al.*, 1969). The ratio of maximal glucose reabsorption (TM_G) to GFR increases only slightly with growth. $Na^+–K^+$ ATPase activity per mg light microsomal protein from kidney cortex and oxygen consumption do not change during growth. These results suggest that in the rat maturation of $Na^+–K^+$ ATPase has reached a maximum by the third week of life, a finding which is temporally comparable to that seen in the rabbit.

The acute and chronic effects of changes in sodium load on renal $Na^+–K^+$

ATPase have also been examined. The effect of changes in dietary sodium on renal Na^+–K^+ ATPase activity has been examined by Paul and Gonick (1968). Studies of enzyme preparations from rats on normal and low salt intake failed to demonstrate any difference in ATPase activity between the two groups. The observed results may be the consequence of the fact that near maximal Na^+–K^+ ATPase activity is present under conditions of normal aldosterone production and excretion. Stimulation of aldosterone production (see Section VI) by a low Na^+ intake might then result in a small increase in Na^+–K^+-activated ATPase which is physiologically important to the organism but not detectable by the methodology utilized in these experiments.

   Katz and Genant (1971) have presented data suggesting that acute volume expansion by isotonic saline infusions increases renal medullary Na^+–K^+ ATPase specific activity while simultaneously decreasing cortical Na^+–K^+ ATPase specific activity. These changes are difficult to reconcile with studies from our laboratory. As shown in Table I, in collaboration with Allen, we were unable to demonstrate changes in either cortical or medullary Na^+–K^+ ATPase isolated from dogs which had undergone acute volume expansion with hypertonic saline. This is despite the fact that in our studies distal sodium reabsorption was most likely higher than that observed by Katz and Genant (1971). Both of these studies, which address themselves to important physiological questions (the role of the enzyme in modulating short- and long-term changes in total body sodium), require further analysis.

   An interesting finding pertaining to the possible role of the enzyme in renal sodium reabsorption is the distribution of activity throughout the nephron. In a technically sophisticated series of studies Schmidt and Dubach (1969; Schmidt *et al.*, 1975) demonstrated that the distal nephron has the highest enzyme activity. Most important was the fact that the greatest percentage of the whole nephron enzyme activity is in the ascending limb of the loop of Henle, particularly the

Table I. Effects of Hypertonic Saline Infusion on Renal Na^+–K^+ ATPase Activity[a]
(n = 6)

	Control kidney	Experimental kidney
A. Na^+–K^+ ATPase activity (μmol Pi/mg protein·hr)		
Cortex	28.2 ± 3.4	28.5 ± 3.2
Medulla	60.4 ± 10.4	61.3 ± 11.1
B. Sodium handling		
Filtered load	4260 ± 135	5248 ± 162
Fractional excretion	1.1 ± 0.3	7.5 ± 1.2

[a] Mean ± S.E. Control values for sodium handling were obtained from both control and experimental kidneys in hydropenic conditions and the values were not different from those shown above for control kidney. The right control kidney was then removed and processed for enzyme isolation and assay as described by Martinez-Maldonado *et al.* (1969, 1970, 1972). An infusion of 2% sodium chloride solution was administered until a volume equalling 5% of body weight was infused. At that point the remaining kidney was removed for Na^+–K^+ ATPase isolation and assay as above.

thick portion. The physiological meaning of this finding has been the subject of debate. A possible explanation may be related to the function of the thick ascending limb. This nephron segment, which may be the most important final regulator of renal sodium excretion, has the capacity to raise its sodium reabsorptive capabilities as the load of NaCl reaching it rises. It is possible that this reabsorptive capacity results from the high enzyme content of this particular nephron segment. Another possibility initially proposed by Martinez-Maldonado and co-workers (1969, 1970) is that sodium chloride transport takes place against a steeper NaCl gradient in the thick ascending limb than in any other portion of the nephron, since urea contributes little to interstitial osmolality in this region. This is the case whether sodium is transported from lumen to interstitium or from cell interior to interstitium. Were the former the case, from the point in the medulla where intraluminal fluid becomes isotonic to plasma to the point where it exits into the distal convolution as hypotonic fluid, all NaCl transport would be against a steeper gradient than anywhere else in the nephron. Should transport occur exclusively from cell interior to interstitium, the gradient would be even steeper if cells in the outer medulla contain the same Na^+ concentration as proximal tubular cells. To sustain intracellular composition their transport capacity would have to be greater. This proposal appears to us worthy of strong consideration and experimental testing. It is also of interest that in the eel (*Amphiuma*), enzyme activity is also highest in the distal nephron (Hendler *et al.*, 1971). Since loops of Henle do not exist in this species, distal nephron reabsorption may be the ultimate determinant of sodium excretion.

Another possibility should be considered. Studies of the isolated rabbit ascending limb of Henle's loop have shown that the luminal side is positively charged, indicating predominant active chloride reabsorption across the tubular membrane (Rocha and Kokko, 1973; Burg and Green, 1973). Such a pump would facilitate passive flux of Na^+ into the cell but should not be regarded as an alternative to a peritubular pump. Most of the tubular energy is probably required for transport of Na^+ against the steep electrochemical gradient over the peritubular membrane where most of the ATPase activity is located. Therefore, increases in the intracellular sodium concentration might stimulate the enzyme. As mentioned before, in view of the sodium reabsorption capacity of the thick ascending limb of Henle, the presence of a Na^+-dependent pump would make it well suited for ultimate regulation of Na^+ transport. If loop cells are similar to red blood cell ghosts (Whittam, 1962), a rise in intracellular Na^+ concentration in the cells of the loop would increase the activity of Na^+–K^+ ATPase and stimulate the outward transport of Na^+; this in turn could account for distal regulation of Na^+ transport and free-water generation. Intraluminal Na^+ concentration falls along the poorly water-permeable ascending limb. Any rise in the delivery of isotonic fluid from the proximal tubules would tend to increase Na^+ concentration along the ascending limb of Henle's loop and raise the passive influx into the cells. In addition, the luminal chloride pump might be activated. A rise in intracellular Na^+ concentration could augment the activity of Na^+–K^+ ATPase and increase Na^+ reabsorption and free-water generation.

An explanation for the differences in specific activity of enzyme isolated from cortex and medulla must lie in some factor determining the characteristic physiological functions of the thick limb since enzyme preparations isolated from cortex and medulla are biochemically similar (Nechay, 1974). Within species, the K_m for Mg^{2+} ATP and Na^+ are identical for enzyme prepared from cortex and medulla and follow similar *in vivo* and *in vitro* biochemical–physiological interrelationships in response to cardiac glycosides (Hendler *et al.*, 1971). Other biochemical characteristics correlate well with physiological observations. Thus in the rat, in which ouabain is a poor diuretic, the I_{50} of ouabain for the renal microsomal enzyme preparation is $6 \times 10^{-3} M$ as compared to $1.6 \times 10^{-6} M$ for canine kidney (which responds to ouabain with a massive natriuresis) when measured under identical conditions (Nechay, 1974).

One conceptual difficulty in relating Na^+–K^+ ATPase to sodium transport by the kidney comes from its close biochemical resemblance to transport ATPase in the human erythrocyte. In red cells, the stoichiometry of the Na^+–K^+ exchange takes place in a 1:1 or 3:2 ratio but must be clearly different in the case of urine dilution (Epstein and Silva, 1974). In isolated rabbit proximal tubule fragments the influx of K^+ is only 1/10 the efflux of Na^+, making it difficult to have a clear understanding of how K^+ is handled in relation to Na^+ and the ATPase system in the renal tubule (Burg and Abramow, 1966; Burg and Orloff, 1966). It may be that the Na^+–K^+ ATPase function in the kidney is the coupled transport of Na^+ and Cl^- instead of Na^+ and K^+. As already alluded to, it is interesting that careful tubular dissection studies (Schmidt and Dubach, 1971) have demonstrated that the enzyme activity is limited to the contraluminal surface of the tubule where active reabsorption of Na^+ is thought to occur. Another piece of circumstantial evidence in favor of important overall Na^+ transport function for Na^+–K^+-ATPase is the low enzyme activity in thin limbs of Henle in the papilla (Bonting *et al.*, 1961; Hendler *et al.*, 1971; Schmidt and Dubach, 1969, 1970; Martinez-Maldonado *et al.*, 1969) which could explain the presence of little or no active reabsorption in this nephron segment (Imai and Kokko, 1974).

C. Biochemical Properties

In recent years four laboratories have reported procedures for the purification of the Na^+–K^+ ATPase: Kyte (1971), Jørgensen *et al.* (1971), and Lane *et al.* (1973) from the outer medulla of mammalian kidney, Hokin *et al.* (1973) from the rectal gland of *Squalus acanthias,* and Dixon and Hokin (1974) from the electric organ of *Electrophorus.* The Na^+–K^+ ATPase fractions prepared by these procedures are quite similar. All are insoluble and consist of a 95,000-dalton protein which is phosphorylated by $[\gamma$-$^{32}P]$ATP in the presence of magnesium and sodium, a glycoprotein of approximately 50,000 daltons, and various lipids. The specific activities of the preparations vary from 10–37 μmol Pi/min mg, with virtually all of the activity inhibitable by ouabain. Three of the preparations have been reported to bind between 3 and 5.7 nmol ouabain/mg protein (Lane *et al.*, 1973; Kyte, 1972a; Jørgensen, 1974a).

To date, the glycoprotein has not been shown to have any catalytic function, and it is not yet known whether it is, in fact, a subunit of the Na^+-K^+ ATPase. The molar ratio of the glycoprotein to the phosphorylatable-protein varies from 0.5 to 1.0 to 2.0 (Kyte, 1972b; Lane *et al.*, 1973; Hokin *et al.*, 1973) in the above preparations, but Kyte (1972b) has suggested that since the two proteins can be covalently cross-linked by dimethylsuberimadate that they must be close to one another in the membrane.

Hokin *et al.* (1973) report that their purified Na^+-K^+ ATPase from rectal gland can exist in the form of vesicles, rods, or rings. The rods are approximately 80 Å in diameter, with projecting knobs of 35–55 Å in diameter. They have suggested that the smaller-diameter projections may be the glycoprotein component.

The *in vivo* function of the Na^+-K^+-ATPase, i.e., the sodium pump, would require the enzyme to traverse the plasma membrane and to have receptor sites on both the interior and exterior surfaces of the membrane. Kepner and Macey (1966), based on their radiation inactivation studies, have calculated a diameter of 85 Å for the Na^+-K^+ ATPase which suggests that the enzyme is large enough to span the membrane. In addition, Ruoho and Kyte (1974) have reported that the larger peptide, which is known to be phosphorylated by ATP (a reaction occurring at the interior surface), can be covalently labeled with an ethyldiazomalonyl derivative of the cardiac glycoside cymarin. Since the cardiac glycoside binding site on the sodium pump is known to be on the exterior surface of the cell membrane, it appears that the larger polypeptide of the Na^+-K^+ ATPase does traverse the plasma membrane.

The final proof that the Na^+-K^+ ATPase is the *in vitro* analog of the sodium pump is the reconstitution of sodium transport from the purified Na^+-K^+ ATPase. Recently, two groups have reported the reconstitution of sodium transport activity in liposomes prepared from phospholipids and cholate-solubilized purified Na^+-K^+ ATPase. Goldin and Tong (1974) first reported the reconstitution of an ATP-dependent, ouabain-inhibitable sodium transport from dog kidney medulla Na^+-K^+ ATPase. However, instead of a countertransport of potassium, the authors found that chloride was either actively pumped or was translocated along with the sodium. Sweadner and Goldin (1975) later found that when a crude dog brain Na^+-K^+ ATPase fraction was incorporated into similar liposomes both sodium and potassium were transported, in a ratio of 3 sodium to 1.8 potassium. Hilden *et al.* (1974; Hilden and Hokin, 1975) have also reported the reconstitution of sodium and potassium transport activity with liposomes prepared similarly from phospholipids and the purified rectal gland Na^+-K^+ ATPase.

It may be that the enzyme in its native state in renal medulla, in contrast to other organs, may not couple pumping of Na^+ to K^+, but instead translocates Na^+ along with Cl^-.

III. IMPORTANCE OF ISOLATION PROCEDURES

Biochemical studies of the properties and characteristics of the enzyme require that the preparation be as pure as possible. The "purity" of the preparation will in turn depend on the methodology of isolation and treatment (Schwartz *et al.*, 1975). These procedures will determine the activity of the enzyme preparation obtained. It is, therefore, necessary to compare the methodology of enzyme isolation and assay conditions when attempting to interpret different studies relating enzyme activity to physiological function. In the rabbit for example, as in the case of canine kidney, different preparations will have different specific activities (Jørgensen and Skou, 1969; Jørgensen, 1974a–c). This also implies that, conceivably, the pharmacological changes induced by cardiac glycosides, hormones, etc., regardless of the dose administered, may be limited or exaggerated by the "purity" of the enzyme preparation isolated for assay. The functional complexity of the kidney may preclude the demonstration of "complete" inhibition of the enzyme when cardiac glycosides or other agents are administered or withdrawn "*in vivo*" or in isolated kidney preparations. It is critical to show, particularly after administration of drugs, what changes, if any, are brought about by examining enzyme preparations of different degrees of purity.[1]

Hokin (1974) has attempted to purify Na^+-K^+ ATPase in order that its biologically active form be available to perform physical and biological studies on the purified molecule. Most efforts of partial purification of the Na^+-K^+ ATPase have attempted to extract impurities with detergents or high salt concentrations from membrane fractions which would yield membrane fragments enriched in Na^+-K^+ ATPase (Hokin, 1974). Hokin's attempt at purification has been based on methodology which pursues solubilization of the enzyme with a noninactivating nonionic detergent (Lubrol WX) and purification of the Na^+-K^+ ATPase starting with the soluble form. Two criteria have been utilized in assessing the purity of a membrane-bound enzyme: (1) specific activity and, (2) polyacrylamide-gel patterns. Both of these are subject to pitfalls in applying specific activity as a criterion for purity, since consideration must be given to activations or inactivations by detergents. In applying polyacrylamide-gel patterns one must take into account the resolving power of the particular gel electrophoresis system.

These procedures may ultimately be necessary in studies attempting to correlate physiological and pharmacological data. It may not be sufficient to have "internal" controls, comparison, let us say, between control and medullary enzyme preparation of right vs. left kidney, but rather isolation procedures which are comparable to those utilized in previous work. The use of detergents in isolation is of particular importance and must be emphasized since the activity measured afterward may represent greater levels than that operative *in vivo*. Purification of the enzyme may eventually provide the answer as to the specific mechanism by which hormones, cardiac glycosides, and other agents inhibit the enzyme.

---

[1] For detailed discussion of isolation procedures and the biochemical characteristics of these preparations the reader is referred to the review by Schwartz, Lindenmayer, and Allen, *Pharmacol. Rev.* 27:3–134, 1975.

IV. INTERACTIONS BETWEEN CARDIAC GLYCOSIDES AND RENAL ATPase

Early studies by Strickler and Kessler (1961) and Cade and co-workers (1961) in the dog and Orloff and Burg (1960) in the chicken established that cardiac glycosides were saluretic and that they probably acted from the basal side of the cell. Initial attempts to establish the site of action of cardiac glycosides in the nephron led to the general suggestion that their primary effect is in the "distal nephron" (Wilde and Howard, 1960). As these results were obtained from stop-flow studies, more precise localization was not possible. Clearance studies in the dog have provided evidence that a major site of action of cardiac glycosides is the ascending limb of Henle's loop (Martinez-Maldonado et al., 1969, 1970, 1972). From the marked rise in distal delivery of fluid it was inferred that a proximal tubular effect also occurred as a result of cardiac glycoside administration (Martinez-Maldonado et al., 1970). More direct evidence for an effect in both the proximal tubule and the ascending limb of Henle's loop comes from miropuncture and isolated tubular segment experiments (Schatzmann et al., 1958; Rocha and Kokko, 1973; Burg and Green, 1973; Györi et al., 1972). It is of interest that in dog the natriuretic effect of cardiac glycosides and the ATPase inhibition have been shown to last for days (Nelson and Nechay, 1970). By contrast, in the isolated tubule of rabbits the inhibitory effect of ouabain is reversible within minutes of application (Chapter 2), suggesting that this species, like the rat, is relatively insensitive to cardiac glycosides (Allen and Schwartz, 1969). Most likely the enzyme–drug complex is more readily reversible and hence higher doses of drug are needed to observe a physiological effect (Schwartz et al., 1974). This may preclude a precise appreciation of the renal effects of cardiac glycosides and their effect on $Na^+–K^+$ ATPase in rat or rabbit kidney.

Studies on the binding of tagged cardiac glycosides to enzyme have helped to clarify some aspects of their relationship. Along these lines, the binding of [^{3}H]ouabain to enzyme isolated from dog kidney after the in vivo infusion of cardiac glycosides has been shown to be directly proportional to the remaining enzyme activity as shown in Figure 1 (Allen et al., 1971). In vivo infusion of [^{3}H]ouabain has corroborated these findings (Torretti et al., 1972). These studies are strong evidence that the $Na^+–K^+$ ATPase is a pharmacological receptor of cardiac glycosides and that its inhibition is directly related to the diuresis. Another important observation pertinent to this association is that when examined in vivo and in vitro the inhibitory effect of ouabain is time dependent (Allen and Schwartz, 1974). At high doses of digoxin (>1.0 μg/kg/min) the onset of diuresis when infused into one renal artery of dog is between 30 and 45 min, but at doses lower than 0.7 μg/kg·min diuresis will not occur until 60–90 min or more have elapsed (Martinez-Maldonado et al., 1972).

Cardiac glycosides such as ouabain or digoxin result in marked impairment in urine concentration and dilution (Martinez-Maldonado et al., 1970; Torretti et al., 1972) which coincides with marked inhibition of the enzyme activity, principally in the outer medulla where the thick portion of the ascending limb of

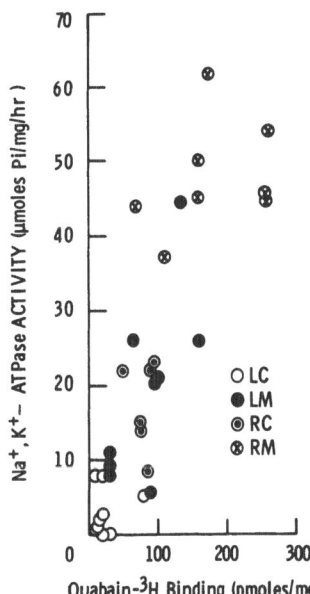

Figure 1. Relationship between Na⁺–K⁺ ATPase activity and *in vitro* binding of [³H] ouabain in all high-dose experiments. LC = left cortex; LM = left medulla; RC = right cortex; RM = right medulla. The regression line is $y = 33.5495 + 2.38816(x)$; the correlation coefficient is 0.693113, significant at a $P < 0.001$.

Henle's loop is located (Rhodin, 1971). This occurs without changes in GFR or renal blood flow and is associated with a proportional reduction in renal oxygen consumption (Fülgraff *et al.*, 1970). Associated with this effect of cardiac glycosides, there is a marked reduction in the disappearance rate of ATP from cortex and medulla of dog kidney (Kessler, 1970). Following glycoside administration the recovery of Na⁺ reabsorption and the enzyme activity are parallel, but cortical enzyme activity returns to control values faster (2 days) than medullary activity (3 days) (Nelson and Nechay, 1970). The characteristic interference of K⁺ with the effect of digitalis on Na⁺–K⁺ ATPase from other organs is also observed with renal enzyme (Nelson and Nechay, 1971). When KCl is simultaneously administered, the reduction in Na⁺ reabsorption which results from ouabain is delayed and so is the inhibition of the enzyme (Nelson and Nechay, 1971).

Some basic questions relative to the interaction of Na⁺–K⁺ ATPase with cardiac glycosides remain to be answered. An important unknown is the total dose of cardiac glycoside required to obtain a maximal diuresis. *In vivo* the maximal effect of ouabain is limited by how much glycoside can be administered. In an ingenious study Nechay (1974) and his collaborators have utilized two dogs connected in series by cross-circulation and have been able to administer into one renal artery ouabain in doses as high as 138 μg/kg while the animals were receiving 10 ml/min of saline. Sodium reabsorption was reduced to an average of 71% of the filtered load, and the enzyme activity was reduced to 11% of the activity seen in control animals. In experiments by Sejersted, Lie, and Kiil (1971) an average inhibition of 17% of the filtered Na⁺ was obtained during the infusion of ouabain and saline at 1 ml/min. Torretti and his collaborators (1972) showed that saline or mannitol–saline loads increased the natriuretic effects of ouabain to 33% and 44% of the filtered load as compared to

25% in hydropenia. In fact, in some experiments as much as 76% of the filtered Na^+, including the osmotic components, has been obtained. These changes have been attributed to shifts of reabsorbed Na^+ from proximal to more distal sites in the nephron. A limiting aspect to the evaluation of the diuresis following intrarenal infusion of ouabain and digoxin is imposed by the resulting vasoconstriction which tends to reduce salt and water excretion. To circumvent this difficulty, Lie *et al.* (1974) infused acetylcholine prior to ouabain infusion and were able to demonstrate that approximately 35% of the filtered Na^+ appears in the urine. In these experiments, the use of the heat-accumulation technique by the insertion of thermistors into the cortex or outer medulla indicated that ouabain infusion during acetylcholine-induced vasodilation reduced cortical and outer medullary metabolic rate, thus indicating that ouabain reduced Na^+ reabsorption, tubular hydrodynamic resistance, and energy requirements in these areas.

A second problem which appears more difficult to solve is whether the degree of inhibition found after *in vivo* ouabain or digoxin infusion is comparable to the one present after *in vitro* assay. In the first place, during the isolation procedure tissue is diluted more than 1:80,000 (Nechay *et al.*, 1967) yet enzyme inhibition continues to be detectable in microsomes prepared from kidneys treated with ouabain. This suggests that the enzyme–ouabain complex is pseudo-irreversible. Were it reversible *in vivo,* the drug would be diluted out during isolation and no inhibition would be detectable since the amount of bound drug is a function of the drug concentration. The concentration of ouabain in the infused kidney after maximally effective doses of the drug is from 10^{-6} to 10^{-5} *M*. Dilution by more than 80,000 would result in concentrations in the order of 10^{-11} or 10^{-10} ouabain which are not inhibitory *in vitro*. Furthermore, fivefold dilutions of microsomes isolated from kidneys inhibited *in vivo* did not alter the degree of inhibition (Nelson and Nechay, 1970). Ackerman–Potter analysis of ouabain inhibition of isolated microsomal preparations reveals that enzyme–drug interaction at first exhibits reversible kinetics, but upon preincubation of the drug with the enzyme, irreversible characteristics are acquired. This indicates that specific binding of the drug to the enzyme *in vivo* is irreversible. It is of interest that if the enzyme in whole kidney homogenates is prepared at various time intervals after removal from the dog, the activity of the enzyme drops and one might miss a difference between the two kidneys after infusion of ouabain (Nechay, 1974).

Another problem which remains to be solved centers around the observation that when digitalis is infused into one renal artery, despite Na^+–K^+ ATPase inhibition of the contralateral kidney, no diuresis results (Nelson and Nechay, 1970; Martinez-Maldonado *et al.,* 1972). This lack of correlation between inhibition of the enzyme and natriuresis may have to do with drug–receptor sites interaction or with tubular mechanisms of sodium reabsorption other than the ATPase system. It is of interest that the faster ouabain is given into one renal artery, the greater the reduction in Na^+ reabsorption and enzyme activity. Furthermore, when the drug is given intravenously instead of into one renal artery, the inhibition of enzyme activity is less, as is the depression in Na^+

reabsorption, but the relationship between the two remains similar. This suggests that the concentration of the drug in peritubular plasma influences the degree of inhibition and is in keeping with the observation that the binding rates of ouabain to Na^+–K^+ ATPase *in vitro* are directly proportional to the concentration of drug (Lindenmayer and Schwartz, 1973). It is possible that compensatory mechanisms insensitive to ouabain are responsible for the conservation of glomerular filtrate. Alternate mechanisms for Na^+ reabsorption surely exist, as ouabain infusion does not inhibit the reabsorption of all filtered Na^+ (Ross *et al.*, 1974). Moreover, frequently, as ouabain diuresis progresses, urine flow from the contralateral kidney slows down and sodium excretion diminishes despite the fact that glomerular filtration rate is unchanged. High infusion rates of saline, mannitol, *p*-aminohippurate, and creatinine solutions reverse the sodium retention and diuresis ensues (Torretti *et al.*, 1972; Nechay, 1974). Whatever the exact mechanisms for these observations, they suggest the participation of other sodium transport systems.

V. INTERACTIONS BETWEEN ETHACRYNIC ACID AND RENAL Na^+–K^+ ATPase

The renal effects of ethacrynic acid occur primarily in the thick ascending limb of Henle's loop (Goldberg *et al.*, 1964). The magnitude of the response suggests a large effect on the mechanism of reabsorption at this site. Accordingly, the possibility that the reduction in sodium reabsorption is the result of Na^+–K^+ ATPase inhibition must be considered. Renal ATPase from heavy microsomal preparations from guinea pig kidney is depressed by ethacrynic acid, but both Na^+–K^+ and magnesium ATPase are inhibited (Davis, 1970). The inhibition is nearly two order of magnitude less than that obtained by equimolar doses of ouabain and *p*-hydroxymercuribenzoate (POMB). Cysteine added to the incubation medium partially blocks ATPase inhibition by either ethacrynic acid or the known sulfhydryl inhibitor POMB. The degree of sulfhydryl reactivity and ATPase inhibition for ethacrynic acid is proportional. Furthermore, increasing the cysteine-to-drug molar ratio leads to a further block of the effect of ethacrynic acid. In contrast to the dissociation of the enzyme–drug complex observed when the reversible inhibitor POMB is used, the ethacrynic acid–enzyme complex is not reversible. This tends to eliminate the possibility that the nature of the interaction of ethyacrynic acid with ATPase *in vitro* accounts for its diuretic activity, since *in vivo* the diuretic effect has brief duration and is rapidly reversible.

The effect of ethacrynic acid on renal protein-bound sulfhydryl groups has also been examined by Komorn and Cafruny (1965). They demonstrated that ethacrynic acid reduces the concentration of stainable protein-bound sulfhydryl groups in renal cells of dogs at a time when diuresis is maximal or increasing. In rats, which respond poorly to the diuretic effects of ethacrynic acid, this does not take place even when the dose administered intravenously is 100 times as large as that effective in dogs. It should be pointed out that some mercurials which react with SH groups are not diuretic, precluding the necessity for reaction with SH groups to occur in order for diuresis to ensue (Kessler *et al.*, 1964).

Charnock *et al.* (1970) also found that ethacrynic acid inhibits a microsomal preparation of $Na^+–K^+$ ATPase from guinea pig cortex. In contrast to ouabain, concentrations of ethacrynic acid less than $10^{-4}\ M$ did not inhibit ATPase. Furthermore, as shown by others, inhibition of Mg^{2+} ATPase is also a feature of the ethacrynic acid effect. As in the case of ouabain, on the other hand, the degree of inhibition of ethacrynic acid was influenced by the concentration of K^+ ion present and was greatest when K^+ ion concentration was lowest. In the presence of 20 mM Na^+, ethacrynic acid did not affect the amount of [^{32}P]phosphoenzyme formed from gamma-labeled [^{32}P]ATP, but did slow considerably the release of inorganic phosphate upon subsequent addition of K^+. This effect was most evident at low K^+ concentrations. It appears that ethacrynic acid inhibits the K^+-dependent dephosphorylation step in the overall mechanism of ATP hydrolysis by this enzyme, offering an explanation for the antogonism between this diuretic agent and K^+ ions. Similar results have been obtained by Banerjee *et al.* (1970). These investigators have shown that ethyacrynic acid affects two different steps of enzyme turnover (Figure 2). First, ethacrynic acid blocked the phosphorylation of $Na^+–K^+$ ATPase but had an insignificant effect upon the dephosphorylation step when the Na^+/K^+ ratio was 10:1. The diuretic also prevented the ADP–ATP exchange reaction. The degree of inhibition by the diuretic of specific activity of the enzyme was closely correlated with the degree of inhibition of phosphorylation at the ADP–ATP exchange step. Second, ethacrynic acid seemed to stabilize the spontaneous disappearance of the phosphorylated intermediate and slightly decreased the apparent affinity for K^+ with respect to hydrolysis of the intermediate. The decrease in apparent affinity for K^+ could not be observed in an assay medium with a Na^+/K^+ ratio of 4:1. When the concentrations of Na^+ and K^+ were changed to those found in extracellular fluid, ethacrynic acid-treated enzyme showed a 20–30% decrease in specific activity as compared to the usual assay system. From these observations the authors concluded that the inhibition of phosphorylation by ethacrynic acid appears to be of significance for inhibition of enzyme activity *in vitro*, while the stabilization of the phosphorylated intermedi-

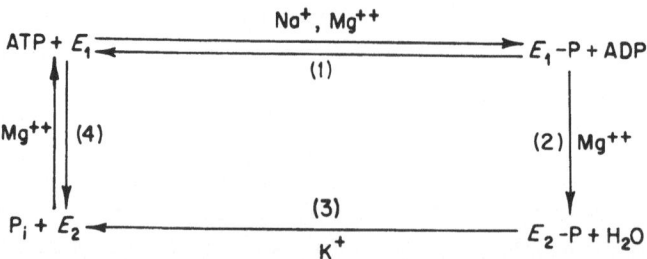

Figure 2. Possible sites for the effect of ethacrynic acid on Na^+K^+ ATPase turnover. (Adapted from Banerjee *et al.*, 1970.)

ate may be involved in drug-induced diuresis. According to the authors, of the two mechanisms only the latter appears to be relevant to the diuretic *in vivo* effects. As in previous studies, the concentration of ethacrynic acid employed to inhibit ATPase *in vitro* was much higher than those required to induce natriuresis and there appeared to be a considerable amount of nonspecific binding. Therefore, unless the kidney has some special mechanism for transporting or concentrating ethacrynic acid at the receptor site, inhibition of phosphorylation is an unlikely biochemical mechanism of production of diuresis by this drug. Since ATP did not phosphorylate the ethacrynic acid-treated enzyme significantly faster than untreated enzyme, the stabilized form must have been E_2P rather than E_1P. Therefore, an alternative mechanism by which ethacrynic acid inhibits Na^+-K^+ ATPase appears to be by slowing down dephosphorylation of the phosphorylated intermediate by K^+. This site of action of ethacrynic acid would be identical to that of ouabain. In addition, there are other common features. Both these inhibitors stabilize the E_2P form and, as already discussed, the degree of inhibition of dephosphorylation is affected by the concentration of K^+. While stabilization of E_2P by ethacrynic acid is a little more marked than by ouabain, its sensitivity to K^+ is less effective. This latter effect probably makes ethacrynic acid a much weaker inhibitor of Na^+-K^+-ATPase than ouabain. Stabilization of the phosphorylated intermediate precedes inhibition of the formation of the phosphorylated intermediate. According to Banerjee *et al.* (1970), stabilization of E_2P may have pharmacological significance. If this type of inhibition occurred in the whole animal, no decrease in Na^+-K^+ ATPase activity would be observed *in vitro* at the Na^+/K^+ concentration ratio of 4 to 10 which has been employed by most workers. However, the enzyme may turn over more slowly *in vivo* since the Na^+/K^+ ratio in the extracellular fluid is 36, and under these conditions inhibition by ethacrynic acid may be more readily observed.

Duggan and Noll (1972), however, have reported that in dog kidneys undergoing ipsilateral diuresis in response to ethacrynic acid, drug-derived radioactivity, approximately 5×10^{-10} M/mg of protein, was found in kidney and that the preparation was significantly inhibited relative to contralateral kidneys removed immediately prior to administration of the diuretic. In their hands and contrary to most other observations, inhibition was specific for the Na^+-K^+ fraction and was not reversed by soluble thiols. Dilution and prolonged incubation also failed to reverse the inhibition. The authors interpreted the lack of correlation between drug concentration and enzyme inhibition as evidence that the cells can indeed concentrate drug disproportionately at the receptor sites. The dosages of ethacrynic acid utilized by these investigators, however, were supermaximal with respect to saluretic effect at 15 min. The large dose and the apparent irreversible nature of enzyme inhibition occurring *in vivo* is inconsistent with the transient aspect of the initial diuretic response.

Despite the suggestion by some, evidence exists against a mechanism leading to concentration of drug at a receptor site. The uptake of labeled ethacrynic acid by rabbit kidney cortex approaches a steady-state level by 1 hr of incubation and is clearly dependent on the external concentration of the compound (Epstein, 1972). Furthermore, uptake is not affected by metabolic inhibitors. Examination of tissue components have demonstrated that 40% of the label could not be washed out; also the same fraction of the label was found in a well-washed tissue solid sedimenting at up to $18,000 \times g$. Thiol reagents such as n-ethylmaleimide, mercuric chloride, and iodoacetic acid did not diminish binding of ethacrynic acid. The uptake and efflux of ethacrynic acid from rabbit kidney cortex are not modified by the presence, in various concentrations, of materials (e.g., ouabain) which presumably associate with sites of active transport of ions and sugars. It is apparent, therefore, that the major part of the binding of ethacrynic acid to rabbit kidney cortex is not specific for either tissue sulfhydryl groups or unique membrane-active transport sites.

Other studies have also purportedly advanced evidence of an *in vivo* effect of ethacrynic acid on Na^+–K^+ ATPase. After administration of a single dose of ethacrynic acid (25 mg/kg) or furosemide (50 mg/kg) to rats, a diuresis is only observed with the latter (Duggan and Noll, 1965). Yet Na^+–K^+ ATPase activity appeared to be inhibited in the kidneys removed after either diuretic. The changes induced by both diuretics were small, and studies with furosemide were performed only in 3 rats. It is not possible to be certain that the ethacrynic acid effect on ATPase was specific. It is also surprising that inhibition was observed with the doses of ethacrynic acid used.

Opposite results have been observed by other investigators. The effects of furosemide and ethacrynic acid on ATPase activity in rat renal plasma membranes *in vivo* and *in vitro* was examined by Ebel *et al.* (1972). Furosemide, although a potent diuretic in the rat, had no influence on renal ATPase activity. Ethacrynic acid, which was active as a diuretic only after intravenous injection of relatively large doses, had no influence on renal Na^+–K^+ ATPase activity after *in vivo* administration. *In vitro* studies showed that furosemide in concentrations of 1 mM had no influence on ATPase activity. In kinetic studies the mechanisms of inhibition of total ATPase were further characterized. No consistent relationship was observed between inhibition of Na^+–K^+ ATPase and inhibition of sodium reabsorption. Thus it was concluded that these diuretics do not act by inhibiting plasma membrane Na^+–K^+ ATPase. The plasma membrane fraction was prepared from rat kidney homogenates. It should be mentioned, however, that in isolated nephron segments an effect of furosemide on renal Na^+–K^+-ATPase has been shown (Schmidt and Dubach, 1970).

Studies of the *in vivo* effects of ethacrynic acid on ATPase on dog and rat have also been performed by Nechay and Contreras (1972). They removed kidneys from dogs 15 min to 2 hr after single intravenous injections (0.2, 1, or 5 mg/kg) of ethacrynic acid. An ATPase which was sensitive to ouabain *in vivo* but had little sensitivity *in vitro* was prepared separately from cortex and outer medulla. Ethacrynic acid inhibited ATPase from both portions in a dose-dependent manner. The time of recovery of the enzyme activity was also dose dependent and was complete for the 5 mg/kg dose in 100 min. If enzyme was pretreated with ouabain, little inhibition resulted from ethacrynic acid, suggesting that it too interacted with Na^+–K^+ ATPase. In the rat, ethacrynic acid did not inhibit the enzyme after 15–25 min of doses of 1–5 mg/kg intravenous), yet the enzyme preparation from rat kidneys was as sensitive to ethacrynic acid *in vitro* as was the preparation from dog kidney. The microsomal preparation which was highly sensitive to ouabain *in vitro* reacted with ethacrynic acid and had irreversible characteristics according to Ackerman–Potter analysis, yet the enzyme from rat kidneys behaved according to the kinetics of reversible inhibition even after the incubation.

Studies on the effects of ethacrynic acid on renal ATPase have been conducted in our laboratory. Extensive *in vivo* and *in vitro* work in association with Tsaparas and Inagaki (Martinez-Maldonado *et al.*, 1974) has demonstrated that the effect of ethacrynic acid, as indicated by previous authors, is nonspecific. Despite the use of varied isolation methodologies, in particular ones similar to those of Duggan and Noll (1972) and Nechay and Contreras (1972), we have not been able to demonstrate (Inagaki *et al.*, 1973) that Na^+–K^+ ATPase is inhibited after *in vivo* administration of ethacrynic acid nor were we able to demonstrate that assay with a sodium-to-potassium ratio of 36:1 made any difference in the demonstration of an *in vivo* ethacrynic acid effect on the enzyme. Nevertheless, by examining the characteristics of cation-mediated [^{3}H]ouabain binding to the enzyme preparations, we were able to demonstrate that ethacrynic acid reduces the usual reactivity of Na^+–K^+ ATPase to ouabain binding in the presence of Na^+ and K^+. The nonspecific binding of ethacrynic acid to membranes reduces the reactivity of the membrane ATPase to some cations, and it may be this aspect of its effect which mediates the observed diuresis. Unfortunately, a kinetic analysis of this reaction could not be made to determine the degree of reversibility and, therefore, to attempt to correlate these results with those observed after administration of diuretic *in vivo*. It is of interest, nevertheless, that the administration of ouabain prevents the complete effect of ethacrynic acid on the ascending limb of the loop of Henle (Martinez-Maldonado *et al.*, 1974). It is not necessary that this be interpreted as an indication that ethacrynic acid and ouabain have identical mechanisms of action. In other words, alteration of membrane conformation, therefore reducing the reactivity of the enzyme to different cations, may result in the diuresis despite the fact that the enzyme is not a pharmacologic receptor for ethacrynic acid.

An alternative explanation to an effect of ethacrynic acid on renal Na^+–K^+ ATPase has been advanced by Wolf *et al.* (1969). These authors have studied the effect of ethacrynic acid on renal oxygen consumption and tubular Na^+ reabsorption in dogs. After the administration of 5 mg/kg of ethacrynic acid, Na^+ reabsorption was depressed from 96 to 71% of the filtered load whereas oxygen consumption remained constant. Mean renal blood flow was increased to 134% of the control level, but the renal arterial–venous difference of oxygen was lowered. Thus, the ratio TN_A/V_{O_2} was decreased significantly. The calculated equations for the regression lines were $V_{O_2} = 0.022TN_A + 0.067$ before and $V_{O_2} = 0.35TN_A + 0.064$ after injection of ethacrynic acid. This led the authors to suggest that ethacrynic acid does not directly inhibit the active Na^+ transport mechanism but rather influences cell membrane permeability.

VI. EFFECT OF ADRENAL STEROIDS ON Na$^+$–K$^+$ ATPase

Evidence exists suggesting that aldosterone regulates Na$^+$ transport through DNA-dependent synthesis of RNA with increases in *de novo* synthesis of proteins. Two important theories have been proposed for the mechanism of action of aldosterone (Sharp and Leaf, 1966; Fanestil, 1969). The energy theory suggests that aldosterone increases the activity of one or several metabolic steps, leading to an increased rate of synthesis of ATP. Alternatively, the permease theory proposes that aldosterone increases *mucosal* surface Na$^+$ permeability by increasing the synthesis of the carrier protein thereby increasing the quantity of Na$^+$ available to a Na$^+$-limited pumping mechanism. They both incorporate the concept of an active Na$^+$ pump that is regulated by increased availability of either Na$^+$ ions and/or ATP. The biochemical manifestation of this active Na$^+$ pump is Na$^+$–K$^+$ ATPase and, therefore, induction of synthesis of Na$^+$–K$^+$ ATPase could constitute a third possible mechanism. Despite the fact that aldosterone increases ATPase in microsomal fraction isolated from adrenalectomized rats, the changes in electrolyte excretion and Na$^+$–K$^+$ ATPase activity following adrenalectomy and aldosterone treatments have not correlated well.

Jørgensen (1969), for example, has examined the effect of aldosterone on the activity of ATPase in kidneys of adrenalectomized rats. Repeated injections of aldosterone increased the activity in the microsomal fraction from whole kidneys after 14 and 24 hr. In this period of time, corticosterone had no effect on enzyme activity while combinations of aldosterone and corticosterone caused a significant increase in activity. After 48 hr corticosterone restored the activity to normal levels while aldosterone, at best, increased the activity to a level midway between the activity of adrenalectomized and normal rats. In an attempt to localize an effect of aldosterone, the activity of ATPase was measured in preparations from subdivisions of the kidney. In physiologic doses aldosterone produced significant increase in activity in the outer medulla where the ascending limbs of Henle predominate. In the inner cortex an increase in activity was observed after treatment with the two higher doses of aldosterone while only insignificant changes were found in the outer cortex. The rise in activity was gradual and first detectable in these experiments only after more than 6 hr of treatment. The results are compatible with an adaptation of the level of Na$^+$–K$^+$ ATPase to the sustained increase in the absorption of Na$^+$ following repeated injections of aldosterone to adrenalectomized rats.

Similar results have been obtained in fetal rat kidney. AT this stage renal Na$^+$–K$^+$ ATPase has been found to be very low on day 17 and 18 of gestation but starts increasing from day 19. The rise does not occur when maternal and fetal sources of adrenal steroids are suppressed by adrenalectomy of the mother or by metapyrone administration (Geloso and Basset, 1974). In these animals aldosterone promptly restores the activity of ATPase to normal levels. These observations are consonant with the ones previously alluded to relating renal function maturation to the activity of the enzyme. Nevertheless, failure to isolate the enzyme in pure form may frequently prevent the proper identification of the changes which are responsible for the increment in Na^+ reabsorption. Adrenalectomized rats maintained on saline solution for 5 days have been shown by Knox and Sen (1974) to sustain a 24% decrease in Na^+-K^+ ATPase activity of heavy microsomal fraction without alterations in magnesium ATPase activity. Aldosterone, in doses of 10 μg had no effect; 20 μg enhanced the activity by 50%. The magnesium ATPase activity, in all groups allowed access to 0.9% NaCl, did not vary from control values. On the other hand, adrenalectomized rats deprived of saline solution showed a significant reduction in both ATPase and magnesium ATPase activity by 47% and 31%, respectively. Within 3 hr of aldosterone treatment, renal Na^+-K^+ ATPase activity had increased. This increment could account for the increased tubular Na^+ uptake that occurred during this time period. Others, as already indicated, have found that several hours must elapse before optimal Na^+ uptake can occur (Chignell and Titus, 1966; Jørgensen, 1968). However, the ATPase activity of the heavy microsomal fractions utilized was several-fold more active than membrane preparations employed by others, allowing for detection of more subtle alterations in enzyme activity. Sucrose-gradient studies demonstrated that the effects of aldosterone were more apparent as the enzyme preparation was progressively purified. Access of the rats to either tap water or saline is of great importance since the increment in renal ATPase activity was substantially greater than that of adrenalectomized rats with access to 0.9% NaCl. Furthermore, it has been demonstrated that the decline in activity is greater when rats are deprived of saline solution for 5 days (Knox and Sen, 1974). Also, when rats are maintained on tap water alone the decline in ATPase microsomal activity is observed more rapidly. Kinetic data reveal that such a decrease in Na^+-K^+ ATPase activity following adrenalectomy results from changes in the level of Na^+-K^+ ATPase since there was no apparent alteration in the K_m for ATP, Na^+, or K^+. The changes which occur when contralateral nephrectomy and high-protein diet are given to increase ATPase activity are noteworthy. These maneuvers increase GFR and enhance Na^+ reabsorption, suggesting that Na^+ itself may somehow trigger the increase in Na^+-K^+ ATPase activity.

Schmidt *et al.* (1974, 1975), utilizing isolated nephron segments, have examined the effect of aldosterone on Na^+-K^+ ATPase. It is of interest that restoration of enzyme activity after one physiological dose of aldosterone given to an adrenalectomized rat, just 90 min before sacrifice, occurred within 1 hr after injection, resulting in a highly significant increase (50%) in enzyme activity, particularly in the thick ascending limb of Henle's loop and the distal convolution. By contrast, microsomal fractions are slower in response to physiological injections of aldosterone. Further discrepancies come from the fact that in tubular portions the enzyme activity in the adrenalectomized rats is 60–80% below the normal activity, while only half of these percentages are found in the microsomal fraction of renal cell homogenates 6 days after adrenalectomy. These changes decrease and increase after adrenalectomy and aldosterone administration, are more pronounced, and occur more rapidly in the distal than in the proximal tubule. Cycloheximide and actinomycin D prevent stimulatory hormonal effect of aldosterone on Na^+–K^+ ATPase activities both in proximal and distal convolutions, as well as in the thick ascending limb. Therefore, it is most likely that the effect of aldosterone is connected with protein synthesis. Rapid restoration of Na^+–K^+ ATPase by aldosterone in the adrenalectomized rat could also be due to an aldosterone effect similar to that of deoxycholate which unmasks the catalytic sites of the enzyme or else a production of a protein which unmasks the activity. Nephrectomy also increases ATPase activity in the distal portions of the tubule and occurs approximately 12 hr after operation. This also takes place faster in isolated tubular segments than in the microsomal fraction of broken renal cells. Conceivably, the difference between these results and total homogenate is that homogenates measure total activity while the tubule segments measure functional activity. It is likely that the aldosterone effect is mediated by *de novo* protein synthesis. However, until now, no aldosterone-induced protein has been isolated or identified. It is nevertheless possible that one of the aldosterone-induced proteins is Na^+–K^+ ATPase. This is evident from the fact that aldosterone can acutely increase the activity of Na^+–K^+ ATPase, that [^{14}C]leucine incorporation into protein correlates with increasingly pure preparations of Na^+–K^+ ATPase, and that aldosterone induces the synthesis of the protein that is localized to the same position on polyacrylamide gel as Na^+–K^+ ATPase (Knox and Sen, 1974). It is not known, however, whether the increase in ATPase activity is due to *de novo* synthesis or a decrease in enzyme breakdown. The increase in synthesis does not exclude the possibility that aldosterone may induce the synthesis of other proteins; also it does not contradict the evidence in support of changes in Na^+–K^+ ATPase that occur when the Na^+ load to the kidney is chronically increased.

Other steroids also appear to affect renal Na^+–K^+ ATPase activity. Hendler *et al.* (1972) examined the effects of adrenalectomy and hormone replacement on renal ATPase. In their hands, adrenalectomy produced a reduction in Na^+–K^+ ATPase of 30–50% in both cortex and red medulla of the kidney unaccompanied by changes in adenyl cyclase or 5′-nucleotidase. The glucocorticoid methylprednisolone restored Na^+–K^+ ATPase to normal, also without changing the other two membrane-bound enzymes. Ouabain binding by microsomes of guinea pig kidney rose in parallel with Na^+–K^+ ATPase activity after treatment with methylprednisolone. These data suggest that adrenal glucocorticoids have a specific influence on Na^+–K^+ ATPase that is not paralleled by changes in other enzymes of the plasma membrane and hence is probably associated with an increased quantity of enzyme per unit of membrane material. Injections of *dl*-aldosterone produced a rise in ATPase of outer medulla after 24 hr, but no effect was seen after deoxycorticosterone or Na^+ deprivation.

Renal enzyme activities have also been measured after adrenalectomy in mice and rats (Suzuki and Ogawa, 1969). In mice, carbonic anhydrase activity in homogenates and microsomal and supernatant fractions was decreased while microsomal Na^+–K^+ ATPase activity was increased after adrenalectomy. In both rats and mice the changes of both enzymatic activities after adrenalectomy were reversible. Changes in carbonic anhydrase after adrenalectomy were restored to normal levels with aldosterone and DOCA replacement, but corticosterone and cortisol had no effect on the enzyme activity in either animal species. The elevation in Na^+-K^+ ATPase activity after adrenalectomy in mice was restored with DOCA and cortisol, but aldosterone had no effect on enzymatic activity. The decline in Na^+-K^+ ATPase activity after adrenalectomy in rats was prevented and approached the normal levels with replacement of both mineralocorticoids and glucocorticoids. The reason for the observed lack of effect of aldosterone in mice remains unexplained, and further functional data in this species are required before they can be interpreted adequately.

VII. EFFECT OF THYROID HORMONE ON Na^+-K^+ ATPase

For several years it has been known that thyroid hormones have an important effect on renal function. The lack or excess of thyroid hormone has been demonstrated to alter renal hemodynamics, urine concentrating and diluting capacities, and overall renal sodium handling in both man (DiScala and Kinney, 1971) and experimental animals (Holmes and DiScala, 1970). The hypothyroid state is of particular interest since it is associated with a profound defect in urine concentration and dilution and is accompanied by marked reductions in medullary Na^+-K^+ ATPase activity at least in the rat (Katz and Lindheimer, 1973). Furthermore, micropuncture studies in the hypothyroid rat have demonstrated that proximal reabsorption is depressed at least 30% (Michael *et al.*, 1972). Since these animals cannot regulate sodium loads normally, controversy has arisen as to whether defective sodium reabsorption is a consequence of intrinsic alterations in tubular transport mechanisms (including Na^+-K^+ ATPase) or if the changes in enzyme, etc., result from diminished load of sodium (Katz and Lindheimer, 1973).

Studies by Edelman (1975) have partially attacked this issue, in addition to attempting to decipher the mechanism of thyroid hormone action on the kidney ATPase system. This author has shown that administration of T_3 (250 mg/100 g body wt) leads to a 68% increase in cortical Na^+-K^+ ATPase by 12 hr; by 48 hr activity peaks at 83%. Only modest and statistically insignificant results were obtained on Mg^{2+} ATPase activity. By comparison, the increment in Na^+-K^+ ATPase in the medulla was, at best, minimal (20%), and no change in papillary ATPase was observed. These results differ from those of Katz and Lindheimer (1973) who noted a significant increase in medullary Na^+-K^+ ATPase activity after replacement therapy in hypothyroid rats. Nevertheless, the results of Edelman (1975) are compatible with the significant improvement in proximal (cortical) reabsorption seen by Michael and his collaborators (1972) in T_3-treated hypothyroid rats. The reasons for the discrepancies between the results of Katz and Lindheimer (1973) and Edelman's group are not apparent. Nevertheless, it appears clear from thyroid hormone effects on renal cortical slices that oxygen consumption and sodium transport are intimately linked.

Studies on kidney slices from euthyroid rats and rabbits demonstrate that 36% of the Q_{O_2} is ouabain-inhibitable, implying that one third of the Q_{O_2} is coupled to active sodium transport under these conditions. The administration of T_3 to euthyroid rats, sufficient to produce modest hyperthyroidism, leaads to a 22% increase in Q_{O_2} and a 28% increase in ouabain-inhibitable respiration, indicating that approximately 46% of the thyroid-induced increase in Q_{O_2} is mediated by increased energy expenditure in active sodium transport (Ismail-Beigi and Edelman, 1971). Kidney slices of thyroidectomized rats injected with thyroid hormone show a 54% increase in Q_{O_2} and a 50% increase in ouabain-inhibitable respiration. The increase in sodium-transport-dependent respiration accounted for 30% of the total increase elicited by the hormone. However, no information is available on the effect of renal Q_{O_2} and sodium transport in intact animals after the administration of thyroid hormones. As pointed out by Edelman (1975), this is necessary, since slice studies only reflect basal oxygen consumption: Sodium and potassium are not transported transtubularly in this model. These results, however, appear to be clearcut evidence that thyroid hormones exert an important effect on Na^+ transport. In view of the changes in Na^+–K^+-ATPase, it would be necessary to elucidate whether the increase in enzyme is the result of the activation of a fixed number of pump sites or of the induction of new sodium pump sites. In the latter case, the affinities for the substrates ATP, sodium, and potassium might change with the activation of the transport enzyme. Thyroidectomized rats, given 50 μg T_3 per hundred grams of body wt on alternate days for a total of 3 injections, had cortical membrane fractions assayed for Na^+–K^+ ATPase activity at various concentrations of ATP in a regenerating system consisting of excess phosphoenolpyruvate and pyruvate kinase. T_3 had no effect on K_m for ATP, sodium, or potassium. In contrast, V_{max} increased 66, 31, and 51% for Na^+, K^+, and ATP, respectively. Results were identical even when activity was calculated on the basis of DNA content in order to see if the change reflected an increase in transport enzyme content per unit renal cell. Therefore, these findings may represent an increase in the biosynthesis of new sodium pumps or the activation of latent pumps by a biochemical pathway. Whichever of these two is taking place, the final net result will be an increase in the number of pump sites per cell. The number of sodium pump sites was determined from the number of phosphorylated intermediates formed by Na^+–K^+ ATPase from [γ-^{32}P]ATP in the presence of sodium and magnesium. The ATPase activity increased 70% as ^{32}P incorporation increased 79%, a relationship of almost 1:1, indicating that thyroid hormone increased the number of transport sites rather than activating a fixed number of sites. Unfortunately, it cannot be said with certainty whether this represents increased synthesis or unmasking of the sites already present. Further studies on this problem are certainly needed.

ACKNOWLEDGMENT

Parts of these studies were supported by U.S.P.H.S. grant AM 15604 and a grant from the American Heart Association, Houston Chapter. We are also grateful to Drs. Jules C. Allen, Lois K. Lane, and Earl T. Wallick for their review of the manuscript and their helpful suggestions. We also thank Ms. Consuelo Lopez for her secretarial assistance.

REFERENCES

Allen, J. C. and Schwartz, A. 1969. A possible biochemical explanation for the insensitivity of the rat to cardiac glycosides. *J. Pharmacol. Exp. Ther.*, *168:*42.

Allen, J. C. and Schwartz, A. 1974. Na$^+$, K$^+$-ATPase, the transport enzyme: Evidence for its proposed role as pharmacologic receptor for cardiac glycosides. *Ann. N.Y. Acad. Sci.*, *242:*646.

Allen, J. C., Martinez-Maldonado, M., Suki, W. N., Eknoyan, G., and Schwartz, A. 1971. Relation between digitalis binding in vivo and inhibition of sodium, potassium adenosine triphosphatase in canine kidney. *Biochem. Pharmacol.*, *20:*73.

Banerjee, S. P., Khanna, V. K., and Sen, A. K. 1970. Inhibition of sodium- and potassium-dependent adenosine triphosphatase by ethacrynic acid: Two modes of action. *Mol. Pharmacol.*, *6:*680.

Bonting, S. L., Simon, K. A., and Hawkins, N. M. 1961. Studies on sodium–potassium activated adenosine triphosphatase 1. Quantitative distribution in several tissues of the cat. *Arch. Biochem. Biophys.*, *95:*416.

Burg, M. B. and Abramow, M. 1966. Localization of tissue sodium and potassium compartments in rabbit renal cortex. *Am. J. Physiol.*, *211:*1011.

Burg, M. B. and Green, N. 1973. Function of the thick ascending limb of Henle's loop. *Am. J. Physiol.*, *224:*659.

Burg, M. B. and Orloff, J. 1966. Effect of temperature and medium K on Na and K fluxes in separated renal tubules. *Am. J. Physiol.*, *211:*1005.

Burg, M. B. and Orloff, J. 1970. Electrical potential difference across proximal convoluted tubules. *Am. J. Physiol.*, *219:*1714.

Cade, J. R., Shalhoub, R. J., Canessa-Fisher, M., and Pitts, R. F. 1961. Effect of strophanthidin on the renal tubules of dogs. *Am. J. Physiol.*, *200:*373.

Charnock, J. S., Potter, H. A., and McKee, D. 1970. Etharcynic acid inhibition of (Na$^+$ + K$^+$)-activated adenosine triphosphatase. *Biochem. Pharmacol.*, *19:*1637.

Chignell, C. F. and Titus, E. 1966. Effect of adrenal steroids on a Na$^+$ and K$^+$-requiring adenosine triphosphatase from rat kidney. *J. Biol. Chem.*, *241:*5083.

Czâky, T. Z., Prachnabmoli, K., Eiseman, B., and Ho, P. M. 1964. The effect of digitalis on the renal tubular transport of glucose in normal and heartless dogs. *J. Pharmacol. Exp. Ther.*, *150:*275.

Dantzler, W. H. 1974. PAH transport by snake proximal renal tubules: Differences from urate transport. *Am. J. Physiol.*, *226:*634.

Davis, P. W. 1970. Inhibition of renal Na$^+$, K$^+$-activated adenosine triphosphatase activity by ethacrynic acid. *Biochem. Pharmacol.*, *19:*1983.

Davis, P. W. and Dixon, R. L. 1971. Selective postnatal development of Na,K-activated-adenosinetriphosphatase in rabbit kidneys. *Proc. Soc. Exp. Biol. Med.*, *136:*95.

DiScala, V. A. and Kinney, M. J. 1971. Effects of myxedema on the renal diluting and concentrating mechanism. *Am. J. Physiol.*, *50:*325.

Dixon, J. F. and Hokin, L. E. 1974. Studies on the characterization of the sodium–potassium transport adenosine triphosphatase. Purification and properties of the enzyme from the electric organ of Electrophorus electricus. *Arch. Biochem. Biophys.*, *163:*749.

Duarte, C. G., Chométy, F., and Giebisch, G. 1971. Effect of amiloride, ouabain and furosemide on distal tubular function. *Am. J. Physiol.*, *221:*632.

Duggan, D. E. and Noll, R. M. 1965. Effects of ethacrynic acid and cardiac glycosides upon a membrane adenosinetriphosphatase of renal cortex. *Arch. Biochem. Biophys.*, *109:*388.

Duggan, D. E. and Noll, R. M. 1972. Effects of ethacrynic acid upon membrane ATPase of dog kidney *in vivo* and *in vitro*. *Proc. Soc. Exp. Biol.Med.*, *139:*762.

Ebel, H., Ehrich, J., De Santo, N. G., and Doerken, U. 1972. Plasma membranes of the kidney: III. Influence of diuretics on ATPase activity. *Pfluegers Arch., 335:*224.

Edelman, I. S. 1975. Thyroidal regulation of renal energy metabolism and (Na$^+$ + K$^+$)-activated adenosine triphosphatase activity. *Med. Clin. N. Am., 59:*605.

Epstein, F. H. and Silva, P. 1974. Role of sodium, potassium-ATPase in renal function. *Ann. N.Y. Acad. Sci., 242:*519.

Epstein, R. W. 1972. The binding of ethacrynic acid to rabbit kidney cortex. *Biochem. Biophys. Acta., 274:*119.

Fanestil, D. D. 1968. Renal Na–K ATPase relationship to total functional renal mass. *Nature, 218:*176.

Fanestil, D. D. 1969. Mechanism of action of aldosterone. *Ann. Rev. Med., 20:*223.

Farber, S. J., Alexander, J. D., Pellegrino, E. D., and Earle, D. P. 1951. The effect of intravenously administered digoxin on water and electrolyte excretion and on renal functions. *Circulation, 4:*378.

Fülgraff, G., Bieg, A., and Wolf, K. 1970. Der renale Sauerstoffverbrauch nach Strophanthin und 6-Aminonicotinamid. *Naunyn-Schmiedeberg's Arch. Pharmakol., 266:*43.

Geloso, J. P. and Basset, J. C. 1974. Role of adrenal glands in development of foetal rat kidney Na-K-ATPase. *Pfluegers Arch., 348:*105.

Goldberg, M., McCurdy, D. K., Foltz, E. L., and Bluemle, L. W., Jr. 1964. Effects of ethacrynic acid (a new saluretic agent) on renal diluting and concentrating mechanisms: Evidence for site of action in the loop of Henle. *J. Clin. Invest., 43:*201.

Goldin, S. M. and Tong, S. W. 1974. Reconstitution of active transport catalyzed by the purified Na and K ion-stimulated adenosine triphosphatase from canine renal medulla. *J. Biol. Chem., 249:*5907.

Gordon, E. E. 1965. Influence of ouabain on metabolism of rat kidney. *Biochim. Biophys. Acta., 104:*606.

Grantham, J., Burg, M. B., and Orloff, J. 1970. The nature of transtubular Na and K transport in isolated rabbit renal collecting tubules. *J. Clin. Invest., 49:*1815.

Györi, A. Z., Brandel, U., and Kinne, R. 1972. Effect of cardiac glycosides and sodium ethacrynate on transepithelial sodium transport *in vivo* micropuncture experiments and on isolated plasma membrane Na–K-ATPase in vitro of the rat. *Pfluegers Arch., 335:*287.

Hendler, E. D., Torretti, J., and Epstein, F. H. 1971. The distribution of sodium–potassium-activated adenosine triphosphatase in medulla and cortex of the kidney. *J. Clin. Invest., 50:*1329.

Hendler, E. D., Torretti, J., Kupor, L., and Epstein, F. H. 1972. Effects of adrenalectomy and hormone replacement on Na–K-ATPase in renal tissue. *Am. J. Physiol., 222:*754.

Hilden, S. and Hokin, L. E. 1975. Active potassium transport coupled to active sodium transport in vesicles reconstituted from purified sodium and potassium ion-activated adenosine triphosphatase from the rectal gland of *Squalus acanthias. J. Biol. Chem., 250:*6296.

Hilden, S., Rhee, H. M., and Hokin, L. E. 1974. Sodium transport by phospholipid vesicles containing purified sodium and potassium ion-activated adenosine triphosphatase. *J. Biol. Chem., 249:*7432.

Hokin, L. E. 1974. Purification and properties of the (sodium + potassium)-activated adenosinetriphosphatase and reconstitution of sodium transport. *Ann. N.Y. Acad. Sci., 242:*12.

Hokin, L. E., Dahl, J. L., Deupree, J. D., Dixon, J. F., Hackney, J. F., and Perdue, J. F. 1973. Studies on the characterization of the sodium–potassium transport adenosine triphosphatase. X. Purification of the enzyme from the rectal gland of *Squalus acanthias. J. Biol. Chem., 248:*2593.

Holmes, E. W., Jr. and DiScala, V. A. 1970. Studies on the exaggerated natriuretic response to a saline infusion in the hypothyroid rat. *J. Clin. Invest., 49:*1224.

Hook, J. B. 1969. A positive correlation between natriuresis and inhibition of renal Na–K adenosine triphosphatase by ouabain. *Proc. Soc. Exp. Biol. Med., 131:*731.

Hyman, A. L., Jacques, W. E., and Hyman, E. S. 1956. Observations on the direct effect of digoxin on renal excretion of sodium and water. *Am. Heart J., 52:*592.

Imai, M. and Kokko, J. P. 1974. Sodium chloride, urea, and water transport in the thin ascending limb of Henle. *J. Clin. Invest., 53:*393.

Inagaki, C., Martinez-Maldonado, M., and Schwartz, A. 1973. Some *in vivo* and *in vitro* effects of ethacrynic acid on renal Na$^+$,K$^+$-ATPase. *Arch. Biochem. Biophys., 158*:421.

Ismail-Beigi, F. and Edelman, I. S. 1971. The mechanism of the calorigenic action of thyroid hormone: Stimulation of Na$^+$ + K$^+$-activated adenosine triphosphatase activity. *J. Gen. Physiol., 57*:710.

Jørgensen, P. L. 1968. Regulation of the (Na$^+$ + K$^+$)-activated ATP hydrolyzing enzyme system in rat kidney. I. The effect of adrenalectomy and the supply of sodium on the enzyme system. *Biochim. Biophys. Acta, 51*:212.

Jørgensen, P. L. 1969. Regulation of the (Na$^+$ + K$^+$)-activated ATP hydrolyzing enzyme system in rat kidney. II. Effect of aldosterone on the activity in kidneys of adrenalectomized rats. *Biochim. Biophys. Acta, 192*:326.

Jørgensen, P. L. 1974a. Purification of (Na$^+$ + K$^+$)-ATPase: Active site determinations and criteria of purity. *Ann. N.Y. Acad. Sci., 242*:36.

Jørgensen, P. L. 1974b. Purification and characterization of (Na$^+$ + K$^+$)-ATPase: III. Purification from the outer medulla of mammalian kidney after selective removal of membrane components by sodium dodecylsulphate. *Biochim. Biophys. Acta, 356*:36.

Jørgensen, P. L. 1974c. Purification and characterization of (Na$^+$ + K$^+$)-ATPase: IV. Estimation of the purity and of the molecular weight and polypeptide content per enzyme unit in preparation from the outer medulla of rabbit kidney. *Biochim. Biophys. Acta, 356*:53.

Jørgensen, P. L. and Skou, J. C. 1969. Preparation of highly active (Na$^+$ + K$^+$)-ATPase from the outer medulla of rabbit kidney. *Biochem. Biophys. Res. Commun., 37*:39.

Jørgensen, P. L., Skou, J. C., and Solomonson, L. P. 1971. Purification and characterization of (Na$^+$ + K$^+$)-ATPase: II. Preparation of zonal centrifugation of highly active (Na$^+$ + K$^+$)-ATPase from the outer medulla of rabbit kidneys. *Biochim. Biophys. Acta, 233*:381.

Katz, A. I. and Epstein, F. H. 1967. The role of sodium–potassium-activated adenosine triphosphatase in the reabsorption of sodium by the kidney. *J. Clin. Invest., 46*:1999.

Katz, A. I. and Genant, H. K. 1971. Effect of extracellular volume expansion on renal cortical and medullary Na$^+$-K$^+$-ATPase. *Pfluegers Arch., 330*:136.

Katz, A. I. and Lindheimer, M. D. 1973. Renal sodium- and potassium-activated adenosine triphosphatase and sodium reabsorption in the hypothyroid rat. *J. Clin. Invest., 52*:796.

Kepner, G. R. and Macey, R. I. 1966. Red cell membrane ATPase: Radiation inactivation estimates of "size." *Biochem. Biophys. Res. Commun., 23*:202.

Kessler, R. H. 1970. The effects of glucose and inhibitor compounds on renal nucleotides *in vivo*. *Proc. IVth Int. Cong. Nephrol., 2*:137.

Kessler, R. H., Weinstein, S. W., Nash, F. D., and Fujimoto, M. 1964. Effects of chlormerodrin, *p*-chloromercuribenzoate and dichlorphenamide on renal. sodium reabsorption and oxygen consumption. *Nephron, 1*:221.

Kinsolving, C. R., Post, R. L., and Beaver, D. L. 1963. Sodium plus potassium transport adenosine triphosphatase activity in kidney. *J. Cell. Comp. Physiol., 62*:85.

Knox, W. H. and Sen, A. K. 1974. Mechanism of action of aldosterone with particular reference to (Na + K)-ATPase. *Ann. N.Y. Acad. Sci., 242*:471.

Kokko, J., Burg, M. B., and Orloff, J. 1971. Characteristics of NaCl and water transport in the renal proximal tubule. *J. Clin. Invest., 50*:69.

Komorn, R. and Cafruny, E. J. 1965. Effects of ethacrynic acid on renal protein-bound sulfhydryl groups. *J. Pharmacol. Exp. Ther., 148*:367.

Kramer, H. J. and Gonick, H. C. 1973. Effect of maleic acid on sodium-linked tubular transport in experimental Fanconi syndrome. *Nephron, 10*:306.

Kramer, J. and Burgard, U. G. 1974. Further studies on epithelial transport defect in experimental and human Fanconi syndrome. *Clin. Chim. Acta, 55*:57.

Kupfer, S. and Kosovsky, J. D. 1965. Effects of cardiac glycosides on renal tubular transport of calcium, magnesium, inorganic phosphate, and glucose in the dog. *J. Clin. Invest., 44*:1132.

Kyte, J. 1971. Purification of the sodium- and potassium-dependent adenosine triphosphatase from canine renal medulla. *J. Biol. Chem., 246*:4157.

Kyte, J. 1972a. The titration of the cardiac glycoside binding site of the (Na$^+$ + K$^+$)-adenosine triphosphatase. *J. Biol. Chem., 247*:7634.

Kyte, J. 1972b. Properties of the two polypeptides of sodium- and potassium-dependent adenosine triphosphatase. *J. Biol. Chem., 247*:7642.

Lane, L. K., Copenhaver, J. H., Jr., Lindenmayer, G. E., and Schwartz, A. 1973. Purification and characterization of and [³H]ouabain binding to the transport adenosine triphosphatase from outer medulla of canine kidney. *J. Biol. Chem., 248*:7197.

Lie, M., Sejersted, O. M., Raeder, M., and Kiil, F. 1974. Comparison of renal responses to ouabain and ethacrynic acid. *Am. J. Physiol., 226*:1221.

Lindenmayer, G. E. and Schwartz, A. 1973. Nature of the transport adenosine triphosphatase digitalis complex. *J. Biol. Chem., 248*:1291.

Martinez-Maldonado, M., Allen, J. C., Eknoyan, G., Suki, W., and Schwartz, A. 1969. Renal concentrating mechanism: Possible role for sodium–potassium activated adenosine triphosphatase. *Science, 165*:807.

Martinez-Maldonado, M., Eknoyan, G., Allen, J. C., Suki, W. N., and Schwartz, A. 1970. Urine dilution and concentration after digoxin infusion into the renal artery of dogs. *Proc. Soc. Exp. Biol. Med., 134*:855.

Martinez-Maldonado, M., Allen, J. C., Inagaki, C., Tsaparas, N., and Schwartz, A. 1972. Renal sodium–potassium-activated adenosine triphosphatase and sodium reabsorption. *J. Clin. Invest., 51*:2544.

Martinez-Maldonado, M., Tsaparas, N., Inagaki, C., and Schwartz, A. 1974. Interactions of digoxin and ethacrynic acid with renal sodium–potassium activated adenosine triphosphatase. *J. Pharmacol. Exp. Ther., 188*:605.

Michael, U. F., Barenberg, R. L., Chavez, R., Vaamonde, C. A., and Papper, S. 1972. Renal handling of sodium and water in the hypothyroid rat. *J. Clin. Invest., 51*:1405.

Nechay, B. R. 1974. Relationship between inhibition of renal Na⁺ plus K⁺-ATPase and natriuresis. *Ann. N.Y. Acad. Sci., 242*:501.

Nechay, B. R. and Contreras, R. R. 1972. In vivo effect of ethacrynic acid on renal adenosine triphosphatase in dog and rat. *J. Pharmacol. Exp. Ther., 183*:127.

Nechay, B. R. and Nelson, J. A. 1970. Renal ouabain-sensitive ATP-ase activity and Na⁺ reabsorption. *J. Pharmacol. Exp. Ther., 175*:717.

Nechay, B. R., Palmer, R. F., Chinoy, A., and Posey, V. A. 1967. The problem of Na⁺ + K⁺ adenosine triphosphatase as the receptor for diuretic action of mercurials and ethacrynic acid. *J. Pharmacol. Exp. Ther., 157*:599.

Nelson, J. A. and Nechay, B. R. 1970. Effect of cardiac glycosides on renal adenosine triphosphatase activity and Na⁺ reabsorption in dogs. *J. Pharmacol. Exp. Ther., 175*:727.

Nelson, J. A. and Nechay, B. R. 1971. Interaction of ouabain and K⁺ in vivo with respect to renal adenosine triphosphatase activity and Na⁺ reabsorption. *J. Pharmacol. Exp. Ther., 176*:558.

Orloff, J. and Burg, M. 1960. Effect of strophanthidin on electrolyte excretion in the chicken. *Am. J. Physiol., 199*:39.

Paul, W. and Gonick, H. C. 1968. Response of rat kidney Na⁺-K⁺-activated adenosine triphosphatase to sodium deprivation. *Proc. Soc. Exp. Biol. Med., 127*:1175.

Potter, D., Jarrah, A., Sakai, T., Harrah, J., and Holliday, M. A. 1969. Character of function and size in kidney during normal growth of rats. *Pediat. Res., 3*:51.

Rhodin, J. A. G. 1971. Structure of the kidney. In *Disease of the Kidney*, 2nd ed., Vol. I, pp. 1–30. Ed. by M. Strauss, and L. Welt, Little, Brown, Boston.

Rocha, A. S. and Kokko, J. P. 1973. Sodium chloride and water transport in the medullary thick ascending limb of Henle. Evidence for active chloride transport. *J. Clin. Invest., 52*:612.

Ross, B., Leaf, A., Silva, P., and Epstein, F. H. 1974. Na-K-ATPase in sodium transport by the perfused rat kidney. *Am. J. Physiol., 226*:624.

Ruoho, A. and Kyte, A. 1974. Photoaffinity labeling of ouabain-binding site on (Na⁺ + K⁺) adenosine triphosphatase. *Proc. Natl. Acad. Sci. U.S.A., 71*:2352.

Schatzmann, H. J., Windhager, E. E., and Solomon, A. K. 1958. Single proximal tubules of Necturus kidney. II. Effect of 2.4-dinitrophenol and ouabain on water reabsorption. *Am. J. Physiol., 195*:570.

Schmidt, U. and Dubach, U. C. 1969. Activity of (Na-K)-stimulated adenosine triphosphatase in the rat nephron. *Pfluegers Arch., 306*:219.

Schmidt, U. and Dubach, U. C. 1970. The behaviour of Na^+K^+-activated adenosine triphosphatase in various structures of the rat nephron after furosemide application. *Nephron, 7*:447.

Schmidt, U. and Dubach, U. C. 1971. Na–K-stimulated adenosine triphosphatase: Intracellular localization within the proximal tubules of the rat nephron. *Pfluegers Arch., 330*:265.

Schmidt, U., Schmid, H., Funk, B., and Dubach, U. C. 1974. The function of Na,K-ATPase in single portions of the rat nephron. *Ann. N.Y. Acad. Sci., 242*:489.

Schmidt, U., Schmid, J., Schmid, H., and Dubach, U. C. 1975. Sodium- and potassium-activated ATPase. A possible target of aldosterone. *J. Clin. Invest., 55*:655.

Schwartz, A., Allen, J. C., Van Winkle, W. B., and Munson, R. 1974. Further studies on the correlation between the inotropic action of ouabain and its interaction with the Na^+, K^+- adenosine triphosphatase: Isolated perfused rabbit and cat hearts. *J. Pharmacol. Exp. Ther., 191*:119.

Schwartz, A., Lindenmayer, G. E., and Allen, J. C. 1975. The sodium–potassium adenosine triphosphatase: Pharmacological, physiological and biochemical aspects. *Pharmacol. Rev., 27*:3.

Sejersted, O. M., Lie, M., and Kiil, F. 1971. Effect of ouabain on metabolic rate in renal cortex and medulla. *Am. J. Physiol., 220*:1488.

Sharp, G. W. G. and Leaf, A. 1966. Mechanism of action of aldosterone. *Physiol. Rev., 46*:593.

Skou, J. C. 1957. The influence of some cations on an adenosine triphosphatase from peripheral nerves. *Biochim. Biophys. Acta, 23*:394.

Skou, J. C. 1960. Further investigations on a Mg^{++} + Na^+ activated adenosine triphosphatase possibly related to the active linked transport of Na^+ and K^+ across the nerve membrane. *Biochim. Biophys. Acta, 42*:6.

Skou, J. C. 1964. Enzymatic aspects of active linked transport of Na^+ and K^+ through the cell membrane. In: *Progress in Biophysics and Molecular Biology*, Vol. 14 pp. 131–166. Ed. by J. A. V. Butler, and H. E. Huxley, Pergamon Press, London.

Skou, J. C. 1965. Enzymatic basis for active transport of Na^+ and K^+ across cell membrane. *Physiol. Rev., 45*:596.

Strickler, J. C. and Kessler, R. H. 1961. Direct renal action of some digitalis steroids. *J. Clin. Invest., 40*:311.

Strieder, N., Khuri, R., Wiederholt, M., and Giebisch, G. 1974. Studies on the renal action of ouabain in the rat. Effects in the non-diuretic state. *Pfluegers Arch., 349*:91.

Suzuki, S. and Ogawa, E. 1969. Experimental studies on the carbonic anhydrase activity-XII. *Biochem. Pharmacol., 18*:993.

Sweadner, K. J. and Goldin, S. M. 1975. Reconstitution of active ion transport by the sodium and potassium ion-stimulated adenosine triphosphatase from canine brain. *J. Biol. Chem., 250*:4022.

Torretti, J., Hendler, E., Weinstein, E., Longnecker, R. E., and Epstein, F. H. 1972. Functional significance of Na–K-ATPase in the kidney: Effects of ouabain inhibition. *Am. J. Physiol., 222*:1398.

Whittam, R. 1962. The asymmetrical stimulation of a membrane adenosine triphosphatase in relation to active cation transports. *Biochem. J., 84*:110.

Wilde, W. S. and Howard, P. J. 1960. Renal tubular action of ouabain on Na and K transport during stop-flow and slow-flow technique. *J. Pharmacol. Exp. Ther., 130*:232.

Wolf, K., Bieg, A., and Fülgraff, G. 1969. On the mode of action of diuretics II. Effects of ethacrynic acid on renal oxygen consumption and tubular sodium reabsorption in dogs. *Eur. J. Pharmacol., 7*:342.

Chapter **8**

Interactions between Vitamin D and the Kidney

Jack W. Coburn, Robert L. Saltzman

Medical and Research Service
V.A. Wadsworth Hospital Center
and Department of Medicine
UCLA School of Medicine
Los Angeles, California

and

Shaul G. Massry

Department of Medicine
Los Angeles County—USC Medical Center
Los Angeles, California

I. INTRODUCTION

The relationship between vitamin D and the kidney will be considered from two aspects: the conversion of vitamin D to its active metabolic form(s) by the kidney and the action of vitamin D or its metabolites on renal tubular function. Vitamin D_3 (cholecalciferol) is relatively inactive itself; the effects attributed to vitamin D_3 occur following its conversion to 1,25-dihydroxycholecalciferol $[1,25(OH)_2 D_3]$, an event occurring exclusively in the kidney (Fraser and Kodicek, 1970). Thus, the kidney acts as an endocrine organ regulating the conversion of a steroid prohormone to its active form and controls a metabolic step which plays an important role in calcium metabolism. Also, vitamin D or one of its metabolic forms may have specific effects on renal metabolism and tubular transport of various ions, such as phosphate, calcium, sodium, and bicarbonate.

II. METABOLISM OF VITAMIN D

A. Sources of Vitamin D

Man acquires vitamin D from two sources: his diet and via the ultraviolet irradiation of the provitamin, 7-dihydrocholesterol in the epidermal layer of his skin (Wheatley and Reinertson, 1958; Rauschkolb et al., 1969). The amount of endogenous vitamin D made is uncertain and probably variable, but it probably averages the minimum daily requirement of 2.5–10.0 μg/day (100–400 IU/day). In the present discussion, quantities of vitamin D and its metabolic forms will be presented in units of microgram (μg) and milligram (mg). The quantitative relationships between vitamin D and its other metabolic forms are summarized in Table I. Dietary vitamin D may be D_3 (cholecalciferol) or D_2 (ergocalciferol); the latter is an artificially produced sterol made from ultraviolet irradiation of the plant steroid, ergosterol. Dietary vitamin D is absorbed in the proximal small bowel (Schachter et al., 1965), carried in plasma bound to an α-globulin (Peterson, 1971), and transported to the liver. It may also be carried to and stored in other sites (Mawer and Schaefer, 1969; Rosenstreich et al., 1971), where it may be available for use when intake is low or exposure to sunlight is inadequate.

B. 25-Hydroxycholecalciferol

Ponchon and DeLuca (1969) found that the liver hydroxylates vitamin D_3 to form 25-hydroxycholecalciferol [25(OH)D_3]. They noted that when radiolabeled D_3 was given intravenously, it disappeared rapidly and 25(OH)D_3 appeared. The latter is the predominant form of circulating vitamin D_3 (Smith and Goodman, 1971; Gray et al., 1974). Disagreement exists about the degree of control of this conversion, with considerable evidence that all vitamin D_3 is not quantitatively converted to 25(OH)D_3. Using tissue homogenates from chicks, Tucker et al. (1973) found no evidence for the regulation of this conversion when the dietary intake of vitamin D_3 was varied within the physiological range. They found that

Table I. Quantitative Considerations of Vitamin D_3 and its Metabolites[a]

	Vitamin D_3 + metabolites			Vitamin D_2 + metabolites		
	D_2	25-OH-D_3	1,25(OH)$_2$$D_3$	D_2	25-OH-D_2	1,25(OH)$_2$$D_3$
Molecular weight	384.6	400.3	416.3	396.6	412.4	428.0
ng/65 pmoles[b]	25.00	26.01	27.06	25.78	26.80	27.8
"Units"/μg	40.0	38.5	37.0	38.8	37.3	35.8

[a] Modified from Coburn et al. (1974).
[b] 1.0 International unit (IU) of Vitamin D_3 (cholecalciferol) has been defined to be 0.025 μg (65.0 pmol) (League of Nations, Health Organization Memorandum, 1935). No official definitions of "units" have been formulated for 25-hydroxycholecalciferol or 1,25-dihydroxycholecalciferol. Some problems related to quantitation of vitamin D are discussed elsewhere (Norman, 1972).

25-hydroxylase activity was also present in renal and intestinal tissue. Bhatta-charyya and DeLuca (1973) found evidence for regulation of $25(OH)D_3$ production in rats whose vitamin D_3 intake was varied over a wider range. Mawer et al. (1971) found that a greater fraction of vitamin D_3 was converted to a metabolite believed to be $25(OH)D_3$ in patients with vitamin D-deficiency than in those receiving ample quantities of the vitamin. These latter two observations suggest the occurrence of regulation of this step. However, the relatively high levels of $25(OH)D$ found in the plasma of lifeguards exposed to sunlight(Haddad and Chyu, 1971b), the seasonal variation in $25(OH)D$ levels (Stamp and Round, 1974), and the tendency for plasma levels of $25(OH)D$ to increase after the administration of vitamin D_3 (Avioli and Haddad, 1973) all suggest that this "regulation" is overcome when the intake or production of vitamin D_3 is substantially increased.

Arnaud et al. (1975) found that a large fraction of the $25(OH)D_3$ produced is excreted into the duodenum via the biliary tract with a large portion subsequently reabsorbed into the enterohepatic circulation. From the liver, $25(OH)D_3$ is carried via a specific binding globulin (Haddad and Chyu, 1971a) to the kidney, where it undergoes further metabolic conversion.

C. Metabolism of 25-Hydroxycholecalciferol

At the time of this writing, at least four other metabolic products of $25(OH)D_3$ have been described: 25,26-dihydroxycholecalciferol [$25,26(OH)_2D_3$], 24,25-dihydroxycholecalciferol [$24,25(OH)_2D_3$], 1,24,25-trihydroxycholecalci-ferol [$1,24,25(OH)_3D_3$], and 1,25-dihydroxycholecalciferol [$1,25(OH_2D_3$]. In later sections, the production and action of $1,25(OH)_2D_3$, the most active form of vitamin D_3, will be discussed at length. The pathways of conversion and chemical structures of these compounds are shown in Figure 1.

1. 25,26-Dihydroxycholecalciferol

Suda et al. (1970) produced and identified $25,26(OH)_2D_3$ in pigs that had been given large doses of radiolabeled vitamin D_3. They found $25,26(OH)_2D_3$ stimulated intestinal calcium absorption but had no effect on bone calcium mobilization in the rat. It had no antirachitic properties, as measured by the line test, in the rat; moreover, its site of production is unknown. Lam et al. (1975) were able to synthesize $25,26(OH)_2D_3$ in vitro and found it able to increase calcium absorption. Its potency was less in anephric animals, suggesting that further metabolism by the kidney, possible 1-hydroxylation, was needed to activate this compound.

2. 24,25-Dihydroxycholecalciferol

This sterol is produced in chick kidneys by the enzyme 25-hydroxycholecal-ciferol-24-hydroxylase (Holick et al., 1972; Knutson and DeLuca, 1974). Tucker et al. (1973) found evidence for the presence of this enzyme in renal and

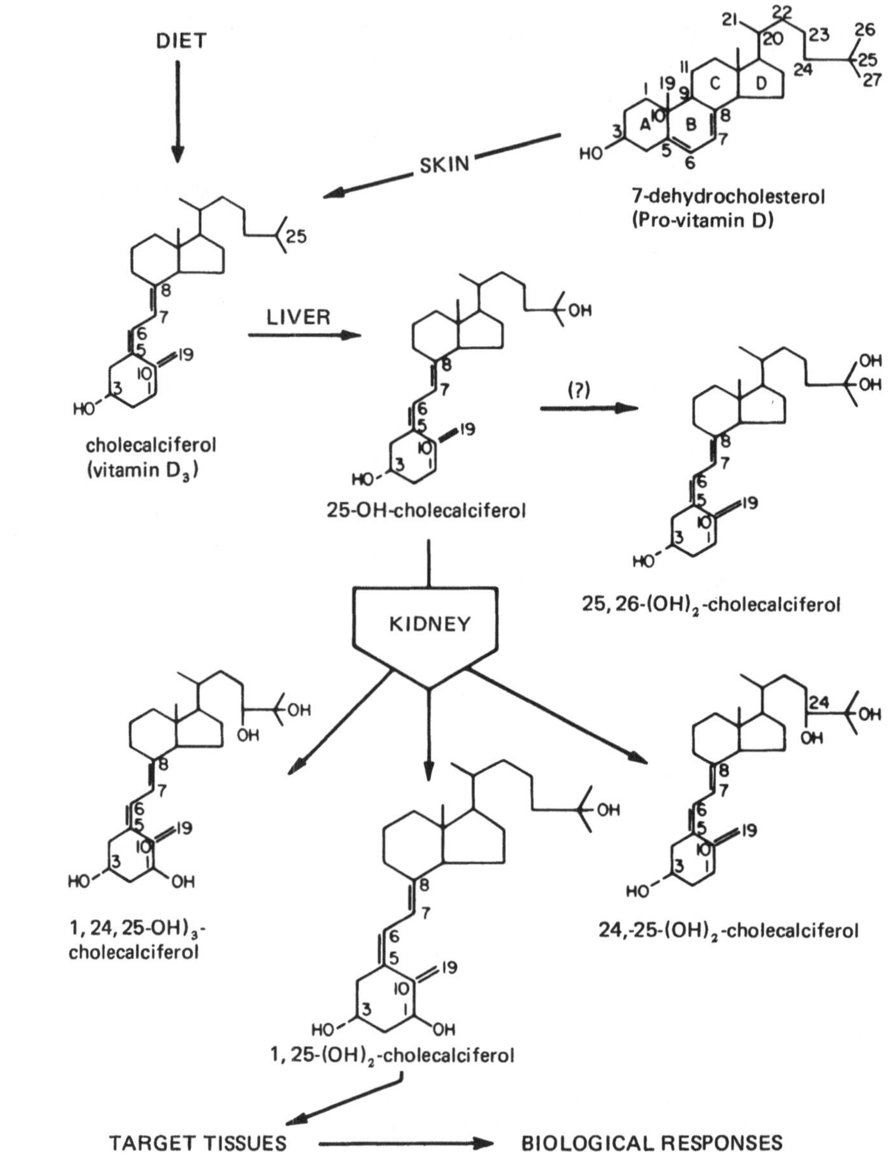

Figure 1. Scheme of vitamin D metabolism. (Reproduced from Coburn *et al.*, 1974, with permission.)

intestinal tissue as well. Unlike 25(OH)D$_3$-1-hydroxylase, which is described subsequently, the enzyme responsible for production of 24,25(OH)$_2$D$_3$ is insensitive to carbon monoxide inhibition (Ghazarian *et al.*, 1974) and is stimulated by conditions which tend to be inhibitory to the 1-hydroxylase system (Boyle *et al.*, 1971). Boyle *et al.* (1973) reported that 24,25(OH)$_2$D$_3$ enhances intestinal calcium transport but is less active in causing bone calcium mobilization. They also found the effects of 24,25(OH)$_2$D$_3$ could be abolished by nephrectomy, implying the need for further metabolism by the kidney. Also, previous feeding with a high-calcium diet abolished the stimulatory effects of $24,25(OH)_2D_3$ on intestinal calcium absorption.

3. 1,24,25-Trihydroxycholecalciferol

This compound can stimulate both intestinal calcium absorption and bone calcium mobilization and has been produced *in vivo* by the rat and *in vitro* using homogenates of chick kidney incubated with $24,25(OH)_2D_3$ (Holick *et al.*, 1973). Whether $1,24,25(OH)_3D_3$ is invariably produced *in vivo* remains unsettled; Friedlander and Norman (1975) could not induce its production in the chick *in vitro*; Gray *et al.* (1974) demonstrated a peak in plasma from normal subjects and anephric humans given ^{3}H-labeled $25(OH)D_3$ which had chromatographic similarities to authentic $1,24,25(OH)_3D_3$.

D. 1,25-Dihydroxycholecalciferol

1. Intestinal Actions of 1,25(OH)₂D₃

A lengthy discussion of the mode of action of vitamin D on its target tissues is beyond the scope of this chapter and reviews of vitamin D action may be found elsewhere (Avioli, 1972; Coburn *et al.*, 1974; Norman and Henry, 1975). It is pertinent to review briefly some of the current knowledge about its action on the intestine, the most extensively studied target tissue. In the intestinal mucosa, $1,25(OH)_2D_3$ becomes bound to a cytosol protein receptor (Haussler and Norman, 1969; Brumbaugh and Haussler, 1974), migrates to the nucleus (Brumbaugh and Haussler, 1973), and then becomes associated with a specific chromatin receptor (Brumbaugh and Haussler, 1975). It is then believed to induce the formation of a messenger RNA, which stimulates new protein synthesis. A specific calcium-binding protein (CaBP) has been identified along the microvillous membrane of intestinal epithelial cells and on goblet cells following treatment with vitamin D (Taylor and Wasserman, 1969). The observations that the action of vitamin D can be blocked by actinomycin D (Norman, 1965; Zull *et al.*, 1965), that the template activity of DNA-directed RNA synthesis is increased (Hallick and DeLuca, 1969), and the [^{3}H]uridine incorporation into nuclear RNA is increased by vitamin D (Chen and DeLuca, 1973) all provide evidence that the action of vitamin D may be similar to that of other steroid hormones.

It is believed that CaBP plays a major role in inducing an increase in transmucosal transport of calcium in chick intestine. A vitamin D-dependent CaBP has been found in chicks (Wasserman and Taylor, 1966), rats (Kallfelz *et al.*, 1967), dogs (Taylor *et al.*, 1968; Sands and Kessler, 1971), and New World primates (Wasserman and Taylor, 1971). The appearance of CaBP precedes and parallels the increase in intestinal calcium absorption induced by vitamin D_3 (MacGregor *et al.*, 1970). The fact that CaBP is found in greater concentrations in those segments of the bowel with the greatest capacity for calcium transport

(Taylor and Wasserman, 1967) and observations that CaBP is increased in situations of calcium deprivation when calcium transport is more efficient (Wasserman and Taylor, 1968; Hurwitz and Bar, 1969) have led to the proposal that CaBP plays a major role in augmenting the entry of calcium in the cell.

Whether CaBP is the rate-limiting factor for the transfer of calcium into the cell remains unanswered; it is possible that CaBP may concentrate calcium and make it available for another process which is rate limiting and involved in the actual transcellular transport of this ion. Once calcium is within the cell, there is evidence that it may be concentrated within certain subcellular compartments, such as the mitochondria (Sampson et al., 1970); moreover, the extrusion of calcium from the serosal borders involves active transport against an electro-chemical gradient (Kimberg et al., 1961). Two separate ATPases have been identified and are believed to be essential for this active movement of calcium from the cell (Schachter et al., 1960; Adams and Norman, 1970; Birge et al., 1972). Martin et al. (1969) and Melancon and DeLuca (1970) have demonstrated a vitamin D-dependent ATPase. A schema showing the postulated events that occur associated with vitamin D-induced intestinal calcium transport is given in Figure 2. It is possible that the mechanisms whereby calcium is actively transported by other calcium transporting tissues, such as bone, kidney, egg

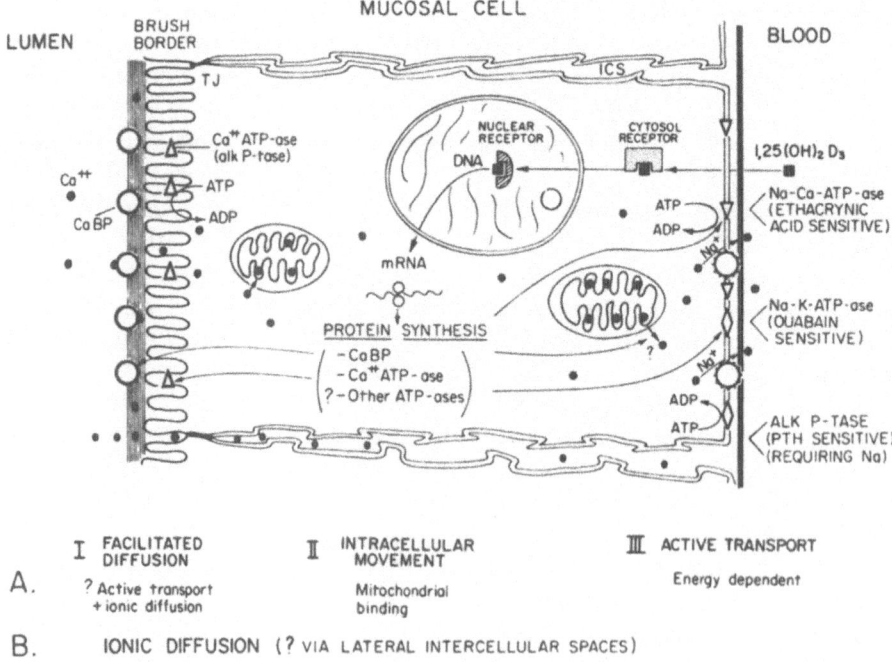

Figure 2. A model showing the events which may occur during vitamin D-stimulated calcium transport across the intestinal epithelium. Abbreviations include: CaBP calcium binding protein; TJ, tight junction; ICS, intercellular space; and alk P-tase, alkaline phosphatase. (Modified from Coburn et al., 1973.)

shell gland, and the mammary gland, may be similar to the process believed to occur in the intestine.

2. Renal Production of 1,25-Dihydroxycholecalciferol

Localization and Characteristics of 25-Hydroxycholecalciferol-1-hydroxylase. Observations that the conversion of $25(OH)_3$ to $1,25(OH)_2 D_3$ is the most closely controlled step in the metabolism of vitamin D have focused attention to the responsible enzyme, namely, 25-hydroxycholecalciferol-1-hydroxylase. This enzyme has been found only in the kidney (Fraser and Kodicek, 1970) and is localized in the mitochondrial fraction of the renal cortex (Gray *et al.*, 1972; Midgett *et al.*, 1973); it requires molecular oxygen, NADPH, and is inhibited by carbon monoxide and metapyrone. The last observation suggests that it is a cytochrome P-450 enzyme (Gray *et al.*, 1972; Ghazarian *et al.*, 1974). Thus, the $25(OH)D_3$-1-hydroxylase has certain similarities to other mixed-function oxidases found in other steroidogenic tissues (Henry and Norman, 1974). This enzyme is also substrate specific in that it will not 1-hydroxylate cholecalciferol or dihydrotachysterol (Gray *et al.*, 1972). Presently, data are not available to indicate the specific cellular distribution of the enzyme in the cortex; thus, the enzyme could be diffusely distributed in cortical tubular cells, may be found only in one part of the tubule (i.e., proximal or distal), or may be limited to specialized cells, such as the juxtaglomerular apparatus.

General Considerations of Enzyme Regulation. Considerable interest has focused on the physiological signals which stimulate or inhibit the conversion of $25(OH)D_3$ to $1,25(OH)_2 D_3$. When one analyzes data concerning the activity of $25(OH)D_3$-1-hydroxylase, they are most often expressed as a function of the quantity of end product, $1,25(OH)_2 D_3$, generated. A change in the production of $1,25(OH)_2 D_3$ could be due to (1) alterations in the balance between synthesis and degradation of enzyme, (2) activation or inactivation of a steady-state quantity of enzyme, or (3) an indirect affect on enzyme activity because of a change in substrate or cofactor availability. In particular, it is possible for the quantity of end product to differ not as a direct effect of the signal, but indirectly because the signal may affect the availability of a cofactor or alter the ionic environment of the enzyme. The fact that the enzyme, $25(OH)D_3$-1-hydroxylase, is present within mitochondria imposes severe restrictions on methods which can be used to study mechanisms of enzyme regulation. Both the cell and the investigator are faced with a signal reaching the surface of the cell and transmitting its message into the cell, to the mitochondria, and finally, into the mitochondrion itself. Changes in the intracellular or intramitochondrial concentrations of calcium, phosphate, or hydrogen ion may comprise the final signals, and possible effectors include parathyroid hormone, calcitonin, vitamin D_3, or one of the latter's metabolic forms. Also, cylic AMP must be considered as a potential mediator. Data reported to support or refute the roles of each of these factors are summarized below.

Most data concerning vitamin D_3 metabolism, whether obtained *in vivo* or *in vitro*, involve the use of animals which are made vitamin D-deficient. The animals are given radiolabeled vitamin D_3 or $25(OH)D_3$, and the metabolic fate of the steroid and the influence of a potential signal can be measured. The vitamin D-deficient state is necessary for several reasons: the available radiolabeled vitamin D_3 or $25(OH)D_3$ is of relatively low specific activity. The amount of radioactivity that can be given must be kept small so that the quantity of vitamin D given is within the "physiological" range. If radiolabeled vitamin D_3 or $25(OH)D_3$ is given to a non-vitamin D-deficient animal, the label becomes diluted in unlabeled, naturally occurring pools of vitamin D_3 and its metabolites, each of unknown size. Estimates of plasma levels and turnover rates of vitamin D_3, $25(OH)D_3$, and $1,25(OH)_2D_3$ in man are summarized in Table II. As will be discussed later, the activity of $25(OH)D_3$-1-hydroxylase is greatest and most accurately measured in the vitamin D-deficient state; thus, only under the circumstances of vitamin D deficiency is the $25(OH)D_3$-1-hydroxylase activity of sufficient magnitude so that measurable amounts of end product are generated. Some of these problems will be obviated when simple and reproducible methods are developed for measuring physiological quantities of nonradioactive $1,25(OH)_2D_3$ and other metabolites in biologic samples and tissue extracts.

Effect of Parathyroid Hormone. One potential modulator of $25(OH)D_3$-1-hydroxylase that has been extensively studied is parathyroid hormone (PTH). Garabedian *et al.* (1972) evaluated the *in vivo* production of $1,25(OH)_2D_3$ from radiolabeled 25-hydroxy D_3 in vitamin D-deficient rats subjected to thyroparathyroidectomy (TPTX). They found reduced quantities of $1,25(OH)_2D_3$ in plasma of TPTX animals and suggested that PTH is a specific trophic factor. However, they gave the TPTX rats small amounts of nonradioactive $1,25(OH)_2D_3$ to prevent fatal hypocalcemia. This maneuver may have influenced the results; the role of vitamin D and its metabolites in affecting the metabolic production of $1,25(OH)_2D_3$ is reviewed below.

Rasmussen *et al.* (1972) studied the conversion of $25(OH)_2D_3$ to $1,25(OH)_2D_3$ in isolated renal tubules from vitamin D-deficient chicks; the rate of

Table II. Approximate Plasma Concentrations and Turnover Times of Vitamin D_3 and Its Metabolites in Man

	Vitamin D_3	$25(OH)D_3$	$1,25(OH)_2D_3$
Turnover Time ($T\frac{1}{2}$)			
Vitamin D-deficient (days)	4.5^a	16^a	<1.0
Vitamin D-replete (days)	4.5^a	$23–30^{a,b}$	<1.0
Plasma Concentrations (pg/ml)	25×10^3 ^{c}	$20–40 \times 10^3$ ^{c,d}	$15–20^e$
Estimated endogenous production rate (μg/day) or intake	$2.5–>20$	$10–20^{a,b}$	$0.5–1.0^f$

[a] From Mawer *et al.* (1971).
[b] From Gray *et al.* (1975).
[c] From Belsey *et al.* (1971).
[d] From Haddad and Stamp (1974).
[e] From Brumbaugh *et al.* (1974).
[f] From Brickman *et al.* (1974).

conversion was enhanced by parathyroid hormone in concentrations of 5 and 50 ng/ml. The conversion was decreased slightly with a concentration of 0.5 ng/ml, and a much higher concentration of 0.5 μg/ml had no effect. Shain (1972), who utilized a similar preparation but a slightly different buffer system, found no effect of purified PTH at 10 μg/ml.

Galante *et al.* (1972) gave parathyroid extract (PTE) in large doses of 8, 40, and 200 units/day for two days to vitamin D-deficient, nonrachitic rats rendered mildly hypercalcemic with a high dietary calcium intake. Following the administration of [^{3}H]25 hydroxycholecalciferol, treatment with PTE was associated with lower quantities of 1,25(OH)$_2$D$_3$ in serum, while the amount of 24,25(OH)$_2$D$_3$ was increased. The hypercalcemia may have been a factor in leading to these results, which differ from those noted above. Fraser and Kodicek (1973) measured the activity of 25(OH)D$_3$-1-hydroxylase in homogenates of whole kidney obtained from vitamin D-deficient chicks. The administration of bovine PTE, in doses of 30 units/100 g body wt every 6 hr for 48 hr, led to an increase in enzyme activity. Moreover, when parathyroidectomy (PTX) was carried out, the activity of the enzyme decreased.

In other experiments, Galante *et al.* (1973) found that the activity of the 25(OH)D$_3$-1-hydroxylase remained high in the kidneys of hypocalcemic chicks given a low-Ca diet and subjected to parathyroidectomy. They concluded that PTH was not essential for the maintenance of high enzyme activity. The hypocalcemia was more marked after PTX, and this may have been a factor preventing a decrease in enzyme activity. Also, Larkins *et al.* (1973) found that parathyroidectomized rats, whose dietary calcium was changed from high to low and dietary phosphate from normal to low, produced increased quantities of 1,25(OH)$_2$D$_3$ from 25(OH)D$_3$. Moreover, a similar reduction in dietary phosphate alone also increased production of 1,25(OH)$_2$D$_3$, although the increment was smaller. It was again concluded that PTH was not essential for the production of 1,25(OH)$_2$D$_3$.

Larkins *et al.* (1974a) studied clumps of viable cells from renal tubules of vitamin D-deficient chicks. When calcium was present in the incubation media at a concentration of 1.2 mM, the addition of PTH slightly reduced the activity of the 25(OH)D$_3$-1-hydroxylase; however, this was only seen if the rates of conversion during the control period were high. Studies carried out with the calcium removed from the media by means of the chelator, ethanedioxy-bis(ethylamine)tetraacetate (EGTA), revealed a slight decrease in the rate of basal conversion of 25(OH)D$_3$ to 1,25(OH)$_2$D$_3$; the addition of PTH, 50 or 500 ng/ml, caused a significant augmentation in production of 1,25(OH)$_2$D$_3$, but the effect was not as great as that caused by adding dibutyryl cyclic AMP. In a study which evaluated the activity of the 25(OH)D$_3$-1-hydroxylase in mitochondria isolated from vitamin D-deficient chicks, Henry *et al.* (1974) found that parathyroidectomy led to a decrease in enzyme activity to a level found in chicks given ample quantities of vitamin D. Moreover, from the effects of cyclohexamide treatment, they suggested that this effect was due to alterations in the rate of biosynthesis of the enzyme.

To provide further evidence for a role of parathyroid hormone in the rate of synthesis of $1,25(OH)_2D_3$, Haussler *et al.* (1975a) reported increased plasma levels of $1,25(OH)_2D_3$, as measured by a competitive binding assay, in the plasma of patients with hyperparathyroidism. Moreover, the administration of parathyroid extract intramuscularly for several days to normal individuals increased the plasma levels of $1,25(OH)_2D_3$. Plasma levels were low in patients with hypoparathyroidism (Haussler *et al.*, 1975b). Evidence in support of a role for the parathyroid glands in mediating changes in production of $1,25(OH)_2D_3$ has been derived from plasma levels of $1,25(OH)_2D_3$ in both intact and thyroparathyroidectomized rats given a low-calcium diet. Thus, Hughes *et al.* (1975) found that TPTX prevented the appearance of the increased plasma $1,25(OH)_2D_3$ that was observed in intact rats fed a low-calcium diet.

Although the results of certain studies evaluating the effect of PTH may seem to be in conflict, data from several independent laboratories and with the use of divergent methodology support the postulate that the production of $1,25(OH)_2D_3$ is enhanced by PTH, while the synthesis of the sterol may be reduced in the absence of PTH. Although the data of MacIntyre *et al.* (1974) may seem contradictory, they emphasize that changes in the production of $1,25(OH)_2D_3$ can occur without alterations in PTH levels. The different results may, as they suggest, be related to variation in the intracellular content of calcium under different study situations.

Effect of Vitamin D Status. There is general agreement that vitamin D_3 or $1,25(OH)_2D_3$ can inhibit the activity of the $25(OH)D_3$-1-hydroxylase. Garabedian *et al.* (1972) found reduced levels of $1,25(OH)_2D_3$ produced *in vivo* from its radiolabeled precurser in TPTX rats given small amounts of unlabeled $1,25(OH)_2D_3$. Although this effect on the enzyme was considered to be related to the absence of PTH, it is possible that the result was due to the administration of $1,25(OH)_2D_3$ itself. Henry *et al.* (1974) reported that the activity of the enzyme studied *in vitro* was highest in tissues from vitamin D-deficient chicks and lower in birds given 0.62 μg vitamin D_3 per day. Similarly, the administration of $1,25(OH)_2D_3$, 0.077 μg/day, suppressed the level of the renal enzyme. When treatment with either vitamin D_3 or $1,25(OH)_2D_3$ was discontinued, enzyme activity increased within 2–3 days. It should be noted that vitamin D-deficient chicks are generally hypocalcemic, and the possibility exists that the inhibition produced by vitamin D_3 or $1,25(OH)_2D_3$ may be due to the changes in the plasma calcium levels. Moreover, Henry *et al.* (1974) reported a highly significant inverse correlation between $25(OH)D_3$-1-hydroxylase activity and the levels of serum calcium. They inferred that the action of vitamin D_3 or $1,25(OH)_2D_3$ was mediated by a change in enzyme synthesis rather than a change in rate of degradation, since the latter, as evaluated by the rate of decrease in enzyme activity following cyclohexamide treatment, was no different in chicks receiving or lacking vitamin D_3. Furthermore, the rate of enzyme synthesis was 4–5 times greater in vitamin D-deficient than vitamin D-replete chicks. Henry and Norman (1974) suggested that the V_{max} of $25(OH)D_3$-1-hydroxylase is also enhanced in rachitic chicks compared to vitamin D-treated birds.

Larkins *et al.* (1974a) utilized suspensions of kidney tubules and found that the conversion of $25(OH)D_3$ to $1,25(OH)_2D_3$ was decreased following preincubation with $1,25(OH)_2D_3$, itself. They propose that this effect of $1,25(OH)_2D_3$ on the enzyme is due to its enhancing influx of calcium into the cell, which, in turn, inhibits the $25(OH)D_3$-1-hydroxylase activity. Pertinent to this suggestion, Larkins *et al.* (1974b) also reported that the inhibitory effect of $1,25(OH)_2D_3$ on $25(OH)D_3$-1-hydroxylase was reduced as the calcium concentration in the incubation media was lowered.

Additional observations in support of an inhibition of the $25(OH)D_3$-1-hydroxylase by vitamin D_3 or $1,25(OH)_2D_3$ were reported by Horiuchi *et al.* (1974). Chicks received a high-calcium intake and either a vitamin D-free diet or varying doses of vitamin D. The high-calcium intake produced hypercalcemia, thereby suppressing the parathyroid glands. The enzyme activity, based on production of $1,25(OH)_2D_3$ *in vitro*, was highest in chicks not pretreated with vitamin D_3 and fell dramatically with even the lowest dose of vitamin $D_3(0.025$ μg/day). Also, there was an increased production of $24,25(OH)_2D_3$ as the generation of $1,25(OH)_2D_3$ fell (Figure 3).

Norman *et al.* (1973) administered vitamin D_3 in daily doses of 0.375, 1.25, or 12.5 μg/day to 4-week-old chicks deprived of vitamin D for 2 weeks. Serum calcium and the activity of the renal $25(OH)D_3$-1-hydroxylase were measured. All doses of vitamin D_3 raised serum calcium to normal, while only the higher doses (1.25 and 12.5 μg/day) completely suppressed the elevated activity of

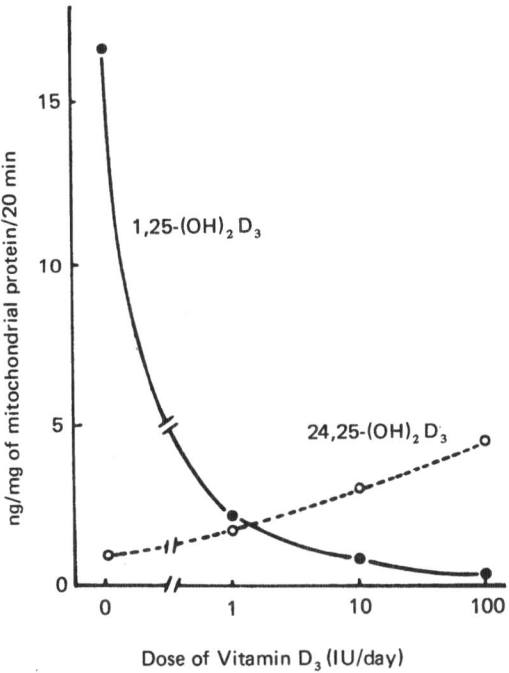

Figure 3. Quantity of either $1,25(OH)_2D_3$ or $24,25(OH)_2D_3$ produced *in vitro* by chick kidneys in relation to vitamin D administration *in vivo*. (From Horiuchi *et al.*, 1974, with permission).

25(OH)D_3-1-hydroxylase. The failure of 0.375 μg/day to suppress the enzyme despite the presence of a normal serum calcium suggests that hypocalcemia may not be necessary to increase the activity of 25(OH)D_3-1-hydroxylase with vitamin D deficiency. The reasons for the apparent discrepancies in the amount of vitamin D_3 required to suppress the 25(OH)D_3-1-hydroxylase in the results of Horiuchi et al. (1974) and Norman et al. (1973) are not apparent. The birds studied by Horiuchi et al. (1974) received a vitamin D-deficient diet from the time of hatching and were presumably smaller than the chicks studied by Norman et al. (1973). The mechanism whereby vitamin D_3 or 1,25(OH)$_2$$D_3$ inhibits the action of renal 25(OH)D_3-1-hydroxylase remains unanswered. Changes in intracellular or mitochondrial Ca^{2+} or HPO_4^{2-} content are likely possibilities, and data concerned with the effect of these ions on vitamin D metabolism are reviewed in a subsequent section.

Effect of Calcitonin. A number of studies have been carried out to evaluate the effect of calcitonin (CT) on the renal enzyme, 25(OH)D_3-1-hydroxylase. Galante et al. (1972) gave varying doses of synthetic salmon calcitonin to vitamin D-deficient, normocalcemic, nonrachitic rats. They evaluated the intestinal content of vitamin D metabolites, believed to be 1,25(OH)$_2$$D_3$ and 24,25(OH)$_2$$D_3$, following the administration of radiolabeled 25(OH)D_3. Using quantities of calcitonin which caused hypocalcemia during the first 24 hr, they found a significant increase in the intestinal content of 1,25(OH)$_2$$D_3$ and a reduction in the quantity of 24,25(OH)$_2$$D_3$. These results were similar to those observed following treatment with a low-calcium diet, and they suggest that calcitonin may exert its effect by causing a reduction in the intracellular concentration of calcium in renal cells. In another study, Larkins et al. (1973) studied the effect of salmon and human calcitonin on the production of 1,25(OH)$_2$$D_3$ by isolated chick renal tubules. The addition of 500 ng/ml salmon calcitonin, but not 50 ng/ml, caused a small but significant increase in synthesis of 1,25(OH)$_2$$D_3$, while human calcitonin, added in the same concentrations, was without effect. There were no changes in the quantities of cyclic AMP produced with these concentrations of calcitonin.

Rasmussen et al. (1972) also evaluated the effects of calcitonin on isolated renal tubules from vitamin D-deficient chicks. In their experimental model, they found that porcine calcitonin, in concentrations of 5–10 ng/ml, inhibited the formation of 1,25(OH)$_2$$D_3$. They also added calcitonin to renal tubules, whose production of 1,25(OH)$_2$$D_3$ was stimulated by parathyroid hormone; under these circumstances, calcitonin did not block the stimulatory effect of PTH.

Effect of Inorganic Phosphate. Inorganic phosphate is among the signals which may affect the activity of the renal 25(OH)D_3-1-hydroxylase. Interest in a possible role of phosphate in vitamin D metabolism first arose because of the similarities between the skeletal lesion of phosphate depletion and those of osteomalacia resulting from vitamin D-deficiency (Day and McCollum, 1939; Lotz et al., 1964). Speculating that phosphate depletion might alter vitamin D metabolism, Haddad et al. (1971) studied the metabolism of either [3H]-labeled vitamin D_3 or [^{3}H]25(OH)D_3 in phosphate-depleted rats receiving ample quantities of vitamin D in their diets. Despite findings of poor growth, hypercalcemia, hypophosphatemia, and florid rickets in the phosphate-depleted animals, the metabolism of vitamin D was not different from controls.

The results of Haddad *et al* (1971) and those of others in man (Lotz *et al.*, 1968) and the rat (Morrissey and Wasserman, 1971; Tanaka *et al.*, 1973) indicate that the intestinal absorption of calcium is increased during phosphate depletion. Moreover, Tanaka and DeLuca (1973) found larger quantities of radiolabeled $1,25(OH)_2D_3$ in the serum of phosphate-depleted, vitamin D-deficient rats compared to results when dietary phosphate was normal. Moreover, the quantity of radiolabeled $1,25(OH)_2D_3$ in serum varied inversely with levels of serum phosphorus, while the amount of $24,25(OH)_2D_3$ varied directly with the serum phosphorus. The results were found to be independent of the presence or absence of the parathyroid glands. Also, the amount of $1,25(OH)_2D_3$ appearing in plasma varied inversely with the inorganic phosphate in renal tissue. They suggested that a reduced renal content of phosphate is an important factor stimulating the activity of renal $25(OH)D_3$-1-hydroxylase and accounting for the increased intestinal absorption of calcium noted in phosphate depletion. These changes occurred despite the presence of hypercalcemia and also without the need for intact parathyroid glands.

Henry *et al.* (1974) studied the regulation of $25(OH)D_3$-1-hydroxylase *in vivo* utilizing mitochondria from chick kidneys. They found that variations in dietary phosphate had no effect on the activity of the enzyme when the chicks were studied following the withdrawal of vitamin D_3. Thus, the activity of $25(OH)D_3$-1-hydroxylase rose after the withdrawal of vitamin D_3, independent of the quantity of phosphate in the diet. In studies carried out in chicks, Bikle and Rasmussen (1975) reduced dietary phosphate intake in vitamin D-deficient chicks. The activity of renal $25(OH)D_3$-1-hydroxylase, studied *in vitro*, was not enhanced by phosphate restriction above the already high levels due to vitamin D deficiency. When dietary phosphate was increased to high levels (3%), there was a fall in enzyme activity (Figure 4). The reason for the apparent difference between the results obtained in the rat by Tanaka *et al.* (1973) and in the chick by both Henry *et al.* (1974) and Bikle and Rasmussen (1975) is uncertain, but it may relate to species differences. In additional studies carried out in the rat, Hughes *et al.* (1975) found that a low-phosphate diet caused an increase in the plasma level of $1,25(OH)_2D_3$ in vitamin D-replete rats, independent of the presence or absence of the parathyroid glands. Thus, their data are consistent with those of Tanaka *et al.* (1973), which suggest a direct role of phosphate in the regulation of the renal enzyme converting $25(OH)D_3$ to $1,25(OH)_2D_3$.

In studies carried out with isolated renal tubules from vitamin D-deficient chicks, Bikle and Rasmussen (1975) found that varying the phosphate concentration, in the presence of 1–2 mM calcium, caused a biphasic effect on enzyme activity. As the phosphate concentration was increased from 0 to 0.6 mM, there was reduced production of $1,25(OH)_2D_3$ by the enzyme; as the concentration of phosphate was increased above 1.2 mM, the enzyme activity increased. In the absence of calcium or with a higher calcium concentration (4 mM), the biphasic effect of varying phosphate concentration did not occur. It is of interest that a decrease in the concentration of phosphate in the incubation media from a value

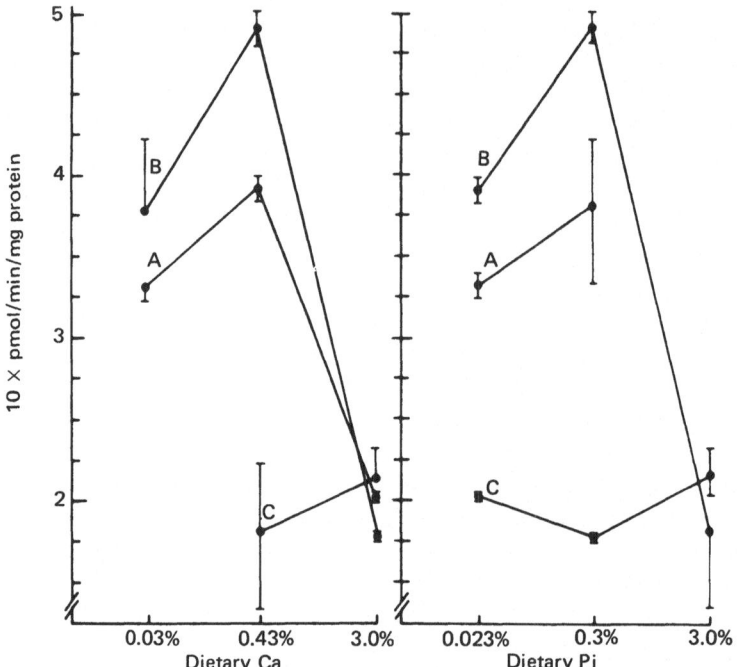

Figure 4. The effect of varying dietary content of phosphate (left) and calcium (right) on the production of 1,25(OH)$_2$D$_3$ by renal tubules from vitamin D-deficient chicks. The designations A (low), B (med), and C (high) refer to the content of either phosphate or calcium superimposed on the quantities of calcium or phosphate, shown on the abscissa. (From Bikle and Rasmussen, 1975, with permission.)

that approximates the physiological extracellular level to a lower concentration was associated with increased enzyme activity, an observation similar to those found *in vivo* with phosphate depletion. In experiments carried out *in vitro*, Henry and Norman (1974) found that phosphate, at a concentration of 5×10^{-3} *M*, produced a 50% inhibition of the 25(OH)D$_3$-1-hydroxylase activity in mitochondria from vitamin D-deficient chicks.

Bikle *et al.* (1975) found that an increase in the concentration of inorganic phosphate from $10^{-3.5}$ to 10^{-3} *M* enhanced the activity of the enzyme in mitochondria from kidneys of vitamin D-deficient chicks; with a further increase in phosphate concentration to $10^{-2.5}$ *M*, the activity decreased. Moreover, in many instances, the effects of calcium and phosphorus were additive, with the highest enzyme activity obtained utilizing a 10^{-5} *M* calcium concentration.

Gray *et al.* (1975) studied vitamin D metabolism in normal humans subjected to phosphate depletion by withdrawal of phosphate from the diet. They evaluated the metabolic fate of injected radiolabeled vitamin D$_3$ or 25(OH)D$_3$ in serial blood samples. With phosphate depletion, calcium absorption increased and the half-time ($t\frac{1}{2}$) of plasma 25(OH)D$_3$ decreased from 23 ± 1.3 days to 14.6 ± 1.3 days (Figure 5). The plasma turnover of 25(OH)D$_3$ increased from 6.2 ± 0.8 n*M*/day to 11.7 ± 1.7 n*M*/day. There was no change in vitamin D_3 excretion or change in total pool size. They could not demonstrate an increase in the amount of plasma radioactivity chromatographically identical to $1,25(OH)_2 D_3$. This was probably due to the small amount of $1,25(OH)_2 D_3$ present and the low specific activity of radiolabeled vitamin D_3 given. However, their observations could be explained by an increased conversion of $25(OH)D_3$ to $1,25(OH)_2 D_3$ (Figure 5).

Effect of Calcium. The possibility that variations in dietary calcium intake, serum calcium, or the intracellular calcium content may affect the activity of the renal $25(OH)D_3$-1-hydroxylase has received considerable attention. Boyle *et al.* (1971) studied the effect of variation in dietary calcium intake on the metabolism of $[^3H]25(OH)D_3$ as studied *in vivo*. Vitamin D-deficient rats which received a very high calcium diet (3%) with added lactose had lower intestinal content of $1,25(OH)_2 D_3$ than rats receiving lower calcium diets. In rats receiving 0.025 $\mu g/$ day of vitamin D_3, the ingestion of a 0.3% calcium diet compared with a 0.47% calcium diet was associated with a greater level of serum $1,25(OH)_2 D_3$. In the absence of dietary vitamin D, a high-calcium diet (3%) without lactose increased serum calcium to or near normal but failed to suppress the high production of $1,25(OH)_2 D_3$. These data suggest that the enzyme activity is altered by variations in calcium intake and in serum calcium (Figure 6), but they also stress that vitamin D itself is a potent inhibitor of the enzyme. In the same study, they found no correlation between the concentration of serum phosphorus and the production of $1,25(OH)_2 D_3$. Also, there was a reciprocal relationship between

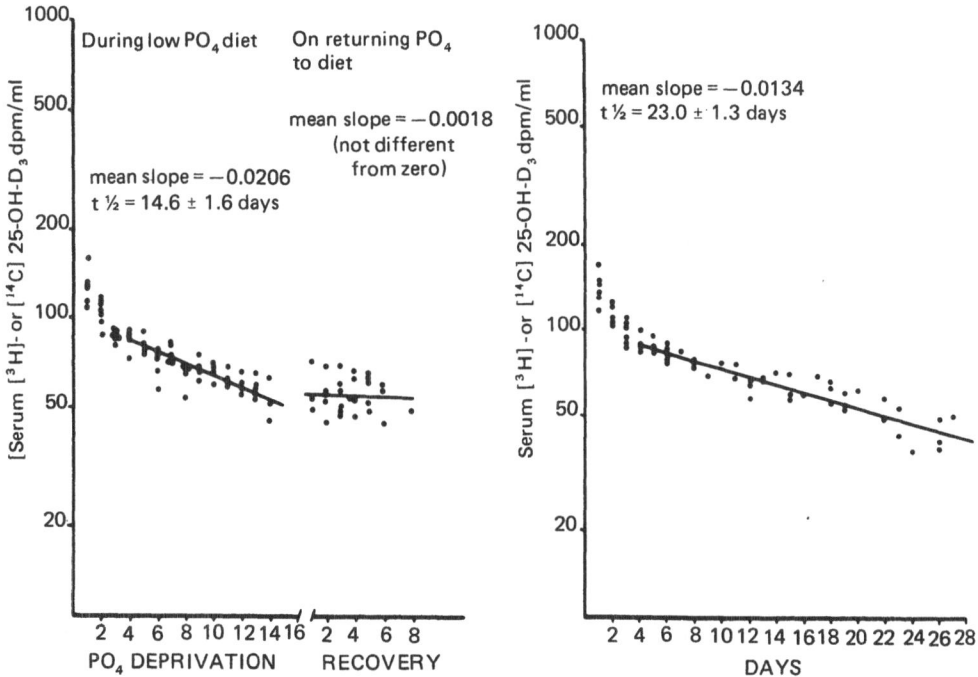

Figure 5. The plasma turnover of $[^3H]$ or $[^{14}C]25(OH)D_3$ in normal man (right) or normal volunteers before and after feeding a low phosphate (PO_4) diet (left). (From Gray *et al.*, 1975, with permission.)

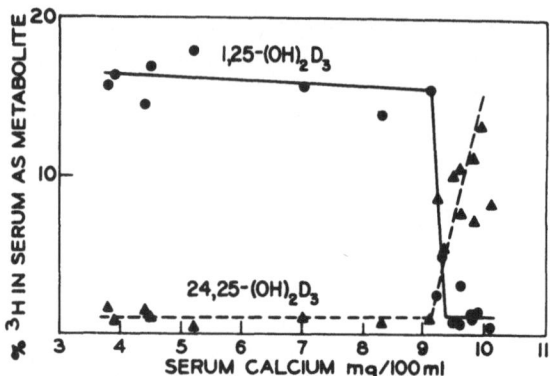

Figure 6. Relation between serum calcium and the percent of ^3H in plasma identified as either 1,25$(OH)_2D_3$ or 24,25$(OH)_2D_3$ in rats receiving varying calcium intakes. (From Boyle et al., 1971, with permission.)

the amount of 1,25$(OH)_2D_3$ present and that of 24,25$(OH)_2D_3$, which was incorrectly identified as 21,25$(OH)_2D_3$.

MacIntyre et al. (1974) also evaluated the effect of a low-calcium diet on the appearance of 1,25$(OH)_2D_3$ in rats. They found that a low-calcium diet favored the production of 1,25$(OH)_2D_3$ over 24,25$(OH)_2D_3$; moreover, rats receiving a maintenance intake of vitamin D_3 were capable of increasing 1,25$(OH)_2D_3$ production when they received a low-calcium diet. This occurred despite the performance of parathyroidectomy. They concluded that changes in activity of 25$(OH)D_3$-1-hydroxylase produced by variations in calcium intake could occur independent of alterations in PTH. On the other hand, Hughes et al. (1975) measured plasma levels of 1,25$(OH)_2D_3$ in vitamin D-replete rats, either with or without their parathyroid glands, while their dietary calcium intake was varied. They found that ingestion of a low-calcium diet was followed by a prompt increase in plasma levels of 1,25$(OH)_2D_3$ in rats with intact parathyroid glands, while TPTX rats showed no increase in plasma levels of 1,25$(OH)_2D_3$. In contrast to the view of MacIntyre et al. (1974), Hughes et al. (1975) concluded that parathyroid hormone was essential in mediating the effect produced by changes in dietary calcium. Using kidney homogenates and mitochondria prepared from chicks which had been fed a diet either high or low in calcium content, Omdahl et al. (1972) found an inverse relationship between dietary calcium and the percent of radioactivity recovered as 1,25$(OH)_2D_3$ following the administration of radiolabeled precursor. Moreover, they found increased amounts of a metabolite chromatographically identical to 24,25$(OH)_2D_3$ in chicks which had received a high-calcium diet and showed low quantities of 1,25$(OH)_2D_3$. Henry et al. (1974) studied the activity of 25$(OH)D_3$-1-hydroxylase in mitochondria from kidneys obtained from chicks receiving varying dietary calcium intakes. In chicks receiving vitamin D_3, 0.62 μg/day, they found an inverse relationship between serum calcium and the activity of the enzyme (Figure 7).

In another study, Larkins et al. (1973) varied dietary calcium in thyroparathyroidectomized, vitamin D-deficient rats and evaluated the metabolites of ^3H-

labeled $25(OH)D_3$ found in intestine and plasma. When dietary calcium was reduced from 3.7% to 0.13%, there was a striking increase in the percent of radioactivity recovered as $1,25(OH)_2D_3$. In order to achieve reasonable survival of the TPTX rats receiving a low-calcium diet, it was necessary to give them a diet low in phosphate. Nonetheless, these workers showed that a decrease in dietary calcium (and a decrease in phosphate) increased the apparent production of $1,25(OH)_2D_3$ independent of changes in the activity of parathyroid hormone.

Bikle and Rasmussen (1975) evaluated the effect of variations in dietary calcium intake on the activity of $25(OH)D_3$-1-hydroxylase, studied in isolated renal tubules obtained from vitamin D-deficient chicks; these circumstances would be expected to result in high levels of enzymatic activity. As dietary calcium intake was increased from 0.4% to 3%, there was a marked inhibition of the activity of the enzyme. The administration of a low-calcium diet did not lead to any further increase in $25(OH)D_3$-1-hydroxylase; indeed, the activity fell slightly. If one evaluates the activity of the enzyme in terms of product formed and relation to serum calcium, there appears to be an inverse relation between the enzyme activity and serum calcium level, particularly if one excludes data from the chicks receiving a very high phosphate intake.

Because of observations which indicate that variations in the calcium needs of the organism can somehow alter the activity of the $25(OH)D_3$-1-hydroxylase,

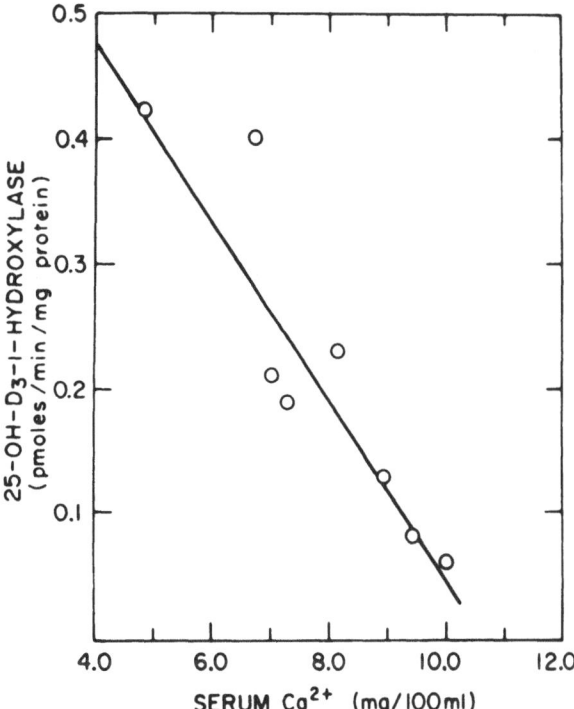

Figure 7. Relation between the activity of the renal enzyme, $25(OH)D_3$-1-hydroxylase, as measured *in vitro* in homogenates of chick kidney, and the plasma calcium concentration, which was varied by altering dietary calcium intake. (From Henry *et al.*, 1974, with permission.)

several investigators have evaluated the effect of changing the calcium concentration in the incubation media used for isolated renal tubules, homogenates of kidney tissues, or mitochondria isolated from kidney cells. At this time, divergent results have been reported, possibly due to variations in the techniques used in preparation of the tubules or cellular subfractions. Also, it is apparent that alterations in the environment external to the cell (i.e., extracellular fluid) may differ considerably from variations in the environment of the intramitochondrial enzyme. Shain (1972) studied the metabolism of $25(OH)D_3$ and the production of $1,25(OH)_2D_3$ in tubules isolated from vitamin D-deficient chicks. He found that variations in the calcium concentration from 0.1 to 2.5 mM had no effect on either the uptake of $25(OH)D_3$ or the production of $1,25(OH)_2D_3$. Also, the effect of parathyroid hormone was not affected by changes in ionic calcium concentration. Henry and Norman (1974) evaluated the conversion of $25(OH)D_3$ to $1,25(OH)_2D_3$ in mitochondria isolated from chick kidneys. The activity of the $25(OH)D_3$-1-hydroxylase fell sharply as the calcium concentration was increased from 0.01 to 0.03 mM; as the calcium concentration was increased further to 0.1 and 1.0 mM, no further change occurred. Horiuchi et al. (1974) found that the production of $1,25(OH)_2D_3$ by mitochondria from chick kidneys increased as the calcium concentration increased from 0 to 0.2 mM and then fell as the concentration was increased to 0.7 mM. They also reported that isolated mitochondria from chicks given vitamin D_3, 2.5 μg/day, showed no change in the production of $1,25(OH)_2D_3$ as the calcium concentration in the media was increased from 0 to 0.1 mM to 0.7 mM.

The reasons for the apparent discrepancy between the results of Horiuchi et al. (1974) and Henry and Norman (1974) are not apparent. In a subsequent communication, Henry and Norman (1975) studied factors affecting the inhibition of $25(OH)D_3$-1-hydroxylase by 0.02 mM calcium. This inhibition occurred independent of whether the hydrogen ion donor was malate or NADPH, was unaffected by a hypotonic media, and persisted after freezing and thawing the mitochondria. Also, the inhibition by 0.02 mM calcium occurred with mitochondria from either vitamin D-deficient or vitamin D-treated chicks. They felt that these observations support the hypothesis that the inhibition of $25(OH)D_3$-1-hydroxylase by calcium was specific and not due to a nonspecific effect of calcium on mitochondrial metabolism.

MacIntyre et al. (1974) studied the conversion of $25(OH)D_3$ to $1,25(OH)_2D_3$ in homogenates of chick kidney; the production of $1,25(OH)_2D_3$ increased as the concentration of calcium was decreased from 0.5 mM to "zero." Moreover, addition of the chelating agent, EGTA, to media containing no calcium caused a fall in metabolic conversion. Larkins et al. (1974a) evaluated the conversion of $25(OH)D_3$ to $1,25(OH)_2D_3$ by isolated kidney tubules; the depletion of calcium in the incubation media by the addition of EGTA caused a decrease in the conversion. This effect is opposite to that seen in homogenates.

Bikle and Rasmussen (1975) also studied the effect of varying the calcium and phosphorus concentration in the incubation media during the evaluation of $1,25(OH)_2D_3$ production in isolated renal tubules. Under these circumstances, the removal of calcium caused a decrease in $1,25(OH)_2D_3$ generated by the enzyme; the optimal calcium concentration ranged from 0.5 to 2.0 mM. The effect of variations in calcium concentration was much more prominent when phosphate was present in the incubation media. Thus, when studies were carried out in the absence of phosphate, enzyme activity rose only slightly with the addition of calcium and did not fall as calcium concentration was increased further.

In a study of the effect of variations in the calcium concentration on the activity of 25(OH)D$_3$-1-hydroxylase in renal mitochondria, Bikle *et al.* (1975) reported somewhat different observations from those described by Colston *et al.* (1973), Fraser and Kodicek (1973), and Henry and Norman (1974). Bikle *et al.* (1975) utilized a system where the calcium level was controlled at variable levels by adding the chelator, EGTA, and sufficient calcium to give a desired free calcium ion concentration. They found that increasing the calcium concentration from 10^{-6} to 10^{-5} M resulted in a fivefold increase in enzyme activity. These observations were made with the pH regulated between 6.5 and 6.9; little effect was seen at a pH of 7.1. The reason for the discrepancy between the results of Bikle *et al.* (1975) and those reported by others is not clear; there may have been differences in pH and in the methods used to control calcium concentration.

Effect of Miscellaneous Factors. In their study of isolated renal tubular cells, Bikle and Rasmussen (1975) evaluated the effect of changes in the pH of the incubation media on the production of 1,25(OH)$_2$D$_3$. As the pH of the media was reduced from 7.4 to 6.7, there was a reduction in enzyme activity; this effect was seen at all levels of calcium concentration between 0 and 4 mM. These observations are of interest in view of the increased loss of skeletal calcium that occurs during chronic acidosis. One might speculate that an increase in production of 1,25(OH)$_2$D$_3$ might occur as a consequence of acidosis. The observations of Bikle and Rasmussen (1975) suggest that enhanced production of 1,25(OH)$_2$D$_3$ is not the cause of skeletal calcium loss during acidosis.

The addition of strontium to the diet effectively reduces the activity of the 25(OH)D$_3$-1-hydroxylase. Omdahl and DeLuca (1972) studied kidney mitochondria from strontium-fed chicks and found decreased production of 1,25(OH)$_2$D$_3$ from 25(OH)D$_3$. This inhibition in conversion was overcome when the dietary calcium was restored to normal.

Administration of the diphosphonate, disodium ethane-1-hydroxyl-1,1-diphosphonate (EHDP), an agent which stabilizes bone crystal, alters the renal production of 1,25(OH)$_2$D$_3$ and the intestinal absorption of calcium. The administration of EHDP, 16 μmol/kg/day, to vitamin D-replete rats stimulated intestinal calcium absorption and increased the intestinal content of 1,25(OH)$_2$D$_3$ following the administration of [³H]25-hydroxylcholecalciferol (Guilland *et al.*, 1975). It had been previously shown that doses of EHDP that were 10 times larger *impaired* intestinal absorption of calcium (Gasser *et al.*, 1972) and blocked the production of 1,25(OH)$_2$D$_3$ in the vitamin D-replete rat (Hill *et al.*, 1973) and in chicks (Baxter *et al.*, 1974). This effect was seen in the vitamin D-treated but not in the vitamin D-deficient state, suggesting that the inhibition of EHDP was overcome by vitamin D deficiency. The doses of EHDP given were sufficient to prevent skeletal retention of calcium (Gasser *et al.*, 1972). Whether this effect of

EHDP on $1,25(OH)_2 D_3$ production represents an effect on the renal tubular cell or occurs because of its effect on the skeleton remains unknown. It is of interest that quantities of EHDP given to patients with Paget's disease were found to enhance the intestinal absorption of calcium (Guncaga et al., 1974).

Summary of Controlling Factors. Present-day knowledge about regulation of the production of the renal hormone, $1,25(OH)_2 D_3$, must be regarded as fragmentary. As reviewed above, considerable data suggest that the intake of a low-calcium diet, the administration of large quantities of parathyroid hormone, removal of vitamin D from the diet, or restriction of dietary phosphate intake can each lead to enhanced renal production of $1,25(OH)_2 D_3$ (Table III). However, most studies which have evaluated changes in production of $1,25(OH)_2 D_3$ were carried out under extremes of pathophysiologic variations. Thus, animals were studied during vitamin D deficiency, following the acute administration of vitamin D_3; after parathyroidectomy, following the administration of substantial quantities of PTH; or while fed diets with extreme variations in calcium or phosphate content. It is not clear whether the altered production of $1,25(OH)_2 D_3$ observed in such studies would also occur during variation in these parameters that occur from day to day.

Vitamin D deficiency or the intake of a low-calcium diet may reduce serum calcium, thereby stimulating the secretion of parathyroid hormone. Each of these factors, individually, has been suggested to increase the renal production of $1,25(OH)_2 D_3$. In the normal animal, which has regulatory processes intact, it is difficult to separate the effect of these variables.

Phosphate depletion, on the other hand, should reduce or inhibit the secretion of PTH; yet, this maneuver has been shown to enhance the production of $1,25(OH)_2 D_3$. These observations have led to the suggestion that reduced serum or intracellular phosphate concentration may control the production of

Table III. Factors Reported to Affect Renal
Production of $1,25(OH)_2 D_3$

I.   Stimulatory:
     A.   Low-calcium diet
     B.   Vitamin D-deficient state
     C.   Low-phosphate diet
     D.   Parathyroid hormone
     E.   Hypocalcemia
II. Inhibitory:
     A.   Treatment with vitamin D
     B.   Parathyroidectomy
     C.   High-phosphate diet
     D.   High-calcium diet
     E.   High-strontium diet
III. Variable effects:
     A.   Calcitonin
     B.   Diphosphonate (EHDP)
     C.   Variations in pH

$1,25(OH)_2D_3$. Whether the changes in extracellular or tissue phosphate concentration that occur as a consequence of normal fluctuation in dietary phosphate intake or as a result in variation in secretion of PTH in various species, including man, can alter vitamin D metabolism is unknown. Generally, the sources of phosphate are so ubiquitous that dietary phosphate deficiency is quite rare.

With these major problems in the understanding of the role of *in vivo* factors in controlling renal production of $1,25(OH)_2D_3$, it is not surprising that study of intracellular or intramitochondrial events that regulate production of the hormone leads to inconclusive results. Also, the specific renal cell responsible for production of $1,25(OH)_2D_3$ remains unknown. It is attractive to consider that transcellular transport of calcium and/or phosphate may be the event leading to variations in production of $1,25(OH)_2D_3$. The reader should note that this suggestion is speculative. Moreover, there may be variation in renal $25(OH)D_3$-1-hydroxylase from species to species, and alterations in production of $1,25(OH)_2D_3$ may be more important in species, such as birds or crustacea, which require rapid mobilization of large quantities of calcium for the generation of an egg shell or chitinous exoskeleton. Finally, it remains uncertain whether the renal production of $1,25(OH)_2D_3$ does play a role in the hour-to-hour homeostasis of plasma calcium in man.

III. VITAMIN D ACTION ON THE KIDNEY

The actions of vitamin D on the kidney may be considered at three levels: first, the effects of physiologic amounts; second, the actions of pharmacologic quantities; third, the action of very large doses which produce toxic manifestations that are usually associated with hypercalcemia. The separation of these effects is difficult and, of necessity, somewhat arbitrary. With knowledge about the metabolic conversion of vitamin D_3 first to $25(OH)D_3$ and then to $1,25(OH)_2D_3$, it is likely that the distinction between these levels of effect may be related both to the dose of vitamin D given and to the rate of its subsequent conversion to $25(OH)D_3$ or to $1,25(OH)_2D_3$.

A. Calcium and Phosphorus Homeostasis

Before considering how vitamin D or its metabolites affect the renal handling of various electrolytes, a review of the kidney's role in the normal homeostasis of calcium and phosphorus is in order. The renal handling of calcium and phosphorus will be emphasized because of the known major role of vitamin D in controlling the metabolism of calcium and phosphorus in other organs. Vitamin D or one of its metabolic forms may also affect the renal handling of sodium, bicarbonate, and amino acids. These possible actions will be briefly reviewed, despite a questionable role of vitamin D in their normal homeostasis.

Several processes are involved in the regulation of the concentrations of calcium and phosphorus in the blood. There is a large store of calcium and phosphate in bone, and the interchange between the skeleton and extracellular fluid plays a major role in determining the concentration of these ions in blood. Second, large quantities of calcium and phosphate are lost from the blood into the glomerular filtrate and then subsequently reclaimed by tubular reabsorption. Alterations in the filtration or tubular reabsorption of these ions could effect their blood levels. Third, a reciprocal interdependence exists between the plasma concentrations of phosphate and calcium in blood, which may be related to their solubility product. Thus, an increase in phosphate concentration causes a fall in that of calcium, presumably due to the deposition of calcium phosphate salts in bone; conversely, a fall in plasma phosphate is associated with enhanced movement of calcium from bone to extracellular fluid and, in some species, a rise in concentration of blood calcium. Also, variations in the intestinal absorption of calcium may affect its blood levels. Finally, there are a number of hormones that control the movement of these ions between extracellular fluid, on the one hand, and the intestinal tract, the skeleton, and the kidney, on the other.

In the case of phosphate, 40–60% of the ingested quantity is absorbed by the intestine, with little relation between the fraction absorbed and the body's needs for phosphate. The inorganic phosphate in the blood is all or nearly all filtered at the glomerulus, and the renal tubule reabsorbs 80–90% of the quantity filtered. Under situations of increased phosphate intake, plasma phosphorus may rise transiently and approach a maximum tubular reabsorption rate (Tm) with additional filtered phosphate appearing in the urine. Dietary phosphate restriction, on the other hand, is associated with complete or nearly complete reabsorption of phosphorus by the renal tubule. Thus, the kidney plays a very major role in regulation of the plasma concentration of phosphorus. Several factors are known to influence the tubular reabsorption of phosphorus: There is a strong interrelationship between phosphate and sodium handling, and the expansion of extracellular volume by the infusion of large quantities of saline causes an increase in phosphorus excretion. Parathyroid hormone, by decreasing tubular reabsorption of phosphate, has a marked phosphaturic action. Changes in blood calcium concentration may also affect the renal handling of phosphate. Thus, the short-term infusion of calcium into one renal artery causes an ipsilateral decrease in urinary phosphorus (Lavender and Pullman, 1963); on the other hand, an increase of serum calcium to normal by a prolonged infusion of calcium chloride in patients with untreated hypoparathyroidism causes an increase in urinary phosphate excretion and a fall in serum phosphorus (Eisenberg, 1965).

The concentration of blood calcium and particularly its ionized form, in contrast to phosphate, is very carefully regulated through complex interactions between (1) the movement of calcium in and out of bone, (2) intestinal absorption of calcium, and (3) the renal tubular reabsorption of calcium lost into the renal tubule by glomerular filtration. In the average man, approximately 11,000 mg of calcium are lost from the plasma into glomerular filtrate each day. However, only 0.5–1.0% of filtered calcium is lost in the urine because of remarkedly effective tubular reabsorption. Several hormonal and nonhormonal factors can alter the renal handling of calcium and change its excretory rate. First, there is a very close association between the renal tubular reabsorption of calcium and that of sodium, and many experimental maneuvers which alter tubular reabsorption of sodium have a similar effect on calcium handling; among such factors are saline infusion, renal vasodilatation, and the administration of certain diuretics, such as furosemide and ethacrynic acid. An increase in urinary excretion of calcium could arise from an increase in filtered load, decreased tubular reabsorption, or both. An increase in filtered load that is produced by an augmentation in glomerular filtration rate has only a small effect on calcium excretion (Massry and Kleeman, 1972), but an increase in the filtered load produced by hypercalcemia may be capable of decreasing tubular reabsorption of calcium more markedly. Under certain circumstances, urinary calcium may increase in association with a small increase in intestinal calcium absorption. This is presumably related to an increase in the filtered load of calcium. Parathyroid hormone (PTH) is one of the hormonal factors which can alter the tubular reabsorption of calcium. Thus, PTH lowers urinary calcium by means of an increase in reabsorption with a tendency to increase the serum level of calcium. As serum calcium increases under the influence of PTH, tubular reabsorption may be inhibited by the hypercalcemia and also because of the increased filtered load of calcium; thus, urinary calcium may increase. A number of other factors affect the renal handling of calcium, including phosphate depletion, acidosis, and the ingestion of carbohydrate. These factors are beyond the scope of this review but are described in detail elsewhere (Walser, 1973; Massry and Coburn, 1973). The relative contribution of the kidney toward the regulation of plasma calcium is somewhat controversial. It is generally believed that the rates of movement of calcium from the skeleton and the gut are the primary determinants of serum calcium, although others maintain that the kidney may be an important regulator of serum calcium concentration (Nordin and Peacock, 1969; Nordin, 1972).

B. Effects on Renal Tubular Function

1. Renal Handling of Phosphate

The results of many early studies on the effect of vitamin D on renal phosphate handling are difficult to interpret because the experimental design did not separate an effect of vitamin D, per se, from an indirect action produced by inhibition of parathyroid hormone secretion. This inhibition could clearly be a consequence of the increase in serum calcium and it might possibly arise via a direct action of vitamin D on the parathyroid gland (Oldham *et al.*, 1974; Henry and Norman, 1975).

Harrison and Harrison (1942) first noted that vitamin D_2, 0.5 mg/day for 3 days, lowered urinary phosphate excretion and caused a rise in the *Tm* for phosphate in vitamin D-deficient dogs with intact parathyroid glands and a single vitamin D-replete animal. A fall in urinary phosphorus excretion and an increase in phosphate *Tm* has been described in rachitic children following treatment with vitamin D (Liu *et al.*, 1940; Klein and Gow, 1953). Under these conditions, the effect of vitamin D might well arise from inhibition of PTH secretion caused by an increase in serum calcium.

Other investigators have reported an increase in urinary phosphate excretion following the administration of either vitamin D_2 or D_3 to parathyroidectomized animals. Ney *et al.* (1968) gave vitamin D_3, 12.5 μg/min intravenously for 2 hr, 2.5 mg intramuscularly once a day, followed by 0.75 mg/day by mouth for 6 days. They noted an increase in urinary phosphorus excretion after 1–5 days. Such observations can be interpreted to indicate an inhibition of phosphate reabsorption. However, "control" observations were made 6 hr following parathyroidectomy. Dogs and rats exhibit avid phosphate reabsorption, which is not readily inhibited by usual measures except by parathyroid extract, in the immediate period after parathyroidectomy (Frick, 1969; Gradowska *et al.*, 1973). Thus, the observations of Ney *et al.* (1968), which show an increase in phosphate excretion after vitamin D, may be explained by a gradual "escape" from the avid phosphate reabsorption that immediately follows PTX. Crawford *et al.* (1955) noted an increase in urinary phosphate excretion in PTX rats given 12.5 mg/day of either vitamin D_2 or D_3. It has been shown that a slow increase in serum calcium from low to normal value causes phosphaturia in humans lacking their parathyroid glands (Eisenberg, 1965), and such a mechanism might account for these results. Gekle *et al.* (1971) studied proximal tubular phosphate reabsorption by micropuncture techniques in both intact and PTX rats, either deficient in or replete with vitamin D. Following an infusion of vitamin D, 0.5–45 μg/100 g body wt per minute, they noted an increase in phosphate reabsorption. Costanzo *et al.* (1974) gave vitamin D_3, 2.5 μg, as a single dose to vitamin D-deficient rats subjected to acute thyroparathyroidectomy; 48 hr later clearance experiments were carried out during phosphate loading. Rats not treated with vitamin D excreted significant quantities of phosphate at low filtered loads (2 μmol/min), while the vitamin D-treated, TPTX rats exhibited no phosphate in the urine despite higher filtered loads (5 μmol/min). It should be noted that serum calcium levels were significantly higher in the vitamin D-treated than in the vitamin D-depleted rats. The experiments described above suffer from the additional problem that the sterol administered was either vitamin D_2 or D_3 rather than one of their subsequent, more active metabolites, such as $25(OH)D_3$ or $1,25(OH)_2D_3$.

Puschett *et al.* (1972a) evaluated the effect of vitamin D_3 and $25(OH)D_3$ on renal phosphate handling in vitamin D-replete dogs that had undergone TPTX 6–7 days previously. Extracellular volume expansion was produced with a saline infusion to decrease tubular phosphate reabsorption and enhance phosphaturia. Under these conditions, the administration of vitamin D_2, 25 μg over 12–13 min, led to a fall in phosphate excretion after 50–60 min. When $25(OH)D_3$, 0.25 to 0.30 μg, was given, phosphate excretion was unaffected, while the infusion of 2.6–3.0 μg produced a fall in phosphate excretion within 30–40 min and a maximum decrease after 90–120 min. The infusion of parathyroid hormone, superimposed on the administration of $25(OH)D_3$, caused a phosphaturic response and obliterated the hypophosphaturic action of $25(OH)D_3$. When $25(OH)D_3$, 1.3–1.5 $\mu g/hr$, was superimposed on a continuous infusion of parathyroid hormone, 10–30 units/hr, phosphate clearance fell. However, $25(OH)D_3$ had no hypophosphaturic effect when it was added to a higher rate of PTH infusion (50–60 units/hr). Puschett et al. (1972b) studied the effect of $1,25(OH)_2D_3$, either 0.625 μg or 0.125 μg, utilizing the same protocol described for $25(OH)D_3$. The lower dose had no effect, while the larger amount caused a reduction in phosphate clearance within 20–30 min. In other experiments in volume-expanded, TPTX dogs, Puschett et al. (1974) studied the interaction between $25(OH)D_3$, on one hand, and cyclic AMP, calcitonin, and an increase in serum calcium to normal, on the other. They found that cyclic AMP produced phosphaturia and obscured the hypophosphaturic action of $25(OH)D_3$. Calcitonin, which was without affect on electrolyte excretion in the dog, also blocked the effect of $25(OH)D_3$ on phosphate transport. Calcium infusion, which increased the ultrafilterable plasma calcium to normal, also prevented the hypophosphaturic action of $25(OH)D_3$.

Popovtzer et al. (1974) studied the effects of $25(OH)D_3$ on the renal handling of phosphorus in the rat. The infusion of $25(OH)D_3$, 1 $\mu g/kg/hr$, into rats with intact parathyroid glands caused a decrease in phosphate excretion. When the same procedure was carried out in rats that had undergone parathyroidectomy 2 days before the study, $25(OH)D_3$ had no effect on phosphate clearance. Correction of hypocalcemia, phosphate loading, and volume expansion with saline did not modify this lack of response. When parathyroid hormone was infused into TPTX rats, the addition of $25(OH)D_3$ inhibited, to a large extent, the phosphaturic action of PTH. This effect of $25(OH)D_3$ was seen within 20 min, and its maximum action on phosphate excretion occurred in 40–60 min. The administration of $25(OH)D_3$ not only blocked the further phosphaturic action of PTH, but it prevented the usual increase in urinary cAMP (Popovtzer and Robinette, 1975); (Figure 8). A similar dose of $1,25(OH)_2D_3$ also reduced urinary phosphate excretion. All the experiments cited above on the action of $25(OH)D_3$ or $1,25(OH)_2D_3$ were carried out in vitamin D-replete animals.

Brickman, Coburn, and Norman (unpublished observations) administered $1,25(OH)_2D_3$, 2.7 μg, to vitamin D-deficient dogs. In approximately two thirds of the experiments, there was a decrease in phosphate excretion following the administration of $1,25(OH)_2D_3$ (Figure 9). This occurred prior to the appearance of changes in plasma concentrations of calcium or phosphorus. In normal man, Coburn et al. (1975) found that the administration of $1,25(OH)_2D_3$, 2.7 μg, in a single dose failed to alter urinary phosphorus excretion over the first 12 hr. During this same period, there was an increase in urinary calcium excretion and a decrease in urinary cAMP. Steele et al. (1975) found that parathyroidectomized, vitamin D-deficient rats receiving a low-phosphate diet showed avid tubular reabsorption of phosphate. Thus, they found no evidence for phosphate wasting in these animals lacking both vitamin D and parathyroid hormone. These observations are somewhat at variance with those of Costanzo et al. (1974).

Rasmussen and Bordier (1974) note that the phosphaturic response to PTH in TPTX, vitamin D-deficient rats is only 30–40% of the effect observed in vitamin D-fed animals. Restoration of serum calcium to normal by feeding a high-calcium diet restored PTH responsiveness, as measured by its phosphaturic action. Rasmussen and Bordier suggest that these observations are consistent with a model in which vitamin D acts to regulate the renal cellular content of calcium and phosphate. When this content is normal, the response to PTH is also normal; however, when the cellular stores are altered or depleted, the physiologic response to PTH is reduced even though the biochemical response, as measured by increases in cAMP concentration, may be enhanced (Nagata and Rasmussen, 1968).

These experiments cited above, which were designed to clarify the effect of vitamin D or its subsequent metabolic forms on phosphate transport by the kidney, must be interpreted with caution. Under certain circumstances there is convincing evidence that vitamin D, or more specifically $25(OH)D_3$ or $1,-25(OH)_2D_3$, can enhance the tubular reabsorption of phosphate. Often this effect can be demonstrated only under conditions which deviate considerably from a normal physiological state. Whether one of these sterols normally plays a regulatory role in the homeostasis of phosphate by the kidney remains speculative. Also, there may be considerable differences in the renal responsiveness to vitamin D from one species to another, as is suggested by the variation in results of Puschett et al. (1972a, b, 1974) in the dog and Popovtzer et al. (1974) and Popovtzer and Robinette (1975) in the rat.

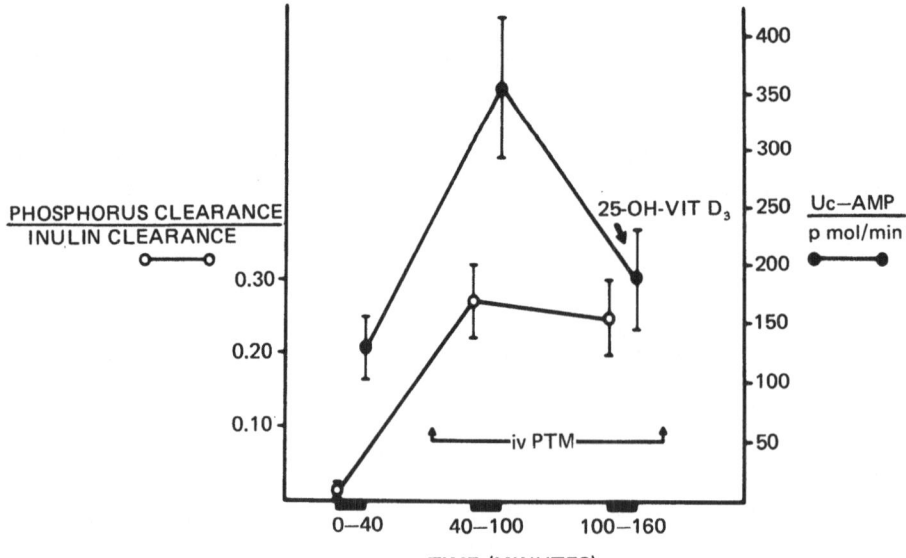

Figure 8. The fractional excretion of phosphate (phosphate clearance/inulin clearance) and urinary excretion of cyclic AMP in parathyroidectomized rats before (1–40 min) and during the infusion of PTH (40–160 min). During the period from 100–160 min they also received $25(OH)D_3$. (Modified from Popovtzer and Robinette, 1975.)

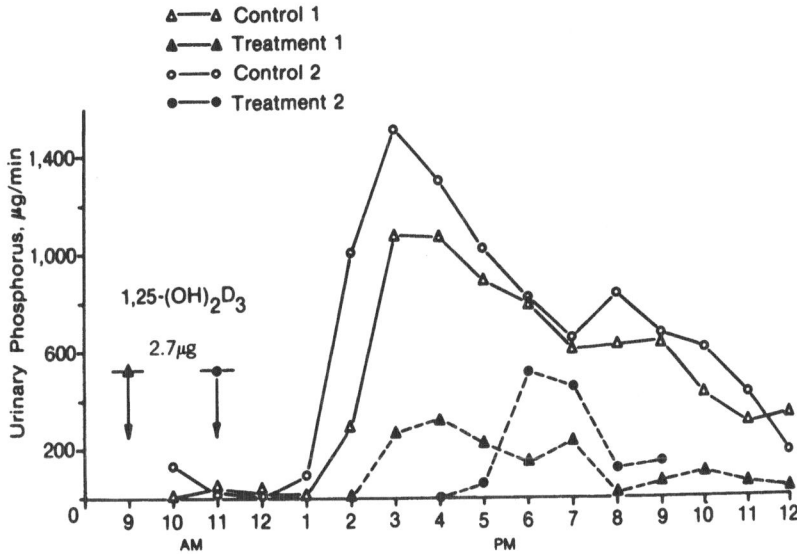

Figure 9. Urinary excretion of phosphate in two vitamin D-deficient dogs studied twice: before (control) and after administration of 1,25(OH)$_2$D$_3$, 2.7 μg, intravenously. (From unpublished observations of Brickman, Coburn, and Norman.)

2. Renal Handling of Calcium

When pharmacologic doses of vitamin D are given, an increase in the urinary excretion of calcium almost invariably occurs (Litvak *et al.*, 1958; Hanna, 1961; Edwards and Hodgkinson, 1965). With such treatment, the intestinal absorption of calcium is augmented, bone resorption increases, and serum calcium rises, thereby enhancing the filtered load of calcium and consequently increasing urinary calcium excretion. It was suggested by Litvak *et al.* (1958) that vitamin D$_3$ may inhibit calcium transport by the nephron. This conclusion was reached on the basis of the finding that vitamin D treatment of patients with hypoparathyroidism produced marked hypercalcuria with only a slight increase of serum calcium. Subsequently, Bernstein *et al.* (1963) compared the renal clearance of calcium in patients with hypoparathyroidism whose serum calcium was increased by either calcium infusion or vitamin D treatment. They found no difference in the fraction of filtered calcium excreted at comparable levels of serum calcium. They concluded that the high rate of calcium excretion in vitamin D-treated patients with hypoparathyroidism was caused by an increase in filtered calcium and parathyroid hormone. Ney *et al.* (1968), in the experiments cited above, found that the administration of vitamin D$_2$, in large doses to vitamin D-deficient, acutely TPTX dogs, was associated with a fall in urinary calcium over the first 2–24 hr. Six days later, urinary calcium was higher at a time when serum calcium levels were increased. In dogs subjected to thyroparathyroidectomy and volume expansion with saline, two maneuvers which inhibit calcium reabsorption, the administration of either 25(OH)D$_3$ or

1,25(OH)$_2$D$_3$ enhanced the tubular reabsorption of calcium (Puschett et al., 1972a, b). Puschett et al. (1974) found that the administration of parathyroid hormone, cAMP, calcitonin, or the infusion of calcium to raise serum calcium to normal each blocked the effect of 25(OH)D$_3$ on tubular reabsorption of calcium. Costanzo et al. (1974) noted that the fractions of filtered calcium excreted were significantly lower in vitamin D-treated than in vitamin D-deficient TPTX rats studied at comparable levels of sodium clearance. The vitamin D treatment consisted of vitamin D$_3$, 2.5 µg, 48 hr prior to the experiment. Also, Steele et al. (1975) noted that the fraction of filtered calcium excreted was significantly lower in animals given 1,25(OH)$_2$D$_3$, (0.25–0.5 µg/rat) than in untreated, vitamin D-deficient controls. Thus, most observations show that vitamin D$_3$, 25(OH)D$_3$, or 1,25(OH)$_2$D$_3$ can augment renal tubular reabsorption of calcium in animals that are hypocalcemic and thyroparathyroidectomized or in animals whose tubular calcium reabsorption was inhibited by volume expansion.

Observations in vitamin D-replete, normocalcemic humans differ considerably. The administration of large doses of vitamin D$_3$ itself (Hall et al., 1969) or 1.0–2.5 µg of 1,25(OH)$_2$D$_3$ to normal man is associated with an increase in urinary calcium (Brickman et al., 1974). This effect can be seen within 7–8 hr after a single dose of 1,25(OH)$_2$D$_3$ (Coburn et al., 1975). Very likely, this action is due to enhanced intestinal calcium absorption which leads to a small increase in the filtered load of calcium and also may inhibit PTH secretion, thereby decreasing tubular reabsorption of calcium.

3. Renal Handling of Sodium

As noted above, the tubular reabsorption of calcium and phosphorus is interrelated with the tubular transport of sodium. Many maneuvers which affect the renal handling of calcium have similar effects on sodium handling. There is little evidence that vitamin D plays any role in sodium homeostasis, and any acute effect observed may be quickly overcome by measures which normally maintain sodium homeostasis. Therefore, studies which evaluate the short-term effects of vitamin D might provide data about an action on sodium transport not seen in long-term studies. For example, Costanzo et al. (1974) noted that the fraction of filtered sodium excreted (C_{Na}/GFR) was similar in vitamin D-deficient rats and animals treated with vitamin D, 25 µg, 48 hr earlier.

Puschett et al. (1972a,b) observed a decrease in both the absolute rate of sodium excretion and the fraction of sodium excreted (C_{Na}/GFR) in dogs given vitamin D, 250 µg; 25(OH)D$_3$, 2.5–3.0 µg; or 1,25(OH)$_2$D$_3$, 0.625 µg. The magnitude of change was similar to the decrease in calcium and phosphorus excretion. As noted above, these studies were carried out during volume expansion, with high baseline rates of sodium excretion. Popovtzer et al. (1974) studied the effect of 25(OH)D$_3$ in vitamin D-replete, TPTX rats undergoing volume expansion; they found no change in the renal handling of sodium, calcium, or phosphate. Puschett et al. (1974) provided further evidence for an association between the action of vitamin D on the renal handling of sodium and that of calcium and phosphorus in the dog; they found that the effects of

$25(OH)D_3$ on the excretion of all three ions were blocked by treatment with calcitonin, cAMP, or the infusion of calcium to raise its concentration to normal.

4. Renal Handling of Bicarbonate

Studies by Siegfried *et al.* (1975) in the dog revealed that $25(OH)D_3$, 0.2 μg/kg/hr, enhanced the renal tubular reabsorption of bicarbonate in the dog. This effect of $25(OH)D_3$ was observed in animals with intact parathyroid glands, in TPTX dogs receiving a constant infusion of parathyroid hormone, but not in TPTX dogs. They concluded that an inhibition of bicarbonate reabsorption by $25(OH)D_3$ requires the presence of PTH.

5. Renal Handling of Potassium

Puschett *et al.* (1974) found that $25(OH)D_3$ decreased urinary excretion of potassium in volume-expanded, TPTX dogs. This effect was blocked by pretreatment with calcitonin or cAMP or correcting the hypocalcemia. As noted below, the administration of toxic doses of vitamin D, which are associated with hypercalcemia, may have an opposite effect on urinary potassium.

6. Renal Handling of Amino Acids

The existence of aminoaciduria has long been known in patients with vitamin D-deficiency; treatment with vitamin D leads to a slow decrease in the excessive rates of amino acid excretion (Jonxis and Huisman, 1953). It was suggested that this phenomenon is related to the attendant secondary hyperparathyroidism (Fraser *et al.*, 1967), and the hyperaminoaciduria in vitamin D-deficient rats has been shown to be dependent on the presence of the parathyroid glands (Grose and Scriver, 1968). Short *et al.* (1974) demonstrated that the administration of parathyroid hormone to normal man increases renal excretion of several amino acids, providing further evidence that the aminoaciduria of vitamin D deficiency may be related to the excessive levels of parathyroid hormone present. It is not known whether the administration of $25(OH)D_3$ or $1,25(OH)_2D_3$ might directly modify the excretion of amino acids, as is the case for phosphate (Popovtzer *et al.*, 1974).

7. Summary of Renal Action

The information cited above suggests that pharmacologic but not toxic quantities of vitamin D, $25(OH)D_3$, or $1,25(OH)_2D_3$ can enhance the renal tubular reabsorption of phosphate and calcium. Moreover, there may be similar actions on sodium and bicarbonate reabsorption. The effect of vitamin D on phosphate transport is opposite to that of parathyroid hormone, and some observations suggest that vitamin D or a related steroid may block the action of PTH on phosphate transport in the renal tubule. Whether this effect of vitamin

D on phosphate and calcium transport in the kidney is of physiologic importance remains unknown. Observations that a low dietary phosphate can stimulate the renal production of $1,25(OH)_2D_3$ raise the possibility that an effect of $1,25(OH)_2D_3$ to enhance renal tubular phosphate reabsorption may be a defense mechanism to prevent the development of more marked phosphate depletion. Vitamin D is known to stimulate the transepithelial transport of calcium and phosphorus in the intestine, and it is possible that the sterol acts in an analogous manner on the kidney. Further information is clearly necessary to clarify a role of vitamin D in normal homeostasis in the kidney.

C. Toxic Effects of Vitamin D on the Kidney

The long-term administration of large quantities of vitamin D leads to hypercalcemia and certain characteristic alterations in renal function. These alterations are probably caused by the hypercalcemia. The effects of hypercalcemia on renal function are reviewed extensively elsewhere (Epstein, 1968, Massry et al., 1973). There are certain physiologic effects which occur as a direct and immediate consequence of hypercalcemia per se. Thus, a high blood calcium level can increase peripheral vascular resistance and hence, elevate the blood pressure (Weidmann et al., 1972). Also, hypercalcemia may directly affect the tubular transport of certain ions; thus, an increase in the level of calcium in the glomerular filtrate inhibits the tubular reabsorption of calcium (Guttman and Gottschalk, 1966) and sodium (Dibona, 1971); acute hypercalcemia reduces the reabsorption of sodium in the loop of Henle (Suki et al., 1969) and in the proximal tubule (Massry et al., 1968). An increase in serum calcium also decreases tubular magnesium reabsorption (Coburn et al., 1970).

One of the earliest clinical manifestations of hypercalcemia is polyuria and impaired urinary concentrating ability; this may occur with little or no change in glomerular filtration rate (GFR). An impaired ability to concentrate urine has been produced in the dog by the administration of large doses of vitamin D (Epstein et al., 1958; Manitius et al., 1960). The degree of the renal concentrating defect appeared to be related to the duration of hyerpcalcemia and degree of nephrocalcinosis rather than to the magnitude of hypercalcemia. However, Bennett (1970) concluded that the impaired concentrating ability produced by chronic hypercalcemia could be accounted for by the decrease in GFR produced.

Epstein et al. (1958) indicated that the renal lesions of vitamin D-induced hypercalcemia were similar to the changes produced by large doses of parathyroid extract. The earliest abnormality consisted of degeneration and necrosis of the tubular epithelium of the ascending limb of the loop of Henle, the distal convoluted tubule, and the collecting duct. Calcification is initially intracellular or intratubular with calcific casts which abstruct the lumen and lead to intrarenal hydronephrosis. With more prolonged hypercalcemia, deposits of calcium appear in the renal interstitium. Urinary tract infection and hypertension are common clinical sequellae of chronic hypercalcemia, and pathologic lesions of nephrosclerosis and chronic pyelonephritis are common. In cases of fatal vitamin D overdosage in man, renal failure is frequently observed (Ziegler and Delling, 1975).

Hypokalemia (Verner *et al.*, 1958) with excessive loss of urinary potassium (Ferris *et al.*, 1961) has been noted with long-standing hypercalcemia produced by vitamin D overdosage. On the basis of these clinical observations, Ferris *et al.* (1962) studied renal potassium handling in rats intoxicated with vitamin D_2, 5 mg/day for 4 days. The vitamin D-treated rats developed hypercalcemia and an impaired ability to conserve potassium when stressed with a low-potassium diet. Also, the urinary excretion of titratable acid was lower in the hypercalcemic rats. They suggested that renal potassium wasting and renal tubular acidosis may be acquired as a result of hypercalcemia due to long-standing vitamin D toxicity.

IV. ADDITIONAL VITAMIN D–KIDNEY INTERACTIONS

A number of interactions between vitamin D and the kidney were noted before 1966, the approximate time of the explosion of current knowledge about the metabolism of vitamin D to its active forms and the probable mode of vitamin D action. Following the administration of large doses of low-specific-activity, radiolabeled vitamin D_3, there was localization of radioactivity in the kidney; also, the effects of vitamin D on intermediary metabolism and mitochondrial function in kidney tissue were studied. Many of these observations are reviewed in detail elsewhere (DeLuca, 1967; Norman, 1968). In light of present-day knowledge and theories about both the action and metabolism of vitamin D_3, the significance of many of these observations is uncertain. Studies of the localization of radiolabeled vitamin D were done utilizing large doses of low specific activity. Under such conditions, only a small fraction of the administered vitamin D_3 would be converted to its more active forms. Also, experiments using isolated mitochondria or tissue homogenates showed almost instantaneous effects upon addition of vitamin D_3, compared to the relatively slow time course observed in a known target organ evaluated *in vivo*. Nonetheless, a brief review of certain of these observations is relevant.

A. Localization of Vitamin D in the Kidney

Following administration of large doses of vitamin D, biologic assays of tissue extracts for vitamin D activity (Morgan and Shimotori, 1943) suggested that it was present in the kidney, heart, intestine, brain, lungs, spleen, muscle, fat, skin, and hair. With the development of [^{3}H]vitamin D of higher specific activity (Norman and DeLuca, 1963), it was found that the administration of 12.5 μg resulted in a rapid accumulation of radioactivity in the liver, with less-generalized distribution in the kidneys, heart, liver, blood, brain, lung, small intestine, muscle, skeleton, and feces. With the use of a 12.5-μg dose, there was no preferential localization in the intestine, skeleton, and kidneys.

Kodicek (1960) carried out radioautographic studies following the administration of radiolabeled vitamin D_3. Radioactivity localized in the liver, proximal tubule of the kidney, and chondrocytes in the metaphyseal area of bone. It should be noted that 0.5–1.0 mg of vitamin D, a pharmacologic quantity, was given in this study. With the administration of much smaller doses (0.125 μg), Haussler and Norman (1967) found that the skeleton had accumulated 0.01 μg; the small intestine, 0.003 μg, the liver, 0.004 μg; and the kidneys, 0.015 μg. Haussler and Rasmussen (1972) found 0.020 μg, 0.032 μg, and 0.018 μg/g tissue of vitamin D_3, 25(OH)D_3, and 1,25(OH)$_2D_3$, respectively, in chick kidney following the administration of 0.5 μg vitamin D_3 to vitamin D-deficient chicks. The quantity of 25(OH)D_3 found in kidney was 68% of that in intestinal mucosa on a weight basis. Both these studies were carried out with vitamin D_3 itself, which presumably was converted to 25(OH)D_3 prior to localizing in the kidney. Studies of tissue localization of 25(OH)D_3 and 1,25(OH)D_3 will be of considerable interest.

B. Citrate Metabolism

Between 1941 and 1957, there was considerable interest and experimental work concerning the interrelation between vitamin D and citrate metabolism, with many studies utilizing kidney tissue. The administration of vitamin D_3 increased serum citrate and urinary citrate excretion in several species (Freeman and Chang, 1950; Bellin and Steenbock, 1952; Harrison et al., 1957) and also the citrate content of the kidney (Steenbock and Bellin, 1953). Subsequent investigation (Norman and DeLuca, 1964; Kunin and Krane, 1965) suggested that vitamin D did not increase citrate synthesis but reduced its rate of conversion to subsequent intermediates in the tricarboxylic acid cycle. Studies of kidney homogenates (DeLuca et al., 1957) and of mitochondrial preparations from kidney, but not liver, indicated that the administration of vitamin D reduced citrate and isocitrate oxidation. This effect was observed instantaneously, after the addition of vitamin D_3, 12.5 mg, to kidney mitochondria from vitamin D-deficient rats (DeLuca and Steenbock, 1957). Electron micrographs of mitochondria isolated from kidneys of vitamin D-deficient rats disclosed gross morphological alterations in the mitochondria with damaged, swollen cristae; treatment with vitamin D in vivo protected against the damage, which was observed only in vitro (DeLuca et al., 1960). The diminished oxidation of citrate after vitamin D treatment might be explained by a reduced penetration of citrate into the normal mitochondria as compared to abnormal mitochondria from vitamin D-deficient animals. In these studies on citrate metabolism, the quantities of vitamin D given were pharmacologic and, as noted above, the effects were almost instantaneous; thus, these results differ considerably from the action of vitamin D in vivo. There is other evidence (Harrison et al., 1957, 1958; Guroff et al., 1963) that the action of vitamin D on extracellular citrate can be prevented by treatment with pantothenic acid, cortisol, or by pyridoxine deficiency; these maneuvers did not interfere with the action of vitamin D in elevating serum calcium. These observations suggest that the action of vitamin D on citrate metabolism is not a primary effect but may occur as a consequence of the action of vitamin D on some other function, such as membrane permeability.

Thompson and DeLuca (1964) reported that vitamin D increased the incorporation of radiolabeled inorganic phosphate, incubated *in vitro*, into phospholipids in kidney slices and intestinal mucosal cells but not in liver slices. These observations may indicate that vitamin D has some fundamental action on the metabolism of phosphorus in target tissues, but it is not clear whether this is independent of or in some fashion coupled with the transport of calcium.

C. Mitochondrial Release of Calcium

Interest has focused on the relationship between vitamin D and the uptake and release of calcium by mitochondria, and mitochondria from the kidney exhibited this "vitamin D effect." Studies done to demonstrate that vitamin D enhances calcium uptake by mitochondria *in vitro* were negative (DeLuca *et al.*, 1962). However, vitamin D had a dramatic effect in causing the release of calcium which had been previously accumulated by mitochondria (Engstrom and DeLuca, 1962, 1964; DeLuca *et al.*, 1962). These actions were obtained with mitochondria from kidney and liver but not from heart; the results were elicited by vitamin D, 50 μg, but not by dihydrotachysterol, an active, vitamin D-related sterol. The release of calcium from mitochondria was instantaneous following the addition of vitamin D *in vitro*. Also, pretreatment with actinomycin D failed to block an effect of vitamin D on calcium release from mitochondria; Actinomycin D, given *in vivo*, blocked the action of vitamin D on intestinal calcium absorption (Zull *et al.*, 1966). Borle (1971) has indicated that treatment with vitamin D increases the mitochondrial pool of calcium *in situ*, and mitochondria isolated from the renal cortex of vitamin D-deficient rats contain only one third as much calcium/mg protein as mitochondria from vitamin D-fed animals (Kimmich and Rasmussen, 1969). The latter observations provide evidence that alterations in the intracellular content of calcium may, indeed, be affected by vitamin D. Whether this effect is related to alterations in metabolism of vitamin D by the kidney or to the physiologic effects of vitamin D on renal tubular transport is unknown. These interactions have been discussed in earlier section of this chapter.

ACKNOWLEDGMENTS

Supported in part by U.S.P.H.S. grants AM 5383 and AM 14-750. VA Study 1490–01.

Valuable secreterial assistance was provided by Eve Miller, Barbara Stabnow, and Harriet Goldware-Sorkin.

REFERENCES

Adams, T. N. and Norman, A. W. 1970. Studies on mechanisms of action of calciferol. I. Basic parameters of vitamin D mediated calcium transport. *J. Biol. Chem., 245*:4421.

Arnaud, S. B., Goldsmith, R. S., Lambert, P. W., and Go, V. L. W. 1975. 25-Hydroxyvitamin D_3: Evidence for an enterohepatic circulation in man. *Proc. Soc. Exp. Bio. Med., 149*:570.

Avioli, L. V. 1972. Intestinal absorption of calcium. *Arch. Intern. Med., 129*:345.

Avioli, L. V. and Haddad, J. G. 1973. Vitamin D: Current concepts. *Metabolism, 22*:507.

Baxter, L. A., DeLuca, H. F., Boujour, J. P., and Fleisch, H. A. 1974. Inhibition of vitamin D metabolism by ethane-1-hydroxy-1,1-diphosphate. *Fed. Proc., 33*:680.

Bellin, S. A. and Steenbock, H. 1952. Vitamin D and citraturia. *J. Biol. Chem., 194*:311.

Belsey, R., DeLuca, H. F., and Potts, J. T. Jr. 1971. Competitive binding assay for vitamin D and 25-OH vitamin D. *J. Clin. Endocrinol., 33*:554.

Bennett, C. M. 1970. Urine concentration and dilution in hypokalemic and hypercalcemic dogs. *J. Clin. Invest., 49*:1447.

Bernstein, D., Kleeman, C. R., and Maxwell, M. H. 1963. The effect of calcium infusions, parathyroid hormone, and vitamin D on renal clearance of calcium. *Proc. Soc. Exp. Biol. Med., 112*:353.

Bhattacharyya, M. and DeLuca, H. F. 1973. The regulation of rat liver calciferol-25-hydroxylase. *J. Biol. Chem., 248*:2969.

Bikle, D. D. and Rasmussen, H. 1975. The ionic control of 1,25-dihydroxy-vitamin D_3 production in isolated chick renal tubules. *J. Clin. Invest., 55*:292.

Bikle, D. D., Murphy, E. W., and Rasmussen, H. 1975. The ionic control of 1,25-dihydroxyvitamin D_3 synthesis in isolated chick renal mitochondria. *J. Clin. Invest., 55*:299.

Birge, S. J. Jr., Gilbert, H. R., and Avioli, L. V. 1972. Intestinal calcium transport; the role of sodium. *Science, 176*:168.

Borle, A. B. 1971. Calcium transport in kidney cells and its regulation. In *Cellular Mechanisms for Calcium Transfer and Homeostasis*, pp. 133–171. Ed. by Nichols, G. Academic Press, New York.

Boyle, I. T., Gray, R. W., and DeLuca, H. F. 1971. Regulation by calcium of "in vivo" synthesis of 1,25-dihydroxycholecalciferol and 21,25-dihydroxycholecalciferol. *Proc. Nat. Acad. Sci. U.S.A., 68*:2131.

Boyle, I. T., Omdahl, J. L., Gray, R. W., and DeLuca, H. F. 1973. The biological activity and metabolism of 24,25-dihydroxyvitamin D_3. *J. Biol. Chem., 248*:4174.

Brickman, A. S., Coburn, J. W., Massry, S. G., and Norman, A. W. 1974. 1,25-Dihydroxy-vitamin D_3 in normal man and patients with renal failure. *Ann. Intern. Med., 80*:161.

Brumbaugh, P. F. and Haussler, M. R. 1973. Nuclear and cytoplasmic receptors for 1,25$(OH)_2 D_3$ in intestinal mucosa. *Biochem. Biophys. Res. Commun., 51*:74.

Brumbaugh, P. F. and Haussler, M. R. 1974. Association of 1α,25-dihydroxycholecalciferol with intestinal mucosa chromatin. *J. Biol. Chem., 249*:1251.

Brumbaugh, P. F. and Haussler, M. R. 1975. Nuclear and cytoplasmic binding components for vitamin D metabolites. *Life Sci., 16*:353.

Brumbaugh, P. F., Haussler, D. H., Bressler, R., and Haussler, M. R. 1974. Radioreceptor assay for 1α,25-dihydroxyvitamin D_3. *Science, 183*:1089.

Chen, T. C. and DeLuca, H. F. 1973. Stimulation of ^{3}H-uridine incorporation into nuclear RNA of rat kidney by vitamin D metabolites. *Arch. Biochem. Biophys., 156*:321.

Coburn, J. W., Massry, S. G., and Kleeman, C. R. 1970. The effect of calcium infusion on renal handling of magnesium with normal and reduced glomerular filtration rate. *Nephron, 7*:131.

Coburn, J. W., Hartenbower, D. L., and Massry, S. G. 1973. Intestinal absorption of calcium and the effect of renal insufficiency. *Kidney Int., 4*:96.

Coburn, J. W., Hartenbower, D. L., and Norman, A. W. 1974. Metabolism and action of the hormone vitamin D. *West. J. Med., 121*:22.

Coburn, J. W., Brickman, A. S., Llach, F., Kurokawa, K., Canterbury, J., Reiss, E., and Norman, A. W. 1975. Acute actions of 1,25 dihydroxy-vitamin D_3 on calcium and on calcium and parathyroid hormone in normal man. *Clin. Res., 23*:134A.

Colston, K. W., Evans, I. M. A., Galante, L., MacIntyre, I., and Moss, D. W. 1973. Regulation of vitamin D metabolism: Factors influencing the rate of formation of 1,25-dihydroxycholecalciferol by kidney homogenates. *Biochem. J., 134*:817.

Costanzo, L. S., Sheehe, P. R., and Weiner, I. M. 1974. Renal actions of vitamin D in D-deficient rats. *Am. J. Physiol., 226*:1490.

Crawford, J. D., Gribetz, D., and Talbot, N. B. 1955. Mechanism of renal tubular phosphate reabsorption and the influence thereon of vitamin D in completely parathyroidectomized rats. *Am. J. Physiol., 180:*156.

Day, H. G. and McCollum, E. V. 1939. Mineral metabolism, growth, and symptomatology of rats on a diet extremely deficient in phosphorus. *J. Biol. Chem., 130*:269.

DeLuca, H. F. 1967. Mechanism of action and metabolic fate of vitamin D. *Vitam. Horm., 25*:315.

DeLuca, H. F. and Steenbock, H. 1957. An in vitro effect of vitamin D on citrate oxidation by kidney mitochondria. *Science, 126*:258.

DeLuca, H. F., Gran, F. C., and Steenbock, H. 1957. Vitamin D and citrate oxidation. *J. Biol. Chem., 224*:201.

DeLuca, H. F., Reiser, S., Steenbock, H., and Kaisberg, P. 1960. Vitamin D and the structure of kidney mitochondria. *Biochim. Biophys. Acta, 40*:526.

DeLuca, H. F., Engstrom, G. W., and Rasmussen, H. 1962. The action of vitamin D and parathyroid hormone in vitro on calcium uptake and release by kidney mitochondria. *Proc. Nat. Acad. Sci. U.S.A., 48*:1604.

Dibona, G. F. 1971. Effect of hypermagnesemia on renal tubular sodium handling in the rat. *Am. J. Physiol., 221*:53.

Edwards, N. A. and Hodgkinson, A. 1965. Metabolic studies in patients with idopathic hypercalciuria. *Clin. Sci., 29*:143.

Eisenberg, E. 1965. Effects of serum calcium level and parathyroid extracts on phosphate and calcium excretion in hypoparathyroid patients. *J. Clin. Invest., 44*:942.

Engstrom, G. W. and DeLuca, H. F. 1962. The action of vitamin D in vivo and in vitro on the release of calcium from kidney mitochondria. *J. Biol. Chem., 237*:974.

Engstrom, G. W. and DeLuca, H. F. 1964. Vitamin D-stimulated release of calcium from mitochondria. *Biochemistry, 3*:203.

Epstein, F. H. 1968. Calcium and the kidney. *Am. J. Med., 45*:700.

Epstein, F. H., Rivera, M. J., and Carone, F. A. 1958. The effect of hypercalcemia induced by calciferol upon renal concentrating ability. *J. Clin. Invest., 37*:1702.

Ferris, T. F., Kasgarian, M., Levitin, H., Brandt, I., and Epstein, F. H. 1961. Renal tubular acidosis and renal potassium wasting acquired as a result of hypercalcemic nephropathy. *N. Engl. J. Med., 265*:924.

Ferris, T. F., Levitin, H., Phillips, E. T., and Epstein, F. H. 1962. Renal potassium-wasting induced by vitamin D. *J. Clin. Invest., 41*:1222.

Fraser, D. R. and Kodicek, E. 1970. Unique biosynthesis by kidney of a biologically active vitamin D metabolite. *Nature, 228:*764.

Fraser, D. R. and Kodicek, E. 1973. Regulation of 25-hydroxycholecalciferol-1-hydroxylase activity in kidney by parathyroid hormone. *Nature (London), New Biol., 241*:163.

Fraser, D., Kooh, S. W., and Scriver, C. R. 1967. Hyperparathyroidism as the cause of hyperaminoaciduria and phosphaturia in human vitamin D-deficiency. *Pediat. Res., 1*:425.

Freeman, S. and Chang. T. S. 1950. Effect of thyroparathyroidectomy and vitamin D on serum calcium and citric acid of normal and nephrectomized dogs. *Am. J. Physiol., 160*:341.

Frick, A. 1969. Mechanism of inorganic phosphate diuresis secondary to saline infusions in the rat. *Pfluegers Arch., 313*:106.

Friedlander, E. J. and Norman, A. W. 1975. Vitamin D: A search *in vitro* and *in vivo* for 1,24,25(OH)$_3$-cholecalciferol, *Arch. Biochem. Biophys., 170*:731.

Galante, L., Colston, K., MacAuley, S., and MacIntyre, I. 1972. Effect of parathyroid extract on vitamin D metabolism. *Lancet, 1*:985.

Galante, L., Colston, K. W., Evans, I. M. A., Byfield, P. G. H., Matthews, E. W., and MacIntyre, I. 1973. The regulation of vitamin D metabolism. *Nature, 244*:438.

Garabedian, M., Holick, M. F., DeLuca, H. F., and Boyle, I. T. 1972. Control of 25-

hydroxycholecalciferol metabolism by parathyroid glands. *Proc. Nat. Acad. Sci. U.S.A.,* *69*:1673.

Gasser, A. B., Morgan, D. B., Fleisch, H. A., and Richelle, L. J. 1972. The influence of two diphosphonates on calcium metabolism in the rat. *Clin. Sci., 43*:31.

Geckle, D., Ströder, J., and Rostock, D. 1971. The effect of vitamin D on renal inorganic phosphate reabsorption in normal rats, parathyroidectomized rats, and rats with ricketts. *Pediat. Res., 5*:40.

Ghazarian, J. G., Jefcoate, C. R., Knutson, J. C., Orme-Johnson, W. H., and DeLuca, H. F. 1974. Mitochondrial cytochrome P-450, a component of chick kidney 25-hydroxycholecaciferol-1α-hydroxylase, *J. Biol. Chem., 249*:3026.

Gradowska, L., Caglar, S., Rutherford, E., Harter, H., and Slatopolsky, E. 1973. On the mechanism of the phosphaturia of extracellular fluid volume expansion in the dog. *Kidney Int., 3*:230.

Gray, R. W., Omdahl, J. L., Ghazarian, J. G., and DeLuca, H. F. 1972. 25-Hydroxycholecalci-ferol-1-hydroxylase. *J. Biol. Chem., 247*:7528.

Gray, R. W., Weber, H. P., Dominguez, J. H., and Lemann, J. 1974. The metabolism of vitamin D_3 and 25-hydroxyvitamin D_3 in normal and anephric humans. *J. Clin. Endocrinol. Metab., 39*:1045.

Gray, R. W., Dominguez, J. H., and Lemann, J. 1975. 25-Hydroxyvitamin D metabolism during dietary phosphate deprivation in humans. In: *Vitamin D and Problems Related to Uremic Bone Disease,*pp. 331–337. Ed. by Norman, A. W., Schaefer, K., Grigoleit, H. G., Herrath, D. V., and Ritz, E. Walter de Gruyter, Berlin.

Grose, J. H. and Scriver, C. R. 1968. Parathyroid dependent phosphaturia and aminoaciduria in the vitamin D-deficient rat. *Am. J. Physiol., 214*:370.

Guilland, D., Trechsel, U., Bonjour, J-P., and Fleisch, H. 1975. Stimulation of calcium absorption and apparent increased intestinal 1,25-dihydroxycholecalciferol in rats treated with low doses of ethane-1-hydroxy-1,1-diphosphonate. *Clin. Sci. Mol. Med., 48*:157.

Guncaga, J., Lauffenburger, T., Lenfner, C., Danbecker, M. A., Haas, H. G., Fleisch, H., and Olah, A. J. 1974. Diphosphonate treatment of Paget's disease of bone. A correlated metabolic calcium kinetic and morphometric study. *Horm. Metab. Res., 6*:62.

Guroff, G., DeLuca, H. F., and Steenbock, H. 1963. Citrate and action of vitamin D on calcium and phosphorus metabolism. *Am. J. Physiol., 204*:833.

Guttman, Y. and Gottschalk, C. Y. 1966. Micropuncture study of the effect of calcium on sodium transport in the rat kidney. *Isr. J. Med. Sc., 2*:243.

Haddad, J. G. and Chyu, K. J. 1971a. 25-Hydroxycholecalciferol-binding globulin in human plasma. *Biochim. Biocphys. Acta, 248*:471.

Haddad, J. G. and Chyu, K. J. 1971b. Competitive protein-binding radioassay for 25-hydroxychole-calciferol. *J. Clin. Endocrinol., 33*:992.

Haddad, J. G. and Stamp, T. C. 1974. Circulating 25-hydroxyvitamin D_3 in man. *Am. J. Med., 57*:57.

Haddad, J. G., Boisseau, V., and Avioli, L. V. 1971. Phosphorus deprivation: The metabolism of vitamin D_3 and 25-hydroxycholecalciferol in rats. *J. Nutr., 102*:269.

Hall, B. D., MacMillan, D. R., and Bronner, F. 1969. Vitamin D resistent rickets and high fecal endogenous calcium output. A report of two cases. *Am. J. Clin. Nutr., 22*:448.

Hallick, R. B. and DeLuca, H. F. 1969. Vitamin D_3-stimulated template activity of chromatin from rat intestine. *Proc. Nat. Acad. Sci. U.S.A., 63*:528.

Hanna, S. 1961. Influence of large doses of vitamin D on magnesium metabolism in rats. *Metabolism, 10*:735.

Harrison, H. E. and Harrison, H. C. 1942. A comparison of the physiologic effects of dihydrotach-ysterol and vitamin D in the rachitic and normal dog. *Am. J. Physiol., 137*:171.

Harrison, H. C., Harrison, H. E., and Park, E. A. 1957. Vitamin D and citrate metabolism: Inhibition of vitamin D effect by cortisol. *Proc. Soc. Exp. Biol. Med., 121*:312.

Harrison, H. C., Harrison, H. E., and Park, E. A. 1958. Vitamin D and citrate metabolism: Effect of vitamin D in rats fed diets adequate in both calcium and phosphorus. *Am. J. Physiol., 192*:432.

Haussler, M. R. and Norman, A. W. 1967. The subcellular distribution of physiological doses of vitamin D_3. *Arch. Biochem. Biophys., 118*:145.

Haussler, M. R. and Norman, A. W. 1969. Chromosomal receptor for a vitamin D metabolite. *Proc. Nat. Acad. Sci. U.S.A., 62*:155.

Haussler, M. R. and Rasmussen, H. 1972. Metabolism of vitamin D_3 in the chick. *J. Biol. Chem., 247*:2328.

Haussler, M. R., Bursac, K. M., Bone, H., and Pak, C. Y. C. 1975a. Increased circulating 1α,25-dihydroxyvitamin D_3 in patients with primary hyperparathyroidism. *Clin. Res., 23*(3):322A.

Haussler, M. R., Lightner, E. S., Brumbaugh, P. F., Hughes, M. R., and Bursac, K. 1975b. 1α,25-Dihydroxyvitamin D_3 in idiopathic hypoparathyroidism: Assay of circulating concentrations and therapeutic effect of the sterol. *Clin. Res., 23*(2):155A.

Henry, H. L. and Norman, A. W. 1974. Studies on calciferol metabolism IX. Renal 25-hydroxy-vitamin D_3-1-hydroxylase. Involvement of cytochrome P-450 and other properties. *J. Biol. Chem., 249*:7529.

Henry, H. L. and Norman, A. W. 1975. Studies on calciferol metabolism XIII. Regulation of 25-hydroxy-vitamin D_3-1-hydroxylase in isolated renal mitochondria. *Arch. Biochem. Biophys.* (in press).

Henry, H. L., Midgett, R. J., and Norman, A. W. 1974. Regulation of 25-hydroxyvitamin D_3-1-hydroxylase in vivo. *J. Biol. Chem., 249*:7584.

Hill, L. F., Lumb, G. A., Mawer, E. B. and Stanbury, S. W. 1973. Indirect inhibition of the biosynthesis of 1,25-dihydroxycholecalciferol in rats treated with a diphosphonate. *Clin. Sci., 44*:335.

Holick, M. F., Schnoes, H. K., DeLuca, H. F., Gray, R. W., Boyle, I. T., and Suda, T. 1972. Isolation and identification of 24,25-dihydroxycholecalciferol, a metabolite of vitamin D_3 made in the kidney. *Biochemistry, 2*:4251.

Holick, M. F., Kleiner-Bossaller, A., Schnoes, H. K., Kasten, P. M., Boyle, I. T., and DeLuca, H. F. 1973. 1,24,25-Trihydroxyvitamin D_3. *J. Biol. Chem., 248*:6691.

Horiuchi, N., Suda, T., and Sasaki, S. 1974. Direct involvement of vitamin D in the regulation of 25-hydroxycholecalciferol metabolism, *FEBS Lett., 43*(3):353.

Hughes, M. R., Haussler, M. R., Wergedal, J., and Baylink, D. J. 1975. Regulation of plasma 1α,25-dihydroxyvitamin D_3 by calcium and phosphate. *Clin. Res., 23*(3):323A.

Hurwitz, H. and Bar, A. 1969. Relationship between the lumen–blood electrochemical difference of calcium, calcium absorption and calcium binding protein in the intestine of fowl. *J. Nutr., 99*:217.

Jonxis, J. H. P. and Huisman, T. H. J. 1953. Aminoaciduria in rachitic children. *Lancet, 2*:428.

Kallfelz, F. A., Taylor, A. N., and Wasserman, R. H. 1967. Vitamin D induced calcium binding factor in rat intestinal mucosa. *Proc. Soc. Exp. Biol. Med., 125*:54.

Kimberg, D., Schachter, D., and Schenker, H. 1961. Active transport of calcium by intestine: Effects of dietary calcium. *Am. J. Physiol., 200*:1256.

Kimmich, G. A. and Rasmussen, H. 1969. Regulation of pyruvate carboxylase activity by calcium in intact rat liver mitochondria. *J. Biol. Chem., 244*:190.

Klein, R. and Gow, R. C. 1953. Interaction of parathyroid hormone and vitamin D on the renal excretion of phosphate. *J. Clin. Endocrinol. Metab., 13*:271.

Knutson, J. C. and DeLuca, H. F. 1974. 25-Hydroxyvitamin D_3-24-hydroxylase. Subcellular location and properties. *Biochemistry, 13*:1543.

Kodicek, E. 1960. The metabolism of vitamin D. *4th Int. Cong. Biochem., 11*:198.

Kunin, A. S. and Krane, S. M. 1965. Utilization of citrate by epiphyseal cartilage of rachitic and normal rats. *Biochim. Biophys. Acta, 3*:32.

Lam, H., Schnoes, H. K., and DeLuca, H. F. 1975. Synthesis and biological activity of 25E,26-dihydroxycholecalciferol. *Steroids, 25*:247.

Larkins, R. G., Colston, K. W., Galante, L. S., MacAuley, S. J., Evans, I. M. A., and MacIntyre, I. 1973. Regulation of vitamin D metabolism without parathyroid hormone. *Lancet, 2*:289.

Larkins, R. G., MacAuley, S. J., Rapoport, A., Martin, T. J., Tulloch, B. R., Byfield, P. G. H., Matthews, E. W., and MacIntyre, I. 1974a. Effects of nucleotides, hormones, ions, and 1,25-dihydroxycholecalciferol on 1,25-dihydroxycholecalciferol production in isolated chick renal tubles. *Clin. Sci. Mol. Med., 46*:569.

Larkins, R. G., MacAuley, S. J., and MacIntyre, I. 1974b. Feedback control of vitamin D metabolism by a nuclear action of 1,25-dihydroxycholecalciferol on the kidney. *Nature, 252*:412.

Lavender, A. R. and Pullman, T. N. 1963. Changes in inorganic phosphate excretion induced by renal artery infusion of calcium. *Am. J. Physiol., 205*:1025.

League of Nations. 1935. *Quarterly Bulletin of Health Organization Memorandum on the International Standard for Vitamin D and Its Application, 4*:540.

Litvak, J., Moldawer, M. P., Forbes,A. P., Henneman, P. H. 1958. Hypocalcemic hypercalciuria during vitamin D and dihydrotachysterol therapy of hypoparathyroidism. *J. Clin. Endocrinol. Metab., 18*:246.

Liu, S. H., Chu, H. I., Su, C. C., Yu, T. F., and Cheng, T. Y. 1940. Calcium and phosphorus metabolism in osteomalacia IX. Metabolic behavior of infants fed on breast milk from mothers showing various states of vitamin D nutrition. *J. Clin. Invest., 19*:349.

Lotz, M., Ney, R., and Bartter, F. C. 1964. Osteomalacia and debility resulting from phosphorus depletion. *Trans. Assoc. Am. Physicans Philadelphia, 77*:281.

Lotz, M., Zisman, E., and Bartter, F. C. 1968. Evidence for a phosphorus depletion syndrome in man. *N. Engl. J. Med., 278*:409.

MacGregor, R. R., Hamilton, J. W., and Cohn, D. V. 1970. The induction of calcium binding protein biosynthesis in intestine by vitamin D_3. *Biochim. Biophys. Acta, 222*:482.

MacIntyre, I., Galante, L. S., Evans, I. M. A., Colston, K. W., Moss, D. W., Matthews, E. W., Byfield, P. G. H., MacAuley, S. J., Larkins, R. G., Hillyard, C. J., and Greenberg, P. B. 1974. The regulation of vitamin D metabolism. In:*Endocrinology 1973*, pp. 26–37. Ed. by Taylor, S. Heinemann Medical Books, London.

Manitius, A., Levitin, H., Beck, D., and Epstein, F. H. 1960. On the mechanism of impairment of renal concentrating ability in hypercalcemia. *J. Clin. Invest., 36*:331.

Martin, D. L., Melancon, M. J., and DeLuca, H. F. 1969. Vitamin D stimulated calcium-dependent adenosine triphosphatase from brush borders of rat small intestine. *Biochem. Biophys. Res. Commun., 35*:819.

Massry, S. G. and Coburn, J. W. 1973. The hormonal and non-hormonal control of renal excretion of calcium and magnesium. *Nephron, 10*:66.

Massry, S. G. and Kleeman, C. R. 1972. Calcium and mangesium excretion during acute rise in glomerular filtration rate. *J. Lab. Clin. Med., 80*:654.

Massry, S. G., Coburn, J. W., Chapman, L. W., and Kleeman, C. R. 1968. Role of serum Ca, parathyroid hormone, and NaCl infusion on renal Ca and Na clearances. *Am. J. Physiol., 214*:1403.

Massry, S. G., Friedler, R. M., and Coburn, J. W. 1973. Excretion of phosphate and calcium: Physiology of their renal handling and its relation to clinical medicine. *Arch. Intern. Med., 131*:828.

Mawer, E. B. and Schaefer, K. 1969. The distribution of vitamin D_3 metabolites in human serum and tissues. *Biochem. J., 114*:74.

Mawer, E. B., Lumb, G. A., Schaefer, K., and Stanbury, S. W. 1971. The metabolism of isotopically labelled vitamin D_3 in man: The influence of the state of vitamin D nutrition. *Clin. Sci., 40*:39.

Melancon, M. J. Jr. and DeLuca, H. F. 1970. Vitamin D stimulation of calcium-dependent adenosine triphosphatase in chick intestinal brush borders. *Biochemistry, 9*:1658.

Midgett, R. J., Spielvogel, A. M., Coburn, J. W., and Norman, A. W. 1973. Studies on calciferol metabolism. VI. The renal production of the biologically active form of vitamin D, 1,25-dihydroxycholecalciferol; species, tissue and subcellular distribution. *J. Clin. Endocrinol. Metab. 36*:1153.

Morgan, A. F. and Shimotori, N. 1943. The absorption and retention by dogs of single massive doses of various forms of vitamin D. *J. Biol. Chem., 147*:189.

Morrissey, R. L. and Wasserman, R. H. 1971. Calcium absorption and calcium-binding protein in chicks on differing calcium and phosphorus diets. *Am. J. Physiol., 220:*1509.

Nagata, N. and Rasmussen, H. 1968. Parathyroid hormone and renal cell metabolism. *Biochem. J., 7*:3728.

Ney, R. L., Kelly, G., and Bartter, F. C. 1968. Actions of vitamin D independent of the parathyroid glands. *Endocrinology, 82*:760.

Nordin, B. E. C. 1972. The relative importance of gut, bone and kidney in the regulation of serum calcium. In: *Calcium, Parathyroid Hormone and the Calcitonins*, pp. 263–272. Ed. by Talmage, R. V., and Munson, P. L. Exerpta Medica, Amsterdam.

Nordin, B. E. C. and Peacock, M. 1969. Role of kidney in regulation of plasma calcium. *Lancet*, *2*:1280.

Norman, A. W. 1965. Actinomycin and the response to vitamin D. *Science*, *149*:184.

Norman, A. W. 1968. The mode of action of vitamin D. *Biol. Rev.*, *43*:97.

Norman, A. W. 1972. Problems relating to the definition of an international unit for vitamin D and its metabolites. *J. Nutr.*, *102*:1234.

Norman, A. W. and DeLuca, H. F. 1963. Chromatographic separation of mixtures of vitamin D_2, ergosterol and tachysterol. *Anal. Biochem.*, *35*:1247.

Norman, A. W. and DeLuca, H. F. 1964. Vitamin D and the incorporation of [1-^{14}C]acetate into the organic acids of bone. *Biochem. J.*, *91*:124.

Norman, A. W. and Henry, H. L. 1974. 1,25-Dihydroxycholecalciferol—A hormonally active form of vitamin D_3. *Recent Prog. Horm. Res.*, *30*:431.

Norman, A. W., Tsai, H. C., Spielvogel, A. M., Henry, H. L., and Midgett, R. J. 1973. Studies on the biological production and mode of action of 1,25-dihydroxycholecalciferol, the hormonally active form of vitamin D. In: *Endocrinology 1973*, pp. 52–65. Ed. by Taylor, S. Heinenman Medical Books, London.

Oldham, S. B., Arnaud, C. C., and Jowsey, J. 1974. The influence of vitamin D on the parathyroid. In: *Endocrinology 1973*, pp. 261–268. Ed. by Taylor, S. Heinemann Medical Books, London.

Omhadl, J. L. and DeLuca, H. F. 1972. Rachitogenic activity of dietary strontium I. Inhibition of intestinal calcium absorption and 1,25-dihydroxycholecalciferol synthesis. *J. Biol. Chem.*, *247*:5520.

Omdahl, J. L., Gray, R. W., Boyle, I. T., Knutson, J., and DeLuca, H. F. 1972. Regulation of metabolism of 25-hydroxycholecalciferol by kidney tissue in vitro by dietary calcium. *Nature (London), New Biol.*, *237*:63.

Peterson, P. A. 1971. Isolation and partial characterization of a human vitamin D binding plasma on protein. *J. Biol. Chem.*, *246*:7748.

Ponchon, G. and DeLuca, H. F. 1969. The role of the liver in the metabolism of vitamin D. *J. Clin. Invest.*, *48*:1273.

Popovtzer, M. M. and Robinette, J. B. 1975. The effect of 25-OH-vitamin D_3 on renal handling of phosphorus:evidence for inhibition of cyclic adenosine monophosphate formation. *Am. J. Physiol.*, *229*:907.

Popovtzer, M. M., Robinette, J. B., DeLuca, H. F., and Holick, M. F. 1974. The acute effect of 25-hydroxycholecalciferol on renal handling of phosphorus; Evidence for a parathyroid hormone-dependent mechanism. *J. Clin. Invest.*, *53*(3):913.

Puschett, J. B., Moranz, J., and Kurnick, W. S. 1972a. Evidence for a direct action of cholecalciferol and 25-hydroxycholecalciferol on the renal transport of phosphate, sodium, and calcium. *J. Clin. Invest.*, *51*:373.

Puschett, J. B., Fernandez, P. C., Boyle, I. T., Gray, R. W., Omdahl, J. L., and DeLuca, H. F. 1972b. The acute renal tubular effects of 1,25-dihydroxycholecalciferol. *Proc. Soc. Exp. Biol. Med.*, *141*:379.

Puschett, J. B., Beck, W. S., Jr., Jelonek, A., and Fernandez, P. C. 1974. Study of the renal tubular interaction of thyrocalcitonin, cyclic adenosine 3',5'-monophosphate, 25-hydroxycholecalciferol, and calcium ion. *J. Clin. Invest.*, *53*:756.

Rasmussen, H. and Bordier, P. 1974. Vitamin D-biochemistry and physiology. In: *The Physiological and Cellular Basis of Metabolic Bone Disease*, pp. 207–249. Ed. by Rasmussen, H., and Bordier, P. Williams and Wilkins, Baltimore.

Rasmussen, H., Wang, M., Bikle, D., and Goodman, D. B. P. 1972. Hormonal control of the renal conversion of 25-hydroxycholecalciferol to 1,25-dihydroxycholecalciferol. *J. Clin. Invest.*, *51*:2502.

Rauschkolb, E. W., Davis, H. W., Fenimore, D. C., Black, H. S., and Fabre, L. F. 1969. Identification of vitamin D_3 in human skin. *J. Invest. Dermatol.*, *53*:289.

Rosenstreich, S. J., Rich, C., and Volwiler, W. 1971. Deposition in and the release of vitamin D_3 from body fat: Evidence for a storage site in the rat. *J. Clin. Invest.*, *50*:679.

Sampson, H. W., Matthews, J. L., Martin, J. H., and Kunin, A. S. 1970. An electron microscopic localization of calcium in the small intestine of normal, rachitic and vitamin D-treated rats. *Calcif. Tissue Res., 5*:305.

Sands, H. and Kessler, R. H. 1971. A calcium binding component of dog kidney cortex and its relationship to calcium transport. *Proc. Soc. Exp. Biol. Med., 137*:1267.

Schachter, D., Dowdle, E. B., and Schenker, T. T. 1960. Accumulation of ^{45}Ca by slices of the small intestine. *Am. J. Physiol., 198*:275.

Schachter, D., Finkelstein, J. D., and Kowarski, S. 1965. Metabolism of vitamin D. I. Preparation of radioactive vitamin D and its intestinal absorption in the rat. *J. Clin. Invest., 43*:787.

Shain, S. A. 1972. The in vitro metabolism of 25-hydroxycholecalciferol to 1,25-dihydroxycholecalciferol by chick renal tubules: Effect of actinomycin D, puromycin, calcium and parathyroid hormone. *J. Biol. Chem., 247*:4404.

Short, E. M., Elsas, L. J., and Rosenberg, L. T. 1974. Effect of parathyroid hormone on renal tubular reabsorption of amino acids. *Metabolism, 23*:715.

Siegfried, J. D., Kumar, R., Kurtzman, N. A., and Pillay, V. K. G. 1975. Parathyroid hormone (PTH) dependence of the effect of 25-hydroxycholecalciferol (25 HCC) on HCO_3 reabsorption (HCO_3R). *Clin. Res., 50*:2159.

Smith, J. E. and Goodman, D. S. 1971. The turnover and transport of vitamin D and of a polar metabolite with the properties of 25-hydroxycholecalciferol in human plasma. *J. Clin. Invest., 50*:2159.

Stamp, T. C. B. and Round, J. M. 1974. Seasonal changes in human plasma levels of 25-hydroxyvitamin D. *Nature, 247*:563.

Steele, T. H., Engle, J. E., Tanaka, Y., Lorenc, R. S., Dudgeon, K. L., and DeLuca, H. F. 1975. On the phosphatemic action of 1,25-dihydroxyvitamin D_3. *Am. J. Physiol., 229*:489.

Steenbock, H. and Bellin, S. 1953. Vitamin D and tissue citrate. *J. Biol. Chem., 205*:985.

Suda, T., DeLuca, H. F., Schnoes, H. K., Tanaka, Y., and Holick, M. F. 1970. 25,26-Dihydroxycholecalciferol, a metabolite of vitamin D_3 with intestinal calcium transport activity. *Biochemistry, 9*:3776.

Suki, W. N., Eknoyan, G., Rector, F. C., and Seldin, D. W. 1969. The renal diluting and concentrating mechanisms in hypercalcemia. *Nephron, 6*:50.

Tanaka, Y. and DeLuca, H. F. 1973. The control of 25-hydroxyvitamin D metabolism by inorganic phosphorus. *Arch. Biochem. Biophys., 159*:566.

Tanaka, Y., Frank, H., and DeLuca, H. F. 1973. Intestinal calcium transport: Stimulated by low phosphorus diets. *Science, 181*:569.

Taylor, A. N. and Wasserman, R. H. 1967. Vitamin D_3-induced calcium-binding protein: Partial purification, electrophoretic visualization, and tissue distribution. *Arch. Biochem. Biophys., 119*:536.

Taylor, A. N. and Wasserman, R. H. 1969. Immunofluorescent localization of vitamin D-dependent calcium-binding protein. *J. Histochem. Cytochem., 18*:107.

Taylor, A. N., Wasserman, R. H., and Jowsey, J. 1968. A vitamin D-dependent calcium-binding protein in canine intestinal mucosa. *Fed. Proc., 27*:2582.

Thompson, V. W. and DeLuca, H. F. 1964. Vitamin D and phospholipid metabolism. *J. Biol. Chem., 239*:984.

Tucker, G., Gagnon, R. E., and Haussler, M. R. 1973. Vitamin D_3-25-hydroxylase: Tissue occurrence and apparent lack of regulation. *Arch. Biochem. Biophys., 155*:47.

Verner, J. V., Engel, F. L., and McPherson, H. T. 1958. Vitamin D intoxication: Report of two cases treated with cortisone. *Ann. Intern. Med., 48*:765.

Walser, M. 1973. Divalent cations: Physicochemical state in glomerular filtrate and urine and renal excretion. In: *Handbook of Physiology*, pp. 555–586. Ed. by Orloff, J. and Berliner, R. W. American Physiological Society, Washington, D. C.

Wasserman, R. H. and Taylor, A. N. 1966. Vitamin D_3-induced calcium binding protein in chick intestinal mucosa. *Science, 152*:791.

Wasserman, R. H. and Taylor, A. N. 1968. Vitamin D-dependent calcium-binding protein. *J. Biol. Chem., 243*:3987.

Wasserman, R. H. and Taylor, A. N. 1971. Evidence for a vitamin D_3-induced calcium-binding protein in New World primates. *Proc. Soc. Exp. Biol. Med., 136*:25.

Weidmann, P., Massry, S. G., Coburn, J. W. Atelson, J. A. Maxwell, M. H., and Kleeman, C. R. 1972. Effect of acute hypercalcemia on blood pressure in patients with chronic renal failure. *Ann. Intern. Med., 76*:741.

Wheatley, V. R. and Reinertson, R. P. 1958. The presence of vitamin D precursors in the human epidermis. *J. Invest. Dermatol., 31*:51.

Ziegler, R. and Delling, G. 1975. Clinical observations in lethal vitamin D or DHT-intoxication. In: *Vitamin D and Problems Related to Uremic Bone Disease*, pp. 689–695. Ed. by Norman, A. W., Schaefer, K., Grigoleit, H. G., Herrath, D. V., and Ritz, E. Walter de Gruyter, Berlin.

Zull, J. E., Czarnowska-Misztal, E., and DeLuca, H. F. 1965. Actinomycin D inhibition of vitamin D action. *Science, 149*:183.

Zull, J. E., Czarnowska-Misztal, E., and DeLuca, H. F. 1966. On the relationship between vitamin D action and actinomycin sensitive processes. *Proc. Nat. Acad. Sci. U.S.A., 55*:177.

Chapter **9**

Drugs Affecting the Renal Handling of Uric Acid

George M. Fanelli, Jr.

Merck Institute for Therapeutic Research
West Point, Pennsylvania

I. INTRODUCTION

The renal handling of urate probably presents more complexities than any other endogenous metabolite or foreign compound (drug) for very well-defined reasons. Uric acid excretion apparently has only been of more than passing interest to relatively few investigators beginning with the classic studies that emanated from the laboratory of the late Alexander B. Gutman. Although earlier studies of Folin *et al.* (1924), Bergland and Frisk (1935), Coombs *et al.* (1940), and Talbott (1943) should be recalled, it was primarily the driving force of Gutman, Yü, and co-workers who laid the foundations upon which all subsequent studies on urate transport have been based.[1] For extremely comprehensive reviews of earlier studies and work up to 1974, the reader is referred especially to the works of Emmerson (1975), Gutman and Yü (1972), Mudge *et al.* (1973), Steele and Rieselbach (1975), Weiner and Fanelli (1974, 1975), Weiner and Mudge (1964), and Wesson (1969).

Gutman and Yü (1961) first proposed the now classic "three-component system" for the renal excretion of uric acid consisting of (1) complete filterability of urate at the glomerulus, (2) subsequent tubular reabsorption, and (3) tubular secretion. The uric acid appearing in the final urine was a combination of

---

[1] The accurate quantitative chemical determination of uric acid was fraught by numerous technical difficulties before the the introduction of the specific uricase procedure by Kalckar (1947). For an historical perspective of uric acid methodology in blood and urine, the reader should consult the concise review by Yü and Gutman (1957).

the secreted fraction plus that which may have escaped tubular reabsorption. The above is no longer an hypothesis but now rests on firm scientific fact.

The transport of urate is via bidirectional transport processes, both of which appear to be specifically mediated, i.e., by active transport. The renal handling of urate is unique, certainly not because of two-way movement in the nephron, but far more importantly because of (1) the tremendous species differences in its net transport, (2) the "paradoxical effect" of certain drugs on its excretion some of which are dose dependent, and because (3) urate shares some but by no means all of the characteristics of the well-known organic acid transport system which encompasses the secretion of p-aminohippurate (PAH), penicillin, probenecid (Benemid), phenol red, etc., together with a variety of other weak organic acids. Thus, urate transport and its modification by certain agents represents a very special case. It should be duly noted that Mudge (1967) and Mudge et al. (1968b), quite accurately presaged our current knowledge regarding the very large magnitude of the urate secretory and reabsorptive fluxes.

This review will endeavor to point out just how our present knowledge came about which has, in the main, resulted from the judicious use of pharmacologic agents on urate transport in various animal species including man.

II. RENAL HANDLING OF URATE AS DEDUCED FROM CLEARANCE TECHNIQUES

The clearance technique so exquisitely formulated and executed by Homer Smith and co-workers still continues to give valuable results, as a first approximation, to the renal transport of any substance (for an excellent review of the clearance technique, see Levinsky and Levy, 1973). In its simplest form and using inulin as the universally accepted standard of reference for the estimation of glomerular filtration rate (GFR), the renal clearance of exogenous, or, more accurately, endogenous urate, the ratio of the clearance of urate to that of GFR (C_{Ur}/GFR) may be readily calculated. If this ratio is less than unity, tubular reabsorption is indicated; if greater than one, then tubular secretion occurs. Naturally, if the clearance ratio equals one, superficially then, the substance in question appears to be handled by filtration alone. These overall ratios can be quite misleading in that they only give the *net* effect on the way the kidney handles urate; it tells absolutely nothing about the processes responsible or the magnitude of the fluxes involved. For example, an observed clearance ratio may be unity, indicative of glomerular filtration alone, but the substance in actuality may be both reabsorbed and secreted to such a modulated degree relative to filtration, thus giving a spurious interpretation.

In most species, the net clearance of urate is usually reabsorptive in direction, with normal man showing avid reabsorption with C_{Ur}/GFR being somewhat less than 0.10 (Gutman and Yü, 1972). The chimpanzee shows control clearance ratios of 0.10 (Fanelli et al., 1971a); the *Cebus* monkey, 0.08–0.11 (Fanelli et al., 1970a,b). Blanchard et al. (1972) reported control urate-to-inulin clearance ratios from *Cebus* of 0.03–0.11; for the mongrel dog C_{Ur}/GFR ranged from approximately 0.60 to 0.80 (Mudge *et al.*, 1968b). Zins and Weiner (1968) similarly reported a mean control C_{Ur}/GFR of 0.68 ± 0.07 for mongrel dogs. For the Dalmatian coach hound, Friedman and Byers (1948) reported values for C_{Ur}/GFR of about unity, and Beyer *et al.* (1951) found similar values. Yü *et al.* (1960) determined under appropriate conditions of either no urate loading or urate loading and osmotic diuresis, C_{Ur}/GFR ratios greater than 1 in both the Dalmatian and non-Dalmatian dog. The Dalmatian presents a curious genetic phenomenon in that it possess a "leaky kidney" to urate, not to mention the inaccessibility of urate to hepatic oxidation (Yü *et al.*, 1971), and as such represents a breed of dog forced up an evolutionary cul-de-sac. Thus, the renal handling of urate by the Dalmatian and drug effects thereon as they relate to other species are merely of academic interest.

At the other extreme, in some Old World nonhuman primates, C_{Ur}/GFR greatly exceeded unity, indicating a predominance of the tubular secretory process (Fanelli and Beyer, 1974; Fanelli *et al.*, 1970a). These values were all obtained by conventional clearance procedures and show a wide range for different species but again tell us nothing concerning the mechanisms involved.

Throughout this discussion, urate in the particular species studied is understood to show little, if any, significant binding to plasma proteins (Gutman and Yü, 1972; Farrell *et al.*, 1971; Sheikh and Møller, 1968; Yü and Gutman, 1953). Conversely, Wolfson *et al.* (1950) and more recently Alvsaker (1965) and Klinenberg and Kippen (1970) reported that at 4°C urate was bound to the extent of about 20% to plasma proteins (for review see Bluestone *et al.*, 1974). If these findings are in fact true at 37°C, and there is some evidence that they are not (Sheikh and Møller, 1968), then the clearance of urate corrected for plasma protein binding and thus the apparent clearance ratios would actually be greater than heretofore reported. According to Gutman and Yü (1972) "the consensus, therefore, is that *in vivo* binding of urate to plasma proteins is so small as to have negligible physiological implications." We shall, therefore, abide by their conclusion.

Although there are inherent pitfalls in clearance methodology (Levinsky and Levy, 1973), much meaningful data has been accumulated. However, one must always be cautious in the strict interpretation of these results.

III. LESSONS FROM COMPARATIVE PHYSIOLOGY

Comparative physiology (and pharmacology) in the past have played a signal role in the elucidation of various phenomena directly applicable to man, especially in the field of renal physiology (Marshall, 1934, 1966; Smith, 1964), although at the time the practicality of the research and the ultimate intimate association and application to man were not readily discernible. The comparative approach continues to be highly productive as is clearly evident by classic examples too numerous to be touched upon here (Schmidt-Nielsen, 1961; Schroder, 1967; Wilbur, 1964).

Since the subject of this chapter is the effects of drugs only on urate movement, I shall try to remain within this constraint and only refer to non-drug-related studies for reasons of continuity and clarity.

In vitro studies employing slices of kidney cortex or isolated tubule perfusion techniques also will not be elaborated upon except to mention that kidney slices from man, mongrel dog, and rat do not accumulate urate (Platts and Mudge, 1961). Mudge *et al.* (1973) exhaustively covered this area and came to the conclusion that when comparing data from different species, a fairly good correlation was noted between the degree of accumulation *in vitro* and the extent to which urate was secreted *in vivo*.

A. Lower Vertebrates up to and Including Avians

1. Teleosts

In the aglomerular kidney of the marine lophobranch fish *Lophius americanus* (goosefish), probenecid and salicylate decreased uric acid secretion (Murdaugh *et al.*, 1965). It should be recalled that the aglomerular kidney is a purely tubular kidney, so that any substance found in the urine results from a secretory process.

2. Amphibians

Bidirectional transport of urate by the frog kidney was first noted by Bornstein and Forster (R. P. Forster, unpublished data and personal communication); these data on urate transport by the amphibian kidney probably represent the first chronological recognition of two-way transport of any substance in the vertebrate nephron. To this author's knowledge, additional studies with drugs on amphibian urate transport systems have not been performed.

3. Reptiles

Historically, Marshall (1932) first showed that the phlorizinized iguana secreted urate to the extent that a calculated C_{Ur}/GFR of 16 was noted. However, it is not known if the use of phlorizin itself had any influence on the urate secretory mechanism.

The alligator is devoid of uricase and secretes urate with C_{Ur}/GFR approximating 6 at plasma levels of 20–70 $\mu g/ml$ (Coulson and Hernandez, 1964; Mudge *et al.*, 1973). Experiments with acetazolamide in the alligator gave some indication of decreased "undetermined anion excretion" (Coulson and Hernandez, 1964); possibly a large proportion of this is uric acid, so one cannot infer that the effect of acetazolamide is unequivocal. Although various diuretic and other agents were injected into the alligator, any effects on uric acid excretion were not specifically recorded.

Dantzler (1968) has demonstrated in the water snake that bicarbonate-induced metabolic alkalosis caused a twofold increase in uric acid excretion whereas acetazolamide had no effect. Probenecid inhibited tubular secretion of urate and PAH *in vivo* and *in vitro* in the water snake, and on the basis of the relative affinities for the transport systems the suggestion was made that the transport mechanisms for these two organic acids may not be the same (Dantzler, 1970).

4. Birds

It has been well known for many years that the chicken lacks uricase and avidly secretes urate with C_{Ur}/GFR reaching values as high as 18 at endogenous plasma urate concentrations (Mudge *et al.*, 1973). Nechay and Nechay (1959) published a very interesting paper in which they showed that probenecid markedly diminished tubular secretion of urate whereas salicylate and 2,4-dinitrophenol (DNP) were less effective. More significantly, they pointed out that large doses of pyrazinamide were without effect. This finding with pyrazinamide was subsequently confirmed by Berger *et al.* (1960). Unfortunately, the active metabolite, pyrazinoate (PZA), a potent inhibitor of urate secretion (Yü *et al.*, 1957; Weiner and Tinker, 1972), was not tested. Therefore, the possibility exists that the chicken is unable to hydrolyze the amide to the free acid. Berger *et al.* (1960) also showed that probenecid, sulfinpyrazone, zoxazolamine, and high doses of phenylbutazone, all uricosuric in man, depressed tubular secretion of urate in the chicken.

So far, only unidirectional transport of urate by the chicken kidney has been the rule, but in two experiments by Berger *et al.* (1960), after large amounts of probenecid, control tubular secretion was reversed to tubular reabsorption. It is, therefore, obvious that only secretory transport is responsible for uric acid excretion in the chicken and that the magnitude of this flux is so large as to overwhelm any reabsorptive component, be it due to carrier mediation or back-diffusion. Recently, Shideman *et al.* (1975) presented data that the simultaneous infusion of uric acid and either ethacrynic acid or furosemide increased the tubular excretion of uric acid by approximately 100%. Superimposing pyrazinoic acid on this experimental protocol significantly decreased uric acid excretion by as much as 60%. The inference was that approximately 40% of the secreted uric acid was reabsorbed. Therefore, bidirectional tubular transport of urate probably does occur in the chicken kidney.

Chlorothiazide has been reported by Castles and Williamson (1963) to inhibit urate secretion, whereas probenecid depresses the tubular secretion of chlorothiazide. Curiously, lactate, which decreases uric acid excretion in man, did not alter its excretion in the chicken (Berger *et al.*, 1960; Mudge *et al.*, 1973, for review).

An interesting study by Quebbemann (1973) using the well-known Sperber preparation has documented renal synthesis of urate; renal excretion of radiolabeled urate during [^{14}C]xanthine infusion was inhibited by probenecid and PAH but not by the organic cation transport inhibitor quinine. Renal urate synthesis was blocked by the xanthine oxidase inhibitor allopurinol.

B. Higher Vertebrates—Mammals Including Nonhuman Primates

1. Rats

At physiological plasma urate levels, urate is reabsorbed as evidenced by C_{Ur}/GFR approximating 0.80 (Boudry, 1971a). Unpublished observations by Mudge upon urate loading indicated C_{Ur}/GFR was about 0.60. Boudry (1971b) also has shown that probenecid at 200 mg/kg intravenously had a marked uricosuric action at low plasma urate concentrations, the effect of which became much less at higher plasma urate values. In the same study, sulfinpyrazone and hydrochlorothiazide were inactive. High doses of PAH and pyrazinamide depressed urate secretion at high plasma urate levels; this effect was much less impressive at low urate concentrations. Chronic administration of intraperitoneal furosemide caused C_{Ur}/GFR to decrease from 0.12 ± 0.006 to 0.08 ± 0.01 (Weinman *et al.*, 1975).

In diabetes insipidus urine flow increased threefold, but urate clearances were about the same as in lithium-treated rats without diabetes insipidus and sodium-injected controls (Steele *et al.*, 1974).

Roch-Ramel *et al.* (1974) have reported that the rat kidney is able to synthesize as well as catabolize urate. Clearance ratios in animals infused with both hypoxanthine and allopurinol were as low as in animals receiving allopurinol alone. Thus, differences in uric acid excretion noted at comparable plasma urate levels were interpreted as arising from differences in urate synthesis.

2. Guinea Pigs

Mudge *et al.* (1968a), in the only published work on uric acid transport in this species, presented C_{Ur}/GFR ratios ranging from 0.6 to 4.0 under conditions of urate loading; these values were interpreted to mean that urate is normally either reabsorbed, secreted, or both. Stop-flow experiments showed only proximal secretion. Probenecid markedly inhibited urate secretion, thus unmasking proximal reabsorption. Pyrazinoate had only a slight inhibitory action on urate secretion whereas chlorothiazide, ouabain, and lactic acid were without significant effect.

3. Rabbits

Poulsen and Praetorius (1954) were the first investigators to publish that urate reabsorption (10–75%) occurs at normal plasma levels (2–5 µg/ml), whereas at artificially elevated urate concentrations (10–30 µg/ml) uric acid is cleared at a rate 25–200% greater than GFR, i.e., net tubular secretion predominates. Subsequently, Poulsen (1955) noted that tubular secretion of urate was depressed at elevated plasma levels by probenecid and to a lesser extent by salicylate. Møller (1965a,b) carried this work further by confirming it and also showing that probenecid definitely had an inhibitory effect on uric acid excretion at endogenous levels of plasma urate; he also localized the site of tubular secretion of urate to the proximal tubule in stop-flow studies and showed that this proximal secretion was almost completely inhibited by probenecid (Møller, 1965c).

Almost simultaneously, Beechwood *et al.* (1964), using the stop-flow technique, demonstrated urate reabsorption in a majority of rabbits under free-flow conditions, although some animals (ca. 20%) showed net proximal secretion. Chlorothiazide, pyrazinoate, creatinine, and lactic acid produced a pronounced increase in the secretory peak; probenecid completely inhibited this secretory peak, resulting in net reabsorption. Thus, the reversal of tubular secretion was taken as evidence for bidirectional transport of urate in this lagomorph. Additional work by Berndt and Beechwood (1965) using stop-flow analysis indicated that the secretory peak for urate was increased by ouabain: when ouabain and probenecid were given at the same time, they concluded that ouabain acted to block urate reabsorption.

In an impressive series of experiments, Møller (1967a,b), using both clearance and stop-flow methods, showed that following PAH and Diodrast administration a reduction in urate excretion occurred; urate was found to be a rather inefficient inhibitor of PAH secretion. In stop-flow studies, proximal urate secretion at maximal PAH and Diodrast secretion was almost completely blocked. Similarly, DNP, fumarate, succinate, salicylate, and probenecid reduced urate and PAH excretion, but urate secretion was apparently more susceptible to depression than that of PAH by these inhibitors. The conclusion reached was that the affinity of urate was less than that of PAH for the transport system.

4. Dogs

The mongrel and Dalmatian dog are relatively poor animals upon which to study urate transport processes because they possess ample amounts of uricase and are notoriously poor responders to uricosuric agents (Mudge *et al.,* 1968b; Maroske and Weiner, 1968). Nevertheless, some insight has been obtained with respect to the nature of the urate transport mechanisms by certain ingeniously designed protocols (Mudge *et al.,* 1968b; Zins and Weiner, 1968). Earlier studies by Miller *et al.* (1951) attached questionable significance to the slight increase in uric acid excretion after intravenously administered Diodrast, salicylate, and the organomercurial diuretic meralluride. These three agents are uricosuric in man (Gutman and Yü, 1972, for review) and in the chimpanzee (Fanelli *et al.,* 1972a,b, 1973a). Under stringent conditions of urate loading and mannitol osmotic diuresis, urate secretion was evident in the mongrel dog ($C_{Ur}/GFR >$ 1.0) by Lathem *et al.* (1960); probenecid, at the height of diuresis reduced urate clearance, suggesting to these authors that probenecid may depress tubular secretion of urate. Kessler *et al.* (1959), using stop-flow analysis, had already determined that probenecid inhibited proximal tubular urate secretion in the Dalmatian; a depression of the proximal reabsorptive trough in the mongrel dogs was also depicted with the same drug. Yü *et al.* (1960) agreed, in general, with and greatly extended the results of Lathem *et al.* (1960) and presented evidence that probenecid and sulfinpyrazone depressed urate secretion; both reabsorption and secretion of urate in the dog were effected mainly by active processes.

Davis *et al.* (1965), with a modification of the stop-flow technique and renal arterial injection of [2-^{14}C]uric acid, localized transtubular movement in the distal nephron in the dog; pyrazinamide apparently inhibited this distal tubular influx of urate. These studies are suspect: The chemical form of urate was not characterized primarily because of the very small number of counts in the distal samples. Only one other study, by Yü *et al.* (1960), showed a distal secretory site for urate in both the Dalmatian and mongrel dog in which both peaks were obliterated by probenecid and massive doses of PAH.

It is generally agreed, however, that the distal tubule is impermeable to urate since no other investigator has been able to duplicate unequivocal distal tubular secretory peaks for urate in the dog.

The studies of Mudge *et al.* (1968b) and Zins and Weiner (1968) substantially expanded on earlier studies. The former authors employed both clearance and stop-flow protocols to demonstrate that (1) pyrazinoate lowered urate concentration in proximal stop-flow samples, (2) probenecid results were unrevealing, and (3) variable results with cortisone, DNP, 2-nitroprobenecid, salicylate, and ouabain were obtained. The paper by Mudge *et al.* (1968b) is very informative because it points out in their Figure 6 that, using the modified stop-flow procedure of Zins and Weiner (1968), urate secretion is most likely proximal to reabsorption and that "it would not be surprising if the unidirectional fluxes, when measured, prove to be quite high." Zins and Weiner (1968) conclusively showed that during stop-flow occlusions, if large amounts of urate and inulin were infused simultaneously into the renal artery, more urate than inulin appeared in proximal tubular samples. Chlorothiazide, salicylate, and PAH reversed this phenomenon leading them to conclude that the secretory flux for urate was effected through the organic anion transport carrier. Bidirectional movement was demonstrated, and both processes were mediated by active transport. This latter work also succinctly summarized previous studies on urate transport in the dog and deserves scrutiny by anyone interested in solid experimental design, execution, and interpretation of results pertaining not only to urate but also to the organic acid transport system as it exists in the dog. Nolan and Foulkes (1971), using a double-indicator dilution technique with [^{3}H]inulin and [^{14}C]urate, determined that the normal secretory flux for urate in a normal steady state must be small. They also showed that this rapid secretory flux could be inhibited by pyrazinoate, probenecid, PAH, chlorothiazide, furosemide, ethacrynic acid, and lactate but not by the mercurial diuretic chlormerodrin.

5. Other Mammalian Species below the Primates

In the goat, Mudge (1965) reported that urate was secreted in the proximal segment in stop-flow experiments and that this secretion was inhibited by probenecid; he also found slight proximal urate reabsorption in the cat but was unable to show convincing drug effects. In the bull calf, probenecid strongly inhibited proximal urate secretion (Mudge, 1967).

6. *Nonhuman Primates*

Because of their close phylogenetic relationship to man, studies on urate transport processes using simple clearance techniques and sometimes micropuncture have been quite revealing (Fanelli and Beyer, 1974, for review). Some insight into the nature of these processes has stemmed not only from earlier, somewhat forgotten, observations in the literature but also by "challenging" these processes with various drugs.

The net renal clearance of uric acid varies widely between the various species of monkey (Fanelli *et al.,* 1970a). In all monkeys examined, with the exception of the New World *Cebus,* spider, and woolly monkeys, urate loading must be resorted to because of the vanishingly low endogenous levels of plasma urate; this is due to the abundant presence of the oxidative enzyme uricase. It is true that the *Cebus* does possess uricase (Simkin, 1971) and that the relatively high circulating level of urate results from far higher rates of urate synthesis and destruction from that which obtains in man. In general, Old World monkeys show net urate secretion and New World species exhibit varying degrees of net tubular reabsorption.

In a great ape species, the chimpanzee lacks uricase and has a relatively high endogenous level of urate (20–50 μg/ml) with an average C_{Ur}/GFR of approximately 0.10 (Fanelli *et al.,* 1971a). Any agent that is uricosuric in man was also uricosuric, if tested, in the chimpanzee, i.e., agents like probenecid, sulfinpyrazone, zoxazolamine, carinamide, etc. (Fanelli *et al.,* 1971b), and the organomercurial diuretics (Fanelli *et al.,* 1973a).

In the *Cebus* monkey, results with known uricosuric agents were somewhat perplexing in that carinamide, sulfinpyrazone, and the potent zoxazolamine were generally inactive even at high doses (Fanelli *et al.,* 1970c). Mersalyl was also virtually inactive as a diuretic and uricosuric agent in the *Cebus* monkey (Fanelli *et al.,* 1973b). The antiuricosuric agent pyrazinamide or its active metabolite pyrazinoate (Weiner and Tinker, 1972) produced urate retention in the *Cebus* as did nicotinic acid (Fanelli *et al.,* 1970b). Probenecid and its 2-nitro, 2-hydroxyl, and 2-chloro analogs were also found to be uricosuric in the *Cebus,* the probenecid analogs exhibiting 10 times the potency of probenecid when compared on the basis of plasma drug levels (Blanchard *et al.,* 1972).

The potent uricosuric agent benziodarone was found to be markedly uricosuric in man and *Cebus* by Lemieux *et al.* (1973a,b), thus confirming earlier results with this drug in the *Cebus* (Fanelli *et al.,* 1970c).

For a comprehensive review of renal urate transport in animal models, the reader is referred to the recent paper by Weiner and Fanelli (1975).

IV. EFFECTS OF CURRENT DRUGS ON NET URATE TRANSPORT

In this section a greater focus will be on man and the chimpanzee and the effects of the organomercurial diuretic mersalyl (Salyrgan), pyrazinoate, and the newer agents, some of which were developed in these laboratories (Fanelli *et al.*, 1974; Cragoe *et al.*, 1975).

Berliner *et al.* (1950) first demonstrated a reabsorptive tubular maximum (*Tm*) for urate in normal man equivalent to 15 mg/min/1.73 m^2 which implied an active transport process. It must be borne in mind that when these results were reported, unidirectional movement was canon law in renal physiology. In the *Cebus*, an apparent reabsorptive *Tm* for urate was elicited at plasma urate concentrations of about 300 μg/ml (Fanelli *et al.*, 1970b). Evidence was presented that this apparent *Tm* for urate was enhanced by PZA, thereby suggesting that PZA increased reabsorption. This explanation has been neither proved nor disproved, but in the light of current knowledge, PZA-induced enhancement of urate reabsorption seems unlikely. Probenecid increased whereas lactate and β-hydroxybutyrate decreased uric acid excretion, confirming the earlier work of Skeith and Healey (1968). Although a secretory flux for urate in the *Cebus* was not demonstrated until the work of Lemieux *et al.* (1973b) appeared, it was strongly believed that one existed because DNP and high doses of PAH had been shown to depress C_{Ur}/GFR (Fanelli *et al.*, 1970b). During stop-flow studies in *Cebus albifrons*, Lemieux *et al.* (1973b) showed that urate-to-inulin U/P ratios in the proximal area rose from 0.30 to 0.99 after benziodarone infusion and from 0.63 to 1.35 at a distal site, thus indicating a distal secretory site for urate corresponding to the sodium minimum. Using a modified stop-flow technique they found that [2-^{14}C]urate preceded that of [^{3}H]inulin over the entire proximal site.

In the chimpanzee, bidirectional tubular transport of urate has been unequivocally demonstrated, albeit quite fortuitously (Fanelli *et al.*, 1973a). The background for this finding originated from an early, unexplained observation by Berliner *et al.* (1948) in which they noted that intravenous mersalyl depressed the T_m for PAH in man but not in the mongrel dog. Because of the phylogenetic proximity of the chimpanzee to man, evidence was sought to see if mersalyl could, indeed, bring about an inhibition of Tm_{PAH} in the chimpanzee. Virtually identical reductions of Tm_{PAH} of 73% were realized in the chimpanzee with mersalyl (Fanelli *et al.*, 1972b); a mean reduction of 76% was reported for man by Berliner *et al.* (1948). Subsequently, it was announced that in the chimpanzee mersalyl, at low doses of PAH (1–2 mg/100 ml), was so markedly uricosuric that apparent net tubular secretion of urate was readily uncovered, i.e., values for $C_{Ur}/GFR > 1.9$ were obtained (Fanelli *et al.*, 1973a). In this same study net urate secretion was demonstrated in 21 out of 22 experiments, and this apparent net secretion was subject to competitive inhibition by probenecid, Diodrast, PAH, phenol red, bromcresol green, salicylate, sulfinpyrazone, and PZA. It is therefore reasonable to say that urate secretory transport is carrier mediated even though saturation of this mechanism has not been demonstrated. Pyrazinoate was clearly found to produce urate retention at plasma PZA levels ranging from 2–600 μg/ml (Figure 1). It will be noted that C_{Ur}/GFR expressed as percent of control is maximally depressed at plasma PZA levels of about 10–200 μg/ml, whereas at plasma PZA concentrations above 600 μg/ml frank uricosuria supervenes. Since it was previously known that PZA completely nullifies

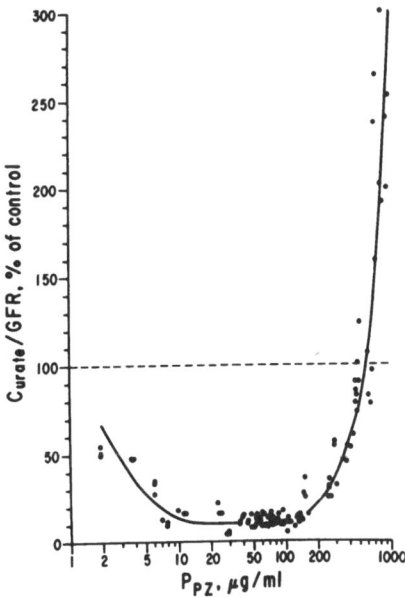

Figure 1. C_{Ur}/GFR (expressed as % of control) plotted as a function of plasma pyrazinoate (P_{PZ}). Twenty-six experiments are included in this figure in which each point represents a single clearance period. (From Fanelli and Weiner, 1973.)

probenecid-induced uricosuria and probenecid is totally unable to overcome PZA-induced urate retention (Fanelli *et al.*, 1971a), Figure 2 attempts to diagramatically explain these observations (Fanelli and Weiner, 1973, 1974). Briefly, scheme A represents a control situation in which the secreted fraction has been assumed to be equal to the filtered load. Basic to this assumption is that secretion is not small compared to urate reabsorption. The magnitude of reabsorption is again arbitrarily set at 189 units in order to have excreted urate equal to 11% of the filtered load. Scheme B depicts partial inhibition of urate secretion and a small reduction in reabsorption; hence under the influence of PZA alone only about 1% of the apparent filtered load reaches the final urine.

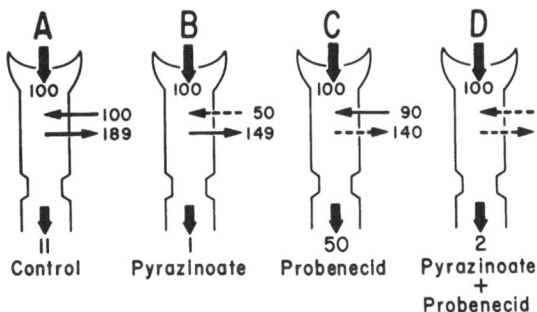

Figure 2. Diagrams of proposals for the action of drugs on urate transport. Solid arrows depict uninhibited transport, dashed arrows partially inhibited urate transport. (From Fanelli and Weiner, 1973.)

The situation that might obtain after probenecid is shown in scheme C, i.e., a small inhibition of secretion accompanied by a greater depression of reabsorption. In scheme D when PZA and probenecid are administered simultaneously the depressions of secretion become additive. Obviously, the above is a gross oversimplification of highly complex events, as numerous other factors no doubt come into play.

The pyrazinamide-suppression test devised by Steele and Rieselbach (1967) as a minimal estimate of urate secretion in man has been employed by many investigators (for review see Steele, 1971, 1973, 1974; Steele and Rieselbach, 1975; Gutman and Yü, 1972). Although the validity of the basic concept has been challenged by Holmes *et al.* (1972) and Fanelli and Weiner (1973, 1974), the test still remains useful as long as its inherent limitations are fully comprehended (Fanelli and Weiner, 1973; Rieselbach and Steele, 1974).

Salicylate exhibits the well-known "paradoxical effect" in man in that low doses produce urate retention and high doses uricosuria (Yü and Gutman, 1959). They postulated that low doses inhibited only urate secretion and that higher doses in addition to secretory inhibition, partially blocked urate reabsorption, with the net effect being uricosuria. Also, and possibly of greater pharmacologic importance, Yü and Gutman (1959) demonstrated in man that alkalosis enhanced the uricosuric action of salicylate; this was the first and still remains the best evidence that the concentration of drug in the tubular fluid was the critical factor in determining uricosuric activity. Alkalosis, itself, showed little if any effect on urate clearance, but in the presence of salicylate plus an alkaline urine, the excretion of salicylate was increased coincident with its enhanced uricosuric action. Therefore, by reducing passive back-diffusion of salicylate, more of the drug remained on the luminal side in order to compete for the active reabsorptive mechanism.

The uricosuric action of probenecid and its therapeutic efficacy in gout are so well documented that reiteration of even a part of its history would be superfluous (Sirota *et al.,* 1952; Gutman, 1966; Fanelli, 1975). The most complete review up to 1966 on various drugs affecting urate transport in man, such as probenecid, sulfinpyrazone, zoxazolamine, etc., together with the history of older agents is that by Gutman (1966).

Other agents that are uricosuric in man are halofenate (Morgan *et al.,* 1971; Ravenscroft *et al.,* 1973) and two benzofuran derivatives from Europe, benziodarone (Lemieux *et al.,* 1973a) and benzbromarone (Jain *et al.,* 1974). The hypoglycemic sulfonylurea acetohexamide (or its metabolic product) reported to be uricosuric in gouty subjects with coexisting diabetes (Yü *et al.,* 1968) was also uricosuric in the chimpanzee at comparable oral doses (unpublished data). In fact, the chimpanzee exhibited a greater sensitivity to acetohexamide than man in that C_{Ur}/GFR increased from 0.069 to 0.218 attaining a peak effect about 2 hr after administration. Mudge (1971) has warned of a possible toxicity factor due to the uricosuric action of certain cholecystographic agents in man.

Various other agents, not organic acids and structurally unrelated such as outdated tetracycline (Funlop and Drapkin, 1965), the tranquilizing agent chlorprothixene (Healey *et al.,* 1965), and zoxazolamine referred to previously, are also uricosuric in man possibly by causing some nonspecific disruption of the reabsorptive function of the proximal tubule although this explanation may not specifically apply to zoxazolamine. Two anticholinergic agents, glycopyrrolate and tridihexethyl chloride, produced a small increase in fractional uric acid excretion in some hyperuricemic subjects but not in normouricemics (Postlethwaite et al., 1974a); these latter two drugs are quaternary ammonium compounds. Also, an expectorant, glyceryl guaicolate, has a mild uricosuric effect in some gouty patients (Ramsdell et al., 1974). It should be noted that the antituberculous agent ethambutol caused hyperuricemia in some tuberculous patients with a mean decrease in C_{Ur}/GFR of 22%. The mechanism of action of ethambutol appears to differ in one or more respects from PZA, diuretics, and ethanol, which also show a similar net reduction on urate clearance (Postlethwaite et al., 1974b). These nonspecific agents increase uric acid excretion by some unknown means and are in all probability unrelated to the mechanisms of action of the specific organic acids which have received considerably greater study.

Kelley (1975) has presented a brief comprehensive review of certain pharmacologic agents that increase uric acid excretion in man.

A. Hyperuricemia Resulting from Chronic Diuretic Therapy

Diuretic-induced hyperuricemia is a well-known phenomenon since it was first reported by Laragh et al. (1958) for chlorothiazide. Since that time, it has become a well-documented side effect characteristic of all the current diuretic agents in man with the possible exception of the antikaluretic drugs amiloride and spironolactone. It is also clearly documented that intravenous chlorothiazide (Demartini et al., 1962) and, to a lesser extent, ethacrynic acid and furosemide (Steele and Oppenheimer, 1969) cause transient uricosuria (for reviews see Bryant et al., 1962; Peters and Roch-Ramel, 1969; Steele and Oppenheimer, 1969).

It has generally been stated by most authors that this diuretic-induced hyperuricemia results from a successful competitive inhibition of tubular secretion of urate by the agent in question as they are all organic acids. We believe this interpretation lacks firm scientific evidence since it has been shown that intravenous mersalyl, an organic acid itself, unmasks frank urate secretion in the chimpanzee (Fanelli et al., 1973a). Also, chlorothiazide and ethacrynic acid at high intravenous priming doses, together with sustaining infusions in "combination experiments" with mersalyl, failed to inhibit mersalyl-induced net urate secretion; ratios of C_{Ur}/GFR were greater than unity in the chimpanzee. We feel that diuretic-induced hyperuricemia results from increased urate reabsorption secondary to contraction of extracellular fluid volume. Fully recognizing that tubular secretion of urate in man may be not as large in magnitude as in the chimpanzee, the secretory mechanism in man may be more susceptible to inhibition. However, certain evidence argues against this, viz., net urate secretion can be demonstrated in normal and gouty man with urate loading, osmotic diuresis, and sulfinpyrazone (Gutman et al., 1959), whereas in the chimpanzee, sulfinpyrazone is apparently able to inhibit the urate secretory flux (Fanelli *et al.*, 1973a). This remains an unexplained species difference.

B. Newer Polyvalent Agents Affecting Uric Acid Excretion

Recently Cragoe *et al.* (1975) and Woltersdorf *et al.* (1975a,b) reported the synthesis of a new class of (1-oxo-2-substituted-5-indanyloxy)acetic acids which possess both inherent uricosuric and saluretic activity. One such compound, (6,7-dichloro-2-methyl-1-oxo-2-phenyl-5-indanyloxy)acetic acid (hereafter referred to as indanone or MK-196, Figure 3), has marked uricosuric–saluretic potency in the chimpanzee following either oral or intravenous administration (Fanelli *et al.*, 1974). Table I summarizes results of experiments with oral administration of indanone and its 2-cyclopentyl-2-methyl analog in the chimpanzee. Inspection of this table shows a marked uricosuric response and saluretic response, especially at the higher doses with the indanone. Significant activity is still evident at oral doses far lower than 0.1 mg/kg. The 2-cyclopentyl-2-methyl analog appears to be substantially less uricosuric and saluretic on a dose basis; with both agents, there is some elevation of potassium excretion.

It is also of considerable pharmacologic interest that the uricosuric action of the indanone is only partially compromised by PZA (Table II) in which the characteristic marked uricosuria, increased urine flow, and saluresis is obtained. Superimposing PZA upon the indanone definitely attenuates the uricosuric response but has no effect whatsoever on the diuresis and saluresis. The reverse experiment is depicted in Table III; the indanone is able to overcome the antiuricosuric action of PZA in that ratios of C_{Ur}/GFR are approximately three times control values although the full expression of the uricosuric response is muted (cf. Table II). PZA definitely does not affect in any apparent manner the diuretic activity of the indanone (Fanelli *et al.*, 1975).

Another uricosuric–diuretic compound, [2,3-dichloro-4-(2-thienylcarbonyl)phenoxy]acetic acid or tienilic acid, has been reported to be active in man although at much higher oral doses than are required for the indanone (Masbernard and Guidicelli, 1974; Stote *et al.*, 1974). There is no doubt that it is an effective uricosuric, but it appears to be only weakly saluretic in man and also in

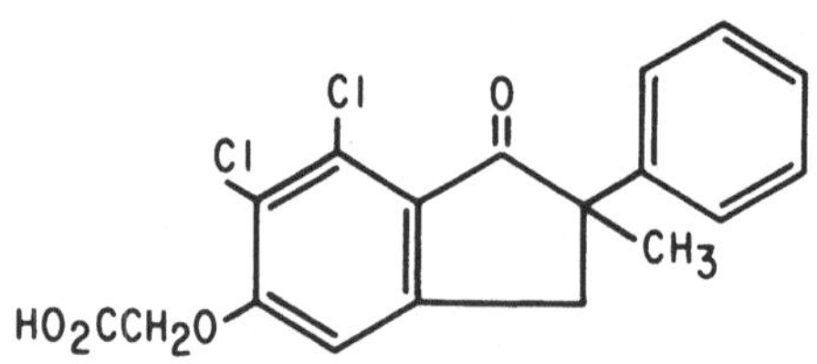

(6,7 - DICHLORO - 2 - METHYL - I - OXO - 2 -
PHENYL - 5 - INDANYLOXY) ACETIC ACID

pKa = 3.67

Figure 3. Chemical structure of a potent uricosuric—saluretic indanone.

Table I. Uricosuric and Diuretic Effects of MK-196 and an Analog in the Chimpanzee

Dose, mg/kg p.o.	Exp. No.	Urine flow, ml/min		GFR, ml/min		C_{Ur}/C_{In}		Na^+, μEq/min		K^+, μEq/min		Cl^-, μEq/min	
		C[a]	E[b]	C	E	C	E	C	E	C	E	C	E
MK-196													
0.0078	1	1.7	0.9	72	78	0.08	0.1	32	47	38	47	19	36
0.0156	4	2.0	1.7	105	111	0.09	0.12	48	108	45	88	34	131
0.0312	2	1.3	1.2	60	68	0.14	0.19	30	105	62	108	47	181
0.0625	4	1.9	3.4	119	117	0.10	0.18	93	384	93	182	109	520
0.125	1	4.9	3.0	118	118	0.07	0.20	69	359	38	96	28	419
0.25	4	1.4	3.4	88	85	0.12	0.25	71	331	78	130	67	422
1.0	1	1.1	4.4	90	87	0.14	0.35	23	318	62	127	44	418
2.5	4	0.9	4.5	86	75	0.10	0.47	24	447	50	135	79	582
5.0	4	1.4	5.0	107	93	0.10	0.43	54	466	61	144	55	609
10.0	4	1.6	8.4	117	103	0.11	0.49	127	924	116	244	138	1220
2-Cyclopentyl-2-methyl analog													
0.25	1	0.9	3.1	90	94	0.11	0.13	77	302	65	86	47	378
1.0	1	5.9	2.4	70	83	0.11	0.15	45	217	29	98	16	309
2.5	2	1.5	2.4	93	95	0.07	0.24	8	140	40	96	23	228
5.0	2	2.2	3.7	124	119	0.07	0.20	49	266	48	98	30	321
10.0	1	2.1	6.7	102	103	0.10	0.29	51	768	64	197	47	1032

[a] Control, average value for 3 clearance periods.
[b] Experimental, average value for 8 clearance periods after treatment.

Table II. Inability of Pyrazinoic Acid to Completely Reverse Indanone-Induced
Uricosuria and Saluresis (Chimpanzee J., Male, 78.0 kg. Expt. No. 590)

Elapsed time, min	Urine flow, ml/min	GFR, ml/min	Urate excretion, mg/min	C_{Ur}/GFR	Na^+ excretion, $\mu Eq/min$	K^+ excretion, $\mu Eq/min$	Cl^- excretion, $\mu Eq/min$
0–20	1.35	157	0.446	0.068	56	62	22
20–40	1.05	164	0.421	0.060	45	68	29
40–60	0.95	148	0.456	0.074	40	71	33
62–66	Prime: Indanone 1 mg/kg i.v.						
65	Infusion II: As I with the indanone 1 mg/kg/hr						
70–85	15.7	157	3.22	0.519	1593	133	1784
85–100	12.7	118	2.95	0.694	1105	115	1354
100–115	15.5	124	3.13	0.719	1519	148	1872
116–121	Prime: Pyrazinoic acid 20 mg/kg i.v.						
120	Infusion III: As II with pyrazinoic acid 60 mg/kg/hr						
125–140	17.6	104	1.26	0.342	1705	157	2052
140–155	16.3	108	1.28	0.342	1642	150	2043
155–170	14.7	129	1.26	0.282	1566	176	1994
170–185	13.9	112	1.30	0.330	1295	162	1676
185–200	13.3	127	1.33	0.308	1325	166	1677
200–215	14.3	121	1.41	0.342	1320	168	1669

the chimpanzee (unpublished observations). From the clinical observations of
Masbernard and Guidicelli (1974), rather severe hypokalemia manifests itself as
a distressing side effect.

C. Sites and Mechanisms of Action

It has been the consensus of many investigators that the site of action of
drugs affecting renal urate handling is at the luminal membrane at some portion
or possibly along the entire length of the proximal tubule. This has unequivocally been shown to be the site of urate reabsorption (and secretion), since the
distal tubule is apparently impermeable to urate (for review see Mudge et al.,
1973; Weiner and Fanelli, 1974, 1975). The mechanism of action of these drugs,
although unproven experimentally, is most probably by competition for the urate
reabsorptive mechanism and the ensuing higher affinity of the drug in question
for the appropriate receptor(s).

V. RENAL HANDLING OF URATE AS DEDUCED FROM MICROPUNCTURE TECHNIQUES

Kramp et al. (1971) reported on intrarenal movement of [2-^{14}C]urate in rats
using the microinjection procedure. They presented data that after proximal
injections, both total and direct recoveries of labeled urate were significantly

greater following probenecid, PAH, or PZA than during saline diuresis. They attributed decreased proximal reabsorption to the effects of the drugs on the luminal membrane; no evidence for urate secretion was found. Similar evidence for net reabsorption of urate in the rat using the microperfusion technique was found by Sonnenberg *et al.* (1965).

In a series of elegant studies from Deetjen's laboratory (Greger *et al.,* 1971, 1974a,b; Lang *et al.*, 1972, 1973) utilizing the microperfusion technique in the rat, it was found (1) that net reabsorption of urate occurs but not in the proximal tubule, (2) net proximal active tubular secretion of urate occurs, and (3) urate is bound to the extent of 35% to plasma proteins and reabsorption occurs as urate is concentrated as it flows down the loop of Henle and passively diffuses into the medullary interstitium where it is trapped in the vasa recta; this passive countercurrent diffusion is highly flow dependent. Greger *et al.* (1974a) have presented data that erythrocytes and to a lesser extent plasma proteins serve as vehicles for urate reabsorption in the kidney medulla. Lang *et al.* (1974) also indicated that the rat kidney has no significant uricase activity and that oxidation of urate to allantoin takes place solely in the liver.

Free-flow micropuncture studies in rats by de Rougemont and Roch-Ramel (1973) indicated net urate reabsorption in certain tubules and net secretion in others, often in the same animals.

In other recent microperfusion studies in rats with [2-^{14}C]urate, chronic furosemide administration resulted in enhanced proximal reabsorption of urate, sodium, and water with no evidence for distal urate reabsorption (Weinman *et al.,* 1975). From the foregoing it is apparent that not all groups are in accord

Table III. Effect of the MK-196 at 1 mg/kg and 1 mg/kg/hr on Pyrazinoic Acid-Induced Urate Retention (Chimpanzee P., Male, 62.2 kg, Expt. No. 591)

Elapsed time, min	Urine flow, ml/min	GFR, ml/min	Urate excretion, mg/min	C_{Ur}/GFR	Na$^+$ excretion, μEq/min	K$^+$ excretion, μEq/min	Cl$^-$ excretion, μEq/min
0–20	4.80	122	0.663	0.135	165	83	241
20–40	4.55	128	0.724	0.140	183	114	304
40–60	3.15	127	0.577	0.112	132	125	245
60–65	Prime: Pyrazinoic acid 20 mg/kg i.v.						
65	Infusion II: As I (inulin) with pyrazinoic acid 60 mg/kg/hr						
70–90	4.65	128	0.076	0.014	215	164	255
90–110	4.88	126	0.096	0.027	181	146	203
110–130	6.90	124	0.134	0.024	415	190	373
130–133	Prime: Indanone 1 mg/kg i.v.						
135	Infusion III as II with the indanone 1 mg/kg/hr						
140–150	26.6	127	1.41	0.268	2631	238	3093
150–170	22.8	108	1.46	0.329	2273	218	2797
170–185	20.6	105	1.42	0.330	2143	218	2648
185–200	16.9	99	1.32	0.331	1753	219	2176
200–215	17.1	94	1.37	0.366	1709	211	2003

concerning secretion and reabsorption of urate and their respective sites. These differences might possibly be due to differences in methodology or chemical techniques or to the strains of rat used.

Free-flow micropuncture studies in the monkey *Cebus albifrons* showed that about 80% of the urate was largely reabsorbed in the proximal tubule with no detectable urate reabsorption in the loops of Henle or surface distal tubules; no evidence for net secretion in this nonhuman primate was uncovered (Roch-Ramel and Weiner, 1973). They also found that proximal net urate reabsorption was inhibited by the powerfully uricosuric agent 2-nitroprobenecid. Also, in free-flow micropuncture collections in the rat with [2-^{14}C]urate, Abramson and Levitt (1974) found net reabsorption of urate in early proximal samples together with net addition of urate to tubular fluid beyond this site. In pyrazinamide-treated rats they found that urate reabsorption and secretion were both inhibited with a predominant effect on secretory inhibition. They also realized that the magnitude of each transport process is far greater than can be determined in control micropuncture experiments.

VI. RELATIVE AFFINITIES OF THE URATE MECHANISMS TO DRUGS IN NONHUMAN PRIMATES AND MAN

Recently, the effects of salicylate, probenecid (Benemid), and pyrazinoate on uric acid excretion were determined in clearance experiments in the chimpanzee and *Cebus* monkey (*C. albifrons* and *C. apella*) (Fanelli and Weiner, 1975). The results were correlated with data from these species in the literature and, where possible, to analogous data in man. With salicylate, the rank order of responsiveness in terms of uricosuric action was chimpanzee > man > *C. albifrons* = *C. apella*. This was true when comparisons were made on the bases of drug concentration in plasma or the rate of drug excretion per ml of glomerular filtrate. A similar rank order was obtained with probenecid except that *C. albifrons* was slightly more responsive than *C. apella*. The latter comparisons were on the basis of plasma concentration of drug. The chimpanzee is more susceptible to the uricosuric action of pyrazinoate than is *C. apella*. With salicylate and pyrazinoate, there was urate retention at levels lower than those required for a uricosuric effect. The results suggest that in comparison with man, the chimpanzee is a hyperresponder to uricosuric drugs and *Cebus* monkeys are hyporesponders. Therefore, caution must be used for extensions of quantitative results from one species to another.

A symposium on the influence of the kidney upon urate homeostasis in man has recently appeared in *Nephron* [*14*(1), 1975] and it is very pertinent to material presented in this chapter.

VII. CONCLUSIONS

This review makes no pretext at being definitive, rather a more simplistic approach has been followed. The complexities of the renal urate transport mechanisms as they appear throughout the vertebrate phylum are great. It is known that bidirectional carrier-mediated or active transport occurs in most species studied and that these mechanisms can be inhibited, one or the other or both, by certain drugs on a dose-dependent competitive basis. Wide species differences play a prominent role in determining net urate transport. Regarding the precise physiologic, pharmacologic, or biochemical nature of these processes, nothing is known.

Teleologically, there is some reason to believe that the renal tubular secretory mechanism, at least for urate, may be being phased out of existence for it must be recalled that the late and prescient E. K. Marshall, Jr., considered tubular secretion to be "a relic of a primitive process."

No doubt, with the strides already realized in the biochemical and pharmacologic disciplines, time can only bring about newer and more refined techniques which may well elucidate the biochemical and biophysical phenomena which continually operate to maintain renal tubular homeostasis or urate and other processes. The record of the past fifteen years speaks for itself.

ACKNOWLEDGMENTS

The author gratefully acknowledges my co-workers D. L. Bohn, C. A. Horbaty, and S. S. Reilly, without whose skilled technical assistance, studies emanating from these laboratories could never have been successfully carried out. The continued support of Drs. J. E. Baer, A. Scriabine, and C. A. Stone is also gratefully acknowledged. Finally, a special debt of gratitude is accorded to my friend and collaborator Professor I. M. Weiner, State University of New York at Syracuse for numerous fruitful discussions on uric acid which have happily persisted and will hopefully continue to persist through the years.

REFERENCES

Abramson, R. G. and Levitt, M. F. 1974. A direct assessment of uric acid transport in the mammalian kidney. *Clin. Res., 22*:571A.

Alvsaker, J. O. 1965. Uric acid in human plasma. III. Investigations on the interaction between urate ion and human albumin. *Scand. J. Clin. Lab. Invest., 17*:467.

Beechwood, E. C., Berndt, W. O., and Mudge, G. H. 1964. Stop-flow analysis of tubular transport of uric acid in rabbits. *Am. J. Physiol., 207*:1265.

Berger, L., Yü, T. F., and Gutman, A. B. 1960. Effect of drugs that alter uric acid excretion in man on uric acid clearance in the chicken. *Am. J. Physiol., 198*:575.

Bergland, H. and Frisk, A. R. 1935. Uric acid elimination in man. *Acta Med. Scand., 86*:233.

Berliner, R. W., Kennedy, T. J., Jr., and Hilton, J. G. 1948. Salyrgan and renal tubular secretion of para-aminohippurate in the dog and man. *Am. J. Physiol., 154*:537.

Berliner, R. W., Hilton, J. G., Yü, T. F., and Kennedy, T. J., Jr. 1950. The renal mechanism for urate excretion in man. *J. Clin. Invest., 29*:396.

Berndt, W. O. and Beechwood, E. C. 1965. Influence of inorganic electrolytes and ouabain on uric acid transport. *Am. J. Physiol., 208*:642.

Beyer, K. H., Russo, H. F., Tillson, E. K., Miller, A. K., Verwey, W. F., and Gass, S. R. 1951.

'Benemid,' *p*-(di-*n*-propylsulfamyl)-benzoic acid: Its renal affinity and its elimination. *Am. J. Physiol., 166*:625.

Blanchard, K. C., Maroske, D., May, D. G., and Weiner, I. M. 1972. Uricosuric potency of 2-substituted analogs of probenecid. *J. Pharmacol. Exp. Ther., 180*:397.

Bluestone, R., Kippen, I., Campion, D., Klinenberg, J., and Whitehouse, M. 1974. Urate binding: A clue to the pathogenesis of gout. *J. Rheumatol., 1*:230.

Boudry, J. F. 1971a. Mécanismes de l'excrétion d'acide urique chez le rat. *Pfluegers Arch., 328*:265.

Boudry, J. F. 1971b. Effet d'inhibiteurs des transports transtubulaires sur l'excrétion rénale d'acide urique chez le rat. *Pfluegers Arch., 328*:279.

Bryant, J. M., Yü, T. F., Berger, L., Schvartz, N., Torosdag, S., Fletcher, L., Jr., Fertig, H., Schwartz, M. S., and Quan, R. F. B. 1962. Hyperuricemia induced by the administration of chlorthalidone and other sulfonamide diuretics. *Am. J. Med., 33*:408.

Castles, T. R. and Williamson, H. E. 1963. The effect of chlorothiazide on the excretion of uric acid and electrolytes by the chicken. *J. Pharmacol. Exp. Ther., 142*:231.

Coombs, F. S., Pecora, L. J., Thorogood, E., Consolazio, W. V., and Talbott, J. H. 1940. Renal function in patients with gout. *J. Clin. Invest., 19*:525.

Coulson, R. A. and Hernandez, T. 1964. *Biochemistry of the Alligator*, pp. 75–84. Louisiana State University Press, Baton Rouge.

Cragoe, E. J., Jr., Schultz, E. M., Schneeberg, J. D., Stokker, G. E., Woltersdorf, O. W., Jr., Fanelli, G. M., Jr., and Watson, L. S. 1975. (1-Oxo-2-substituted-5-indanyloxy)acetic acids, a new class of potent renal agents possessing both uricosuric and saluretic activity. *J. Med. Chem., 18*:225.

Dantzler, W. H. 1968. Effect of metabolic alkalosis and acidosis on tubular urate secretion in water snakes. *Am. J. Physiol., 215*:747.

Dantzler, W. H. 1970. Comparison of renal tubular transport of urate and PAH in water snakes: Evidence for differences in mechanisms and sites of transport. *Comp. Biochem. Physiol., 34*:609.

Davis, B. B., Field, J. B., Rodnan, G. P., and Kedes, L. H. 1965. Localization and pyrazinamide inhibition of distal trans-tubular movement of uric acid-2-C^{14} with a modified stop-flow technique. *J. Clin. Invest., 44*:716.

Demartini, F. E., Wheaton, E. A., Healey, L. A., and Laragh, J. H. 1962. Effect of chlorothiazide on the renal excretion of uric acid. *Am. J. Med., 32*:572.

de Rougemont, D. and Roch-Ramel, F. 1973. Renal uric acid excretion studied by free-flow micropuncture in the rat. *Kidney Int., 5*:309.

Emmerson, B. T. 1975. Effect of drugs on the renal handling of uric acid. In: *Drugs and the Kidney*, pp. 142–152. Ed. by Edwards, K. D. G., S. Karger, Basel.

Fanelli, G. M., Jr., 1975. Uricosuric agents. *Arthritis Rheum., 18*:853.

Fanelli, G. M., Jr., and Beyer, K. H., Jr. 1974. Uric acid in nonhuman primates with special reference to its renal transport. *Annu. Rev. Pharmacol., 14*:355.

Fanelli, G. M., Jr., and Weiner, I. M. 1973. Pyrazinoate excretion in the chimpanzee. Relation to urate disposition and the actions of uricosuric drugs. *J. Clin. Invest., 52*:1946.

Fanelli, G. M., Jr., and Weiner, I. M. 1974. Bidirectional renal urate transport in the chimpanzee. In: *Drugs and the Kidney*, pp. 163–173. Ed. by Edwards, K. D. G., S. Karger, Basel.

Fanelli, G. M., Jr., and Weiner, I. M. 1975. Species variations among primates in responses to drugs which alter the renal excretion of uric acid. *J. Pharmacol. Exp. Ther., 193*:363.

Fanelli, G. M., Jr., Bohn, D. L., and Russo, H. F. 1970a. Renal clearance of uric acid in nonhuman primates. *Comp. Biochem. Physiol., 33*:459.

Fanelli, G. M., Jr., Bohn, D., and Stafford, S. 1970b. Functional characteristics of renal transport in the *Cebus* monkey. *Am. J. Physiol., 218*:627.

Fanelli, G. M., Jr., Bohn, D. L., and Reilly, S. S. 1970c. Renal effects of uricosuric agents in the *Cebus* monkey. *J. Pharmacol. Exp. Ther., 175*:259.

Fanelli, G. M., Jr., Bohn, D. L., and Reilly, S. S. 1971a. Renal urate transport in the chimpanzee. *Am. J. Physiol., 220*:613.

Fanelli, G. M., Jr., Bohn, D. L., and Reilly, S. S. 1971b. Renal effects of uricosuric agents in the chimpanzee. *J. Pharmacol. Exp. Ther., 177*:591.

Fanelli, G. M., Jr., Bohn, D. L., and Reilly, S. S. 1972a. Renal excretion and uricosuric properties of halofenate, a hypolipidemic-uricosuric agent, in the chimpanzee. *J. Pharmacol. Exp. Ther., 180:*377.

Fanelli, G. M., Jr., Bohn, D. L., and Reilly, S. S. 1972b. Effects of mercurial diuretics on the renal tubular transport of *p*-aminohippurate and Diodrast in the chimpanzee. *J. Pharmacol. Exp. Ther., 180:*759.

Fanelli, G. M., Jr., Bohn, D. L., Reilly, S. S., and Weiner, I. M. 1973a. Effects of mercurial diuretics on renal transport of urate in the chimpanzee. *Am. J. Physiol., 224:*985.

Fanelli, G. M., Jr., Bohn, D. L., and Reilly, S. S. 1973b. Effects of mercurial diuretics on renal transport of urate and *p*-aminohippurate in the *Cebus* monkey. *Am. J. Physiol., 224:*993.

Fanelli, G. M., Jr., Bohn, D. L., Horbaty, C. A., Beyer, K. H., Jr., and Scriabine, A. 1974. A new uricosuric–saluretic agent (6,7-dichloro-2-methyl-1-oxo-2-phenyl-5-indanyloxy) acetic acid (Indanone): Evaluation in the chimpanzee. *Kidney Int., 6:*40A.

Fanelli, G. M., Jr., Bohn, D. L., Horbaty, C. A. and Scriabine, A. 1975. Renal interaction between a uricosuric saluretic agent and a urate retaining drug, pyrazinoate, in the chimpanzee. *Pharmacologist, 17:*252.

Farrell, P. C., Popovich, R. P., and Babb, A. L. 1971. Binding levels of urate ions in human serum albumin and plasma. *Biochem. Biophys. Acta, 243:*49.

Folin, O., Bergland, H., and Derick, C. 1924. The uric acid problem. An experimental study on animals and man, including gouty subjects. *J. Biol. Chem., 60:*361.

Friedman, M. and Byers, S. O. 1948. Observations concerning the causes of the excess excretion of uric acid in the Dalmatian dog. *J. Biol. Chem., 175:*727.

Funlop, M. and Drapkin, A. 1965. Potassium-depletion syndrome secondary to nephropathy apparently caused by "outdated tetracycline." *N. Engl. J. Med., 272:*986.

Greger, R., Lang, F., and Deetjen, P. 1971. Handling of uric acid by the rat kidney. I. Microanalysis of uric acid in proximal tubular fluid. *Pfluegers Arch., 324:*279.

Greger, R., Lang, F., and Deetjen, P. 1974a. Urate handling by the rat kidney. IV. Reabsorption in the loops of Henle. *Pfluegers Arch., 352:*115.

Greger, R., Lang, F., Puls, F., and Deetjen, P. 1974b. Urate interaction with plasma proteins and erythrocytes. Possible mechanism for urate reabsorption in kidney medulla. *Pfluegers Arch., 352:*121.

Gutman, A. B. 1966. Uricosuric drugs, with special reference to probenecid and sulfinpyrazone. *Adv. Pharmacol., 4:*91.

Gutman, A. B. and Yü, T. F. 1961. A three-component system for regulation of renal excretion of uric acid in man. *Trans. Assoc. Am. Physicians, 74:*353.

Gutman, A. B. and Yü, T. F. 1972. Renal mechanisms for regulation of uric acid excretion, with special reference to normal and gouty man. *Sem. Arthritis Rheum., 2:*1.

Gutman, A. B., Yü, T. F., and Berger, L. 1959. Tubular secretion of urate in man. *J. Clin. Invest., 38:*1778.

Healey, L. A., Harrison, M., and Decker, J. L. 1965. Uricosuric effect of chlorprothixene. *N. Engl. J. Med., 272:*526.

Holmes, E. W., Kelley, W. N., and Wyngaarden, J. B. 1972. The kidney and uric acid excretion in man. *Kidney Int., 2:*115.

Jain, A. K., Ryan, J. R., McMahon, F. G., and Noveck, R. J. 1974. Effect of single oral doses of benzbromarone on serum and urinary uric acid. *Arthritis Rheum., 17:*149.

Kalckar, H. M. 1947. Differential spectrophotometry of purine compounds by means of specific enzymes. I. Determination of hydroxypurine compounds. *J. Biol. Chem., 167:*429.

Kelley, W. N. 1975. Pharmacologic approach to the maintenance of urate homeostasis. *Nephron, 14:*99.

Kessler, R. H., Hierholzer, K., and Gurd, R. S. 1959. Localization of urate transport in the nephron of mongrel and Dalmatian dog kidney. *Am. J. Physiol., 197:*601.

Klinenberg, J. R. and Kippen, I. 1970. The binding of urate to plasma proteins as determined by equilibrium dialysis. *J. Lab. Clin. Med., 75:*503.

Kramp, R. A., Lassiter, W. E., and Gottschalk, C. W. 1971. Urate-2-^{14}C transport in the rat nephron. *J. Clin. Invest., 50:*35.

Lang, F., Greger, R., and Deetjen, P. 1972. Handling of uric acid by the rat kidney. II. Microperfusion studies on bidirectional transport of uric acid in the proximal tubule. *Pfluegers Arch., 335*:257.

Lang, F., Greger, R., and Deetjen, P. 1973. Handling of uric acid by the rat kidney. III. Microperfusion studies on steady state concentration of uric acid in the proximal tubule. Consideration of free flow conditions. *Pfluegers Arch., 338*:295.

Lang, F., Greger, R., and Deetjen, P. 1974. *In vivo* studies on uricase activity in the rat. *Pfluegers Arch., 351*:323.

Laragh, J. H., Heinemann, H. O., and Demartini, F. F. 1958. Effect of chlorothiazide on electrolyte transport in man. *J. Am. Med. Assoc., 166*:145.

Lathem, W., Davis, B. B., and Rodnan, G. P. 1960. Renal tubular secretion of uric acid in the mongrel dog. *Am. J. Physiol., 199*:9.

Lemieux, G., Gougoux, A., Vinay, P., and Michaud, G. 1973a. Uricosuric effect of benziodarone in man and laboratory animals: A comparative study. *Am. J. Physiol., 224*:1431.

Lemieux, G., Vinay, P., Gougoux, A., and Michaud, G. 1973b. Nature of the uricosuric action of benziodarone. *Am. J. Physiol., 224*:1440.

Levinsky, W. G. and Levy, M. 1973. Clearance techniques. In: *Handbook of Physiology*, Section 8, Renal Physiology, pp. 103–117. Ed. by Orloff, J. and Berliner, R. W. Williams & Wilkins, Baltimore.

Maroske, D. and Weiner, I. M. 1968. The renal handling of zoxazolamine (Flexin). *J. Pharmacol. Exp. Ther., 159*:409.

Marshall, E. K., Jr. 1932. Kidney secretion in reptiles. *Proc. Soc. Exp. Biol. Med., 29*:971.

Marshall, E. K., Jr. 1934. The comparative physiology of the kidney in relation to theories of renal secretion. *Physiol. Rev., 14*:133.

Marshall, E. K., Jr. 1966. Two lectures on renal physiology. *Physiologist, 9*:367.

Masbernard, A. and Guidicelli, C., 1974. Étude clinique de l'action antihypertensive de l'acide chloro-2,3-(thienyl-2-ceto)-phenoxyacetique en administration prolongée. *Lyon Med., 232*:165.

Miller, G. E., Danzig, L. S., and Talbott, J. H. 1951. Urinary excretion of uric acid in the Dalmatian and non-Dalmatian dog following administration of Diodrast, sodium salicylate and a mercurial diuretic. *Am. J. Physiol., 164*:155.

Møller, J. V. 1965a. Clearance experiments on the effect of probenecid on urate excretion in the rabbit. *Acta Pharmacol. Toxicol., 23*:321.

Møller, J. V. 1965b. The tubular site of urate transport in the rabbit kidney, and the effect of probenecid on urate secretion. *Acta Pharmacol. Toxicol., 23*:329.

Møller, J. V. 1965c. Tubular site of urate secretion in the rabbit. *Nature, 208*:492.

Møller, J. V. 1967a. The relation between secretion of urate and *p*-aminohippurate in the rabbit kidney. *J. Physiol., 192*:505.

Møller, J. V. 1967b. The renal accumulation of urate and *p*-aminohippurate in the rabbit. *J. Physiol., 192*:519.

Morgan, J. P., Bianchine, J. R., Hsu, T.-H., and Margolis, S. 1971. Hypolipidemic, uricosuric, and thyroxine-displacing effects on MK-185 (halofenate). *Clin. Pharmacol. Ther., 12*:517.

Mudge, G. H. 1965. The renal tubular transport of urate. *Arthritis Rheum., 8*:686.

Mudge, G. H. 1967. Two-way traffic in the renal tubule. *Dartmouth Med. School Q., 4*:20.

Mudge, G. H. 1971. Uricosuric action of cholecystographic agents. *N. Engl. J. Med., 284*:929.

Mudge, G. H., McAlary, B., and Berndt, W. O. 1968a. Renal transport of uric acid in the guinea pig. *Am. J. Physiol., 214*:875.

Mudge, G. H., Cucchi, J., Platts, M., O'Connell, J. M. B., and Berndt, W. O. 1968b. Renal excretion of uric acid in the dog. *Am. J. Physiol., 215*:404.

Mudge, G. H., Berndt, W. O., and Valtin, H. 1973. Tubular transport of urea, glucose, phosphate, uric acid, sulfate, and thiosulfate. In: *Handbook of Physiology*, Section 8, Renal Physiology, pp. 587–652. Ed. by Orloff, J. and Berliner, R. W. Williams & Wilkins, Baltimore.

Murdaugh, H. V., Robin, E. D., and Drewry, W. F. 1965. Uric acid transport by the aglomerular kidney of *Lophius americanus*. *Bull. Mt. Desert Island Biol. Lab., 5*:40.

Nechay, B. R. and Nechay, L. 1959. Effects of probenecid, sodium salicylate, 2,4-dinitrophenol and pyrazinamide on renal secretion of uric acid in chickens. *J. Pharmacol. Exp. Ther., 126*:291.

Nolan, R. P. and Foulkes, E. C. 1971. Studies on renal urate secretion in the dog. *J. Pharmacol. Exp. Ther., 179*:429.

Peters, G. and Roch-Ramel, F. 1969. Ethacrynic acid and related drugs. In: *Handbach der experimentellen Pharmakologie,* Bd. XXIV, Diuretica pp. 406–435. Ed. by Herken, H. Springer-Verlag, Berlin.

Platts, M. M. and Mudge, G. H. 1961. Accumulation of uric acid by slices of kidney cortex. *Am. J. Physiol., 200*:387.

Postlethwaite, A. E., Ramsdell, C. M., and Kelley, W. N. 1974a. Uricosuric effect of an anticholinergic agent in hyperuricemic subjects. *Arch. Intern. Med., 134*:270.

Postlethwaite, A. E., Bartel, A. G., and Kelley, W. N. 1974b. Hyperuricemia induced by ethambutol. In: *Advances in Experimental Medicine and Biology, Purine Metabolism in Man,* Vol. 41B, pp. 763–767. Ed. by Sperling, O., De Vries, A., and Wyngaarden, J. B. Plenum Press, New York.

Poulsen, H. 1955. Inhibition of uric acid in rabbits given probenecid or salicylic acid. *Acta Pharmacol. Toxicol., 11*:277.

Poulsen, H. and Praetorius, E. 1954. Tubular excretion of uric acid in rabbits. *Acta Pharmacol. Toxicol., 10*:371.

Quebbemann, A. J. 1973. Renal synthesis of uric acid. *Am. J. Physiol., 224*:1398.

Ramsdell, C. M., Postlethwaite, A. E., and Kelley, W. N. 1974. Uricosuric effect of glyceryl guaicolate. *J. Rheumatol., 1*:114.

Ravenscroft, P. J., Sands, J. M., and Emmerson, B. T. 1973. Studies on the uricosuric action of the hypolipidemic drug halofenate. *Clin. Pharmacol. Ther., 14*:547.

Rieselbach, R. E. and Steele, T. H. 1974. Influence of the kidney upon urate homeostasis in health and disease. *Am. J. Med., 56*:665.

Roch-Ramel, F. and Weiner, I. M. 1973. Excretion of urate by the kidneys of *Cebus* monkeys: A micropuncture study. *Am. J. Physiol., 224*:1369.

Roch-Ramel, F., de Rougemont, D., and Peters, G. 1974. Mechanisms of renal excretion of urate in the rat. In: *Advances in Experimental Medicine and Biology. Purine Metabolism in Man,* Vol. 41B, pp. 789–790. Ed. by Sperling, O., De Vries, A., and Wyngaarden, J. B. Plenum Press, New York.

Schmidt-Nielsen, B. 1961. Choice of experimental animals for research. *Fed. Proc., 20*:902.

Schroder, C. R. 1967. Potential species new to laboratory investigation. *Fed. Proc., 26*:1157.

Sheikh, M. I. and Møller, J. V. 1968. Binding of urate to proteins of human and rabbit plasma. *Biochem. Biophys. Acta, 158*:456.

Shideman, J. R., Zmuda, M. J., and Quebbemann, A. J. 1975. The effects of ethacrynic acid (ECA), furosemide (F), and pyrazinoate (PA) on the renal tubular excretion of ^{14}C-urate (UA) in the chicken: Evidence for urate reabsorption. *Pharmacologist, 17*:252.

Simkin, P. A. 1971. Uric acid metabolism in *Cebus* monkeys. *Am. J. Physiol., 221*:1105.

Sirota, J. H., Yü, T. F., and Gutman, A. B. 1952. Effect of Benemid (p-[di-n′-propylsulfamyl]-benzoic acid) on urate clearance and other discrete renal functions in gouty subjects. *J. Clin. Invest., 31*:692.

Skeith, M. D. and Healey, L. A. 1968. Urate clearance in *Cebus* monkeys. *Am. J. Physiol., 214*:582.

Smith, H. W., 1964, Renal physiology. In: *Circulation of the Blood—Men & Ideas,* pp. 545–606. Ed. by Fishman A. P. and Richardson, D. W. Oxford University Press, New York.

Sonnenberg, H., Oetert, H., and Baumann, K. 1965. Proximal tubular reabsorption of some organic acids in the rat kidney in vivo. *Pfluegers Arch., 286*:171.

Steele, T. H. 1971. Control of uric acid excretion. *N. Engl. J. Med., 284*:1193.

Steele, T. H. 1973. Urate secretion in man: The pyrazinamide suppression test. *Ann. Intern. Med., 79*:734.

Steele, T. H. 1974. Studies on urate handling in man utilizing pyrazinamide. In: *Recent Advances in Renal Physiology and Pharmacology,* pp. 361–373. Ed. by Wesson, L. G. and Fanelli, G. M. Jr. University Park Press, Baltimore.

Steele, T. H. and Boner, G. 1973. Origins of the uricosuric response. *J. Clin. Invest., 52*:1368.

Steele, T. H. and Oppenheimer, S. 1969. Factors affecting urate excretion following diuretic administration in man. *Am. J. Med., 47*:564.

Steele, T. H. and Rieselbach, R. E. 1967. The renal mechanism for urate homeostasis in normal man. *Am. J. Med., 43*:868.

Steele, T. H. and Rieselbach, R. E. 1975. Renal urate excretion in normal man. *Nephron, 14*:21.

Steele, T. H., Underwood, J. L., and Dudgeon, K. L. 1974. Urate excretion and urine flow in a lithium-induced diabetes insipidus rat model. *Pfluegers Arch., 346*:205.

Stote, R. M., Cherrill, D. A., Erb, B. B., and Alexander, F. 1974. Site of action of SK&F 62698, a new diuretic-uricosuric agent. *Clin. Res., 22*:721A.

Talbott, J. H. 1943. *Gout.* Oxford University Press, New York.

Weiner, I. M. and Fanelli, G. M., Jr. 1974. Bidirectional transport: Urate and other anions. In: *Recent Advances in Renal Physiology and Pharmacology,* pp. 53–68. Ed. by Wesson, L. G. and Fanelli, G. M., Jr. University Park Press, Baltimore.

Weiner, I. M. and Fanelli, G. M., Jr. 1975. Renal urate excretion in animal models. *Nephron, 14*:33.

Weiner, I. M. and Mudge, G. H. 1964. Renal tubular mechanisms for excretion of organic acids and bases. *Am. J. Med., 36*:743.

Wiener, I. M. and Tinker, J. P. 1972. Pharmacology of pyrazinamide: Metabolic and renal function studies related to drug-induced urate retention. *J. Pharmacol. Exp. Ther., 180*:411.

Weinman, E. J., Eknoyan, G., and Suki, W. N. 1975. The influence of extracellular fluid volume on the tubular reabsorption of uric acid. *J. Clin. Invest., 55*:283.

Wesson, L. G., Jr. 1969. *Physiology of the Human Kidney.* Grune & Stratton, New York.

Wilber, C. G. 1964. Some contributions of exotic animals to biomedical research. *Bioscience, 14*:21.

Wolfson, W. Q., Cohn, C., and Shore, C. 1950. The renal mechanisms for urate excretion in the Dalmatian coach-hound. *J. Exp. Med., 92*:121.

Woltersdorf, O. W., Jr., Cragoe, E. J., Jr., Watson, L. S., and Fanelli, G. M., Jr. 1975a. Synthesis and evaluation of (1-oxo-2-substituted-5-indanyloxy)-acetic acids as novel uricosuric diuretics. *169th Am. Chem. Soc. Meet.,* Philadelphia.

Woltersdorf, O. W., Jr., Schneeberg, J. D., Cragoe, E. J., Jr., Schultz, E. M., Stokker, G. E., Watson, L. S., and Fanelli, G. M., Jr. 1975b. 1-Oxo-2,2-dialkyl- and 1-oxo-2-alkyl-2-aryl-5-indanyloxyacetic acids. A new class of polyvalent saluretics. *169th Am. Chem. Soc. Meet.,* Philadelphia.

Yü, T. F. and Gutman, A. B. 1953. Ultrafilterability of plasma urate in man. *Proc. Soc. Exp. Biol. Med., 84*:21.

Yü, T. F. and Gutman, A. B. 1957. Quantitative analysis of uric acid in blood and urine. Methods and interpretation. *Bull. Rheum. Dis., 7*:S-17.

Yü, T. F. and Gutman, A. B. 1959. Study of the paradoxical effects of salicylate in low, intermediate and high dosage on the renal mechanisms for excretion of urate in man. *J. Clin. Invest., 38*:1298.

Yü, T. F., Berger, L., Stone, D. J., Wolf, J., and Gutman, A. B. 1957. Effect of pyrazinamide and pyrazinoic acid on urate clearance and other discrete renal functions. *Proc. Soc. Exp. Biol. Med., 96*:264.

Yü, T. F., Berger, L., Kupfer, S., and Gutman, A. B. 1960. Tubular secretion of urate in the dog. *Am. J. Physiol., 199*:1199.

Yü, T. F., Berger, L., and Gutman, A. B. 1968. Hypoglycemic and uricosuric properties of acetohexamide and hydroxyhexamide. *Metabolism, 17*:309.

Yü, T. F., Gutman, A. B., Berger, L., and Kaung, C. 1971. Low uricase activity in the Dalmatian dog simulated in mongrels given oxonic acid. *Am. J. Physiol., 220*:973.

Zins, G. R. and Weiner, I. M. 1968. Bidirectional urate transport limited to the proximal tubule in dogs. *Am. J. Physiol., 215*:411.

Chapter **10**

Drugs and Other Agents Affecting the Renal Adenylate Cyclase System

Thomas P. Dousa

Department of Physiology and Biophysics
and Division of Nephrology, Department of Medicine
Mayo Clinic and Mayo Foundation
Department of Medicine and of Physiology
Mayo Medical School
Rochester, Minnesota

I. INTRODUCTION

The major responsibility of the kidney, homeostasis of the internal environment, can be accomplished only if the kidney function is finely regulated and is coordinated with that of other organ systems. Although neural regulation has a distinct role in certain aspects of kidney function, such as control of renal blood flow, most of the regulation is apparently humoral since the completely denervated kidney, either by transplantation or by other means (Cizek, 1968), retains its function almost intact. Studies of the mechanism of hormonal regulation of kidney function at the cellular level are critical not only for basic understanding of the regulation but also for development of agents that may substitute for or inhibit the action of the hormone.

The major single advance in molecular endocrinology in recent years was the discovery that a number of hormones act on their respective target organs through the mediation of a specific nucleotide, adenosine cyclic 3',5'-monophosphate (cyclic AMP) (Sutherland and Rall, 1960). This is the "second messenger" mechanism. Briefly, this mechanism proposes that the hormone molecule approaches the cell from the extracellular fluid and combines with a specific receptor on the outer surface of the membrane of its target cell. The receptor is associated with an enzyme, adenylate cyclase, located in the inner surface of the membrane. The hormone–receptor interaction stimulates the activity of the adenylate cyclase and results in an increased rate of cyclic AMP formation within the cell.

Increases in the cyclic AMP concentration within the cell elicit biochemical or biophysical changes that are the molecular background for the hormonal responses observed in the intact tissue or organ as a change in function. Cyclic AMP formed within the cell can (1) undergo hydrolysis to 5′-AMP and subsequent metabolic products, (2) be bound to intracellular proteins, or (3) escape to the extracellular fluid. The majority of known hormonal responses involve stimulation of cyclic AMP formation and an increase in its intracellular concentration. Some hormones appear to affect the cell by decreasing the cyclic AMP formation. Often, these opposing effects of hormonal agents on cyclic AMP metabolism are reflected in the opposing functional responses to these hormones. Nonhormonal substances, such as natural or synthetic drugs, that have the ability to influence cyclic AMP metabolism or kinetics can mimic or antagonize the action of hormones that operate through cyclic AMP metabolism. The basic scheme of hormone action through cyclic AMP mediation is outlined in Figure 1.

The principles of investigations on the involvement of cyclic AMP in the regulatory function of various hormones were summarized recently (Robison *et al.*, 1971), and similar principles apply to the studies of cyclic AMP in the kidney. In general, the conclusion that cyclic AMP mediates the action of a specific hormone depends on fulfilling the following criteria, outlined by Robison, Butcher, and Sutherland (1971):

1. The hormone stimulates adenylate cyclase activity in cell-free preparations from the target tissue.
2. Treatment of the target tissue *in vivo* or *in vitro* with the hormone leads to an increase in the intracellular concentration of cyclic AMP.
3. Inhibitors of cyclic AMP phosphodiesterase, by virtue of inhibition of

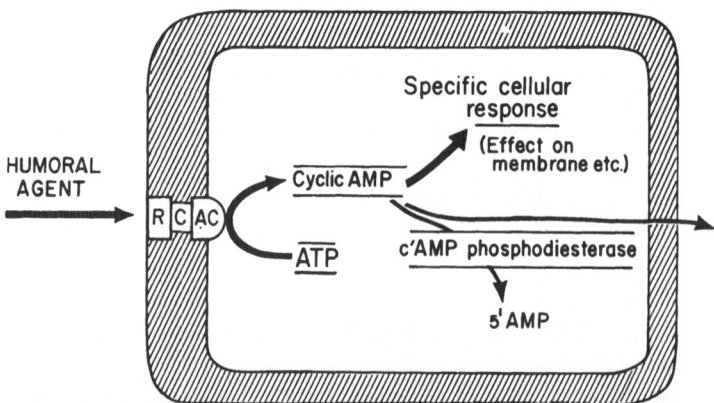

Figure 1. General scheme of action of humoral agent on kidney cell through mediation of cyclic AMP. R = receptor; C = coupling mechanism; AC = adenylate cyclase.

    cyclic AMP breakdown and accumulation of intracellular cyclic AMP, can mimic the specific hormonal effect.

4. Hormonal response can be elicited by exogenously applied cyclic AMP or its analogs.

Criteria 3 and 4 are of limited value because of the complexities in these experimental approaches, but they are useful if combined with other approaches. By using these experimental approaches and these criteria, it can be learned whether a particular hormone or drug produces a change in cyclic AMP metabolism with a consequent change in kidney function. Most kidney functions regulated by hormones through the mediation of cyclic AMP are membrane phenomena—transport or permeability processes.

The mechanism by which cyclic AMP formed within the cells influences these membrane phenomena is largely unknown at the present time. Therefore, the present chapter is focused on methodologic approaches and findings dealing with the actions of various agents on cyclic AMP metabolism rather than with the still highly hypothetical mechanisms by which cyclic AMP might elicit the final functional response.

Many features of cyclic AMP metabolism in kidney are similar to those found in other tissues. Nevertheless, some features are specific to this organ. In mammalian species, the kidney can be grossly subdivided into several zones: cortex, medulla, and papilla. This gross anatomic subdivision can help to localize cyclic AMP-mediated responses to certain structures of the kidney. Nevertheless, the enormous complexity of the structure in those gross anatomic zones still requires that the fine localization of hormone–responsive systems in individual segments of nephron be established in experiments with isolated structures (microdissection, microperfusion, and micropuncture studies of nephron segments) or by immunocytochemical (Steiner *et al.*, 1975) and histochemical methods (these later methods appear to be still in the early developmental stage) (Lemay and Jarett, 1975).

By perfusing the kidney from one artery, one can apply drugs and hormones selectively into one kidney *in vivo*, keeping the other kidney as a control. Also, at least in some species, such as man (Broadus *et al.*, 1970a; Kaminsky *et al.*, 1970a,b; Chase *et al.*, 1969) or rat (Chase and Aurbach, 1967) but apparently not dog (Blonde *et al.*, 1974; Davis *et al.*, 1969), a sizable proportion of the cyclic AMP formed within the kidney tissue is excreted into the urine, adding "nephrogenous" (Kaminsky *et al.*, 1970b) cyclic AMP to that filtered by the glomeruli. Cyclic AMP is also apparently taken up by the tubules from peritubular circulation (Coulson and Bowman, 1974; Coulson *et al.*, 1974). Therefore, in appropriately designed experiments, changes in the urinary excretion of cyclic AMP can indirectly, and at least qualitatively, reflect hormonal effects on cyclic AMP metabolism and could be used as a noninvasive technique for studies of the kidney in intact organisms (Chase *et al.*, 1969). However, it should be taken into account that some of the cyclic AMP can be taken up by organic acid transport system from blood (Coulson and Bowman, 1974; Coulson *et al.*, 1974), and also that tubular handling of cyclic AMP may be influenced by pH of the urine (Czekalski *et al.*, 1974). Finally, some cyclic AMP-mediated hormonal effects on transport processes in distal segments of the mammalian nephron and the amphibian urinary bladder are very similar; therefore, the latter tissue can serve as a model, to a certain degree, for hormonal action on cyclic AMP metabolism in the kidney (Handler and Orloff, 1973).

The following text will first review some methodologic approaches used in studies on cyclic AMP involvement in the action of humoral agents on the kidney. Subsequent sections will review some basic findings resulting from application of these methods.

II. METHODS FOR STUDY OF EFFECT OF HORMONES AND DRUGS ON CYCLIC AMP METABOLISM IN KIDNEY

A. Method for Adenylate Cyclase in Cell-Free Systems

1. Enzyme Preparation

Experimental evidence indicates that the adenylate cyclase in kidney is localized predominantly in the plasma membranes (Barnes *et al.*, 1975c; Schwartz *et al.*, 1974; Bockaert *et al.*, 1973; Neer, 1973b; Campbell *et al.*, 1972; Forte, 1972, Marx *et al.*, 1972; Fitzpatrick, 1969). However, this enzyme can be studied in various cell-free preparations ranging from crude homogenates (Marumo and Edelman, 1971) to partially purified membrane fractions (Dousa *et al.*, 1971; Chase and Aurbach, 1968; Dousa and Rychlik, 1968c; Brown *et al.*, 1963) to plasma membrane fractions. Although adenylate cyclase can be measured in homogenates this preparation has certain disadvantages. The high content of enzymes that catabolize cyclic AMP, ATP, proteins, and test agents in this preparation makes it relatively insensitive to changes due to the test agents.

A sensitive preparation (especially to hormones) is the membrane fraction of homogenate obtained by sedimentation at low gravitational forces (Figure 2, *upper panel*). This contains plasma membrane fragments and has proved to be a useful and sensitive material for assaying adenylate cyclase activity (Rajerison *et al.*, 1974; Dousa *et al.*, 1971; Chase and Aurbach, 1968; Dousa and Rychlík, 1968a). Extensive washing of such membranes, especially with hypotonic buffers (Rajerison *et al.*, 1974; Bockaert *et al.*, 1972, 1973; Dousa and Rychlík, 1968a, 1970a), removes cyclic AMP phosphodiesterase (which is mostly in the soluble fraction; Figure 2, *lower panel*) and a number of other hydrolytic enzymes.

To prepare a more purified plasma membrane fraction, several methods are available (Barnes *et al.*, 1975c; Schwartz *et al.*, 1974; Neer, 1973b; Campbell *et al.*, 1972; Marx *et al.*, 1972). A frequently used and relatively simple procedure was designed by Fitzpatrick (1969) and has been applied to the preparation of plasma membrane from whole kidney (Fitzpatrick, 1969), cortex (Di Bella *et al.*, 1974; Forte, 1972), and medulla (Barnes *et al.*, 1975c; Forte, 1972). A special feature of this procedure is the relatively short time between homogenization

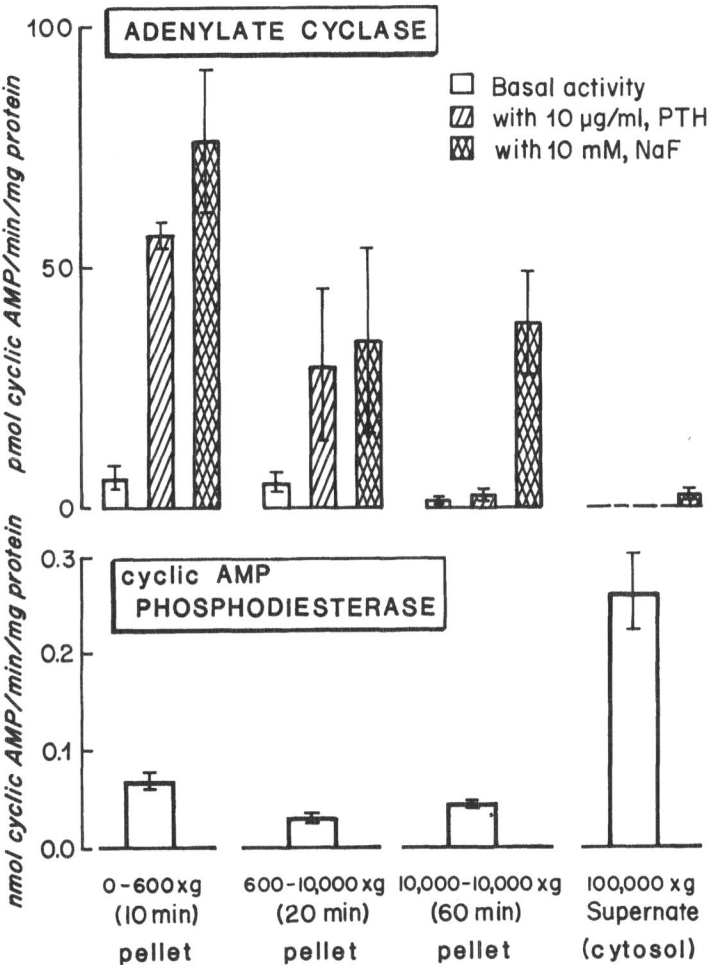

Figure 2. Subcellular distribution of adenylate cyclase and cyclic AMP phosphodiesterase in fractions of homogenate from human renal cortex. Conditions for preparation of fractions are at the bottom of the figure. *Upper Panel,* Adenylate cyclase. PTH = parathyroid hormone. *Lower Panel,* Cyclic AMP phosphodiesterase (10^{-6} M cyclic AMP served as a substrate).

and final preparation. Partially purified membrane preparations of renal adenylate cyclase are very stable when quickly frozen and stored at $-80°C$ (Barnes *et al.*, 1975c). Plasma membrane preparations are also relatively stable for many hours if kept at $0°C$ (Barnes *et al.*, 1975c).

Morel and associates developed a technique which allows measurement of adenylate cyclase in dissected segments of rabbit nephron (Chambardès *et al.*, 1975b; Imbert *et al.*, 1975a,b). By this method, tissue is not homogenized mechanically, but the exposure to hypotonic media and subsequent quick freezing makes the adenylate cyclase in nephron segments accessible to substrate ATP. This preparation appears to be very sensitive to hormonal stimulation (Chambardès *et al.*, 1975b; Imbert *et al.*, 1975a).

2. Assay

Although many different methods of assaying adenylate cyclase in kidney are now in use, the most convenient at the present time appears to be one based on measuring the rate of formation of cyclic [^{32}P]AMP from [α-^{32}P]ATP. This substrate is generally preferred to ^{14}C- or ^{3}H-labeled ATP because it minimizes formation of possible radioactive by-products in the form of nucleotides and bases. The concentration of the ATP substrate usually ranges from 0.1 to 3.2 mM. Because the action of some agents on adenylate cyclase activity depends on the presence or the concentration of nucleotides such as ATP and GTP (Birnbaumer, 1973; Bockaert et al., 1972), it may be preferable to test the system at several different ATP concentrations when exploring the effect of a new agent. Another critical component in the incubation assay is magnesium; it should be present in molar excess to ATP.

Because ATPases are always present in the adenylate cyclase preparations, a constant level of ATP should be maintained by inclusion of an ATP-regenerating system (from either creatine phosphate or phosphopyruvate; the former system may be preferred because of the more favorable equilibrium constant for the ATP-regenerating reaction). If an ATP-regenerating system should be avoided for some reason, an adenylylimidodiphosphate (AMP–PNP) (Rodbell et al., 1971) labeled with ^{32}P at α position (now commercially available) can be used as a substrate; this compound is not destroyed by ATPases. The preferred method for preventing hydrolysis of newly formed radioactive cyclic AMP by cyclic AMP phosphodiesterase is inclusion of unlabeled cyclic AMP at 0.5–1 mM (Bär and Hechter, 1969). The adenylate cyclase incubation is usually stopped by heating after addition of excess chelating agent (such as EDTA) to prevent nonenzymatic formation of cyclic AMP (Bär, 1975).

To separate the newly formed cyclic AMP from the substrate and other ^{32}P-labeled substances, there are three methods that are most frequently applied to the kidney preparations: (1) precipitation of contaminants with BaSO$_4$ followed by separation by ion-exchange column chromatography (Krishna et al., 1968); (2) separation on alumina oxide columns (White and Zenser, 1971; Ramachandran and Lee, 1970); and (3) separation by thin-layer chromatography on plates of polyimine-modified cellulose (Bär, 1975; Bär and Hechter, 1969).

All three methods are relatively quick (results can be obtained within several hours after incubation) and reliable. Advantages of the thin-layer chromatography method are that the separation of cyclic AMP is visually controlled on thin-layer plates and, if both ATP and cyclic AMP spots are counted, cyclic AMP recovery need not be measured by inclusion of cyclic AMP labeled by different isotopes (^{3}H, ^{14}C), thus avoiding double isotope counting (Bär, 1975; Bär and Hechter, 1969).

The method using separation on alumina oxide columns has been scaled down to extremely small volume of incubation mixture and was successfully used for measurement of adenylate cyclase in individual segments of the nephron (Chambardès et al., 1975b; Imbert et al., 1975a,b).

When any of these methods is used for studies of new and unknown agents, certain precautions should be taken. The linearity of cyclic AMP formation in relation to time and to enzyme protein should be ascertained. The new agent should be carefully checked for interference with ATP regeneration or with the separation procedure for isolation of cyclic AMP.

B. Measurement of Cyclic AMP Formation in Intact Cells

The relative rate of formation of cyclic AMP in intact cells (in cell suspension or tissue slices) can be measured by prelabeling the intracellular pool of ATP by preincubation of the cell with radioactive adenine or adenosine. Then, the formation of new cyclic AMP from ATP is measured by the increase in radioactivity in the cyclic AMP (Kebabian *et al.,* 1972). This method has been used only a few times in kidney preparations (Kacew and Singhal, 1974; Kuehl *et al.,* 1972; Ohsawa and Endo, 1972). However, it appears to be a good approach for the measurement of the rate of cyclic AMP formation with other cellular components intact. Also, in this method, the effect of newly tested agents on the prelabeling of ATP should be carefully checked.

C. Measurement of Cyclic AMP Tissue Levels in Kidney

Several methods are now available for measuring cyclic AMP in body fluids or tissue extracts. In the kidney, two methods have been used most frequently under various experimental conditions. One method (Brown *et al.,* 1972; Gilman, 1972; Brostrom and Kon, 1974) uses a specific cyclic AMP-binding protein prepared from beef muscle (or other tissues) and is based on competition for binding between radioactive and unlabeled cyclic AMP. This method, which can detect less than 1 pmole of cyclic AMP, has been applied, sometimes with modifications, to preparations from kidney, apparently with effective results. The other method is a specific radioimmunoassay for cyclic AMP developed by Steiner and associates (1969, 1972b). Although both assays are very specific for cyclic AMP, some substances present in tissue extracts (such as salts or other nucleotides) may interfere and it is recommended that tissue extracts be purified prior to the assay.

Because the tissue levels of cyclic AMP can fluctuate considerably (Kimura *et al.,* 1974; Goldberg and O'Toole, 1971) it is recommended that the tissue be quickly frozen and kept at deep subzero temperature until the cyclic AMP-forming and -catabolizing enzymes are inactivated by homogenization with a deproteinizing agent (Kimura *et al.,* 1974; Goldberg and O'Toole, 1971). Decapitation of the animal tends to increase the kidney cyclic AMP level, and anesthesia with pentobarbital decreases it (Kimura *et al.,* 1974); the preferred method is anesthesia with ether (Kimura *et al.,* 1974), then clamping the kidney between blocks of stainless steel precooled in liquid nitrogen (Goldberg and O'Toole, 1971) and immersion in liquid nitrogen. The frozen tissue is then very quickly homogenized in cold 5% trichloroacetic acid (Kimura *et al.,* 1974).

When cyclic AMP is measured in tissue slices (or cell suspensions) incubated in an *in vitro* medium, at the end of the incubation the tissue slices usually are homogenized, with or without the medium, in trichloroacetic acid (Dousa *et al.*, 1975; Kurokawa and Massry, 1973b; Steiner *et al.*, 1972a). The trichloroacetic acid is removed by extraction with water-saturated ether (Kimura *et al.*, 1974; Gilman, 1972; Chase and Aurbach, 1967) or on ion-exchange column (Omachi *et al.*, 1974), and extracts are further purified, usually on small ion-exchange columns (Kimura *et al.*, 1974; Omachi *et al.*, 1974; Murad *et al.*, 1971). One method, which has proved useful in our laboratory, is purification on a small Dowex AG-1-X8 column in the formate cycle (Kimura *et al.*, 1974; Murad *et al.*, 1971); recovery is measured by adding trace amounts of cyclic [^{3}H]AMP to the homogenate.

D. Cytochemical Localization of Adenylate Cyclase in Kidney

The first attempts have been made to localize adenylate cyclase within different cellular and subcellular elements in the kidney. Stability of adenylate cyclase during fixation cannot be ascertained at the present time. A surprising finding was the high activity of PTH-sensitive adenylate cyclase in the brush border of proximal tubules, even in the absence of adenylate cyclase in the distal portions of the tubules (Jande and Robert, 1974). In another study, adenylate cyclase was detected in microvilli of proximal tubules and also in distal nephrons and, in remarkably high activity, in the glomerulus (Sato *et al.*, 1974). Such histochemical methods were subjected to criticism for their unspecificity (Lemay and Jarett, 1975).

E. Immunocytotopic Localization of Cyclic AMP

Steiner, Ong, and Wedner (in press) and Steiner *et al.* (1975) developed a method for detecting immunoactive cyclic AMP in the cells by using fluorescein-tagged antibody using an immunocytochemical technique. This method was used to detect the presence of cyclic AMP in different cell types in toad bladder in response to vasopressin (Goodman *et al.*, 1975) and for detection of cyclic AMP in kidney cortex in response to PTH (Barnes *et al.*, 1975b). This approach is a promising new way to determine actual accumulation of cyclic AMP in subcellular structures and/or in different cell types. Such an approach will be helpful especially in the kidney, an organ with diverse cell type population.

F. Cyclic AMP in Urine and Plasma

Cyclic AMP and cyclic GMP are present in the urine in appreciable quantities (Murad, 1973). Chances of interference by other substances are minimal in diluted urine samples, and the measurement could be made directly by any assay, but certain precautions should be taken. It has been reported (Goldberg and O'Toole, 1971) that significant cyclic AMP phosphodiesterase activity is present in the urine of some species (Goldberg and O'Toole, 1971) and, therefore, inactivation of it by short heating immediately after collecting the specimens is recommended. Collection in cooled containers or addition of preservatives to prevent bacterial contamination is recommended when urine is collected for prolonged periods (Murad, 1973). When the urine is stored at $-20°C$, the cyclic AMP is stable for more than a year (Murad, 1973).

The cyclic AMP concentration in plasma is much lower than that in urine. To prevent enzymatic degradation of cyclic AMP, inclusion of EDTA to final concentration of 6–7 mM has been recommended (Murad, 1973). Concentration and further purification on ion-exchange columns (such as with tissue extracts) are recommendable.

G. Measurement of Cyclic AMP Breakdown

1. Assay for Cyclic AMP Phosphodiesterase Activity

Cyclic AMP phosphodiesterase can be measured by the rate of formation of its primary product, 5'-AMP. However, in cruder preparations of kidney as well as in other tissues, 5'-AMP is quickly dephosphorylated to nucleosides. Therefore, the most widely used and convenient method is a two-step reaction: Enzyme is first incubated with cyclic AMP; then this reaction is stopped, usually by short heating, and the 5'-AMP produced by the first reaction is converted to the nucleoside by incubation with excess of 5'-nucleotidase (by using preparations of snake venom with high content of this enzyme). A product of this second reaction, inorganic phosphate (P_i) (Dousa and Rychlik, 1970b; Butcher and Sutherland, 1962) or nucleoside (Thompson and Appleman, 1971a), is actually measured. Measurement of P_i has analytic limitations. Therefore, when the cyclic AMP substrate is at low concentration, the preferred method is to use cyclic [³H]AMP (labeled on the nucleoside moiety) with high specific radioactivity as substrate. The total radioactivity of nucleoside at the termination of the second incubation, usually separated from the nucleotide by ion-exchange resin, is measured (Barnes et al., 1975c; Thompson and Appleman, 1971a,b). Recently it was noted that the method using separation of nucleosides from nucleotides by simple addition of ionex resin (Thompson and Appleman, 1971a,b) may underestimate the absolute cyclic AMP phosphodiesterase activity since a certain portion of nucleosides remains bound on the resin (Boudreau and Drummond, 1975; Lynch and Cheung, 1975; Rutten et al., 1973). We observed the same phenomenon when measuring renal cortical or renal medullary enzyme activities. Separation of nucleosides from nucleotides on small columns of QAE-Sephadex, described by Schultz, Böhme, and Hardman (1974), avoids this problem of underestimation of cyclic AMP phosphodiesterase activity (Wells et al., 1975), and the method is applicable to kidney (Barnes, Kim, Harkcom, and Dousa, unpublished observations).

Kidney is similar to other tissues in that it contains several cyclic AMP phosphodiesterases with different K_m's for cyclic AMP (Barnes et al., 1975c; Thompson and Appleman, 1971b; Jard and Bernard, 1970). Although the low-K_m enzymes seem to be more bound to membrane particles (Barnes et al., 1975c; Appleman et al., 1973), they can be solubilized by sonication (Thompson and Appleman, 1971b). The functional significances of the low- and high-K_m phosphodiesterases are not yet elucidated, and when the effect of a new agent is tested it is advisable to evaluate its effect on cyclic AMP phosphodiesterase at several levels of substrate. Also, appropriate controls should be included to show that the tested agent does not inhibit the determination of products or the activity of 5'-nucleotidase, if the two-step incubation method is utilized. Also, linearity with protein enzyme and with time should be checked. One report describes application of the two-step method for histochemical detection of phosphodiesterase in kidney (Shanta *et al.*, 1966).

2. Use of Cyclic AMP Phosphodiesterase Inhibitors

Drugs that inhibit cyclic AMP phosphodiesterase, in general, should mimic the action of hormones acting on the kidney through cyclic AMP accumulation, or at least they should potentiate the hormone's effects.

Use of cyclic AMP phosphodiesterase inhibitors should be undertaken with several precautions. First, some of the most frequently used inhibitors, the methylxanthines, have been shown to have other biochemical and pharmacologic effects unrelated to the inhibition of cyclic AMP phosphodiesterase, such as inhibition of adenylate cyclase (Jakobs *et al.*, 1972; Sheppard, 1971), protein synthesis (Halkerston *et al.*, 1966), and other reactions (Appleman *et al.*, 1973) or effect on cyclic AMP permeation out of cell (Urakabe *et al.*, 1975). Also, if applied to the whole kidney, inhibitors can act simultaneously on several segments of the nephron, producing final effects that are difficult to interpret.

The methylxanthines are competitive inhibitors of cyclic AMP phosphodiesterase (Appleman *et al.*, 1973; Dousa and Rychlík, 1970b; Orloff and Handler, 1967). One of them, theophylline, has been used in isolated tissue systems such as tubule suspensions (Kurokawa and Massry, 1973a) or toad bladder (Omachi *et al.*, 1974; Handler and Orloff, 1973; Orloff and Handler, 1967; Handler *et al.*, 1965). Some synthetic methylxanthine derivatives (Beavo *et al.*, 1970) are much more potent than theophylline or caffeine (Figure 3) and may be preferred in the

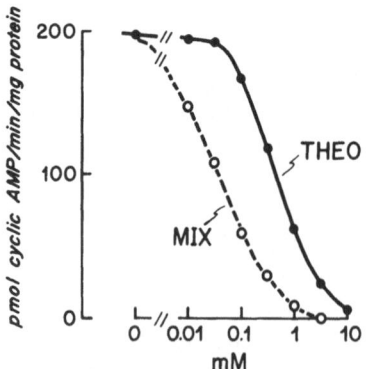

Figure 3. Comparison of inhibitory action of theophylline (THEO) and 1-methyl-3-isobutylxanthine (MIX) on cyclic AMP phosphodiesterase activity in bovine renal medullary cytosol. Substrate (cyclic AMP) level was 5×10^{-6} M. Ordinate: cyclic AMP hydrolyzed; abscissa: concentration of MIX or theophylline.

future. Some synthetic analogs of cyclic AMP are being developed as specific inhibitors of cyclic AMP phosphodiesterase (Simon *et al.*, 1973).

Inhibitors of cyclic AMP phosphodiesterase are useful, although indirect, tools in studies of cyclic AMP in kidney function. If specific inhibitors, acting preferentially on the kidney or some of its structures, can be developed in the future, they might find use as therapeutic agents in states of deficient responsiveness of the kidney to certain hormones or for influencing other kidney function.

H. Use of Exogenous Cyclic AMP and Its Analogs to Mimic Kidney Function

In principle, exogenous cyclic AMP should mimic the effect of those hormones that are mediated through its action (Robison *et al.*, 1971; Sutherland and Rall, 1960). However, many problems are encountered with use of exogenous cyclic AMP and its analogs. As is the case with many other nucleotides, cyclic AMP penetrates the cell membranes poorly, and higher concentrations, by several orders of magnitude, of exogenous cyclic AMP or its analogs should be used to increase the intracellular level (Robison *et al.*, 1971). Fast inactivation of cyclic AMP by cyclic AMP phosphodiesterase further complicates the situation.

For these reasons, some analogs of cyclic AMP were developed specifically for better penetration of membranes and resistance to inactivation by cyclic AMP phosphodiesterases (Meyer and Miller, 1974; Simon *et al.*, 1973; Posternak *et al.*, 1962). The most popular of these is N^6-2'-O-dibutyryl cyclic AMP (DBcAMP) (Posternak *et al.*, 1962). It appears that DBcAMP itself is not very active in mimicking cyclic AMP (Barnes *et al.*, 1975b; Simon *et al.*, 1973) and probably is first deacylated at the 2'-carbon to N^6-monobutyryl cyclic AMP (Neelon and Birch, 1973). Such acylases are relatively abundant in kidney tissue, in both the cortex and the medulla (Blecher and Hunt, 1972). When using DBcAMP, an appropriate control should be included to ascertain that the observed effect is caused by cyclic AMP or its active derivative and not to released butyrate, a metabolic substrate.

Recently, a major effort was made (Meyer and Miller, 1974; Simon *et al.*, 1973) to prepare analogs of cyclic AMP that would be more active than cyclic AMP itself and possibly also more specific in target tissues and more resistant to inactivation. It appears that C-8 substituents of cyclic AMP (Meyer and Miller, 1974; Simon *et al.*, 1973), now commercially available, might be better experimental tools than the currently used DBcAMP, because of their pronounced ability to activate the protein kinase from some tissues *in vitro* and their resistance to breakdown by rabbit kidney cyclic AMP phosphodiesterase (Meyer and Miller, 1974; Simon *et al.*, 1973).

In our recent study we compared DBcAMP, cyclic AMP, and 8-(pCl-phenyl-thio)-cyclic AMP (ClPhScAMP) using activation of renal medullary protein kinase in intact cells of renal medulla as a test system. We found that

DBcAMP was almost inactive in terms of activation of protein kinase in cell-free extracts and completely inactive when used with unbroken cells. On the other hand, ClPhScAMP appeared to penetrate to cells much better than cyclic AMP itself and to activate protein kinase in relatively low concentrations (Dousa and Valtin, in press; Barnes *et al.*, 1975b). Although both DBcAMP and ClPhScAMP are potent inhibitors of cyclic AMP phosphodiesterase, the stimulatory effect of ClPhScAMP is not due to inhibition of cyclic AMP breakdown but to the direct effect of the compound itself. ClPhScAMP is also completely resistant to enzymatic breakdown in renal medullary extracts (Dousa, Barnes, and Hui, unpublished data). ClPhScAMP is much more effective to mimic the vasopressin action in microperfused collecting tubules (D. Hall and J. J. Grantham, personal communication). It appears thus that ClPhScAMP and similar cyclic AMP analogs may be useful as a tool to investigate cyclic AMP-dependent kidney function in the future.

1. Use of Cyclic AMP Analogs Applied to Whole Kidney

This experimental approach is often plagued by uncertainties stemming from the fact that, when injected intravenously or intraperitoneally, exogenous cyclic AMP or its analogs may mimic any cyclic AMP-mediated process in any cell of the kidney as well as in extrarenal tissues. Injection or infusion of cyclic AMP directly into one renal artery can decrease the possibility of extrarenal effects (Martinez-Maldonado *et al.*, 1971) but hardly can be expected to mimic one single renal function without affecting others. This possibility is especially encountered when kidney function is measured by the whole-kidney clearance technique (Martinez-Maldonado *et al.*, 1974; Stavroulaki-Tsapara *et al.*, 1974; Levine, 1968; Alexander, 1965). If kidney function is studied by using micropuncture techniques (Kuntziger *et al.*, 1974; Lorenz, 1974; Agus *et al.*, 1971) and is limited to certain segments of the nephron, a more definite conclusion can be achieved.

2. Use of Cyclic AMP and Its Analogs in Isolated Tissue Systems

Much more consistent data have been obtained by using cyclic AMP or its analogs in isolated tissues such as microperfused segments of renal tubules (Hamburger *et al.*, 1974; Grantham, 1970; Grantham and Orloff, 1968; Grantham and Burg, 1966) or toad bladder (Handler and Orloff, 1973). As in other tissue systems, the concentrations of exogenous cyclic AMP used were usually very high and sometimes exogenous cyclic AMP was combined with cyclic AMP phosphodiesterase inhibitors (Grantham, 1970). Use of new analogs such as ClPhScAMP may be of great advantage in future studies (Dousa and Valtin, in press; Barnes *et al.*, 1975b).

III. HORMONES AND OTHER HUMORAL AGENTS ACTING ON RENAL CYCLIC AMP METABOLISM

A. Parathyroid Hormone (PTH)

The first indication that cyclic AMP plays a role in the renal actions of PTH was provided by Chase and Aurbach (1967) who showed that injection of PTH into the rat is followed by a striking increase in the urinary excretion of cyclic AMP preceding the phosphaturia. Discovery of an adenylate cyclase in rat renal cortex that was stimulated by PTH in dose-dependent fashion (Chase and Aurbach, 1968; Dousa and Rychlík, 1968c) quickly followed. Adenylate cyclase was found in membranous preparations from cortex derived from a number of mammals (Di Bella *et al.*, 1974; Streeto, 1969; Chase and Aurbach, 1968) including man (Kim *et al.*, 1976; DiBella *et al.*, 1975; Arnaud *et al.*, 1973; Marcus *et al.*, 1971), as well as from birds (Dousa, 1974b; Martin *et al.*, 1974) and reptiles (Dousa, 1974b), but not from kidneys of lower vertebrates (Dousa, 1974b). Studies performed with purified preparations of plasma membranes suggest that PTH-sensitive adenylate cyclase is probably localized at the antiluminal portion of the cortical tubular cells (Di Bella *et al.*, 1974; Shlatz *et al.*, 1973; Marx *et al.*, 1972) rather than in the brush border (Wilffong and Neville, 1970).

Studies on the relationship between the structure of PTH and its ability to stimulate adenylate cyclase are in the initial stage. The active NH_2-terminal 1–34 fragment (Potts *et al.*, 1971) of bovine PTH is active also in humans *in vivo* (Czekalski *et al.*, 1974) and has higher affinity for both human (DiBella *et al.*, 1975) and rat (Martin *et al.*, 1974) renal cortical adenylate cyclase than analogous fragments of human hormone (DiBella *et al.*, 1975; Martin *et al.*, 1974). No such difference was observed in chicken (Martin *et al.*, 1974). The penultimate NH_2-terminal 2–34 fragment appears to be an inhibitor of PTH stimulation (Martin *et al.*, 1974). Probably only some species of circulating PTH are capable of stimulating adenylate cyclase (Canterbury *et al.*, 1973).

In agreement with findings on adenylate cyclase, PTH was observed to increase the cyclic AMP level in isolated cells (Michelakis, 1970) and in isolated tubules (Kurokawa *et al.*, 1974; Kurokawa and Màssry, 1973a; Melson *et al.*, 1970; Nagata and Rasmussen, 1970) prepared from renal cortex, in isolated tissue slices (Beck *et al.*, 1972a; Steiner *et al.*, 1972b; Murad *et al.*, 1970a), and in renal cortical tissue *in situ* (Kurokawa *et al.*, 1974; Aurbach *et al.*, 1969; Nagata and Rasmussen, 1968). The majority of cells containing adenylate cyclase sensitive to PTH were always found in the cortical region (Kurokawa *et al.*, 1974; Kurokawa and Massry, 1973a; Melson *et al.*, 1970; Chase and Aurbach, 1968). Because some PTH stimulation of cyclic AMP formation frequently was found also in medullary preparations (Melson *et al.*, 1970; Chase and Aurbach, 1968) (including the human kidney; Dousa, unpublished observations), the presence of PTH-sensitive elements in medullary structures cannot be discounted at the present time. Chambardès *et al.* (1975b) found in a recent study the PTH-sensitive adenylate cyclase in the cortex not only in proximal but also in some distal segments of the tubular system.

Cyclic AMP phosphodiesterase, probably localized closer to the apical portion of cells of proximal convoluted tubules (Shanta et al., 1966), is not influenced by PTH (Chase and Aurbach, 1968; Dousa and Rychlík, 1968a) but is strongly inhibited by theophylline (Dousa and Rychlík, 1968a). In the presence of theophylline, the accumulation of cyclic AMP after stimulation with PTH is much greater (Kurokawa et al., 1974).

Two major functional effects of PTH in kidney are phosphaturia and hypocalciuria. Both these effects were reported to be elicited by administration of theophylline (Rasmussen et al., 1968). Exogenous cyclic AMP and its dibutyryl analog (DBcAMP) frequently have been used to mimic renal actions of PTH, sometimes with variable results. In micropuncture experiments, DBcAMP was demonstrated to inhibit proximal tubular reabsorption of phosphate (Agus et al., 1971), and infusion of cyclic AMP or its analog produced phosphaturia quite consistently, whether administered systemically or into a renal artery (Kuntziger et al., 1974; Bell et al., 1972; Butlen and Jard, 1972; Martinez-Maldonado et al., 1971; Rasmussen et al., 1968). On the other hand, the hypocalciuric effect of PTH was not reproduced under carefully controlled conditions (Kuntziger et al., 1974; Butlen and Jard, 1972).

Experimental evidence to date appears, therefore, rather suggestive that at least some renal effects of PTH, such as phosphaturia, are mediated through the action of cyclic AMP formed under the influence of PTH, although exceptions may exist (Dousa et al., 1976) and many aspects of the PTH effect on kidney function remain unsolved at the present time.

One prominent feature of the PTH effect on renal function is that, at least in some species, cyclic AMP formed under the influence of PTH appears in considerable quantities in urine (Butlen and Jard, 1972; Steiner et al., 1972b; Kaminsky et al., 1970b; Aurbach et al., 1969; Chase and Aurbach, 1967; Williams et al., 1972) and to a lesser degree also in plasma (Kaminsky et al., 1970b). Increase in urinary excretion in the rat was found to be dependent on the dose of PTH (Aurbach et al., 1972). Other species in which increases in urinary cyclic AMP after PTH were found include the hamster (Dousa et al., in press, b) and the gerbil (Dousa and Knox, unpublished data). The most pronounced increases in cyclic AMP in the urine were observed in man (Murad, 1973; Steiner et al., 1972a; Kaminsky et al., 1970b; Aurbach et al., 1969; Chase et al., 1969; Williams et al., 1972). On the other hand, an increase in urinary cyclic AMP was not observed after administration of PTH to dogs (Blonde et al., 1974; Davis et al., 1969; Knox, Schneider, and Dousa, unpublished observation).

The change in urinary cyclic AMP concentration in response to acute administration of PTH in man has been used successfully as a test for certain forms of pseudohypoparathyroidism (Murad, 1973; Aurbach et al., 1970, 1969; Chase et al., 1969). The daily total excretion of cyclic AMP (especially when related to excretion of creatinine or renal clearance of cyclic AMP) is potentially useful in evaluation of hyperparathyroidism, hypoparathyroidism, and related disorders (Murad, 1973).

B. Calcitonin

The physiologic role of calcitonin in the regulation of kidney function is not yet clearly established, but it is obvious that this agent, at least in high doses, stimulates cyclic AMP formation in mammalian kidney (Dousa et al., in press, b; Dousa 1974b; Heersche et al., 1974; Kurokawa et al., 1974; Marx et al., 1972; Melson et al., 1970; Murad et al., 1970a). Calcitonins from various sources were found to produce dose-dependent stimulation of renal cortical and medullary adenylate cyclase in the rat (Heersche et al., 1974; Marx et al., 1972; Murad et al., 1970a), hamster (Dousa et al., in press, b), and in man (Mulvehill and Dousa, unpublished observation). On the other hand, no effect of calcitonin on cyclic AMP metabolism in nonmammalian vertebrates was detected (Dousa, 1974b; Larkis et al., 1974; Martin et al., 1974).

Calcitonin was reported to increase cyclic AMP levels in kidney in situ (Kurokawa et al., 1974) as well as in suspensions of renal tubules (Kurokawa et al., 1974) or slices (Dousa et al., 1976; Murad et al., 1970a), and its effect was potentiated by theophylline (Kurokawa et al., 1974; Murad et al., 1970a). The greatest stimulation of adenylate cyclase by calcitonin was found in membranes isolated from the corticomedullary junction (Marx et al., 1972). Calcitonin did not stimulate the adenylate cyclase from avian kidney (Dousa, 1974b; Larkis et al., 1974; Martin et al., 1974).

There is no clear explanation why calcitonin would have some effects opposite to those of PTH—e.g., on calcium excretion—and at the same time have some effects similar to those of PTH—e.g., phosphaturia and stimulation of cyclic AMP formation in kidney. A tentative explanation may be the possibility that PTH and calcitonin act on different cell populations. Both additive (Murad et al., 1970a) and nonadditive (Kurokawa et al., 1974; Melson et al., 1970) effects with PTH have been reported. In parathyroidectomized rats, humans, dogs, or hamsters, calcitonin did not increase the renal excretion of cyclic AMP (Murad, 1973; Chase and Aurbach, 1967); in another study (Kurokawa et al., 1974) a significant increase occurred in thyroparathyroidectomized rats and hamsters (Dousa et al., 1976).

C. Vasopressin

Vasopressin was one of the first hormones for which the mediating role of cyclic AMP was discovered, in toad bladder (Orloff and Handler, 1961) and in mammalian kidney (Brown et al., 1963). Vasopressin-sensitive adenylate cyclase has been found in medullary preparations from all mammalian species studies so far, including man (Dousa, 1974a,c; Dousa et al., 1971; Brown et al., 1963); in nonmammalian vertebrates, stimulation by vasopressin (Dousa, 1974b) was found only in amphibian kidney and is very prominent in the epithelium of amphibian urinary bladder (Hynie and Sharp, 1971a; Bär et al., 1970).

Renal medullary adenylate cyclase is stimulated by vasopressin analogs in general agreement with their potency in vivo (Dousa and Valtin, in press; Beck et al., 1974b; Rajerison et al., 1974; Bockaert et al., 1972; Dousa et al., 1971; Bär et al., 1970). Analogs that inhibit vasopressin-sensitive adenylate cyclase in vivo also inhibit the adenylate cyclase in vitro (Walter et al., 1972a,b; Dousa et al., 1970). Adenylate cyclase was found predominantly in renal medulla and in the plasma membrane fraction (Barnes et al., 1975c; Schwartz et al., 1974; Bockaert et al., 1972, 1973; Neer, 1973b; Campbell et al., 1972; Forte, 1972). Highest activity of vasopressin-sensitive adenylate cyclase was found in collecting ducts, but stimulation was also detected in the ascending limb of Henle's loop in rabbits (Imbert et al., 1975a). It was demonstrated that vasopressin increases cyclic AMP levels in tissue slices (Dousa et al., 1975; Steiner et al., 1972a; Beck et al., 1971a) or suspensions of tubular fragments or isolated cells (Kurokawa et al., 1974; Kurokawa and Massry, 1973b; Ohsawa and Endo, 1972). A phosphodiesterase inhibitor, theophylline, potentiates such cyclic AMP accumulation (Kurokawa et al., 1974) and also can mimic vasopressin's effect in isolated perfused tubules (Grantham, 1970; Grantham and Orloff, 1968) or amphibian membranes (Orloff and Handler, 1961). Also, in these isolated systems, high concentrations of cyclic AMP or DBcAMP can mimic the vasopressin effect on water permeability (Grantham, 1970; Grantham and Orloff, 1968; Grantham and Burg, 1966; Orloff and Handler, 1961).

In sharp contrast to the isolated systems, it was impossible to mimic conclusively the antidiuretic effect of vasopressin by using theophylline in the whole kidney. Also, exogenous cyclic AMP or its analogs, injected into the systemic circulation or directly into a renal artery, gave variable results (Stavroulaki-Tsapara et al., 1974; Martinez-Maldonado et al., 1971, 1974; Barraclough and Jones, 1970; Abe et al., 1968; Levine, 1968; Alexander, 1965). Renal response to exogenous cyclic AMP has been reported to range from mild antidiuresis to no response to a clearly diuretic response. A probable cause of these disparate results is the fact that cyclic AMP acts on extrarenal hormone-responsive tissues or on segments of nephron that anatomically and functionally precede the collecting ducts—the target tissue for antidiuretic hormone (ADH).

In an obvious contrast to PTH, physiologic doses of ADH apparently did not produce consistent increases in urinary cyclic AMP excretion (Murad, 1973; Kaminsky et al., 1970a; Chase et al., 1969). Some laboratories have reported small increases in urinary cyclic AMP after ADH in man (Fichman and Brooker, 1972; Avery et al., 1971; Takahashi, 1971; Pawlson et al., 1970); other laboratories (including ours) have been unable to confirm these findings (Murad, 1973; Williams et al., 1972; Kaminsky et al., 1970a,b). Similar apparently discrepant results were found in rats in which both increase (Beck et al., 1974b) and no change (Butlen and Jard, 1972) in urinary cyclic AMP have been found after administration of vasopressin. One feature that makes it difficult to evaluate such observations is that plasma levels of cyclic AMP were not always measured simultaneously with urinary excretion. Lacking this information, it is difficult to ascertain whether the observed small increases in urinary cyclic AMP excretion are of renal origin.

D. Glucagon

Besides a slight increase in glomerular filtration rate, glucagon has been shown to produce a number of tubular effects both in experimental animals (Butlen and Jard, 1972; Pullman *et al.*, 1967) and in man (Butturini and Bonomini, 1958; Elrick *et al.*, 1958). These effects include diuresis and increased excretion of Na, K, and PO_4 (Butlen and Jard, 1972; Pullman *et al.*, 1967; Butturini and Bonomini, 1958; Elrick *et al.*, 1958).

Glucagon increases the activity of adenylate cyclase in preparations from rat (Melson *et al.*, 1970; Murad *et al.*, 1970a); no stimulation was found in a preparation from bovine kidney cortex but stimulation by glucagon occurred in the medullary preparation from the same species (Marcus and Aurbach, 1969). In recent experiments we found a prominent dose-dependent stimulation of renal cortical (Kim *et al.*, 1976) adenylate cyclase and even more prominent stimulation of renal medullary adenylate cyclase by glucagon in human kidney (Mulvehill *et al.*, 1976).

Administration of glucagon to the whole organism produced marked increases in urinary phosphate excretion in man (Butturini and Bonomini, 1958; Elrick *et al.*, 1958) and in experimental animals (Butlen and Jard, 1972; Pullman *et al.*, 1967). In parathyroidectomized rats, glucagon produced phosphaturia and a decrease in calcium excretion, an effect similar to that of PTH (Butlen and Jard, 1972); the response to exogenous cyclic AMP was only phosphaturia. It was proposed that glucagon can produce renal tubular effects through action of cyclic AMP formed extrarenally and filtered into urine in high quantity. The presence of glucagon-sensitive adenylate cyclase in kidney suggests that the effects on tubular function may be direct, mediated by cyclic AMP formed in the kidney. Both in man (Broadus *et al.*, 1970b) and in the rat (Butlen and Jard, 1972) the increase in urinary excretion of cyclic AMP after glucagon was apparently of extrarenal origin.

E. Other Polypeptides

Other polypeptide hormones almost invariably have had no effect on the renal adenylate cyclase system. In recent communications, insulin was reported to inhibit PTH-stimulated adenylate cyclase from beef kidney (Sutcliffe *et al.*, 1973). Secretin slightly stimulated human renal medullary adenylate cyclase (Mulvehill and Dousa, unpublished results). Based on indirect experiments on toad bladder, it was suggested that angiotensin acts through adenylate cyclase (Coviello, 1973). No increase in cyclic AMP level after angiotensin was observed in toad bladder (Handler *et al.*, 1965). In very high concentration, angiotensin produced a small stimulation of renal medullary adenylate cyclase (Bockaert *et al.*, 1973). In our present experiments, 5×10^{-8} M angiotensin II did not increase tissue level of cyclic AMP in renal medulla.

F. Prostaglandins

Prostaglandins, mostly of the E type, were shown to exert various effects on the cyclic AMP system in kidney. However, the physiologic role of these effects observed under various experimental situations is unclear at the present time.

Prostaglandins were found to stimulate the basal activity of adenylate cyclase derived from renal medulla (Birnbaumer, 1973; Dousa, 1973; Kuehl *et al.*, 1972; Beck *et al.*, 1971a; Murad *et al.*, 1970a) or toad bladder (Lipson *et al.*, 1971) and also were found to increase the intracellular level of cyclic AMP in the outer renal medulla of the rat (Beck *et al.*, 1971a), the inner medulla of the dog (Beck *et al.*, 1972b), the whole kidney (Besley and Snart, 1973), and the toad bladder (Omachi *et al.*, 1974; Lipson and Sharp, 1971; Lipson *et al.*, 1971). On the other hand, numerous reports indicate that prostaglandins can inhibit cyclic AMP accumulation after submaximal stimulation with vasopressin (Omachi *et al.*, 1974; Besley and Snart, 1973; Beck *et al.*, 1971a) and can inhibit ADH-stimulated adenylate cyclase *in vitro* (Kalisker and Dyer, 1972; Beck *et al.*, 1971a; Lipson *et al.*, 1971; Marumo and Edelman, 1971). The results showing inhibition of the adenylate cyclase stimulated by submaximal doses of vasopressin appear to be in good agreement with the observations on isolated perfused collecting ducts: Prostaglandin itself slightly increased water permeability (an effect potentiated by theophylline) but inhibited the increase in water permeability induced by vasopressin (Grantham and Orloff, 1968). It can be tentatively stated that prostaglandins (probably E type) exert a modulatory effect on vasopressin-sensitive adenylate cyclase in the mammalian kidney related to the control of water permeability. The molecular nature of this interaction is unclear at the present time.

Another report indicates a similar relationship between E-type prostaglandins and renal cortical adenylate cyclase: They did not inhibit the basal activity of adenylate cyclase or the basal level of cyclic AMP in cortical slices but blunted the stimulation of both by PTH (Beck *et al.*, 1972a). On the other hand, in rabbit kidney cortex, PGE_1 increased the level of cyclic AMP in the tissue and the activity of stimulated adenylate cyclase (Chase, 1975). PGE_1 and PGE_2 also had a stimulating effect in the human renal cortex (Kim *et al.*, 1976).

In the toad bladder the situation appears to be more complex than in the kidney. There appear to be two adenylate cyclase systems and two cyclic AMP pools. One is related to water permeability, and in this a relatively low concentration of prostaglandins inhibits vasopressin-stimulated adenylate cyclase (analogous to kidney). In the other, related to control (stimulation) of sodium transport, higher concentrations of prostaglandins stimulated cyclic AMP formation (Omachi *et al.*, 1974; Lipson *et al.*, 1971). It is quite possible that effects ascribed to prostaglandins are sometimes results of the action of their precursors, prostaglandin endoperoxides, as discussed in a recent review (Dousa and Valtin, in press).

G. Catecholamines

Catecholamine-sensitive adenylate cyclase has been found in almost all mammalian tissues (Robison *et al.,* 1971), and kidney is no exception. Melson *et al.* (1970) described stimulation of adenylate cyclase from rat cortical tubules by epinephrine; this stimulation was blocked by propranolol but not phentolamine. In contrast to this, no stimulation by epinephrine was found in bovine cortical or medullary adenylate cyclase (Marcus and Aurbach, 1969). Stimulation of renal cortical adenylate cyclase by isoproterenol, a predominantly β-adrenergic agent, was reported for rat (Bell, 1974; Kurokawa and Massry, 1973b; Marx *et al.,* 1972; Handler *et al.,* 1968) and dog (Beck *et al.,* 1972b) and also occurs in human kidney (Kim *et al.,* 1976). As expected, this stimulation is blocked by propranolol. Stimulation of rat cortical adenylate cyclase by isoproterenol and norepinephrine was dose dependent and additive to stimulation by PTH (Kurokawa and Massry, 1973a). In the renal medulla of the dog, β-adrenergic stimuli increased cyclic AMP formation (Beck *et al.,* 1972b), and a similar effect of isoproterenol and norepinephrine was found for renal medullary tissue from human kidney (Mulvehill *et al.,* 1976). On the other hand, no stimulatory effect of isoproterenol was found in isolated rat renal medullary tubules although, in the same study, β-adrenergic stimulation was found in dog medulla (Kurokawa and Massry, 1973b). Also, no increase in renal medullary cyclic AMP *in situ* was found after administration of isoproterenol to rats with hypothalamic diabetes insipidus (McDonald *et al.,* 1974).

Catecholamine, an α-adrenergic agent, specifically inhibited cyclic AMP increase due to vasopressin in dog renal medulla (Kurokawa and Massry, 1973b; Beck *et al.,* 1972b). α-Adrenergic agents did not influence the increase in cyclic AMP after PTH in dog cortex or after prostaglandin in outer medulla (Beck *et al.,* 1972b). At the present time, we have only preliminary information on which cell population has the catecholamine-sensitive renal adenylate cyclase and on the relationship between catecholamine receptors and other hormone-sensitive renal adenylate cyclase systems. In rabbit kidney, the isoproterenol-sensitive adenylate cyclase was confined to certain segments of distal nephrons (Chambardès *et al.,* 1975a). Norepinephrine, which blocked the increase in water permeability in toad bladder in response to vasopressin (Handler *et al.,* 1968), also inhibited the increase of cyclic AMP level in the toad bladder due to vasopressin (Omachi *et al.,* 1974).

H. Steroid Hormones

According to our present knowledge, the action of steroid hormones is not usually directly mediated by cyclic nucleotides. However, steroid hormones can significantly influence the effect of other hormones on the adenylate cyclase system. In rats, although adrenalectomy did not modify the basal activity of renal medullary cyclase or its stimulation by sodium fluoride (Rajerison *et al.*, 1974; Lang and Edelman, 1972) or the PTH stimulation of renal cortical adenylate cyclase (Rajerison *et al.*, 1974), it did decrease the maximal stimulation by vasopressin in preparations from the renal medulla; it did not modify the apparent K_m for vasopressin. This inhibition of vasopressin stimulation was probably due to deficiency in the receptor–adenylate cyclase coupling; in addition to this, there was small reduction in vasopressin binding capacity in renal medullary membranes (Rajerison *et al.*, 1974). Treatment with dexamethasone reversed both defects; treatment with aldosterone reversed only the defect in vasopressin binding (Rajerison *et al.*, 1974). The steroid hormones had no effect if added to the enzyme directly *in vitro*. These results suggest that adrenal steroids have at least specific modulatory effects on vasopressin-stimulated adenylate cyclase without an effect on the PTH-sensitive system of the kidney.

In another study, no effect of adrenalectomy or administration of aldosterone on vasopressin-stimulated adenylate cyclase was observed (Lang and Edelman, 1972); however, this study focused on basal and fluoride-stimulated adenylate cyclase. In the urinary toad bladder, pretreatment with aldosterone led to increased accumulation of cyclic AMP after both vasopressin and theophylline treatment (Stoff *et al.*, 1972). Further analysis has shown that pretreatment with aldosterone decreased cyclic nucleotide phosphodiesterase activity in the urinary toad bladder, thus probably increasing the cellular accumulation of nucleotide by decreasing breakdown (Stoff *et al.*, 1973).

These results, in both mammalian and nonmammalian systems, indicate that, although adrenal steroids may not directly interact with adenylate cyclase, they can influence (probably through their effect on RNA or protein synthesis) one or more critical components in renal cyclic AMP systems.

Another steroid agent—vitamin D—was shown to modulate the PTH-responsive adenylate cyclase system in the kidney. In vitamin D-deficient rats, the stimulation of renal cortical adenylate cyclase by PTH was markedly decreased. This defect can be corrected by administration of vitamin D. Vitamin D does not appear to affect adenylate cyclase itself but rather PTH binding or receptor-adenylate cyclase coupling (Forte *et al.*, 1976).

I. Thyroxin

Thyroid hormones appear to have a profound effect on renal cyclic AMP systems. Hypothyroid rats had lower activity of renal medullary adenylate cyclase and higher activity of phosphodiesterase (Harkcom *et al.*, 1976b). Both changes were reversed by treatment with thyroxine (Harkcom *et al.*, 1976b). On the other hand, in the renal cortex, thyroid hormones had no distinct effect on cyclic AMP phosphodiesterase; stimulation of cortical adenylate cyclase by PTH is diminished in the hypothyroid state and this defect is not corrected by short-term treatment with thyroxine (Harkcom *et al.*, 1976a).

IV. DRUGS AND OTHER AGENTS ACTING ON RENAL CYCLIC AMP METABOLISM

A. Diuretics and Related Drugs

Although many pharmacologic agents promote excretion of water and electrolytes, the cellular mode of action by which these agents exert their renal effects is largely unknown. A number of studies have tried to explore the possibility that various diuretics influence renal cell function through an effect on cyclic AMP synthesis or action.

1. Ethacrynic Acid

This diuretic is probably the one most actively studied in terms of its action on the renal adenylate cyclase–cyclic AMP system. It was found to inhibit basal and hormone-stimulated adenylate cyclase in the plasma membrane fractions both in rat renal cortex and in rat renal medulla; in concentrations of 10^{-4}–10^{-3} M, it sharply decreased stimulation by PTH and ADH (Jakobs *et al.*, 1972). Inhibitory action of ethacrynic acid was partially prevented by addition of dithioerythol (Jakobs *et al.*, 1972). Similar effects of ethacrynic acid were found in homogenate from cortex or outer medulla (Ebel, 1974). In plasma membranes from canine renal medulla, ethacrynic acid produced dose-dependent inhibition of basal and vasopressin-stimulated adenylate cyclase.

Dihydroethacrynic acid, a derivative of ethacrynic acid that is unable to react with SH groups, and cysteine ethacrynate had a qualitatively similar, but quantitatively less, inhibitory effect on dog renal medullary adenylate cyclase (Barnes *et al.*, 1975a). These results indicate that reaction with SH groups is not necessary for inhibition of renal medullary adenylate cyclase by ethacrynic acid. When the tissue slices were preincubated with ethacrynic acid or dihydroethacrynic acid and then washed before the adenylate cyclase activity was measured, the same inhibition was observed, indicating that the drug can bind and penetrate into the renal cells (Barnes *et al.*, 1974). Inhibition with ethacrynic acid appears to be predominantly noncompetitive in nature (Barnes *et al.*, 1974). Cyclic AMP phosphodiesterase from the renal medulla was not substantially inhibited by relatively high concentrations of ethacrynic acid (Barnes *et al.*, 1974), and injection of ethacrynic acid did not substantially inhibit phosphodiesterase activity in the rat kidney (Senft *et al.*, 1968).

These findings appear to be in reasonable agreement with studies on isolated microperfused tubules (Abramow, 1974) or amphibian toad bladder (Bentley, 1969a) in which ethacrynic acid blocked the response to vasopressin but not that to exogenous cyclic AMP. However, it is difficult at the present time to relate these biochemical actions of ethacrynic acid to its pharmacologic effect on the kidney *in vivo*. These findings taken together may suggest that ethacrynic acid can inhibit the cellular action of vasopressin in the collecting duct of mammalian kidney; there is no indication as to how the effect of ethacrynic acid on cyclic AMP metabolism could possibly inhibit chloride transport in the ascending limb of Henle's loop, a major site of the saluretic effect of this drug.

2. Other Diuretics

Variable results were obtained with another "loop" diuretic, furosemide. Although different conditions were used, stimulation (Dousa and Rychlík, 1968b), inhibition (Ebel, 1974), and no effect (Jakobs *et al.*, 1972) on the renal adenylate cyclase were observed. After injection of furosemide, cyclic AMP phosphodiesterase activity was found to be decreased only in the cortical region of the rat kidney (Senft *et al.*, 1968). Of the other diuretic agents, only mercurial diuretics have been reported to inhibit adenylate cyclase activity (Jakobs *et al.*, 1972; Dousa and Rychlík, 1968c). Amiloride (Ebel, 1974; Jakobs *et al.*, 1972) and chlorothiazide (Jakobs *et al.*, 1972; Dousa and Rychlík, 1968b) had no effect on activity of renal adenylate cyclase; however, chlorothiazide blocked the hydroosmotic effect of vasopressin but not that of exogenous cyclic AMP on toad bladder (Scott and Sapirstein, 1972). Hydrochlorothiazide, when injected into rats, inhibited cyclic AMP phosphodiesterase in the inner medulla (Senft *et al.*, 1968). Acetazolamide had no effect on cyclic AMP phosphodiesterase (Rodriguez *et al.*, 1974; Senft *et al.*, 1968); it apparently specifically inhibited the hydroosmotic effect of oxytocin but not of cyclic AMP or caffeine in the toad bladder (Scott and Sapirstein, 1972). Recently a stimulation of renal cortical adenylate cyclase by this drug was reported (Rodriguez *et al.*, 1974), an observation deserving further analysis.

The present results with these diuretics do not permit conclusions as to whether the described effects on the enzymes of cyclic AMP metabolism could contribute to their pharmacologic effects on the kidney *in vivo*. However, because many functions in kidney are controlled by cyclic AMP-dependent systems, it is possible that the relationship between the action on cyclic AMP metabolism and diuretic action will be clarified in future studies.

3. Chlorpropamide and Related Compounds

It is recognized that chlorpropamide promotes release of endogenous vasopressin and also potentiates the peripheral renal effect of this hormone (Moses *et al.*, 1973). The vasopressin-potentiating effect was demonstrated both in mammals (Brendt *et al.*, 1970; Miller and Moses, 1970) and in toad bladder (Ingelfinger and Hays, 1969; Mendoza, 1969). Depending on the concentration of chlorpropamide used, the drug may increase water permeability itself (Mendoza and Brown, 1974; Urakabe and Shirai, 1971; Urakabe *et al.*, 1970) or potentiate the submaximal effects of vasopressin (Mendoza and Brown, 1974; Ingelfinger and Hays, 1969) or the effect of theophylline (Mendoza and Brown, 1974; Mendoza, 1969).

On the other hand, chlorpropamide does not increase (Ingelfinger and Hays, 1969), and even decreases (Mendoza and Brown, 1974; Lozada *et al.*, 1972;

Mendoza, 1969), the response to exogenous cyclic AMP. A plausible explanation would be that chlorpropamide facilitates accumulation of cyclic AMP in a vasopressin-dependent pool in the target cells in the kidney or amphibian bladder. Because addition of chlorpropamide to adenylate cyclase *in vitro* did not increase its activity or its response to vasopressin (Beck *et al.,* 1974c; Chandhuri and Winer, 1971) and because chlorpropamide decreased the activity of renal medullary cyclic AMP phosphodiesterase *in vitro* (Brooker and Fichman, 1971; Chandhuri and Winer, 1971), it was proposed that its potentiating effect was due to its inhibition of cyclic AMP phosphodiesterase. In a recent study (Beck *et al.,* 1974c), it was found that several days of pretreatment with chlorpropamide increased the response of renal medullary adenylate cyclase to a submaximal concentration of vasopressin and also increased the accumulation of cyclic AMP resulting from treatment with vasopressin in medullary slices; there was no difference in activity of cyclic AMP phosphodiesterase. In contrast, the increase of tissue cyclic AMP in toad bladder in response to a submaximal dose of vasopressin was diminished by chlorpropamide (Omachi *et al.,* 1974). If chlorpropamide sensitizes adenylate cyclase, the mechanism may be indirect—for example, through action of a chlorpropamide metabolite.

It has been suggested that chlorpropamide can antagonize the inhibitory action of prostaglandin on vasopressin-sensitive adenylate cyclase (Ozer and Sharp, 1973); another laboratory has reported that the inhibitory effect of prostaglandin was potentiated (Lozada *et al.,* 1972).

A quite different effect of chlorpropamide on the cyclic AMP system in the renal cortex in rats and man was reported recently (Coulson and Moses, 1975; Numann *et al.,* 1974). Pretreatment with chlorpropamide produced a slight phosphaturia and did not alter the increase in urinary P_i after PTH, but it did diminish the increase in urinary cyclic AMP and in renal tissue cyclic AMP after administration of PTH (Numann *et al.,* 1974). Also, in parathyroidectomized man, pretreatment with chlorpropamide diminished the PTH-induced increase in urinary cyclic AMP but did not alter phosphaturia (Coulson and Moses, 1975). Other compounds producing antidiuretic action are phenylacetamides. Their vasopressin-potentiating effect may be related to inhibition of cyclic AMP phosphodiesterase (Lozada *et al.,* 1972).

B. Antibiotics and Chemotherapeutics

Demeclocycline (Declomycin) causes vasopressin-resistant impairment of the renal concentrating ability without influencing other kidney functions (Singer and Rotenberg, 1973; Wilson *et al.,* 1973; Castell and Sparks, 1965). Results of several studies both *in vivo* and *in vitro* indicate that the drug interferes with renal cyclic AMP metabolism. It inhibited the hydroosmotic response of toad bladder to vasopressin and to cyclic AMP (Feldman and Singer, 1974; Singer and Rotenberg, 1973). In preparations from human renal medulla, this drug inhibited both basal activity of adenylate cyclase and activity stimulated by vasopressin and sodium fluoride (Dousa and Wilson, 1974). It also inhibited protein kinase activity and had only a small effect on cyclic AMP phosphodiesterase activity (Dousa and Wilson, 1974). Because some other tetracyclines that do not produce diabetes insipidus have the ability to interfere with adenylate cyclase and protein kinase, other factors probably would determine why only demeclocycline is effective *in vivo*. A recent report suggests that the capacity to bind to protein may be such a factor (Feldman and Singer, 1974).

Puromycin inhibited stimulation of the renal cortical adenylate cyclase by PTH but did not influence the basal activity of this enzyme (Fratkin *et al.*, 1972) or of renal medullary adenylate cyclase. In other tissues, puromycin was reported to inhibit cyclic AMP phosphodiesterase (Appleman *et al.*, 1973). Valinomycine was reported to block the hydroosmotic effect of vasopressin but not of cyclic AMP in toad bladder, a result interpreted as inhibition of adenylate cyclase (Bentley, 1969b). Microtubule-disrupting alkaloids (colchicine and vinblastine) in low concentrations did not influence enzymes of cyclic AMP metabolism *in vitro* (Dousa and Barnes, 1974) or after pretreatment *in vivo* (Dousa and Barnes, unpublished results). However, colchicine administered in higher doses to rats caused diminished response of renal cortical adenylate cyclase to PTH (Dousa *et al.*, in press, a). Cytochalasin B, an antibiotic that disrupts microfilaments, decreased the accumulation of cyclic AMP in toad urinary bladder in response to ADH (Davis *et al.*, 1974). Indomethacin, an antiinflammatory drug (and inhibitor of prostaglandin synthetase), is a potent inhibitor of cyclic AMP phosphodiesterase from the toad bladder (Flores and Sharp, 1972).

C. Ions and Other Solutes

1. Monovalent Cations

When added to membrane preparations from the renal medulla, sodium had a biphasic effect (Dousa, 1972; Dousa and Hechter, 1970): in lower concentrations (usually less than 100 mM) the activity of adenylate cyclase was increased (Dousa, 1972, 1974c); at higher concentrations the activity decreased (this included basal, vasopressin-stimulated, and fluoride-stimulated activities) (Dousa, 1972). Potassium appears to have similar effects (Dousa, 1972). In a renal cortical adenylate cyclase, sodium concentrations of 50 mM did not have any effect on basal or PTH- or fluoride-stimulated activities, potassium increased basal and PTH-stimulated activity but only in preparations from male rats, and rubidium behaved in the same way as potassium (Marcus and Aurbach, 1971).

Lithium salts are known to produce a vasopressin-resistant diabetes insipidus in man and experimental animals (Forrest *et al.*, 1974; Singer *et al.*, 1972) and to inhibit the hydroosmotic effect of vasopressin on toad urinary bladder (Harris and Jenner, 1972; Singer *et al.*, 1972). In relatively low concentrations, lithium can inhibit the adenylate cyclase from renal medulla of rabbit (Dousa and Hechter, 1970) or man (Dousa, 1974c). This inhibition is especially prominent in the presence of higher concentrations of renal medullary solutes (Dousa, 1974c; Dousa and Hechter, 1970) and appears to be specific for vasopressin-stimulated adenylate cyclase and noncompetitive in nature (Dousa, 1974c). Cyclic AMP phosphodiesterase was not inhibited by lithium salts (Dousa, 1974c). This differential effect on enzymes can be expected to lead to decreased accumulation of cyclic AMP in renal medulla in response to vasopressin; such a finding was reported (Beck *et al.*, 1971b). Divergent results were reported from rats pretreated with lithium *in vivo*. In one study, the basal and fluoride-stimulated renal adenylate cyclase activities from rats with lithium-induced polyuria were not different from controls, but stimulation with vasopressin was significantly decreased (Geisler *et al.*, 1972). In another study, basal activity of renal medullary adenylate cyclase from lithium-treated rats was low, but vasopressin responsiveness was maintained (Eknoyan *et al.*, 1974).

The findings that lithium inhibited, in part, the antidiuretic response to DBcAMP (Forrest *et al.*, 1974) and the hydroosmotic effects of exogenous cyclic AMP (Harris and Jenner, 1972) in toad urinary bladder suggest that lithium could act also in steps subsequent to cyclic AMP generation. In renal cortical adenylate cyclase, lithium at 50 mM will inhibit the basal activity in female rats and the PTH-stimulated activity in males (Marcus and Aurbach, 1971).

Although adenylate cyclase and cyclic AMP phosphodiesterase both have characteristic pH optima, the amount of cyclic AMP in renal cortex slices was not changed significantly by metabolic acidosis or alkalosis (Goodman *et al.*, 1972).

2. Monovalent Anions

Fluoride, as in many other eukaryotic tissues (Robison *et al.*, 1971), stimulates a cell-free renal adenylate cyclase system (Marcus and Aurbach, 1971; Dousa and Rychlik, 1970a) and has a mild inhibitory effect on cyclic AMP phosphodiesterase (Dousa and Rychlík, 1970a). It also increases tissue level of cyclic AMP in toad bladder, but blocks the effect of vasopressin, probably in steps distal to cyclic AMP generation (Urakabe *et al.*, 1975).

3. Divalent Cations

Calcium. When tested in cell-free membrane preparations, addition of calcium, usually in a concentration range of 10^{-5}–10^{-3} M or more, inhibited adenylate cyclase from renal cortex (Beck *et al.*, 1974a; Marcus and Aurbach, 1971; Streeto, 1969), renal medulla (Beck *et al.*, 1974b; Campbell *et al.*, 1972; Marumo and Edelman, 1971), or toad urinary bladder (Bockaert *et al.*, 1972; Hynie and Sharp, 1971a). The inhibitory effect of calcium was less prominent or absent with fluoride-stimulated adenylate cyclase (Bockaert *et al.*, 1972; Campbell *et al.*, 1972; Hynie and Sharp, 1971a; Marumo and Edelman, 1971), possibly because of direct interaction of calcium with fluoride. On the other hand, very low concentrations of calcium might be important for hormonal stimulation because addition of a molar excess of chelator (EGTA) in some experiments abolished stimulation by vasopressin (Bockaert *et al.*, 1972; Campbell *et al.*,

1972), but this was not observed in other studies (Dousa, 1972; Bär *et al.*, 1970). Incubation of toad bladder with 10 mM Ca itself did not change cyclic AMP levels but decreased the increase of the nucleotide in response to vasopressin (Omachi *et al.*, 1974). In cortical slices from hypercalcemic rats, the increase in cyclic AMP content in response to PTH was less than that in controls (Beck *et al.*, 1974a); in medullary slices the increase in cyclic AMP in response to vasopressin was also lower in hypercalcemic animals (Beck *et al.*, 1974b). Cyclic AMP phosphodiesterase was reported to be not influenced by addition of calcium (Beck *et al.*, 1974a,b); in our own experiments there was a slight stimulation of cyclic AMP phosphodiesterase from bovine or rat medullary extracts by this cation (Barnes and Dousa, unpublished results).

It appears that calcium is potentially an important modulating factor of the cyclic AMP system in the kidney, but the exact role of this modulatory effect and the relative influences of extracellular and intracellular calcium or of free and bound calcium remain to be established.

Magnesium. This cation is an essential cofactor for both adenylate cyclase and cyclic AMP phosphodiesterase (Robison *et al.*, 1971) in all tissues. The effects of different agents may depend on the concentration of Mg^{2+} in the incubation mixture, especially with prostaglandins (Birnbaumer, 1973; Zarday *et al.*, 1972). Mn^{2+}, and to a lesser degree Co^{2+} (Forte, 1972), can partially replace Mg^{2+} in the renal adenylate cyclase system (Forte, 1972; Marcus and Aurbach, 1971).

Mn^{2+} caused inhibition of renal cortical adenylate cyclase in the presence of optimal concentrations of Mg^{2+} (Marcus and Aurbach, 1971). Of considerable interest is the finding that Mn^{2+} blocked the activation of the adenylate cyclase by vasopressin but not by fluoride in toad bladder (Hynie and Sharp, 1971b). Sr^{2+} had no apparent effect on renal medullary adenylate cyclase (Dousa and Hechter, unpublished observations).

Of the nonionic solutes, urea was found to inhibit the activity of renal medullary adenylate cyclase at rather high concentrations; glucose was without apparent effect (Dousa, 1972).

D. Other Drugs and Agents

There are numerous sporadic reports about the action of various agents on the renal adenylate cyclase system.

2-Amino-4,5-diphenylthiazole hydrochloride (BAX 49) is an experimental drug that induces a renal concentration defect and, after prolonged administration, cystic changes in the kidney. In rats fed this drug, stimulation by vasopressin is decreased, but basal and fluoride-sensitive activities were normal and there were no differences in renal cortical adenylate cyclase stimulated by PTH (Dousa *et al.*, 1973).

1,1,1-Trichloro-2,2-bis(p-chlorophenyl)ethane (p,p-DDT) and some other insecticides stimulated adenylate cyclase, both in intact renal cortex and in cell-free systems, and inhibited cyclic AMP phosphodiesterase with resulting accumulation of cyclic AMP (Kacew and Singhal, 1974).

In an *in vivo* study, administration of inorganic pyrophosphate to rats blocked the renal effect of PTH (Delong *et al.,* 1971). In another study, pyrophosphate was found to inhibit renal cortical adenylate cyclase (Pilczyk *et al.,* 1972); in preparation from the whole kidney, pyrophosphate also inhibited cyclic AMP phosphodiesterase (Dousa and Rychlik, 1970b). It is possible that there is an association between the pyrophosphate effect on cyclic AMP metabolism and the renal PTH-blocking effect observed *in vivo.*

The effect of phosphonates, compounds now considered for treatment of bone disorders, on renal cortical adenylate cyclase was also tested. When added directly into the cell-free system, dichloromethylenediphosphonate (Cl_2DP) and ethane-1-hydroxy-1,1-diphosphonate (EHDP) both inhibited the activity of adenylate cyclase stimulated by PTH or fluoride (Pilczyk *et al.,* 1972). On the other hand, prolonged *in vivo* administration of phosphonates did not change the responsiveness of rat renal cortical adenylate cyclase to PTH (O'Hara *et al.,* unpublished observations).

Anesthetics such as pentobarbital, thiopentone, and chloralose were reported to diminish the increase in the permeability of toad bladder in response to vasopressin, but the increase in the permeability in response to exogenous cyclic AMP was also depressed (Grey and Ullmann, 1974). Results with pentobarbital may correspond to the decreased level of cyclic AMP found in rat kidney after pentobarbital anesthesia (Kimura *et al.,* 1974). Anesthetic doses of ethanol did not influence the cyclic AMP or ATP in the kidney (Volicer, 1971).

Cysteine inhibited the hydroosmotic response to vasopressin and theophylline but not of cyclic AMP in toad bladder (Handler and Orloff, 1964). On the other hand, cysteine enhanced the stimulation of renal medullary adenylate cyclase by vasopressin or fluoride (Barnes *et al.,* 1975a). Cholera toxin, an agent reported previously to stimulate the adenylate cyclase in several other tissues, was reported to stimulate the adenylate cyclase preparations in the renal cortex and produce accumulation of cyclic AMP (Kurokawa *et al.,* 1975).

Various detergents have been used in attempts to solubilize membrane-bound adenylate cyclase (Neer, 1973a; Forte, 1972; Marcus and Aurbach, 1971), a procedure that frequently led to complete or at least partial loss of responsiveness to hormone, with basal and fluoride-stimulated activities largely preserved. Removal of the detergent partially restored the sensitivity to hormone (Neer, 1973a). This and recently reported (Roy *et al.,* 1975) results on dissociation of vasopressin receptor and adenylate cyclase suggest that phospholipids are critical in coupling the hormone receptors to adenylate cyclase, at least in renal medulla. It appears that calcitonin-sensitive renal cortical adenylate cyclase from pork kidney is especially resistant to detergents during solubilization (Queener *et al.,* 1975).

Various naturally occurring metabolites have been reported to have an effect on the renal cyclic AMP system. Lactate, but not pyruvate, apparently specifically stimulates renal cortical adenylate cyclase and increases cyclic AMP (Rodgers *et al.,* 1974). Treatment of rats with folic acid in preliminary experiments slightly increased tissue levels of cyclic AMP in kidney; however, this appears to be a consequence of acute renal failure rather than the drug itself

(Barnes *et al.*, in press). Various modulatory effects of nucleotides, nucleosides, and bases on toad bladder (Bockaert *et al.*, 1972) and renal medullary adenylate cyclase (Brinbaumer, 1973) were reported. GPPNHP (5'-guanylyl imidophosphate) stimulated adenylate cyclase also in human renal cortical (Kim *et al.*, 1976). ATP and ADP inhibited both renal and toad bladder cyclic AMP phosphodiesterase (Gulyassy, 1971; Dousa and Rychlik, 1970b), and the same effect was observed for adenine and adenosine in toad bladder (Gulyassy, 1971). On the other hand, adenosine increased cyclic AMP phosphodiesterase activity in the kidney (Dousa and Rychlik, 1970b). Of considerable interest is the report showing that guanosine cyclic 3',5'-monophosphate (cyclic GMP) is a potent inhibitor of cyclic AMP breakdown and can cause accumulation of cyclic AMP in rat kidney cortex (Murad *et al.*, 1970b).

V. CONCLUDING REMARKS

The enormous knowledge on the role of cyclic nucleotides in kidney function that has accumulated in the recent years is a result of the progress in this field of research in general. This field probably will develop rapidly, and several yet unexplored areas will be approached.

One such area is the role of cyclic GMP and other cyclic 3',5'-nucleotides in the regulation of renal function. Observations that the kidney is one of the organs most active in cyclic GMP metabolism (Nakazawa and Sano, 1974; Goldberg *et al.*, 1973) make this prediction especially attractive. Attention so far has been focused mostly on the role of cyclic AMP in the mechanisms of hormonal regulation of kidney function. However, there are other areas in which cyclic AMP and other cyclic nucleotides may play a critical role, and these are almost unexplored at the present time. These areas include the regulation of normal or malignant renal growth (Kim *et al.*, 1976), regulation of the regeneration of kidney tissue after injury (Barnes *et al.*, in press; Schlondorff *et al.*, 1975), and possible roles in renal inflammatory and immune reactions associated with the development of parenchymal renal disease.

Basic and applied research on the role of cyclic 3',5'-nucleotides in kidney physiology and pathology not only will elucidate the underlying processes in normal as well as in diseased kidney but also will serve as a rational basis for new therapeutic approaches to kidney disease and the development of new drugs, effective through their action on cyclic 3',5'-nucleotide metabolism, that will be used specifically for testing of renal function and treating renal diseases.

ACKNOWLEDGMENTS

Experimental work from this laboratory reported in this article was supported by U.S. Public Health Service grant AM 16105 and General Research Support Grant 5S01-RR-05530, by a grant from the American Heart Association with funds contributed by the Minnesota Heart Association, and by the Mayo Foundation. The author is an Established Investigator of the American Heart

Association. The author's experimental work was done in part in collaboration with Dr. Larry D. Barnes, Dr. Jin K. Kim, and Mr. Thomas M. Harkcom and Mr. John B. Mulvehill, students of Mayo Medical School. Excellent technical assistance was provided by Mrs. Y. S. F. Hui, Mrs. Denise M. Heublein, and Mr. Christopher Wilson.

REFERENCES

Abe, Y., Morimoto, S., Yamamoto, K., and Ueda, J. 1968. Effects of dibutyryl cyclic 3′,5′-adenosine monophosphate on the renal function. *Jpn. J. Pharmacol., 18:*271.

Abramow, M. 1974. Effects of ethacrynic acid on the isolated collecting tubule. *J. Clin. Invest., 53:*796.

Agus, Z. S., Puschett, J. B., Senesky, D., and Goldberg, M. 1971. Mode of action of parathyroid hormone and cyclic adenosine 3′,5′-monophosphate on renal tubular phosphate reabsorption in the dog. *J. Clin. Invest., 50:*617.

Alexander, C. S. 1965. The effect of 3′,5′-cyclic AMP and other nucleotides on urine flow and hemodynamics in the rat. *J. Clin. Invest., 44:*1025 (abstract).

Appleman, M. M., Thompson, W. J., and Russell, T. R. 1973. Cyclic nucleotide phosphodiesterases. *Adv. Cyclic Nucleotide Res., 3:*65.

Arnaud, C. D., Dousa, T., Sizemore, G. W., Rittel, W., Fairwell, T., Ronan, R., and Brewer, B. 1973. Amino terminal human parathyroid hormone (PTH 1–34): Biological properties and specific radioimmunoassay. *J. Clin. Invest., 52:*5a (abstract).

Aurbach, G. D., Potts, J. T., Jr., Chase, L. R., and Melson, G. L. 1969. Polypeptide hormones and calcium metabolism. *Ann. Intern. Med., 70:*1243.

Aurbach, G. D., Marcus, R., Winickoff, R. N., Epstein, E. H., Jr., and Nigra, T. P. 1970. Urinary excretion of 3′,5′-AMP in syndromes considered refractory to parathyroid hormone. *Metabolism, 19:*799.

Aurbach, G. D., Keutmann, H. T., Niall, H. D., Tregear, G. W., O'Riordan, J. L. H., Marcus, R., Marx, S. J., and Potts, J. T., Jr. 1972. Structure, synthesis, and mechanism of action of parathyroid hormone. *Recent Prog. Horm. Res., 28:*353.

Avery, S., Clark, C. M., Jr., Trygstad, C., and Bell, N. H. 1971. Effects of cyclic adenosine monophosphate (AMP) and dibutyryl cyclic AMP in antidiuretic hormone-deficient and antidiuretic hormone-resistant diabetes insipidus. *J. Clin. Invest., 50:*3a (abstract).

Bär, H.-P. 1975. Measurement of adenyl cyclase and cyclic AMP. *Methods Pharmacol., 3:*593.

Bär, H.-P. and Hechter, O. 1969. Adenyl cyclase assay in fat cell ghosts. *Anal. Biochem., 29:*476.

Bär, H.-P., Hechter, O., Schwartz, I. L., and Walter, R. 1970. Neurohypophyseal hormone-sensitive adenyl cyclase of toad urinary bladder. *Proc. Natl. Acad. Sci. U.S.A., 67:*7.

Barnes, L. D., Hui, Y. S. F., and Dousa, T. P. 1974. Effects of ethacrynic acid (EA) and its derivatives on enzymes mediating the action of vasopressin (VP). *Clin. Res., 22:*515A (abstract).

Barnes, L. D., Hui, Y. S. F., and Dousa, T. P. 1975a. Interaction of ethacrynic and cysteine with renal medullary adenylate cyclase. *Life Sci., 16:*255.

Barnes, L. D., Hui, Y. S. F., and Dousa, T. P. 1975b. Effect of cyclic 3′,5′ AMP (cAMP) analogs on the activation of protein kinase (PK) in intact renal medullary cells. *Kidney Int., 8:*466.

Barnes, L. D., Hui, Y. S. F., Frohnert, P. P., and Dousa, T. P. 1975c. Subcellular distribution of the enzymes related to the cellular action of vasopressin in renal medulla. *Endocrinology, 97:*119.

Barnes, L. D., Heublein, D. M., and Dousa, T. P. 1976. Relationship of tissue cyclic AMP levels and DNA synthesis in renal hyperplasia in course of folic acid (FA)-induced acute renal failure. *Clin. Res., 24:*392A.

Barraclough, M. A. and Jones, N. F. 1970. Effects of adenosine 3′,5′-monophosphate on renal function in the rabbit. *Br. J. Pharmacol., 40:*334.

Beavo, J. A., Rogers, N. L., Crofford, O. B., Hardman, J. G., Sutherland, E. W., and Newman, E. V. 1970. Effects of xanthine derivatives on lipolysis and on adenosine 3',5'-monophosphate phosphodiesterase activity. *Mol. Pharmacol., 6:*597.

Beck, N. P., Kaneko, T., Zor, U., Field, J. B., and Davis, B. B. 1971a. Effects of vasopressin and prostaglandin E on the adenyl cyclase-cyclic 3',5'-adenosine monophosphate system of the renal medulla of the rat. *J. Clin. Invest., 50:*2461.

Beck, N. P., Reed, S. W., and Davis, B. B. 1971b. Effects of lithium (Li) on renal concentration of cyclic AMP (CAMP). *Clin. Res., 19:*684 (abstract).

Beck, N. P., DeRubertis, F. R., Michelis, M. F., Fusco, R. D., Field, J. B., and Davis, B. B. 1972a. Effect of prostaglandin E₁ on certain renal actions of parathyroid hormone. *J. Clin. Invest., 51:*2352.

Beck, N. P., Reed, S. W., Murdaugh, H. V., and Davis, B. B. 1972b. Effects of catecholamines and their interaction with other hormones on cyclic 3',5'-adenosine monophosphate of the kidney. *J. Clin. Invest., 51:*939.

Beck, N., Singh, H., Reed, S., and Davis, B. B. 1974a. Direct inhibitory effect of hypercalcemia on renal actions of parathyroid hormone. *J. Clin. Invest., 53:*717.

Beck, N., Singh, H., Reed, S. W., Murdaugh, H. V., and Davis, B. B. 1974b. Pathogenic role of cyclic AMP in the impairment of urinary concentrating ability in acute hypercalcemia. *J. Clin. Invest., 54:*1049.

Beck, N. P., Kim, K. S., and Davis, B. B. 1974c. Effect of chlorpropamide on cyclic AMP in rat renal medulla. *Endocrinology, 96:*771.

Bell, N. H. 1974. Evidence for a separate adenylate cyclase system response to beta-adrenergic stimulation in the renal cortex of the rat. *Acta Endocrinol. (Copenhagen), 77:*604.

Bell, N. H., Avery, S., Sinha, T., Clark, C. M., Jr., Allen, D. O., and Johnston, C., Jr. 1972. Effects of dibutyryl cyclic adenosine 3',5'-monophosphate and parathyroid extract on calcium and phosphorus metabolism in hypoparathyroidism and pseudohypoparathyroidism. *J. Clin. Invest., 51:*816.

Bentley, P. J. 1969a. Actions of vasopressin and aldosterone on the toad bladder: inhibition by ethacrynic acid. *J. Endocrinol., 43:*347.

Bentley, P. J. 1969b. The effect of valinomycin on the toad bladder: Antagonism to vasopressin and aldosterone. *J. Endocrinol., 45:*287.

Besley, G. T. N. and Snart, R. S. 1973. Effect of prostaglandins on cyclic AMP concentrations in toad bladder and rat kidney. *FEBS Lett., 31:*269.

Birnbaumer, L. 1973. Hormone-sensitive adenylyl cyclases: Useful models for studying hormone receptor functions in cell-free systems. *Biochim. Biophys. Acta, 300:*129.

Blecher, M. and Hunt, N. H. 1972. Enzymatic deacylation of mono- and dibutyryl derivatives of cyclic adenosine 3',5'-monophosphate by extracts of rat tissues. *J. Biol. Chem., 247:*7479.

Blonde, L., Wehmann, R. E., and Steiner, A. L. 1974. Plasma clearance rates and renal clearance of ³H-labeled cyclic AMP and ³H-labeled cyclic GMP in the dog. *J. Clin. Invest., 53:*163.

Bockaert, J., Roy, C., and Jard, S. 1972. Oxytocin-sensitive adenylate cyclase in frog bladder epithelial cells: Role of calcium, nucleotides, and other factors in hormonal stimulation. *J. Biol. Chem., 247:*7073.

Bockaert, J., Roy, C., Rajerison, R., and Jard, S. 1973. Specific binding of [³H]lysine-vasopressin to pig kidney plasma membranes: Relationships of receptor occupancy to adenylate cyclase activation. *J. Biol. Chem., 248:*5922.

Boudreau, R. J. and Drummond, G. I. 1975. A modified assay of 3':5'-cyclic-AMP phosphodiesterase. *Anal. Biochem., 63:*388.

Brendt, W. O., Miller, M., Kettyle, W. M., and Valtin, H. 1970. Potentiation of the antidiuretic effect of vasopressin by chlorpropamide. *Endocrinology, 86:*1082.

Broadus, A. E., Kaminsky, N. I., Hardman, J. G., Sutherland, E. W., and Liddle, G. W. 1970a. Kinetic parameters and renal clearances of adenosine 3',5'-monophosphate and guanosine 3',5'-monophosphate in man. *J. Clin. Invest., 49:*2222.

Broadus, A. E., Kaminsky, N. I., Northcutt, R. C., Hardman, J. G., Sutherland, E. W., and Liddle, G. W. 1970b. Effects of glucagon on adenosine 3',5'-monophosphate and guanosine 3',5'-monophosphate in human plasma and urine. *J. Clin. Invest., 49:*2237.

Brooker, G. and Fichman, M. 1971. Chlorpropamide and tolbutamide inhibition of adenosine 3',5' cyclic monophosphate phosphodiesterase. *Biochem. Biophys. Res. Commun., 42:824.*

Brostrom, C. O. and Kon, C. 1974. An improved protein binding assay for cyclic AMP. *Anal. Biochem., 58:459.*

Brown, B. L., Ekins, R. P., and Albano, J. D. M. 1972. Saturation assay for cyclic AMP using endogenous binding protein. *Adv. Cyclic Nucleotide Res., 2:25.*

Brown, E., Clarke, D. R., Roux, V., and Sherman, G. H. 1963. The stimulation of adenosine 3,5-monophosphate production by antidiuretic factors. *J. Biol. Chem., 238:852.*

Butcher, R. W. and Sutherland, E. W. 1962. Adenosine 3',5'-phosphate in biological materials. I. Purification and properties of cyclic 3',5'-nucleotide phosphodiesterase and use of this enzyme to characterize adenosine 3',5'-phosphate in human urine. *J. Biol. Chem., 237:1244.*

Butlen, D. and Jard, S. 1972. Renal handling of 3'-5'-cyclic AMP in the rat: The possible role of luminal 3'-5'-cyclic AMP in the tubular reabsorption of phosphate. *Pfluegers Arch., 331:172.*

Butturini, U. and Bonomini, V. 1958. Über die Wirkung von Glukagon und Insulin auf Nierenfunktion, Harnausscheidung der Phosphat-, Bicarbonat- und Ammoniakionen und titrierbare Acidität beim Menschen. *Helv. Med. Acta, 25:617.*

Campbell, B. J., Woodward, G., and Borberg, V. 1972. Calcium-mediated interactions between the antidiuretic hormone and renal plasma membranes. *J. Biol. Chem., 247:6167.*

Canterbury, J. M., Levey, G. S., and Reiss, E. 1973. Activation of renal cortical adenylate cyclase by circulating immunoreactive parathyroid hormone fragments. *J. Clin. Invest., 52:524.*

Castell, D. O. and Sparks, H. A. 1965. Nephrogenic diabetes insipidus due to demethylchlortetracycline hydrochloride. *J. Am. Med. Assoc., 193:237.*

Chambardès, D., Imbert, M., and Morel, F. 1975a. Presence and localization of β-adrenergic receptors along the nephron (abstract). Proceedings of the VI International Congress of Nephrology, no. 47.

Chambardès, D., Imbert, M., Clique, A., Montégut, M., and Morel, F. 1975b. PTH sensitive adenyl cyclase activity in different segments of the rabbit nephron. *Pfluegers Arch., 354:229.*

Chandhuri, T. K. and Winer, N. 1971. Effects of chlorpropamide on renal phosphodiesterase. *J. Lab. Clin. Med., 76:863.*

Chase, L. R. 1975. Selective proteolysis of the receptor for parathyroid hormone in renal cortex. *Endocrinology, 96:70.*

Chase, L. R. and Aurbach, G. D. 1967. Parathyroid function and the renal excretion of 3',5'-adenylic acid. *Proc. Natl. Acad. Sci. U.S.A., 58:518.*

Chase, L. R. and Aurbach, G. D. 1968. Renal adenyl cyclase: Anatomically separate sites for parathyroid hormone and vasopressin. *Science, 159:545.*

Chase, L. R., Melson, G. L., and Aurbach, G. D. 1969. Pseudohypoparathyroidism: Defective excretion of 3',5'-AMP in response to parathyroid hormone. *J. Clin. Invest., 48:1832.*

Cizek, L. J. 1968. The kidney. In: *Medical Physiology,* Vol. 1, 12th ed., pp. 307–349. Ed. by Mountcastle, V. B., C. V. Mosby, St. Louis.

Coulson, R. and Bowman, R. H. 1974. Excretion and degradation of exogenous adenosine 3',5'-monophosphate by isolated perfused rat kidney. *Life Sci., 14:545.*

Coulson, R. and Moses, A. M. 1975. Effect of chlorpropamide on renal response to parathyroid hormone in normal subjects and in patients with hypoparathyroidism and pseudohypoparathyroidism. *J. Pharmacol. Exp. Ther., 194:603.*

Coulson, R., Bowman, R. H., and Roch-Ramel, F. 1974. The effects of nephrectomy and probenecid on *in vivo* clearance of adenosine-3',5'-monophosphate from rat plasma. *Life Sci., 15:877.*

Coviello, A. 1973. Hydrosmotic effect of angiotensin II in the toad bladder: Role of cyclic AMP. *Acta Physiol. Lat. Am., 23:350.*

Czekalski, S., Loreau, N., Paillard, F., Ardaillou, R., Fillastre, J.-P., and Mallet, E. 1974. Effect of bovine parathyroid hormone 1–34 fragment on renal production and excretion of adenosine 3',5' monophosphate in man. *Eur. J. Clin. Invest., 4:85.*

Davis, B., Zor, U., Kaneko, T., Mintz, D. H., and Field, J. B. 1969. Effects of parathyroid extract (PTE), arginine vasopressin (AVP) and prostaglandin E_1 (PGE_1) on urinary and renal tissue cyclic 3'5' adenosine monophosphate (CAMP). *Clin. Res., 17:458.*

Davis, W. L., Goodman, D. B. P., Schuster, R. J., Rasmussen, H., and Martin, J. H. 1974. Effects of cytochalasin B on the response of toad urinary bladder to vasopressin. *J. Cell Biol., 63:*986.

Delong, A., Feinblatt, J., and Rasmussen, H. 1971. The effect of pyrophosphate infusion on the response of the hormone and adenosine-3′,5′-cyclic monophosphate. *Calcif. Tissue Res., 8:*87.

Di Bella, F. P., Dousa, T. P., Miller, S. S., and Arnaud, C. D. 1974. Parathyroid hormone receptors of renal cortex: Specific binding of biologically active, ^{125}I-labeled hormone and relationship to adenylate cyclase activation. *Proc. Natl. Acad. Sci. U.S.A., 71:*723.

DiBella, F. P., Arnaud, C. D., Brewer, H. B., Jr., and Dousa, T. P. 1975. Relative biologic activities of human and bovine parathyroid hormones: Dependence on assay system used. *Fed. Proc., 34:*336 (abstract).

Dousa, T. P. 1972. Effect of renal medullary solutes on vasopressin-sensitive adenyl cyclase. *Am. J. Physiol., 222:*657.

Dousa, T. P. 1973. Effect of prostaglandins on adenylate cyclase from human renal medulla. In: *Prostaglandins and Cyclic AMP: Biological Actions and Clinical Applications,* pp. 155–181. Ed. by Kahn, R. H. and Lands, W. E. M. Academic Press, New York.

Dousa, T. P. 1974a. Cellular action of antidiuretic hormone in nephrogenic diabetes insipidus. *Mayo Clin. Proc., 49:*188.

Dousa, T. P. 1974b. Effects of hormones on cyclic AMP formation in kidneys of nonmammalian vertebrates. *Am. J. Physiol., 226:*1193.

Dousa, T. P. 1974c. Interaction of lithium with vasopressin-sensitive cyclic AMP system of human renal medulla. *Endocrinology, 95:*1359.

Dousa, T. P. and Barnes, L. D. 1974. Effects of colchicine and vinblastine on the cellular action of vasopressin in mammalian kidney: A possible role of microtubules. *J. Clin. Invest., 54:*252.

Dousa, T. P. and Hechter, O. 1970. The effect of NaCl and LiCl on vasopressin-sensitive adenyl cyclase. *Life Sci., 9* (Part 1):765.

Dousa, T. P. and Rychlík, I. 1968a. The effect of parathyroid hormone on adenyl cyclase in rat kidney. *Biochim. Biophys. Acta, 158:*484.

Dousa, T. P. and Rychlík, I. 1968b. Adenyl cyclase and adenosine 3′,5′-cyclic phosphate phosphodiesterase in the receptor tissues of neurohypophysial hormones. *Life Sci., 7* (Part 2):1039.

Dousa, T. P. and Rychlík, I. 1968c. The effect of diuretics on adenyl cyclase in the rat kidney. *Physiol. Bohemoslov., 17:*457 (abstract).

Dousa, T. P. and Rychlík, I. 1970a. The metabolism of adenosine 3′,5′-cyclic phosphate. I. Method for the determination of adenyl cyclase and some properties of the adenyl cyclase isolated from the rat kidney. *Biochim. Biophys. Acta, 204:*1.

Dousa, T. P. and Rychlik, I. 1970b. The metabolism of adenosine 3′,5′-cyclic phosphate. II. Some properties of adenosine-3′,5′-cyclic-phosphate phosphodiesterase from the rat kidney. *Biochim. Biophys. Acta, 204:*10.

Dousa, T. P. and Valtin, H. In press. Cellular actions of vasopressin in mammalian kidney. *Kidney Int. 10.*

Dousa, T. P. and Wilson, D. M. 1974. Effects of demethylchlortetracycline on cellular action of antidiuretic hormone *in vitro. Kidney Int., 5:*279.

Dousa, T. P., Hechter, O., Walter, R., and Schwartz, I. L. 1970. [8-Arginine]-vasopressinoic acid: An inhibitor of rabbit kidney adenyl cyclase. *Science, 167:*1134.

Dousa, T. P., Hechter, O., Schwartz, I. L., and Walter, R. 1971. Neurohypophyseal hormone-responsive adenylate cyclase from mammalian kidney. *Proc. Natl. Acad. Sci. U.S.A., 68:*1693.

Dousa, T. P., Rowland, R. G., and Carone, F. A. 1973. Renal medullary adenylate cyclase in drug-induced nephrogenic diabetes insipidus. *Proc. Soc. Exp. Biol. Med., 142:*720.

Dousa, T. P., Hui, Y. S. F., and Barnes, L. D. 1975. Effect of vasopressin (VP) on *in situ* activation and translocation of protein kinase (PK) in renal medulla. *Clin. Res., 23:*542A.

Dousa, T. P., Preiss, J., Hui, Y. S. F., and Knox, F. G. 1976. Dissociation of cAMP formation and phosphaturia following parathyroid hormone (PTH) and calcitonin (CT) in hamster. *Clin. Res., 24:*36A.

Dousa, T. P., Duarte, C. G., and Knox, F. G. In press (a). Effect of colchicine on urinary phosphate and regulation by parathyroid hormone. *Am. J. Physiol. 230.*

Dousa, T. P., Preiss, J., Kim, J. K., Hui, Y. S. F., and Knox, F. G. In press (b). Activation of cyclic AMP system and protein hormone by parathyroid hormone and calcitonin without phosphaturia. *Clin. Res.*

Ebel, M. 1974. Effect of diuretics on renal NaK-ATPase and adenyl cyclase. *Naunyn-Schmiedeberg's Arch. Pharmacol., 281:*301.

Eknoyan, G., Corey, G. R., Loomis, J., Suki, W. N., and Martinez-Maldonado, M. 1974. Lithium (Li$^+$) induced diabetes insipidus: Effect on urinary cyclic AMP (cAMP) excretion and renal tissue adenylate cyclase (AC) activity. *Clin. Res., 22:*524A (abstract).

Elrick, H., Huffman, E. R., Hlad, C. J., Jr., Whipple, N., and Staub, A. 1958. Effects of glucagon on renal function in man. *J. Clin. Endocrinol. Metab., 18:*813.

Feldman, H. A. and Singer, I. 1974. Comparative effects of tetracyclines on water flow in toad urinary bladders. *Clin. Res., 22:*525A (abstract).

Fichman, M. P. and Brooker, G. 1972. Deficient renal cyclic adenosine 3'-5'-monophosphate production in nephrogenic diabetes insipidus. *J. Clin. Endocrinol. Metab., 35:*35.

Fitzpatrick, D. F. 1969. Characterization of plasma membrane proteins in mammalian kidney. I. Preparation of a membrane fraction and separation of the protein. *J. Biol. Chem., 244:*3561.

Flores, A. G. A. and Sharp, G. W. G. 1972. Endogenous prostaglandins and osmotic water flow in the toad bladder. *Am. J. Physiol., 233:*1392.

Forrest, J. N., Jr., Cohen, A. D., Torretti, J., Himmelhoch, J. M., and Epstein. F. H. 1974. On the mechanism of lithium-induced diabetes insipidus in man and the rat. *J. Clin. Invest., 53:*1115.

Forte, L. R. 1972. Characterization of the adenyl cyclase of rat kidney plasma membranes. *Biochim. Biophys. Acta, 266:*524.

Forte, L. R., Nickols, G. A., and Anast, C. S. 1976. Renal adenylate cyclase and the interrelationship between parathyroid hormone and vitamin D in regulation of urinary phosphate and adenosine cyclic 3',5'-monophosphate excretion. *J. Clin. Invest., 57:*559.

Fratkin, M., Smith, P., and Estep, H. 1972. Specific inhibition of parathyroid hormone (PTH) response renal adenyl cyclase. *Clin. Res., 20:*426 (abstract).

Geisler, A., Wraae, O., and Olesen, O. V. 1972. Adenyl cyclase activity in kidneys of rats with lithium-induced polyuria. *Acta Pharmacol. Toxicol., 31:*203.

Gilman, A. G. 1972. Protein binding assays for cyclic nucleotides. *Adv. Cyclic Nucleotide Res., 2:*9.

Goldberg, N. D. and O'Toole, A. G. 1971. Analysis of cyclic 3',5'-adenosine monophosphate and cyclic 3',5'-guanosine monophosphate. In: *Methods of Biochemical Analysis*, Vol. 20, pp. 1–39. Ed. by Glick, J. Wiley, New York.

Goldberg, N. D., O'Dea, R. F., and Haddox, M. K. 1973. Cyclic GMP. *Adv. Cyclic Nucleotide Res., 3:*155.

Goodman, A. D., Steiner, A. L., and Pagliara, A. S. 1972. Effects of acidosis and alkalosis on 3',5'-GMP and 3',5'-AMP in renal cortex. *Am. J. Physiol., 223:*620.

Goodman, D. B. P., Bloom, F. E., Battenberg, E. R., Rasmussen, H., and Davis, W. L. 1975. Immunofluorescent localization of cyclic AMP in toad urinary bladder: Possible intercellular transfer. *Science, 188:*1023.

Grantham, J. J. 1970. Vasopressin: Effect on deformability of urinary surface of collecting duct glands. *Science, 168:*1093.

Grantham, J. J. and Burg, M. B. 1966. Effect of vasopressin and cyclic AMP on permeability of isolated collecting tubules. *Am. J. Physiol., 211:*255.

Grantham, J. J. and Orloff, J. 1968. Effect of prostaglandin E$_1$ on permeability response of isolated collecting tubule to vasopressin adenosine 3',5'-monophosphate and theophylline. *J. Clin. Invest., 47:*1154.

Grey, D. and Ullmann, E. 1974. The influence of anaesthetics on the increase in the water permeability of the toad bladder induced by vasopressin. *Br. J. Pharmacol., 50:*131.

Gulyassy, P. F. 1971. Inhibition of cyclic 3',5'-nucleotide phosphodiesterase by adenine compounds. *Life Sci., 10* (Part 2):451.

Halkerston, I. D., Feinstein, M., and Hechter, O. 1966. An anomalous effect of theophylline on ACTH and adenosine 3',5'-monophosphate stimulation. *Proc. Soc. Exp. Biol. Med., 122:*896.

Hamburger, R. J., Lawson, N. L., and Dennis, V. W. 1974. Effects of cyclic adenosine nucleotides on fluid absorption by different segments of proximal tubule. *Am. J. Physiol., 227:*396.

Handler, J. S. and Orloff, J. 1964. Cysteine effect on toad bladder response to vasopressin, cyclic AMP, and theophylline. *Am. J. Physiol., 206:*505.

Handler, J. S. and Orloff, J. 1973. The mechanism of action of antidiuretic hormone. In: *Handbook of Physiology. Section 8, Renal Physiology,* pp. 791–814, Ed. by Orloff, J., Berliner, R. W., and Geiger, S. R. American Physiological Society, Washington, D.C.

Handler, J. S., Butcher, R. W., Sutherland, E. W., and Orloff, J. 1965. The effect of vasopressin and of theophylline on the concentration of adenosine 3′,5′-phosphate in the urinary bladder of the toad. *J. Biol. Chem., 240:*4524.

Handler, J. S., Bensinger, R., and Orloff, J. 1968. Effects of adrenergic agents on toad bladder response to ADH, 3′,5′-AMP, and theophylline, *Am. J. Physiol., 215:*1024.

Harkcom, T. M., Palumbo, P. J., Hui, Y. S. F., Kim, J. K., and Dousa, T. P. 1976a. Differential effect of thyroid hormones on renal and liver hormone-sensitive adenylate cyclase (AC). *58th Annual Meeting of the Endocrine Society,* July, San Francisco (abstract 625, p. 369).

Harkcom, T. M., Kim, J. K., Hui, Y. S. F., Palumbo, P. J., and Dousa, T. P. 1976b. Defect in cellular action of vasopressin (VP) in hypothyroidism and its correction by thyroxin (T_4) treatment. *Clin. Res., 24:*401A.

Harris, C. A. and Jenner, F. A. 1972. Some aspects of the inhibition of the action of antidiuretic hormone by lithium ions in the rat kidney and bladder of the toad *Bufo marinus. Br. J. Pharmacol., 44:*223.

Heersche, J. N. M., Marcus, R., and Aurbach, G. D. 1974. Calcitonin and the formation of 3′,5′-AMP in bone and kidney. *Endocrinology, 94:*241.

Hynie, S. and Sharp, G. W. G. 1971a. Adenyl cyclase in the toad bladder. *Biochim. Biophys. Acta, 230:*40.

Hynie, S. and Sharp, G. W. G. 1971b. Inhibition by manganese of the action of antidiuretic hormone on adenyl cyclase in toad bladder. *J. Endocrinol., 50:*231.

Imbert, M., Chambardès, D., Montégut, M., Clique, A., and Morel, F. 1975a. Vasopressin dependent adenylate cyclase in single segments of rabbit kidney tubule. *Pfluegers Arch., 357:*173.

Imbert, M., Chambardès, D., Montégut, M., Clique, A., and Morel, F. 1975b. Adenylate cyclase activity along the rabbit nephron as measured in single isolated segments. *Pfluegers Arch., 354:*213.

Ingelfinger, J. R. and Hays, R. M. 1969. Evidence that chlorpropamide and vasopressin share a common site of action. *J. Clin. Endocrinol. Metab., 29* 738.

Jakobs, K. H., Schultz, K., and Schultz, G. 1972. Hemmung von Adenyl-Cyclase-Präparationen aus der Rattenniere durch Calciumionen und verschiedene Diuretica. *Naunyn-Schmiedeberg's Arch. Pharmacol., 273:*248.

Jande, S. S. and Robert, P. 1974. Cytochemical localization of parathyroid hormone activated adenyl cyclase in rat kidney. *Histochemistry, 40:*323.

Jard, S. and Bernard, M. 1970. Presence of two 3′-5′-cyclic AMP phosphodiesterases in rat kidney and frog bladder epithelial cells extracts. *Biochem. Biophys. Res. Commun., 41:*781.

Kacew, S. and Singhal, R. L. 1974. Effect of certain halogenated hydrocarbon insecticides on cyclic adenosine 3′,5′-monophosphate-^{3}H formation by rat kidney cortex. *J. Pharmacol. Exp. Ther., 188:*265.

Kalisker, A. and Dyer, D. C. 1972. Inhibition of the vasopressin-activated adenyl cyclase from renal medulla by prostaglandins. *Eur. J. Pharmacol., 20:*143.

Kaminsky, N. I., Ball, J. H., Broadus, A. E., Hardman, J. G., Sutherland, E. W., and Liddle, G. W. 1970a. Hormonal effects on extracellular cyclic nucleotide in man. *Trans. Assoc. Am. Physicians, 83:*235.

Kaminsky, N. I., Broadus, A. E., Hardman, J. G., Jones, D. J., Jr., Ball, J. H., Sutherland, E. W., and Liddle, G. W. 1970b. Effects of parathyroid hormone on plasma and urinary adenosine 3′,5′-monophosphate in man. *J. Clin. Invest., 49:*2387.

Kebabian, J. W., Kuo, J. F., and Greengard, P. 1972. Determination of relative levels of cyclic AMP in tissues or cells prelabeled with radioactive adenine. *Adv. Cyclic Nucleotide Res., 2:*131.

Kim, J. K., Dousa, T. P., Barnes, L. D., Hui, Y. S. F., Farrow, G. M., and Frohnert, P. P. 1976. Enzymes of cyclic AMP metabolism in renal cell carcinoma. *Clin. Res., 24:*468A.

Kimura, H., Thomas, E., and Murad, F. 1974. Effects of decapitation, ether and pentobarbital on guanosine 3',5'-phosphate and adenosine 3',5'-phosphate levels in rat tissues. *Biochim. Biophys. Acta, 343:*519.

Krishna, G., Weiss, B., and Brodie, B. B. 1968. A simple, sensitive method for the assay of adenyl cyclase. *J. Pharmacol. Exp. Ther., 163:*379.

Kuehl, F. A., Jr., Humes, J. L., Cirello, V. J., and Ham, E. A. 1972. Cyclic AMP and prostaglandins in hormone action. *Adv. Cyclic Nucleotide Res., 1:*493.

Kuntziger, H., Amiel, C., Roinel, N., and Morel, F. 1974. Effects of parathyroidectomy and cyclic AMP on renal transport of phosphate, calcium, and magnesium. *Am. J. Physiol., 227:*905.

Kurokawa, K. and Massry, S. G. 1973a. Interaction between catecholamines and vasopressin on renal medullary cyclic AMP of rat. *Am. J. Physiol., 225:*825.

Kurokawa, K. and Massry, S. G. 1973b. Evidence for two separate adenyl cyclase systems responding independently to parathyroid hormone and β-adrenergic agents in the renal cortex of the rat. *Proc. Soc. Exp. Biol. Med., 143:*123.

Kurokawa, K., Nagata, N., Sasaki, M., and Nakane, K. 1974. Effects of calcitonin on the concentration of cyclic adenosine 3',5'-monophosphate in rat kidney *in vivo* and *in vitro*. *Endocrinology, 94:*1514.

Kurokawa, K., Friedler, R. M., and Massry, S. G. 1975. Renal action of cholera toxin. II. Effects on adenylate cyclase-cyclic AMP system. *Kidney Int., 7:*137.

Lang, M. A. and Edelman, I. S. 1972. Effects of aldosterone and vasopressin on adenyl cyclase activity of rat kidney. *Am. J. Physiol., 222:*21.

Larkis, R. G., MacAuley, S. J., Rapoport, A., Martin, T. J., Tulloch, B. R., Byfield, P. G. H., Matthews, E. W., and MacIntyre, I. 1974. Effects of nucleotides, hormones, ions and 1,25-dihydroxycholecalciferol on 1,25-dihydroxycholecalciferol production in isolated chick renal tubules. *Clin. Sci. Mol. Med., 46:*569.

Lemay, A. and Jarett, L. 1975. Pitfalls in the use of lead nitrate for the histochemical demonstration of adenylate cyclase activity. *J. Cell Biol., 65:*39.

Levine, R. A. 1968. Antidiuretic responses to exogenous adenosine 3',5'-monophosphate in man. *Clin. Sci., 34:*253.

Lipson, L. C. and Sharp, G. W. G. 1971. Effect of prostaglandin E₁ on sodium transport and osmotic water flow in the toad bladder. *Am. J. Physiol., 220:*1046.

Lipson, L., Hynie, S., and Sharp, G. 1971. Effect of prostaglandin E₁ on osmotic water flow and sodium transport in the toad bladder. *Ann. N.Y. Acad. Sci., 180:*261.

Lorenz, W. B., Jr. 1974. The effect of cyclic AMP and dibutyryl cyclic AMP on the permeability characteristics of the renal tubule. *J. Clin. Invest., 53:*1250.

Lozada, E. S., Gouaux, J., Franki, N., Appel, G. B., and Hays, R. M. 1972. Studies of the mode of action of the sulfonylureas and phenylacetamides in enhancing the effect of vasopressin. *J. Clin. Endocrinol., 34:*704.

Lynch, T. J. and Cheung, W. Y. 1975. Underestimation of cyclic 3',5'-nucleotide phosphodiesterase activity by a radioisotopic assay using an anionic-exchange resin. *Anal. Biochem., 67:*130.

Marcus, R. and Aurbach, G. D. 1969. Bioassay of parathyroid hormone *in vitro* with a stable preparation of adenyl cyclase from rat kidney. *Endocrinology, 85:*801.

Marcus, R. and Aurbach, G. D. 1971. Adenyl cyclase from renal cortex. *Biochim. Biophys. Acta, 242:*410.

Marcus, R., Wilber, J. F., and Aurbach, G. D. 1971. Parathyroid hormone-sensitive adenyl cyclase from the renal cortex of a patient with pseudohypoparathyroidism. *J. Clin. Endocrinol. Metab., 33:*537.

Martin, T. J., Vakakis, N., Eisman, J. A., Livesey, S. J., and Tregear, G. W. 1974. Chick kidney adenylate cyclase: Sensitivity to parathyroid hormone and synthetic human and bovine peptides. *J. Endocrinol., 63:*369.

Martinez-Maldonado, M., Eknoyan, G., and Suki, W. N. 1971. Natriuretic effects of vasopressin and cyclic AMP: Possible site of action in the nephron. *Am. J. Physiol., 220:*2013.

Martinez-Maldonado, M., Stavroulaki-Tsapara, A., and Eknoyan, G. 1974. Renal effects of cyclic AMP in normal and congenital diabetes insipidus rats. *Life Sci., 14:*2025.

Marumo, F. and Edelman, I. S. 1971. Effects of Ca^{++} and prostaglandin E$_1$ on vasopressin activation of renal adenyl cyclase. *J. Clin. Invest., 50:*1613.

Marx, S. J., Fedak, S. A., and Aurbach, G. D. 1972. Preparation and characterization of a hormone-responsive renal plasma membrane fraction. *J. Biol. Chem., 247:*6913.

McDonald, K. M., Kuruvila, K. C., Aisenbrey, G. A., and Schrier, R. W. 1974. Effect of beta-adrenergic stimulation on water excretion and medullary tissue cyclic AMP in intact and diabetes insipidus rats. *Kidney Int., 6:*70A (abstract).

Melson, G. L., Chase, L. R., and Aurbach, G. D. 1970. Parathyroid hormone-sensitive adenyl cyclase in isolated renal tubules. *Endocrinology, 86:*511.

Mendoza, S. and Brown, C. F., Jr. 1974. Effect of chlorpropamide on osmotic water flow across toad bladder and the response to vasopressin, theophylline and cyclic AMP. *J. Clin. Endocrinol. Metab., 38:*883.

Mendoza, S. A. 1969. Effect of chlorpropamide on the permeability of the urinary bladder of the toad and the response to vasopressin, adenosine-3',5'-monophosphate and theophylline. *Endocrinology, 84:*411.

Meyer, R. B., Jr. and Miller, J. P. 1974. Analogs of cyclic AMP and cyclic GMP: General methods of synthesis and the relationship of structure to enzymic activity. *Life Sci., 14:*1019.

Michelakis, A. M. 1970. Hormonal effects on cyclic AMP in a renal-cell suspension system. *Proc. Soc. Exp. Biol. Med., 135:*13.

Miller, M. and Moses, A. M. 1970. Potentiation of vasopressin action by chlorpropamide *in vivo. Endocrinology, 86:*1024.

Moses, A. M., Numann, P., and Miller, M. 1973. Mechanism of chlorpropamide-induced antidiuresis in man: Evidence for release of ADH and enhancement of peripheral action. *Metab. Clin. Exp., 22:*59.

Mulvehill, J. B., Hui, Y. S., Barnes, L. D., Palumbo, P. J., and Dousa, T. P. 1976. Glucagon sensitive adenylate cyclase in human renal medulla. *J. Clin. Endocrinol. Metab., 42:*348.

Murad, F. 1973. Clinical studies and applications of cyclic nucleotides. *Adv. Cyclic Nucleotide Res., 3:*355.

Murad, F., Brewer, H. B., Jr., and Vaughan, M. 1970a. Effect of thyrocalcitonin on adenosine 3':5'-cyclic phosphate formation by rat kidney and bone. *Proc. Natl. Acad. Sci. U.S.A., 65:*446.

Murad, F., Manganiello, V., and Vaughan, M. 1970b. Effects of guanosine 3',5'-monophosphate on glycerol production and accumulation of adenosine 3',5'-monophosphate by fat cells. *J. Biol. Chem., 245:*3352.

Murad, F., Manganiello, V., and Vaughan, M. 1971. A simple sensitive protein-binding assay for guanosine 3':5'-monophosphate, *Proc. Natl. Acad. Sci. U.S.A., 68:*736.

Nagata, N. and Rasmussen, H. 1968. Parathyroid hormone and renal cell metabolism. *Biochemistry, 7:*3728.

Nagata, N. and Rasmussen, H. 1970. Renal gluconeogenesis: Effects of Ca^{2+} and H$^+$. *Biochim. Biophys. Acta, 215:*1.

Nakazawa, K. and Sano, M. 1974. Studies on guanylate cyclase: A new assay method for guanylate cyclase and properties of the cyclase from rat brain. *J. Biol. Chem., 249:*4207.

Neelon, F. A. and Birch, B. M. 1973. Cyclic adenosine 3':5'-monophosphate-dependent protein kinase: Interaction with butyrylated analogues of cyclic adenosine 3':5'-monophosphate. *J. Biol. Chem., 248:*8361.

Neer, E. J. 1973a. Vasopressin-responsive, soluble adenylate cyclase from the rat renal medulla. *J. Biol. Chem., 248:*3742.

Neer, E. J. 1973b. The vasopressin-sensitive adenylate cyclase of the rat renal medulla. *J. Biol. Chem., 248:*4775.

Numann, P., Coulson, R., and Moses, A. 1974. Chlorpropamide-induced inhibition of the action of parathyroid hormone. *J. Clin. Invest., 53:*57a (abstract).

Ohsawa, M. and Endo, H. 1972. Level of newly synthesized cyclic AMP in the isolated rat kidney cells and its changes by vasopressin. *Endocrinol. Jpn., 19:*251.

Omachi, R. S., Robbie, D. E., Handler, J. S., and Orloff, J. 1974. Effects of ADH and other agents on cyclic AMP accumulation in toad bladder epithelium. *Am. J. Physiol., 226:*1152.

Orloff, J. and Handler, J. S. 1961. Vasopressin-like effects of adenosine 3',5'-phosphate (cyclic 3',5'-AMP) and theophylline in the toad bladder. *Biochem. Biophys. Res. Commun., 5:*63.

Orloff, J. and Handler, J. 1967. The role of adenosine 3',5'-phosphate in the action of antidiuretic hormone. *Am. J. Med., 42:*757.

Ozer, A. and Sharp, G. W. G. 1973. Modulation of adenyl cyclase action in toad bladder by chlorpropamide: Antagonism to prostaglandin E_1. *Eur. J. Pharmacol., 22:*227.

Pawlson, L. G., Taylor, A., Mintz, D. H., Field, J. B., and Davis, B. B. 1970. Effect of vasopressin on renal cyclic AMP generation in potassium deficiency and patients with sickle hemoglobin. *Metab. Clin. Exp., 19:*694.

Pilczyk, R., Sutcliffe, H., and Martin, T. J. 1972. Effects of pyrophosphate and diphosphonates on parathyroid hormone- and fluoride-stimulated adenylate cyclase activity. *FEBS Lett., 24:*225.

Posternak, T., Sutherland, E. W., and Henion, W. F. 1962. Derivatives of cyclic 3',5'-adenosine monophosphate. *Biochim. Biophys. Acta, 65:*558.

Potts, J. T., Jr., Tregear, G. W., Keutmann, H. T., Niall, H. D., Sauer, R., Deftos, L. J., Dawson, B. F., Hogan, M. L., and Aurbach, G. D. 1971. Synthesis of a biologically active N-terminal tetratriacontapeptide of parathyroid hormone. *Proc. Natl. Acad. Sci. U.S.A., 68:*63.

Pullman, T. N., Lavender, A. R., and Aho, I. 1967. Direct effects of glucagon on renal hemodynamics and excretion of inorganic ions. *Metab. Clin. Exp., 16:*358.

Queener, S. F., Fleming, J. W., and Bell, N. H. 1975. Solubilization of calcitonin-responsive renal cortical adenylate cyclase. *J. Biol. Chem., 250:*7586.

Rajerison, R., Marchetti, J., Roy, C., Bockaert, J., and Jard, S. 1974. The vasopressin-sensitive adenylate cyclase of the rat kidney: Effect of adrenalectomy and corticosteroids on hormone receptor-enzyme coupling. *J. Biol. Chem., 249:*6390.

Ramachandran, J. and Lee, V. 1970. Divergent effects of *o*-nitrophenyl sulfenyl ACTH on rat and rabbit fat cell adenyl cyclases. *Biochem. Biophys. Res. Commun., 41:*358.

Rasmussen, H., Pechet, M., and Fast, D. 1968. Effect of dibutyryl cyclic adenosine 3',5'-monophosphate, theophylline, and other nucleotides upon calcium and phosphate metabolism. *J. Clin. Invest., 47:*1843.

Robison, G. A., Butcher, R. W., and Sutherland, E. W. 1971. *Cyclic AMP.* Academic Press, New York.

Rodbell, M., Birnbaumer, L., Pohl, S. L., and Krans, H. M. J. 1971. The glucagon-sensitive adenyl cyclase system in plasma membranes of rat liver. V. An obligatory role of guanyl nucleotides in glucagon action. *J. Biol. Chem., 246:*1877.

Rodgers, G. M., Fisher, J. W., and George, W. J. 1974. Lactate stimulation of renal cortical adenylate cyclase: A mechanism for erythropoietin production following cobalt treatment or hypoxia. *J. Pharmacol. Exp. Ther., 190:*542.

Rodriguez, H. J., Wells, J., Yates, J., and Klahr, S. 1974. Effects of acetazolamide on the urinary excretion of cyclic AMP and on the activity of renal adenyl cyclase. *J. Clin. Invest., 53:*122.

Roy, C., Rajerison, R., Bockaert, J., and Jard, S. 1975. Solubilization of the [8-lysine]vasopressin receptor and adenylate cyclase from pig kidney plasma membranes. *J. Biol. Chem., 250:*7885.

Rutten, W. J., Schoot, B. M., and De Pont, J. J. H. H. M. 1973. Adenosine 3',5'-monophosphate phosphodiesterase assay in tissue homogenates. *Biochim. Biophys. Acta, 315:*378.

Sato, T., Garcia-Bunuel, R., and Brandes, D. 1974. Ultrastructural cytochemical localization of adenylate cyclase in the rat nephron. *Lab. Invest., 30:*222.

Schlondorff, D., Weber, H., and Trizna, W. 1975. Cyclic nucleotide metabolism in compensatory renal hypertrophy. *Physiologist, 18:*381.

Schultz, G., Böhme, E., and Hardman, J. G. 1974. Separation and purification of cyclic nucleotides by ion-exchange resin column chromatography. In *Methods in Enzymology,* Vol. 38, pp. 9–20. Ed. by Hardman, J. G. and O'Malley, B. W. Academic Press, New York.

Schwartz, I. L., Shlatz, L. J., Kinne-Saffran, E., and Kinne, R. 1974. Target cell polarity and membrane phosphorylation in relation to the mechanism of action of antidiuretic hormone. *Proc. Natl. Acad. Sci. U.S.A., 71:*2595.

Scott, W. N. and Sapirstein, V. S. 1972. Effects of Diamox and chlorothiazide on toad bladder adenyl cyclase: Evidence for different receptors for hydro-osmotic and sodium fluxes. *Physiologist, 15:*260.

Senft, G., Munske, K., Schultz, G., and Hoffmann, M. 1968. Der Einfluss von Hydrochlorothiazid und anderen sulfonamidierten Diuretica auf die 3',5'-AMP-Phosphodiesterase-Aktivität in der Rattenniere. *Naunyn-Schmiedeberg's Arch. Pharmakol. Exp.Pathol., 259:*344.

Shanta, T. R., Woods, W. D., Waitzman, M. B., and Bourne, G. H. 1966. Histochemical method for localization of cyclic 3',5'-nucleotide phosphodiesterase. *Histochemie, 7:*177.

Sheppard, H. 1971. Inhibition of norepinephrine stimulated adenyl cyclase by theophylline. *Nature (London), 228:*567 (letter to the editor).

Shlatz, L. J., Kinne, R., Kinne-Saffran, E., and Schwartz, I. L. 1973. Plasma membrane polarity of proximal tubule and collecting duct cells of rat and bovine kidney in relation to the mechanism of action of PTH and ADH. *Physiologist, 16:*451 (abstract).

Simon, L. N., Shuman, D. A., and Robins, R. K. 1973. The chemistry and biological properties of nucleotides related to nucleoside 3',5'-cyclic phosphates. *Adv. Cyclic Nucleotide Res., 3:*225.

Singer, I. and Rotenberg, D. 1973. Demeclocycline-induced nephrogenic diabetes insipidus: In-vivo and in-vitro studies. *Ann. Intern. Med., 79:*679.

Singer, I., Rotenberg, D., and Puschett, J. B. 1972. Lithium-induced nephrogenic diabetes insipidus: In vivo and in vitro studies. *J. Clin. Invest., 51:*1081.

Stavroulaki-Tsapara, A., Haley, D., Eknoyan, G., and Martinez-Maldonado, M. 1974. Changes in electrolyte excretion following intraperitoneal injection of dibutyryl cyclic AMP in the Brattleboro rat. *Life Sci., 14:*2031.

Steiner, A. L., Kipnis, D. M., Utiger, R., and Parker, C. 1969. Radioimmunoassay for the measurement of adenosine 3',5'-cyclic phosphate. *Proc. Natl. Acad. Sci. U.S.A., 64:*367.

Steiner, A. L., Wehmann, R. E., Parker, C. W., and Kipnis, D. M. 1972a. Radioimmunoassay for the measurement of cyclic nucleotides. *Adv. Cyclic Nucleotide Res., 2:*51.

Steiner, A. L., Pagliara, A. S., Chase, L. R., and Kipnis, D. M. 1972b. Radioimmunoassay for cyclic nucleotides. II. Adenosine 3',5'-monophosphate and guanosine 3',5'-monophosphate in mammalian tissues and body fluid. *J. Biol. Chem., 247:*1114.

Steiner, A. L., Whitley, T. H., Ong, S. H., and Stowe, N. W. 1975. Cyclic AMP and cyclic GMP: Studies utilizing immunohistochemical techniques for the localization of the nucleotides in tissue. *Metabolism, 24:*419.

Steiner, A. L., Ong, S. H., and Wedner, H. J. In press. Cyclic nucleotide immunocytochemistry. *Adv. Cyclic Nucleotide Res.*

Stoff, J. S., Handler, J. S., and Orloff, J. 1972. The effect of aldosterone on the accumulation of adenosine 3':5'-cyclic monophosphate in toad bladder epithelial cells in response to vasopressin and theophylline. *Proc. Natl. Acad. Sci. U.S.A., 69:*805.

Stoff, J. S., Handler, J. S., Preston, A. S., and Orloff, J. 1973. The effect of aldosterone on cyclic nucleotide phosphodiesterase activity in toad urinary bladder. *Life Sci., 13:*545.

Streeto, J. M. 1969. Renal cortical adenyl cyclase: Effect of parathyroid hormone and calcium. *Metab. Clin. Exp., 18:*968.

Sutcliffe, H. S., Martin, T. J., Eisman, J. A., and Pilczyk, R. 1973. Binding of parathyroid hormone to bovine kidney-cortex plasma membranes. *Biochem. J., 134:*913.

Sutherland, E. W. and Rall, T. W. 1960. The relation of adenosine-3',5'-phosphate and phosphorylase to the actions of catecholamines and other hormones. *Pharmacol. Rev., 12:*265.

Takahashi, K. 1971. Effects of vasopressin, water load and aminophylline on adenosine 3',5'-phosphate in human urine. *Kobe J. Med. Sci., 17:*17.

Thompson, W. J. and Appleman, M. M. 1971a. Multiple cyclic nucleotide phosphodiesterase activities from rat brain. *Biochemistry, 10:*311.

Thompson, W. J. and Appleman, M. M. 1971b. Characterization of cyclic nucleotide phosphodiesterases of rat tissues. *J. Biol. Chem., 246:*3145.

Urakabe, S. and Shirai, D. 1971. Effect of vasopressin, cyclic 3',5'-AMP, and chlorpropamide on water permeability of toad urinary bladder. *Med. J. Osaka Univ., 21:*151.

Urakabe, S., Shirai, D., Ando, A., Takamitsu, Y., Orita, Y., and Abe, H. 1970. Effect of sulfonylureas on the permeability to water and electrical properties of the urinary bladder of the toad. *Jpn. Circ. J., 34:*595.

Urakabe, S., Handler, J. S., and Orloff, J. 1975. Release of cyclic AMP by toad urinary bladder. *Am. J. Physiol., 228:*954.

Volicer, L. 1971. Effect of ethanol on adenosine 3',5'-monophosphate (cyclic AMP) in rat tissues *in vivo. Pharmacologist, 13:*218 (abstract).

Walter, R., Schwartz, I. L., Hechter, O., Dousa, T., and Hoffman, P. L. 1972a. Bromoacetyl-oxytocin, an irreversible inhibitor of neurohypophyseal hormone-stimulated adenylate cyclase, and a possible affinity label for hormone receptors. *Endocrinology, 91:*39.

Walter, R., Kirchberger, M. A., and Hruby, V. J. 1972b. Competitive inhibitor of neurohypophyseal hormones on adenylate cyclase from the toad urinary bladder. *Experientia, 28:*959.

Wells, J. N., Baird, C. E., Wu, Y. J., and Hardman, J. G. 1975. Cyclic nucleotide phosphodiesterase activities of pig coronary arteries. *Biochim. Biophys. Acta, 384:*430.

White, A. A. and Zenser, T. V. 1971. Separation of cyclic 3',5'-nucleoside monophosphates from other nucleotides on aluminum oxide columns: Application to the assay of adenyl cyclase and guanyl cyclase. *Anal. Biochem., 41:*372.

Wilffong, R. F. and Neville, D. M., Jr. 1970. The isolation of a brush border membrane fraction from rat kidney. *J. Biol. Chem., 245:*6106.

Williams, R. H., Barish, J., and Ensinck, J. W. 1972. Hormone effects upon cyclic nucleotide excretion in man. *Proc. Soc. Exp. Biol. Med., 139:*447.

Wilson, D. M., Perry, H. O., Sams, W. M., Jr., and Dousa, T. P. 1973. Selective inhibition of human distal tubular function by demeclocycline. *Curr. Ther. Res. Clin. Exp., 15:*734.

Zarday, A., Gonaux, J., and Hays, R. 1972. Inhibition of toad bladder adenyl cyclase by prostaglandin E_1(PGE_1): The critical role of magnesium on the PGE_1/vasopressin ratio. *5th Int. Congr. Nephrol.* 620, p. 113 (abstract).

IV

Organic Acid

Chapter **11**

Proximal Tubular Transport and Renal Metabolism of Organic Cations and Catechol

Barbara R. Rennick

Department of Pharmacology and Therapeutics
Medical School
State University of New York
Buffalo, New York

I. INTRODUCTION

Renal excretion of drugs and autopharmacologic agents which are strong organic cations is regulated by glomerular filtration of the ions not bound to protein in the plasma or by tubular mechanisms. An active excretory transport from peritubular blood to urine has been demonstrated for many strong organic cations (bases). Table I presents lists of cations demonstrated to be excreted by the renal tubule. The transported cations are both autopharmacologic agents and drugs. During excretory active transport of these organic cations, renal metabolism may alter the excretory transport rate by the formation of polar anionic conjugates such as glucuronides which are avidly transported, or by the formation of metabolites which are less well transported than the parent compound. Several reviews of renal tubular transport mechanisms have appeared in the last few years (Forster, 1967; Peters, 1960; Rennick, 1972, 1974; Rennick and Quebbemann, 1971; Schanker, 1972; Sperber, 1959; Torretti *et al.*, 1962; Weiner, 1973, 1971, 1967; Weiner and Mudge, 1964).

Table I. Organic Cations Excreted by the Proximal Renal Tubule

Autopharmacologic agents	Drugs
Acetylcholine (Acara and Rennick, 1972a)	Atropine (Acara and Rennick, 1972a)
Choline (Acara and Rennick, 1972b; Rennick, 1958)	Hexamethonium (Rennick, 1958)
Creatinine (Rennick, 1967)	
Dopamine (Rennick, 1968)	Mecamylamine (Baer et al., 1956)
Epinephrine (Rennick and Yoss, 1962)	Mepiperphenidol (Beyer et al., 1953)
Histamine (Lindahl and Sperber, 1956)	Morphine (May et al., 1967)
Isoproterenol (Quebbemann and Rennick, 1969; Lifschitz et al., 1973)	Neostigmine (Roberts et al., 1965)
N'-Methylnicotinamide (Sperber, 1948; Beyer et al., 1950)	Quinine (Torretti et al., 1962)
Norepinephrine (Rennick and Pryor, 1965)	Tetraethylammonium (Rennick et al., 1947, 1954)
Serotonin (Sanner and Wortman, 1962)	
Thiamine (Rennick, 1958)	Tolazoline (Orloff et al., 1953)
Tyramine (Quebbemann and Rennick, 1969)	Amprolium (Beyer and Gelarden, 1975)

II. METHODS TO STUDY RENAL TUBULAR TRANSPORT AND METABOLISM *IN VIVO*

A. Sperber Technique in Chickens

An accessory renal portal circulation in birds makes it possible to administer substances to the renal tubules of one kidney and to recognize tubular secretion rate without concern for plasma protein binding or glomerular filtration rate. Sperber (1946; 1947; 1948a,b; Lindahl and Sperber, 1956) designed this *in vivo* experimental technique in chickens in which substrates are infused directly into a saphenous vein in the leg. The saphenous blood goes to the renal portal circulation and bathes the renal tubules on the infused side (Figure 1). Urine is collected separately from each kidney. Any infused substrate which enters the ipsilateral renal portal circulation and which is secreted by the renal tubules will appear in the urine from the ipsilateral kidney in excess of that appearing in the urine from the contralateral kidney. The expression for the excess excreted from the infused kidney was described by Sperber in the following way: *ATEF* (apparent tubular excretion fraction) = $(E - C)/I$, where E is the rate of excretion from infused kidney, C is that excreted from the control kidney, and I is the rate of infusion. If the infused substance is excreted by the renal tubules, there will be a greater amount in the urine from the infused kidney than from the uninfused kidney. Any infused substance that escapes excretion from the infused kidney tubules will enter the systemic circulation and be recirculated to both kidneys equally. The amount excreted by the control kidney is subtracted from the infused-kidney excretion, and the difference is the minimal amount excreted by the tubules of the infused kidney. This correction takes care of the amount

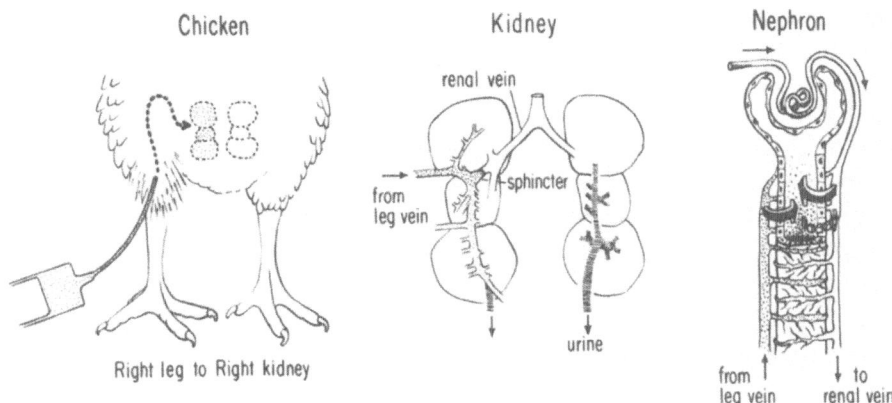

Figure 1. Infusion into a leg vein will flow to the kidney of the infused side. Infusion will then bathe the peritubular capilary network of that kidney. Transportable substrates will enter the urine on the infused side. The infused substance will not reach the glomerulus of the infused kidney. (Reprinted from Acara *et al.*, 1973.)

added by glomerular filtration and any tubular contribution to the control urine. The excess recovered from the infused kidney was added by the tubule and plasma protein binding is of no concern. No plasma assays are necessary. Experimentally it is necessary to coadminister a marker to determine the amount of infusion reaching the kidney. For example, if one is studying the transport of an experimental organic cation, the simultaneous transport of an organic anion such as PAH is measured. A selective inhibition of the cation by a cation competitor, while the anion continues to be transported, indicates that there is a selective effect on tubular transport of the cation and no decrease in blood supply. However, if both the organic cation and organic anion transports are inhibited, it is not possible to distinguish between an inhibition of transport and a diversion of the infusion through a venous bypass away from the kidney.

The Sperber technique provides some unique advantages. Studies can be performed with infusion of extremely small amounts of very potent physiologically active substances. For example, radioactively labeled norepinephrine can be administered in amounts of 10^{-9} mol per minute and its tubular transport can be measured without complicating cardiovascular effects. In this *in vivo* system the material is infused into a sequestered pool where the material moves from the saphenous vein directly to the renal parenchyma and out through the renal pelvis to be excreted. Hence, little of the infused material is available to the central circulation, and the low concentrations used do not produce any untoward effects on the renal circulation. Thus, it is possible to investigate such things as norepinephrine transport *in vivo* without its disturbing circulatory effects.

Another unique advantage of this preparation relates to the study of renal metabolism *in vivo*. The ATEF gives a measure of the substrate which is transported by the renal tubule of the infused kidney when the substrate makes its first trip through that kidney. The subtraction of the excretion from the contralateral or control uninfused kidney ensures that the remainder represents only the substrate transported by the ipsilateral renal tubule on the first trip past the tissue. When the urine is examined for the infused substrate and its metabolites, the metabolites excreted in excess on the infused side represent only the metabolites produced intrarenally. No consideration of extrarenal metabolites complicates this observation. Furthermore, it is possible to secure information about the capacities *in vivo* of certain renal metabolic pathways and to assess the effects of drugs and chemicals on the activity of certain renal enzymes.

B. Intrarenal Artery Injection in the Dog

Infusion of substrates into one renal artery, with collection of urine from the kidneys separately, permits the study of renal metabolism of the substrates. If inulin and PAH are simultaneously infused, comparison of the excretion of the test substrate with these markers of filtration and renal plasma flow will permit easy recognition of tubular excretion (Rennick *et al.*, 1947). Metabolites recovered from the urine from the infused kidney in excess of those from the control urine represent metabolites formed by the kidney. A word of caution: Mixing of the infusion stream with the renal blood stream may be incomplete. Brand and Cohen (1972) have observed that complete mixing occurred in dogs only at infusion rates into the renal artery above 50 ml/min.

C. Stop-Flow Pattern

The site along the nephron at which transport is occurring may be identified by stop-flow techniques. To avoid extrarenal metabolism and systemic effects of the substrate, the test substance is injected into the renal artery during ureteral occlusion (Rennick and Moe, 1960). (See the Chapter 12 for discussion of this method.)

III. RENAL TUBULAR EXCRETION AND METABOLISM OF BIOGENIC CATIONS

A. Catecholamines: Epinephrine, Norepinephrine, Dopamine, Isoproterenol

Many observations have been published on the excretion of catecholamines and their metabolites into the urine under varying conditions. The catecholamines are cations at body pH with pK's around 9. The mechanisms for excretion include glomerular filtration and active proximal tubular excretion. Passive diffusion from lumen to blood of these cations in the distal tubule would be unlikely. This discussion will focus on the evidence for the mechanisms which regulate catecholamine excretion by the kidney and the renal pathways for metabolism of catecholamines.

First, evidence that the catecholamines are excreted by the proximal renal tubule actively as cations will be presented. Using the Sperber technique in unanesthetized chickens, there was evidence *in vivo* that epinephrine, norepinephrine, dopamine, and isoproterenol were actively excreted by the renal tubule when infused intravenously into the renal portal circulation to steady state at loads of 1×10^{-9} mol/min (0.07 μg/kg·min) (Table II) (Quebbemann and Rennick, 1969; Rennick and Yoss, 1962; Rennick *et al.*, 1965). The rate of tubular transport was about 65% that of PAH being transported simultaneously. Competitive inhibition studies revealed that the active transport mechanism was that for the organic cation. Cyanine-863 and quinine, two cations which are selective and potent competitive inhibitors of the organic cation transport system, inhibited catecholamine excretion.

A study of the metabolites in the urine following [^{14}C]epinephrine infusion into the renal portal circulation in chickens revealed that about 75% of the epinephrine was secreted by the infused kidney without being metabolized (Rennick *et al.*, 1965). Simultaneously, *O*-methylated, deaminated, and conjugated metabolites were excreted in excess by the infused kidney in small amounts. This was evidence that these metabolites were formed by the infused kidney. Similar results occurred during norepinephrine infusion.

Binding of these catecholamines to plasma protein was studied by ultrafiltration (Rennick, 1968). Binding was quantitatively similar in dog and chicken plasma. The values for binding were: Dopamine, 50%; epinephrine, 22%; norepinephrine, 35%; tetraethylammonium was not bound. The plasma binding of catecholamines will reduce the filtered load of catecholamines. Thus, tubular active secretion becomes a greater portion of the observed excretion rate.

During dopamine infusion into one renal artery in a dog at 9×10^{-10} mol/min (0.016 μg/kg·min) (Table II) (Rennick, 1968), the infused kidney excreted dopamine at a rate 50% that of simultaneously infused *p*-aminohippuric acid. If

Table II. Studies of Renal Tubular Excretion of Catecholamines

Investigator	Administration Route	Rate, μg/kg·min[a]	Evidence for renal tubular excretion
Jones and Blake, 1958	i.v., dog	1.7, E	+
Rennick and Yoss, 1962	renal–portal, chicken	0.24, E	+
Overy *et al.*, 1967	i.v., dog	0.00003, NE	0
Rennick, 1968	Renal artery	0.016, D	+
Quebbemann and Rennick, 1969	renal–portal, chicken	0.07, E, NE, D	+
Gryglewski and Vane, 1970	Aorta, dog	1.7, Iso	+
Lifschitz *et al.*, 1973	Renal artery, dog	0.009, Iso	+
Hempel *et al.*, 1973	Renal artery, dog, stop-flow	0.36, E, NE, D	0
Hempel *et al.*, 1974	Renal artery dog, single injection	0.33, E, total	+

[a] E = epinephrine; NE = norepinephrine; D = dopamine; Iso = isoproterenol.

the filtration fraction were 0.2, and the plasma binding of dopamine were 50%, about 45% of the excreted dopamine must have been derived from the tubules. This constituted evidence that dopamine was excreted by the renal tubules in the dog. Under similar experimental conditions epinephrine was excreted at a rate 60% that of simultaneous PAH excretion.

Schrier has studied the mechanism of the renal clearance of isoproterenol in the dog in some detail. In his studies of the role of the β-adrenergic receptor in salt and water excretion by the kidney, he observed that isoproterenol caused an increase in cardiac output when given intravenously, but the same dose of isoproterenol caused no change in cardiac output when given into the renal artery (Schrier *et al.*, 1972). This suggested that isoproterenol was in large part either metabolized or excreted in one passage through the kidney. Similarly Gryglewski and Vane (1970) (Table II), in studying the inactivation of noradrenaline, epinephrine, and isoproterenol in various vascular beds in dogs, concluded that when infusions were made just before the renal arteries there was a much greater removal of catecholamines from the circulation than when they were introduced at other points in the circulation. Schrier's group (Lifschitz *et al.*, 1973) studied the mechanism of isoproterenol excretion in dogs. They found that the renal clearance of isoproterenol was greater than the clearance of inulin but less than that of PAH. They infused 0.009 μg/kg·min (Table II) of isoproterenol into one renal artery. The ratio of renal clearance of isoproterenol to inulin was 1.38. The renal venous extraction of isoproterenol was 0.64. Studies with cocaine, a cationic competitor for transport (Quebbemann and Rennick, 1970), indicated that isoproterenol was being transported by the organic cation mechanism. Since isoproterenol is bound to plasma protein, the actual tubular contribution is greater than indicated by the clearance ratio. The metabolites of isoproterenol were not identified. These *in vivo* experiments clearly indicated renal tubular transport of catecholamines.

Recently Hempel *et al.* (1973) have measured the excretion of catecholamines using a modified stop-flow technique. During occlusion of the ureter, catecholamines were infused into the renal artery at a rate of 0.26–0.47 μg/kg·min (Table II) along with inulin. The ureter was released after 2 min, and fractional urine collections were made for the ensuing 8 min. The catecholamine infusion was continued throughout the collections. The extraction of unmetabolized catecholamines into the urine never exceeded the rate of extraction of inulin. The percent of unmetabolized dopamine and adrenaline excreted from the infused, ureter-occluded kidney was equal to the inulin excretion. The percent of dopamine and adrenaline excreted as *O*-methylated metabolites was twice that of those unmetabolized. These findings were interpreted to mean the following:

1. The dog kidney showed no net tubular excretion of unmetabolized catecholamines.
2. The infused kidney metabolized a large part of the catecholamines to *O*-methylated metabolites.
3. These metabolites entered the urine readily.
4. Only renal metabolites are excreted into the urine by the tubule.

Other aspects which were not considered were:

1. Any binding to plasma proteins would enhance the fraction of the catecholamine clearance that was a function of tubular excretion.
2. A product made by the tubule cell cannot properly be proposed as a simple tubular transport function. A new species made in the tubule cell might diffuse out since it will necessarily have a downhill gradient from cell to urine.

Hempel's group explored tubular transport of catecholamines in another group of experiments using dogs (Hempel *et al.*, 1974). Injections of [^{14}C]adrenaline and [^{3}H]inulin were given into both renal arteries. Injections were completed in 15 sec. Adrenaline was given in a dose of 9.3 μg as free base. Urine was analyzed for catecholamines, both unmetabolized and metabolized. In the chicken it was clear that the kidney tubule actively excreted unmetabolized catecholamines at a high rate, nearly as great as PAH. The mammal may have a high catechol-*O*-methyltransferase (COMT) activity in the kidney. In these experiments Hempel infused a COMT inhibitor to reduce metabolism.

The excretion of unmetabolized adrenaline increased several-fold after COMT inhibitors were given, and metanephrine excretion decreased. Since the COMT inhibitor did not affect glomerular filtration rate, it was concluded that the increased excretion of unmetabolized adrenaline was occurring by tubular excretion. They concluded that *O*-methylation cannot be a prerequisite for tubular excretion of catecholamines.

These results suggest tubular excretion of free catecholamines but did not provide data showing free catecholamine extraction greater than inulin extraction.

There are a few technical features that might be considered:

1. The single-shot technique of administration may be less satisfactory than a constant infusion to a steady state. The catecholamines are avidly taken up by tissues and metabolized, and during the rapidly changing levels brought about by a single injection, these simultaneous dispositions are going on at varying rates.
2. No consideration was given to plasma protein binding, which affects glomerular filtration of catecholamines.
3. COMT inhibitors may affect the tubular transport rate of the unmetabolized catecholamines.
4. Anesthesia may affect the excretion of catecholamines.

The earliest observation of tubular excretion of catecholamines in the dog was made by Jones and Blake, (1958). They infused *l*-epinephrine intravenously at rates of 0.87–2.67 μg/kg·min (Table II). They measured the urinary clearance of epinephrine by a fluorometric method and found it to be greater than the simultaneous clearance of exogenous creatinine. The clearance ratio of epinephrine to inulin was 1.64 ± 0.08 in nine experiments in six dogs.

Overy *et al.* (1967) studied norepinephrine clearance in dogs following intravenous infusion of 0.00003 μg/kg·min (Table II). They found norepinephrine clearance to be 64% of glomerular filtration rate when they extracted free catecholamine in urine and plasma using alumina columns. The monoamine oxidase inhibitor, Catron, and exogenous creatinine were added in their experiments. Catron is capable of inhibiting the renal tubular transport of norepinephrine in the chicken (Rennick and Pryor, 1965). Caution is necessary in using exogenous creatinine since it is transported itself by the organic cation transport mechanism (Rennick, 1967) and can inhibit tubular excretion of catecholamines. Overy *et al.* (1967) reported that there was no plasma binding of norepinephrine. The amount of norepinephrine infused was exceedingly small and would probably be subjected to extensive deposition and metabolism. They found only 9% of the administered label as unmetabolized norepinephrine in the urine.

B. Plasma Protein Binding of Catecholamines

Catecholamines interact at various sites, such as receptor sites in effector cells, in transport systems, on membranes, and on enzymes. Catecholamines may also react at nonaction sites such as those on serum and tissue proteins, with the result that these sites regulate the rate of transport of catecholamines to various tissues and the rate of elimination from the body (Gillette, 1973).

Understanding the mechanism of renal excretion of catecholamines will ultimately depend on the ability to measure with confidence catecholamines that are plasma protein bound and hence not filterable so that a value may be assigned to the fraction that is transported by the tubules. Another aspect of protein binding that may be related to the transport function of the tubules is the ability of plasma protein-bound catecholamines to dissociate while passing the proximal tubule cells to enter into the tubular excretory transport pathway. Such functional details are not yet certain, even for well-studied molecules such as PAH and phenol red (Goldstein *et al.,* 1974).

There is growing evidence that catecholamines bind to plasma protein or to protein fractions. The experimental data is of such a varied nature that it cannot with certainty be applied to the present physiological problem, which is to specify the amount of binding of catecholamines to plasma protein *in vivo* that will prevent filtration or that will affect dissociation at the peritubular site of the proximal tubule. In Table III data from the literature is summarized to describe plasma binding of catecholamines. Various techniques were applied and various goals were given attention in these studies. The only generalization that might be plucked from the data in Table III that will begin to elucidate that problem of catecholamine filtration rate is the fact that values from 12 to 50% are reported for binding of epinephrine and norepinephrine to whole plasma. The various species and experimental techniques make real quantitative comparisons impossible at the present.

If, as suggested by this data, catecholamines are bound to plasma proteins, tubular excretion of catecholamines may account for a significant fraction of excretion, since the filtered load of catecholamines becomes a diminished portion of the catecholamine excretion.

To summarize the situation concerning renal tubular excretion of catechola-

Table III. Catecholamine Binding Studies

Investigator	Catecholamine binding, %[a]	Experimental concentration, M	Species
Antoniades et al., 1958			Human
Mirkin et al., 1966	NE		Human
Rennick, 1968	E (22), NE (35), D (50), TEA (0)	10^{-10}	Dog, chicken
Cohen et al., 1968	E, NE	10^{-6}	Rabbit
Franksson and Anggaard, 1970	E (23), NE (12), D, MET, NMET	10^{-6}	Human
Bryson and Bishoff, 1970	D	10^{-5}	
Zia et al., 1971	E	10^{-1}	BSA
Danon and Sapira, 1972	E, NE, D, ISO	10^{-6}–10^{-8}	HSA
Russell and Doty, 1972	E (50), NE	10^{-9}	Human
Russel and Doty, 1973	E, NE, D	10^{-9}	Human
May et al., 1974	NE	10^{-8}	Human
Branco et al., 1974	NE (57–67)	10^{-6}	Dog

[a] Same as Table II and in addition: TEA = tetraethylammonium; MET = metanephrine; NMET = normetanephrine.

mines, it can be said that catecholamines are excreted by the renal tubule when the catecholamines are administered into the renal artery in dogs or into the renal portal circulation in chickens. Renal metabolism of catecholamines occurs simultaneously to a variable extent depending on the loads offered. The polar anionic metabolites are excreted by the renal tubule by the anion transport system.

Some confusion arose in the past when the identification of the transport mechanisms was investigated by the use of competitive blocking agents. The catecholamine molecule is a zwitterion, existing as a cation at body pH. Studies in which probenecid was found to block the tubular transport of catecholamines were misinterpreted to mean that the catecholamine was being transported as an anion perhaps at the catechol end of the molecule. A more likely explanation is that a portion of the catecholamine was deaminated to an anion or conjugated with glucuronides to form polar anions. These anionic fractions were being transported across the renal tubule and were being blocked by probenecid, the anionic blocker. When amounts of catecholamine are administered to the kidney that are transported predominantly without metabolism or conjugation, the catecholamines are transported as cations and are inhibited only by competitors of cationic transport.

To be able to define the relative proportion of glomerular filtration of catecholamines and tubular active transport depends on reliable values for plasma protein binding to assess the filtered load of catecholamines. The few studies now available give evidence of some plasma protein binding of catecholamines. Further careful studies will be necessary to give reliable values. The plasma binding of catecholamines *in vivo* and then the proportion of tubular excretion may be assigned. From the studies now available in chicken and dog, it is certain that tubular excretion of catecholamines is a major route of excretion when sufficient unmetabolized catecholamine is administered to the renal circulation to exceed metabolism. The studies on isoproterenol provided a clearcut demonstration of tubular excretion of cationic isoproterenol. The metabolic fate of catecholamines will need to be studied for each catecholamine at various exogenous loads. Conway *et al.* (1968) have examined isoproterenol metabolism in a thorough fashion, but they did not differentiate between metabolites formed by the kidney and metabolites formed extrarenally. Such studies, although tedious, will provide an interesting picture of the dynamics of renal transport and renal metabolism.

C. Choline

Choline, a quaternary ammonium ion, is a biologically active cationic substance which is freely filterable and may be excreted by the renal tubule. The renal clearance of free choline at endogenous plasma levels of about $2 \times 10^{-5} M$ was only 1/30 that of the glomerular filtration rate in dogs, chickens, rats, and humans. The response of the kidney tubule to exogenous loads of choline was studied using the Sperber technique in hens (Acara and Rennick, 1972a). At low infusion rates of [^{14}C]choline, the ^{14}C label was not excreted by the renal tubule attached to choline. Analysis of the urine during infusions of choline revealed that at low loads, the infused choline has been largely metabolized by the kidney to betaine and another unidentified metabolite. Betaine is produced by the action of choline oxidase and betaine aldehyde dehydrogenase. When betaine itself was infused, it was not excreted by the renal tubules. As the rate of choline infusion was increased, tubular excretion of choline began when the plasma choline concentration was doubled. Increasing loads of choline resulted in proportionally more tubular transport of choline until, at plasma levels that were ten times that of the endogenous levels, the tubular transport system for choline was saturated and a *Tm* (transport maximum) was apparent. The *Tm* for choline was reached at infusion loads of 2×10^{-6} mol/kg·min, and the amount transported at the *Tm* was 1.2×10^{-6} mol/kg·min. It was clear from these results that the kidney reduces the level of plasma choline by tubular transport when choline levels in plasma are elevated.

Qualitatively and quantitatively similar results were obtained in experiments on dogs with intrarenal artery infusions of [^{14}C]choline (Acara and Rennick, 1973).

To summarize: At endogenous levels of plasma choline most of the filtered choline is reabsorbed by the nephron. The label from tracer amounts of choline infused into the renal portal circulation appeared in the urine only as renal metabolites. The disposition of the choline reabsorbed from the filtrate cannot at the present time be described.

When the plasma choline level doubles, renal tubular excretion occurs in addition to glomerular filtration. At plasma levels 10-fold greater than endogenous levels, a T_m for choline is reached. Thus it is apparent that renal excretory regulation is a homeostatic control to stabilize plasma choline levels *in vivo*. As the plasma choline level rises, the urinary clearance of choline rises, demonstrating a negative feedback to maintain a stable plasma choline level.

Furthermore, the extraurinary clearance decreases as this level rises, indicating a positive feedback. A possible explanation for this seemingly inappropriate regulating mechanism is that the proportion of choline metabolized and taken up by tissues falls as choline levels rise (Acara, 1975).

IV. BIDIRECTIONAL TUBULAR TRANSPORT OF CHOLINE

Studies on the excretion of choline at varying plasma choline levels suggested that choline may be actively transported in both the direction of excretion and reabsorption; this was referred to as bidirectional transport (Acara and Rennick, 1973). Bidirectional transport has been demonstrated for several anions. Uric acid (Zins and Weiner, 1968a), m-hydroxybenzoate, (May and Weiner, 1970), and taurocholate (Zins and Weiner, 1968b) gave experimental evidence in dogs of bidirectional transport. It was suggested that PAH is transported bidirectionally in *Necturus* and in rats (Tanner, 1966; Baines and Gottschalk, 1968). Recent evidence suggests that amino acids share bidirectional transport in the rat kidney (Their, 1974).

Bidirectional transport of choline was evident from the following experimental findings. Secretory transport was demonstrated in the loading studies in chickens and dogs. Reabsorptive transport was demonstrated by clearance measurements in dogs, chickens, rats, and humans. At endogenous levels of free choline, the renal clearance of choline was only 1/30 that of the GFR. Filtered choline is always ionized at body pH because the pK_a choline is 13.4. Choline is not bound to plasma protein and is freely filterable. Thus the removal of choline from the filtrate must occur by active transport out of the lumen.

Such bidirectional transports may operate as part of a feedback system to maintain a relatively constant concentration of plasma choline. At elevated plasma choline levels the tubule can excrete additional choline to reduce the plasma choline level, and at low plasma choline levels the tubule recaptures filtered choline to be returned to body stores.

In support of this concept, it is known that endogenous plasma levels of free choline are maintained at a stable level of about 2×10^{-5} M in several species (Bligh, 1952). This constant value was maintained in the face of attempts to load the animals with choline (Bligh, 1953). In this homeostatic regulation of plasma choline levels it is clear from recent observations that the kidney plays a role. Reid Hunt (1915) was aware of the rapid disposition of exogenous choline when injected intravenously. Gardiner and Paton (1972) observed plasma disappearance rates in the cat.

The concept of bidirectional transport of choline may explain a rather unexpected experimental finding. During the administration of a load of choline, which is near the load producing maximum transport, the infusion of an extremely small load of another cation in the amount of 1×10^{-15} mol/min produced an increase in the rate of choline excretion of about 25–30%. One group of experiments demonstrated enhanced choline excretion during the addition of the cation, hemicholinium (HC-3) (Acara *et al.,* 1973). One means of explaining this enhanced choline excretion is based on the bidirectional movement of choline. If the reabsorptive transport were more sensitive to inhibition, the low amounts of added HC-3 would enhance the excretion of choline. HC-3 at low loads enhanced choline excretion and at high loads inhibited choline excretion (Trimble *et al.,* 1974). HC-3 will also enhance the excretion of acetycholine. Triethylcholine (TEC), (triethylethanolamine) will enhance the excretion of choline or acetycholine when added at the lower loads of 1×10^{-15} mol/min and conversely will decrease the excretion of choline and acetycholine when administered at loads of 1×10^{-6} mol/min (Acara *et al.,* 1975).

The analogy of these responses to that which occurs with uric acid bidirectional transport is apparent. Uric acid excretion is reduced with addition of low loads of other anions, such as probenecid or salicylates, and is increased with large loads. The common interpretation is that the uric acid is subject to bidirectional transport. The secretory transport is thought to be inhibited selectively at the lower loads of added anion thus reducing the excretion. Higher loads of added anion also block the reabsorptive transport and result in enhanced excretion, called the uricosuric effect. The response of choline excretion to low and high loads of another cation is reversed, low doses increase excretion and high doses inhibit excretion. Figure 2 compares in graphic form the relation of excretion of uric acid and choline to various loads of another substrate.

V. TUBULAR EXCRETION AND RENAL METABOLISM OF MORPHINE

Using the Sperber technique in chickens, the cationic drug morphine was actively transported by the proximal tubule and a morphine metabolite was formed during transport by the infused kidney (May *et al.,* 1967). Fujimoto and Haarstad (1969) characterized the metabolite as morphine ethereal sulfate (MES). A cationic competitor, cyanine-863, inhibited the tubular transport of morphine and simultaneously reduced the excretion of the anionic metabolite. Probenecid, the anion competitor, had no effect on the transport of either the morphine or its anion metabolite (Watrous *et al.,* 1970). This led to the interpretation that the morphine was transported into the cell as a cation and that the cationic competitor cyanine-863 blocked the entry into the cell and resulted in a reduced synthesis of the metabolite, MES (Figure 3).

MES was prepared and infused into the renal portal circulation of a chicken. It was transported actively by a probenecid-sensitive transcellular transport but was not inhibited by cationic competitors. Thus the MES was traversing an anionic transport system. It was concluded that probenecid must act on the peritubular side of the cell, since it blocked transtubular transport of infused

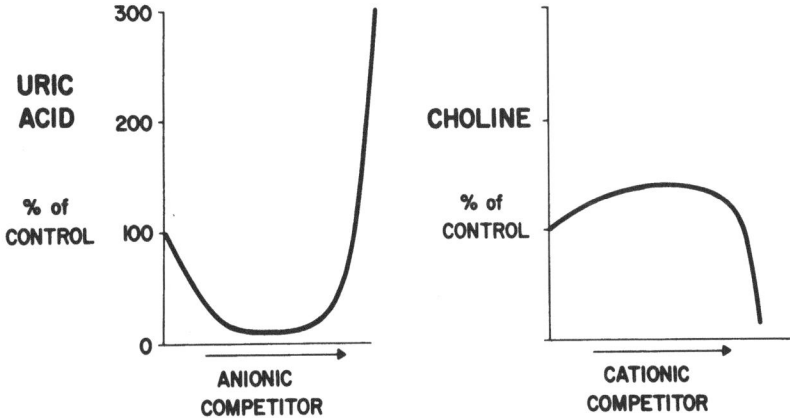

Figure 2. Biphasic response of renal clearance at high and low loads of competitor. The drawing on the left is redrawn from Fanelli and Weiner, 1973. The choline curve on the right is our own data. The anionic competitor was pyrazinamide. The cationic competitor was triethylethanolamine (TEC) triethylcholine.

MES but did not block luminal transport of MES formed within the renal cell from morphine (Watrous *et al.*, 1970).

Hakim and Fujimoto (1971) reported that β-diethylaminoethyl diphenylpropylacetate (SKF 525A) and *N*-methyl-3-piperidyl-*N'*,*N'*-diphenylcarbamate (MPDC) blocked the transport of morphine into the renal tubule cell with the

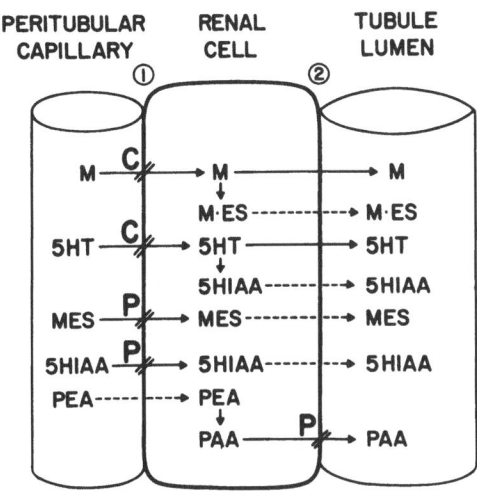

Figure 3. A summary of the data cited in the text. A transport step may occur at sites 1 and 2. The transport of the cations M (morphine) and 5HT (5-hydroxytryptamine) is blocked by C (cyanine-863, a cationic competitor). C did not block the transport of the cation PEA (phenylethylamine). The anionic metabolite of PEA was PAA (phenylacetic acid). The exit of PAA from the site of synthesis in the cell was blocked by the anionic competitor P (probenecid). This suggests that a transport step exists for anions on the luminal side of the proximal renal tubule cell. Probenecid failed to block the exit of MES (morphine ethereal sulfate) and 5HIAA (5-hydroxyindolacetic acid) from the site of synthesis in the cell, but probenecid did block the transcellular transport of MES and 5HIAA, indicating a transport block at the peritubular side of the cell.

result that excretion of morphine and MES was reduced. Diethylaminoethanol also decreased the transport of morphine into the renal cell and thus reduced the excretion of MES formed in the kidney (Fujimoto *et al.*, 1972).

A similar model was developed for 5-hydroxytryptamine (5-HT) (Figure 3). Sanner and Wortman (1962) described the tubular transport of 5-HT using the Sperber technique. Hakim *et al.* (1970) established that 5-HT transport occurred by a cationic mechanism and that the renal cell metabolized a considerable part of the 5-HT to 5-hydroxyindolacetic acid (5-HIAA). Anionic competitors blocked the tubular transport of 5-HIAA infused into the renal portal circulation, but they did not block the excretion of 5-HIAA formed within the renal cell, again suggesting that the transport site was on the peritubular side of the cell.

Novobiocin acted as an anionic competitor for the transtubular transport of MES and 5-HIAA, but had no blocking effect on these substances when formed in the renal cell (Fujimoto *et al.*, 1973). Furthermore, novobiocin had no effect on the tubular transport of morphine or 5-HT, but it did block PAH transport. These findings suggested that novobiocin acts similarly to probenecid in that it blocks the transtubular transport of anions, but not the exit of anions formed in the tubular cell, again suggesting that the transport step for anions is on the peritubular side of the cell.

Other studies using the Sperber technique suggest a different location for the anion transport step. Infusion of the cation [^{14}C]phenylethylamine resulted in active transport of the attached label. Probenecid inhibited this transport, but quinine did not (Quebbemann and Rennick, 1970) (Figure 3). Urine analysis revealed that the renal tubule had metabolized most of the PEA to the anion, phenylacetic acid (PAA). This evidence that intrarenally formed anionic PAA is sensitive to inhibition by probenecid indicates a transport step for anions at the luminal border. An attractive argument to support the idea that there is an active transport site for anions on the luminal side of the cell is based on findings that anion conjugates, such as glucuronides which are formed in the renal cell, have been associated with accelerated excretion from the body. It would seem inefficient to produce a detoxifying conjugate within the cell and then to have a barrier on the luminal border to reduce its exit.

Thus it can be concluded that there is evidence for anionic transport sites on the peritubular side of the cell in the case of exogenously administered MES and 5-HIAA and on the luminal side of the cell in the case of intrarenally formed PAA. It could be that there are anion transport steps on both sides of the cell. Perhaps the transport capacity of the renal cell is greater for some substrates at the luminal border, and this would make it more difficult to reach the saturating concentration with the competitor to result in inhibition of transport.

VI. TUBULAR EXCRETION AND RENAL METABOLISM OF CATECHOL

Sperber (1948a) demonstrated renal formation and excretion of sulfate and glucuronide conjugates of 1,2-dihydroxybenzene (catechol) in the chicken. In an attempt to identify the structural factors which produced differences in transport of catecholamines, Quebbemann and Rennick (1968) investigated the renal transport of catechol. Using the Sperber technique in hens, the ^{3}H label from infused [^{3}H]catechol was actively excreted into the urine. The excess ^{3}H label appearing in the urine from the infused kidney was identified as being two thirds glucuronide and one third sulfate conjugates. The excess of conjugates on the infused side indicated that the kidney was the site of glucuronide and sulfate conjugation. Organic cation and organic anion transport inhibitors had no effect on the formation and excretion of these renal conjugates. However, when preformed catechol glucuronide and catechol sulfate were infused into the renal portal circulation, their excretory transports were inhibited by probenecid. Catechol is a weak acid with a pK_a of 9.85 and would not be ionized at cell or urine pH. Entry into the renal cell by organic ion transport is therefore not possible. The fact that probenecid blocks the transcellular transport of pre- formed catechol glucuronide and catechol sulfate, but not the transport across the luminal membrane of catechol glucuronide and sulfate formed within the proximal renal tubule cell, may be interpreted as evidence for a probenecid- sensitive active transport step for anions at the peritubular membrane.

Experiments in dogs, in which catechol was injected into the renal artery, indicated that the dog kidney excretes catechol only after conjugating it to the ethereal sulfate. In stop-flow experiments in which radiolabeled catechol and phenol were injected into the renal artery during ureteral occlusion, radioactive catechol sulfate and phenyl sulfate were excreted at a tubular site distal to the excretory site for simultaneously administered PAH. In contrast, preformed catechol glucuronide and preformed catechol sulfate were excreted at a site identical to that for PAH excretion (Rennick and Quebbemann, 1970).

Further studies on the renal excretion of catechol analogs, phenol (pK_a 9.89) and p-nitrophenol (PNP) (pK_a 7.15), revealed that these compounds were also conjugated to the glucuronide and sulfate and excreted as the conjugate by the chicken kidney (Quebbemann and Anders, 1971, 1973). Phenol does not appear to occupy either the organic cation or the organic anion excretory transport system and appears to be handled in a manner similar to that of catechol. Renal excretion of PNP was not altered by the organic cation inhibitor, quinine, but was decreased by organic anion inhibitors. High doses of probenecid, which completely blocked PAH excretion, produced a maximum inhibition of approximately 50% of PNP excretion. This was quantitatively similar to the maximum inhibition of PNP excretion produced by high doses of PAH. It was not possible to completely block the excretion of PNP with either of these inhibitors.

Studies on the competition of catechol, phenol, PNP, and morphine for renal conjugation have shown that catechol, phenol, and PNP compete with each other for conjugation. These studies also show that phenol or PNP can completely block the renal conjugation of morphine but that morphine blocks only a portion of PNP conjugation and has virtually no effect on the conjugation of phenol. The small and insignificant effect of morphine on phenol conjugation and excretion is similar to the lack of effect of morphine on catechol conjugation and excretion reported by Watrous and Fujimoto (1971).

Quebbemann and Anders (1971, 1973) proposed a model as a possible explanation for (1) the differences in inhibition by transport competitors of renal excretion of weak organic anions which are conjugated within renal tubular cells, (2) the differences in competition between ionized and un-ionized substrates for renal sulfate and glucuronide conjugating mechanisms, and (3) the differences in the site of excretion of un-ionized catechol and phenol from the site of excretion of organic ions in stop-flow experiments in the dog. The model assumes (a) that organic anion and organic cation excretory transports are located at the peritubular membrane, (b) that un-ionized molecules enter the renal tubular cells by mechanisms which are separable from organic ion transports, and (c) that sulfate and glucuronide conjugations in the renal tubule are not limited to the cells having organic ion excretory transports at their peritubular membrane.

Figure 4 illustrates the proposed movement of the weak organic anions catechol, phenol, and PNP, as well as the organic cation morphine, across the peritubular border into the renal cell. According to this model, diffusion of un-ionized molecules and active transport of ionized molecules of the same drug would coexist in cell having organic ion excretory transports at the peritubular membrane (cell type I). Cells not having organic ion excretory transports at the

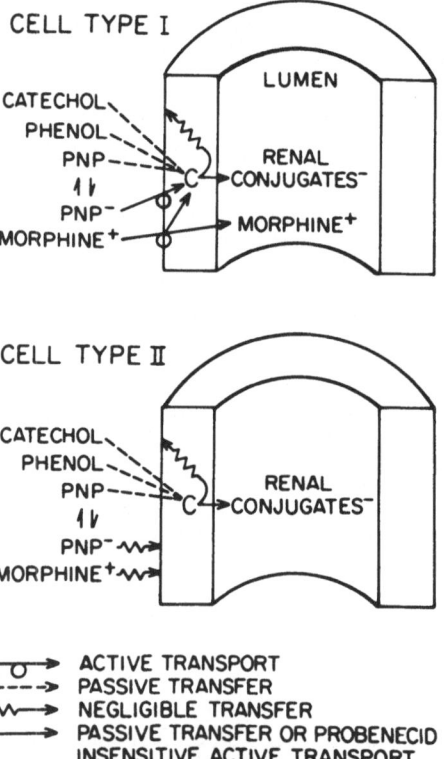

Figure 4. Renal excretory transfer of ionized and un-ionized substrates for sulfate- and glucuronide-conjugating enzymes (C) in renal tubular cells which have organic ion excretory transports at the peritubular membrane (cell type I) and in cells which lack these transports (cell type II). (From Quebbemann and Anders, 1973.)

peritubular membrane (cell type II) would only permit the passive entry of un-ionized molecules. Weak anions which are partially ionized at physiologic pH might use both active and passive processes to move across the peritubular membrane. Phenol and catechol, which are less than 1% ionized at the pH of blood in the chicken, would enter the cell almost entirely by diffusion. PNP is approximately 71% ionized at this pH and, therefore, a larger fraction could enter the cell by occupying an active organic anion transport mechanism. Morphine, which is essentially entirely ionized at physiological pH, would enter the cell only by the organic cation transport system.

The lack of effect of probenecid on catechol and phenol excretion as well as the selective inhibition of PNP excretion by probenecid and PAH may be explained on the basis that movement of weak anions into the renal tubular cells at the peritubular border may be different for the ionized and un-ionized forms of the test compound. A weak organic anion such as PNP may enter the renal cells at the peritubular membrane as organic anions and independently by some other mechanism. The latter mechanism may be passive diffusion of the un-ionized form of the compound and, as such, would not be subject to inhibition by organic ion transport inhibitors acting at the peritubular membrane. The differences in the inhibition of renal conjugating enzymes by catechol, morphine, phenol, and PNP may be explained by assuming separate mechanisms for entry into the cell for ionized and un-ionized molecules at the peritubular membrane. Un-ionized catechol and phenol theoretically could enter cells which have organic ion transports as well as cells which lack these transports. Morphine, present in blood almost entirely as a cation, would primarily enter the cells having organic cation transport and consequently would compete effectively for conjugation with only a portion of catechol. the greater effect of morphine on PNP conjugation and excretion than on phenol or catechol conjugation and excretion can be explained by the fact that both organic cations and organic anions are known to be actively transported in the direction of excretion in the proximal tubule (Wilde and Malvin, 1958; Rennick and Moe, 1960). The ionized fraction of PNP would ensure a higher concentration of PNP in cells having organic ion transports than in cells lacking them. Presumably, cationic morphine would be transported selectively into these same cells resulting in a greater inhibition of PNP conjugation and excretion than that observed for phenol.

The differences in the apparent site of excretion of catechol and phenol from the site of excretion of organic ions in stop-flow experiments support the concept that conjugation and excretion of un-ionized compounds may occur in a portion of the tubule distal to that for organic ion excretion.

The model suggests that the peritubular membrane is relatively impermeable to the exit of sulfate and glucuronide conjugates formed within the renal tubular cells and that there exists a probenecid-insensitive transport mechanism at the luminal membrane which actively extrudes the renal conjugates. The concept that the peritubular membrane is less permeable than the luminal membrane to the exit of sulfate and glucuronide conjugates is supported by the fact that probenecid does not inhibit the excretion of renal sulfate and glucuronide conjugates of phenol and catechol. If the exit of conjugates from the renal tubular cells could occur freely both into urine and blood, appreciable amounts of renal conjugates of these compounds would be released from the cells back into the circulation, and their subsequent renal excretory transport would be inhibited by probenecid.

VII. ISOLATION OF A RENAL CARRIER PROTEIN FOR ORGANIC CATIONS

Active-site labeling of organic cation transport has been explored by the use of irreversible inhibitors (Ross *et al.*, 1968). Two β-haloalkylamines, dibenamine and dibenzyline, were found to be specific inhibitors of the renal uptake *in vitro* of the organic cation N'-methylnicotinamide (NMN) and tetraethylammonium (TEA). The blockade of uptake was found to be irreversible. In order to label the renal carrier for organic bases, dog renal cortical slices were allowed to react with unlabeled dibenamine under conditions in which the presumed carrier was protected by the presence of substrates for transport such as NMN or TEA. During this incubation dibenamine is binding to sites other than specific transport sites. After washing out the reversibly bound cations, NMN or TEA, [^{14}C]dibenamine is added to the slice and should now specifically label the protein fractions representing the NMN and TEA carrier. It was concluded that the protein fraction does indeed contain a carrier-like protein (Ross *et al.*, 1969; Magour *et al.*, 1969).

Ross studied the binding of the cation NMN and the anion PAH to particulate fractions from dog renal cortex (Holohan *et al.*, 1975). The bound and free forms of the ligand were separated by centrifugation through a gel matrix. Binding of NMN and PAH were specific for kidney tissue. Binding was pH, time, temperature, protein-concentration, and ligand-concentration dependent. Saturation of binding for either ligand was observed at concentrations greater than 50 mM suggesting the two systems share many features in common.

ACKNOWLEDGMENTS

This work was supported in part by NIH grants AM-10429 and HL-14092.

REFERENCES

Acara, M. 1975. The role of the kidney in the regulation of plasma choline in the chicken. *Am. J. Physiol., 228*:645.

Acara, M. and Rennick, B. 1972a. Renal tubular transport of choline; modifications caused by intrarenal metabolism. *J. Pharmacol. Exp. Ther., 182*:1.

Acara, M. and Rennick, B. 1972b. Renal tubular transport of acetylcholine and atropine: Enhancement and inhibition. *J. Pharmacol. Exp. Ther., 182*:14.

Acara M. and Rennick, B. 1973. Regulation of plasma choline by the renal tubule: Bidirectional transport of choline. *Am. J. Physiol., 225*:1123.

Acara, M., Kowalski, M., and Rennick, B. 1973. Enhancement by hemicholinium-3 of choline and acetylcholine excretion by the renal tubule of the chicken. *J. Pharmacol. Exp. Ther., 185*:254.

Acara, M., Rennick, B., Hemsworth, B., and Kowalski, M. 1975. Renal tubular excretion of triethylcholine (TEC) in the chicken: Enhancement and inhibition of renal excretion of choline and acetylcholine by TEC. *Brit. J. Pharmacol. Chemother. 54*:41.

Antoniades, H. N., Goldfien, A., Zileli, S., and Elmadjian, F. 1958. Transport of epinephrine and norepinephrine in human plasma. *Proc. Soc. Exp. Biol. Med., 97*:11.

Baer, J. E., Paulson, S. F., Russo, H. F., and Beyer, K. H. 1956. Renal elimination of 3-methylaminoisocamphane hydrochloride (mecamylamine). *Am. J. Physiol., 186*:180.

Baines, A. D. and Gottschalk, C. W. 1968. Microinjection study of *p*-aminohippurate excretion by rat kidneys. *Am. J. Physiol., 214*:703.

Beyer, K. H., Jr. and Gelarden, R. T. 1975. Functional characteristic of the renal tubular secretion of amprolium, a quaternary ammonium base. *J. Pharmacol. Exp. Ther., 195*:194.

Beyer, K. H., Russo, H. F., Gass, S. R., Wilhoyte, K. M., and Pitt, A. A. 1950. Renal tubular elimination of N'-methylnicotinamide. *Am. J. Physiol., 160*:311.

Beyer, K. H., Tillson, E. K., Russo, H. F., and Paulson, S. F. 1953. Physiological economy of darstine, 5-methyl-4-phenyl-1-(1-piperidyl)-3-hexanol methobromide, visceral anticholinergic agent. *Am. J. Physiol., 175*:39.

Bligh, J. 1952. The level of free choline in plasma. *J. Physiol., 117*:234.

Bligh, J. 1953. The role of the liver and the kidneys in the maintenance of the level of free choline in plasma. *J. Physiol., 120*:53.

Branco, D., Torrinha, J. F., and Osswald, W. 1974. Binding of exogenous noradrenaline by the proteins of dog plasma. *Naunyn Schmiedeberg's Arch. Pharmacol., 285*:367.

Brand, P. H. and Cohen, J. J. 1972. Effect of renal arterial infusion rate on distribution of radioisotopes in kidney. *J. Appl. Physiol., 33*:627.

Bryson, G. and Bishoff, F. 1970. Dopamine transport in human blood. *Clin. Chem., 16*:312.

Cohen, Y., Bralet, J., and Rousselet, J. P. 1968. *In vitro* binding of adrenaline-^{14}C and noradrenaline-^{14}C to rabbit serum proteins. *C.R. Soc. Biol. (Paris), 162*:62.

Conway, W. D., Minatoya, H., Lands, A. M., and Shekosky, J. M. 1968. Absorption and elimination profile of isoproterenol III: The metabolic fate of *dl*-isoproterenol-7-3H in the dog. *J. Pharm. Sci., 57*:1135.

Danon, A. and Sapira, J. D. 1972. Binding of catecholamines to human serum albumin. *J. Pharmacol. Exp. Ther., 182*:295.

Fanelli, G. M. and Weiner, I. M. 1973. Pyrazinoate excretion in the chimpanzee. Relation to urate disposition and the actions of uricosuric drugs. *J. Clin. Invest., 53*:1946.

Forster, R. P. 1967. Renal transport mechanisms. *Fed. Proc., 26*:1008.

Franksson, G. and Anggaard, E. 1970. The plasma protein binding of amphetamine, catecholamines and related compounds. *Acta Pharmacol. (Kbh.), 28*:209.

Fujimoto, J. M. and Haarstad, V. B. 1969. The isolation of morphine ethereal sulfate from urine of the chicken and cat. *J. Pharmacol. Exp. Ther., 165*:45.

Fujimoto, J. M., Hakim, R., and Zamiatowski, R. 1972. Inhibition of renal tubular transport of morphine by diethylaminoethanol in the chicken. *Biochem. Pharmacol., 21*:2877.

Fujimoto, J. M., Lech, J. J., and Zamiatowski, R. 1973. A site of action of novobiocin in inhibiting renal tubular transport of drugs in the chicken. *Biochem. Pharmacol., 22*:971.

Gardiner, J. E. and Paton, W. D. M. 1972. The control of the plasma choline concentration in the cat. *J. Physiol., 227*:71.

Gillette, J. R. 1973. Overview of drug-protein binding. *Ann. N.Y. Acad. Sci., 226*:6.

Goldstein, A., Aronow, L., and Kalman, S. M. 1974. The binding of drugs to plasma protein. In: *The Principles of Drug Action*, pp. 158–164. John Wiley and Sons, New York.

Gryglewski, R. and Vane, J. R. 1970. The inactivation of noradrenaline and isoprenaline in dogs. *Br. J. Pharmacol., 39*:573.

Hakim, R. and Fujimoto, J. M. 1971. Inhibition of renal tubular transport of morphine by β-diethylaminoethyl diphenylpropylacetate in the chicken. *Biochem. Pharmacol., 20*:2647.

Hakim, R., Watrous, W. M., and Fujimoto, J. M. 1970. The renal tubular transport and metabolism of serotonin (5-HT) and 5-hydroxyindoleacetic acid (5-HIAA) in the chicken. *J. Pharmacol. Exp. Ther., 175*:749.

Hempel, K., Lange, H. W., Kayser, E. F., Roger, L., Hennemann, H., and Heidland, A. 1973. Role of *O*-methylation in the renal excretion of catecholamines in dogs. *Naunyn-Schmiedeberg's Arch. Exp. Pathol. Pharmakol., 277*:373.

Hempel, K., Carle, W., and Heidland, A. 1974. Effect on COMT-inhibition on the renal excretion of plus or minus-adrenaline in dogs. *Naunyn-Schmiedeberg's Arch. Exp. Pathol. Pharmakol., 282*:107.

Holohan, P. D., Pessah, N. I., and Ross, C. R. 1975. Binding of N'-methylnicotinamide and *p*-aminohippuric acid to a particulate fraction from dog kidney. *J. Pharmacol. Exp. Ther., 195*:22.

Hunt, R. 1915. A physiological test for choline and some of its applications. *J. Pharmacol. Exp. Ther., 7*:301.

Jones, R. T. and Blake, W. D. 1958. Renal excretion of *l*-epinephrine in the dog. *Am. J. Physiol., 193*:371.

Lifschitz, M. D., Keller, D., Goldfien, A., and Schrier, R. W. 1973. Mechanism of renal clearance of isoproterenol. *Am. J. Physiol., 224*:733.

Lindahl, K. M. and Sperber, I. 1956. Some characteristics of the renal tubular transport mechanism for histamine in the hen. *Acta Physiol. Scand., 42*:166.

Magour, S., Farah, A., and Sroka, A. 1969. The partial purification of a carrier-like protein for organic bases from the kidney. *J. Pharmacol. Exp. Ther., 167*:243.

May, D. G. and Weiner, I. M. 1970. Bidirectional active transport of *m*-hydroxybenzoate in proximal tubules of dogs. *Am. J. Physiol., 218*:430.

May, D. G., Fujimoto, J. M., and Inturrisi, C. E. 1967. The tubular transport and metabolism of morphine-N-methyl-C^{14} by the chicken kidney. *J. Pharmacol. Exp. Ther., 157*:626.

May, P., Sanders, F. J., and Donabedian, R. K. 1974. Binding of catechol derivatives to human serum proteins. *Experientia, 30*:304.

Mirkin, B. L., Brown, D. M., and Ulstrom, R. A. 1966. Catecholamine binding protein: Binding of tritium to a specific protein fraction of human plasma following *in vitro* incubation with tritiated noradrenaline. *Nature, 212*:1270.

Orloff, J., Aronow, L., and Berliner, R. W. 1953. The transport of priscoline by the renal tubules. *J. Pharmacol. Exp. Ther., 109*:214.

Overy, H. R., Pfister, R., and Chidsey, C. A. 1967. Studies on the renal excretion of norepinephrine. *J. Clin. Invest., 46*:482.

Peters, L. 1960. Renal tubular excretion of organic bases. *Pharmacol. Rev., 12*:1.

Quebbemann, A. J. and Anders, M. W. 1971. Renal tubular conjugation and excretion (RTCE) of *p*-nitrophenol-^{14}C (PNP) in the chicken. *Pharmacologist, 13*:226.

Quebbemann, A. J. and Anders, M. W. 1973. Renal tubular conjugation and excretion of phenol and *p*-nitrophenol in the chicken: Differing mechanisms of renal transfer. *J. Pharmacol. Exp. Ther., 184*:695.

Quebbemann, A. J. and Rennick, B. R. 1968. Catechol transport by the renal tubule in the chicken. *Am. J. Physiol., 214*:1201.

Quebbemann, A. J. and Rennick, B. R. 1969. Effects of structural modifications of catecholamines on renal tubular transport in the chicken. *J. Pharmacol. Exp. Ther., 166*:52.

Quebbemann, A. and Rennick, B. 1970. Inhibition of renal tubular transport of catecholamines by cocaine; an organic base mechanism. *J. Pharmacol. Exp. Ther., 175*:248.

Rennick, B. R. 1958. The renal tubular excretion of choline and thiamine in the chicken. *J. Pharmacol. Exp. Ther., 122*:449.

Rennick, B. 1967. Transport mechanisms for renal tubular excretion of creatinine in the chicken. *Am. J. Physiol., 212*:1131.

Rennick, B. R. 1968. Dopamine: Renal tubular transport in the dog and plasma binding studies. *Am. J. Physiol., 215*:532.

Rennick, B. R. 1972. Renal excretion of drugs: Tubular transport and metabolism. *Annu. Rev. Pharmacol., 12*:141.

Rennick, B. R. 1974. Choline and the organic cation transport system. In: *Recent Advances in Renal Physiology and Pharmacology*, pp. 81–99. Ed. by Wesson, L. G. and Fanelli, G. M. University Park Press, Baltimore.

Rennick, B. R. and Moe, G. K. 1960. Stop-flow localization of renal tubular excretion of tetraethylammonium. *Am. J. Physiol., 198*:1267.

Rennick, B. R. and Pryor, M. Z. 1965. Effects of autonomic drugs on renal tubular transport of catecholamines in the chicken. *J. Pharmacol. Exp. Ther., 148*:262.

Rennick, B. and Quebbemann, A. 1970. Site of excretion of catechol and catecholamines: Renal metabolism of catechol. *Am. J. Physiol., 218*:1307.

Rennick, B. and Quebbemann, A. 1971. Renal tubular excretion of drugs: Proximal tubule secretion and metabolism. In: *Renal Pharmacology*, pp. 67–84. Ed. by Fisher, J. W. and Cafruny, E. J. Appleton-Century-Crofts, New York.

Rennick, B. and Yoss, N. 1962. Renal tubular excretion of *dl*-epinephrine-2-^{14}C in the chicken. *J. Pharmacol. Exp. Ther., 138*:347.

Rennick, B. R., Moe, G. K., Lyons, R. H., Hoobler, S. W., and Neligh, R. 1947. Absorption and renal excretion of the tetraethylammonium ion. *J. Pharmacol. Exp. Ther., 91*:210.

Rennick, B. R., Calhoon, D. M., Gandia, H., and Moe, G. K. 1954. Renal tubular secretion of tetraethylammonium in the dog and the chicken. *J. Pharmacol. Exp. Ther., 110*:309.

Rennick, B. R., Pryor, M. Z., and Basch, B. G. 1965. Urinary metabolites of epinephrine and norepinephrine in the chicken. *J. Pharmacol. Exp. Ther., 148*:270.

Roberts, J. B., Thomas, B. H., and Wilson, A. 1965. Distribution and excretion of (^{14}C)-neostigmine in the rat and hen. *Br. J. Pharmacol. Chemother., 25*:234.

Ross, C. R., Pessah, N. I., and Farah, A. 1968. Inhibitory effects of beta-haloalkylamines on the renal transport of *N*-methylnicotinamide. *J. Pharmacol. Exp. Ther., 160*:375.

Ross, C. R., Pessah, N. I., and Farah, A. E. 1969. Attempts to label the renal carrier for organic bases with dibenamine. *J. Pharmacol. Exp. Ther., 167*:235.

Russell, J. C. and Doty, D. M. 1972. Plasma-protein binding of epinephrine. *Scand. J. Clin. Lab. Invest., 29*:1414.

Russell, J. C. and Doty, D. M. 1973. Plasma-protein binding of epinephrine. *Physiol. Chem. Phys., 5*:75.

Sanner, E. and Wortman, B. 1962. Tubular excretion of serotonin (5-hydroxytryptamine) in the chicken. *Acta Physiol. Scand., 55*:319.

Schanker, L. S. 1972. Transport of drugs. In: *Metabolic Pathways, VI*, p. 543. Ed. by Hokin, L. Academic Press, New York.

Schrier, R. W., Lieberman, R. A., and Ufferman, R. C. 1972. Mechanisms of antidiuretic effect of beta-adrenergic stimulation. *J. Clin. Invest., 51*:97.

Sperber, I. 1946. A new method for the study of renal tubular excretion in birds. *Nature, 158*:131.

Sperber, I. 1947. The mechanism of renal excretion of some 'detoxication products' in the chicken. *Proc. Int. Physiol. Congr., 17*:217.

Sperber, I. 1948a. The excretion of some glucuronic acid derivatives and phenol sulphuric esters in the chicken. *Lantbrukshogskol. Ann., 15*:317.

Sperber, I. 1948b. The excretion of piperidine, guanidine, methylguanidine and N′-methylnicotinamide in the chicken. *Lantbrukshogskol. Ann., 16*:49.

Sperber, I. 1959. Secretion of organic anions in the formation of urine and bile. *Pharmacol. Rev., 11*:109.

Tanner, G. A. and Kinter, W. B. 1966. Reabsorption and secretion of *p*-aminohippurate and diodrast in *Necturus* kidney. *Am. J. Physiol., 210*:221.

Their, S. O. 1974. Amino acid transport in the renal tubule cell. In:*Recent Advances in Renal Physiology and Pharmacology*, p. 39. Ed. by Wesson, L. G. and Fanelli, G. M. University Park Press, Baltimore.

Trimble, M. E., Acara, M., and Rennick, B. 1974. Effect of hemicholinium-3 on tubular transport and metabolism of choline in the perfused kidney. *J. Pharmacol. Exp. Ther., 189*:570.

Torretti, J., Weiner, I. M., and Mudge, G. H. 1962. Renal tubular secretion and reabsorption of organic bases in the dog. *J. Clin. Invest., 41*:793.

Watrous, W. M. and Fujimoto, J. M. 1971. Inhibition of morphine metabolism by catechol in the chicken kidney. *Biochem. Pharmacol., 20*:1479.

Watrous, W. M., May, D. G., and Fujimoto, J. M. 1970. Mechanism of the renal tubular transport of morphine and morphine ethereal sulfate in the chicken. *J. Pharmacol. Exp. Ther., 172*:224.

Weiner, I. M. 1967. Mechanisms of drug absorption and excretion. The renal excretion of drugs and related compounds. *Annu. Rev. Pharmacol., 7*:39.

Weiner, I. M. 1971. Excretion of drugs by the kidney. In: *Handbook of Experimental Pharmacology*, pp. 329–353. Ed. by Brodie, B. B. and Gillette, J. R. Springer-Verlag, Berlin.

Weiner, I. 1973. Transport of weak acids and bases. In: *Handbook of Physiology, Renal Physiology*, pp. 521–555. Ed. by Orloff, J. and Berliner, R. W. American Physiological Society, Washington, D.C.

Weiner, I. M. and Mudge, G. H. 1964. Renal tubular mechanisms for excretion of organic acids and bases. *Am. J. Med., 36*:743

Wilde, W. and Malvin, R. 1958. Graphical placement of transport segments along the nephron from urine concentration pattern developed with stop-flow technique. *Am. J. Physiol., 195*:153.

Zia, H., Cox, R. H., and Luzzi, L. A. 1971. *In vitro* binding study of epinephrine and bovine serum albumin. *J. Pharm. Sci., 60*:89.

Zins, G. R. and Weiner, I. M. 1968a. Bidirectional urate transport limited to the proximal tubule in dogs. *Am. J. Physiol., 215*:411.

Zins, G. R. and Weiner, I. M. 1968b. Bidirectional transport of taurocholate by the proximal tubule of the dog. *Am. J. Physiol., 215*:840.

Chapter **12**

The Renal Excretion of Drugs

Jorge Torretti and I. M. Weiner

Department of Pharmacology
State University of New York
Upstate Medical Center
Syracuse, New York

I. INTRODUCTION

The role of renal excretion in the overall disposition of drugs varies greatly depending on the particular compound under consideration. Moreover, with a single compound there may be great variation in the contribution of the kidney to its disposition depending on disease states, physiological variables, or the presence of other drugs. Obviously any compound in the circulation is exposed to the kidney, but this exposure may or may not result in its appearance in the urine. The kidney may, in addition, cause the metabolic transformation of the drug, with or without the appearance of the metabolites in the urine. Finally a drug may be accumulated in one or another part of the kidney either in the tubular cells or in the interstitium.

The literature on this subject is sufficiently extensive as to prevent an attempt at comprehensive coverage in the space alloted. Despite its large size, the literature is quite incomplete in terms of description of mechanisms for the renal excretion of many drugs in current use, even at the level permitted in relatively unsophisticated laboratories.

The aims of this chapter are to describe the various mechanisms which play roles in the renal disposition of drugs, to consider the methods of study, and to provide examples of drugs whose excretion patterns illustrate the operations of the various mechanisms, singly and in combination. For the most part we will concentrate on drugs which are not organic bases since the latter are covered in Chapter 11.

II. THE INTRARENAL DISPOSITION OF DRUGS

The following are recognized as major mechanisms affecting the renal disposition of drugs: (1) glomerular filtration, (2) secretion into tubular fluid by active (and possibly passive) transport, (3) reabsorption from tubular fluid by both active and passive mechanisms, (4) accumulation in tubular cells as a result of active transport into cells or binding to cellular components or both, and (5) metabolic conversion of drugs. A particular compound may be affected by one or several of these processes.

A. Glomerular Filtration

The process of glomerular filtration has been fairly well characterized (Renkin and Gilmore, 1973). The mechanism is one of ultrafiltration driven by the hydrostatic pressure in glomerular capillaries. The latter force is opposed by intratubular pressure and the oncotic pressure attributable to plasma proteins. In some (Brenner *et al.,* 1972) but not all physiological conditions (Maddox *et al.,* 1975), filtration equilibrium obtains; that is, the net driving force for ultrafiltration at the distal end of glomerular capillaries is zero. The membranes of the glomerulus are such that molecules of molecular weight 5000 or less are freely filterable, i.e., their concentrations in the filtrate are the same as their concentrations in the plasma water. The foregoing statement must be modified for compounds which are ions at physiological pH. Because of the Donnan phenomenon, concentration of cations will be higher and concentration of anions lower in the glomerular filtrate than in plasma. For univalent ions the deviations from the concentrations in plasma water will be small, approximately 5% in ordinary circumstances. On the other hand, the extent to which drugs of small molecular weight are bound to the macromolecules in plasma is as important a variable in determining their filtration as is the volume of fluid filtered. For the most part the major binding constituent in plasma is albumin. Drugs vary greatly in their affinity for albumin such that at one extreme there may be virtually no binding while at the other more than 99% of a drug may be bound to protein. It is important to recognize that the extent of protein binding may be modified by physiological factors (Goldstein, 1949). Among the major physiological variables are the concentration of albumin in plasma and the pH of plasma. In addition, the presence of a second drug may modify the extent of binding of the first, i.e., some drugs compete with one another for binding (Dayton and Perel, 1971). Hence for the most precise work it is necessary to estimate the fractional binding of drugs in each experiment.

B. Active Secretion

There appear to be at least three active transport mechanisms in the proximal tubule capable of causing the secretion of organic compounds: the organic anion, the organic cation, and the urate mechanisms. The most thoroughly studied of these is the system largely responsible for the secretion of anionic substances such as *p*-aminohippurate (PAH), penicillin G, and salicylate. Since many of the characteristics of this system are analogous to those of the other systems, it is pertinent to outline them here.

The organic anion mechanism is capable of uphill transport; i.e., it can transfer material from a solution of lower concentration (plasma) to a solution of higher concentration (tubular fluid) (e.g., Tune *et al.*, 1969). This transfer is not supported by any known physical factors. The transepithelial electrical potentials in the proximal tubules are small (Seely and Chirito, 1975) and when oriented in the proper direction (lumen positive) are not sufficient to sustain the observed concentration differences. The pH difference across the proximal tubule is small and under normal conditions is opposite to that required for trapping anions in the lumen by a nonionic diffusion mechanism (Gottschalk *et al.*, 1960).

The mechanism is saturable; i.e., there is a maximum concentration of transportable substrate above which an increase in its concentration does not result in enhanced transport. This saturability is thought to arise from a limiting quantity of a specific membrane component (carrier) which effects the transfer of the drug. Within the limits of experimental determinations the kinetics of the system are similar to the Michaelis–Menten model of enzyme reactions (Shannon, 1939; Cho *et al.*, 1960; Kiil, 1961; Huang and Lin, 1965; Kinter, 1966; Tune *et al.*, 1969; Dantzler, 1974a).

The transport mechanism is inhibited by metabolic poisons (see review by Weiner, 1973). Transport against an unfavorable electrochemical potential ultimately requires metabolic energy. However, the exact energy-yielding reactions for the maintenance of this transport system are not known. Indeed it is conceivable that energy transfer to organic anion secretion is indirect. For example, it has been proposed that PAH transport is a consequence of inorganic electrolyte transport (Vogel and Kroger, 1965; Vogel and Stoekert, 1966; Burg and Orloff, 1962a).

There appears to be competition for transport. For example, high concentrations of PAH inhibit the secretion of penicillin (Beyer *et al.*, 1944). There are numerous examples of one organic anion inhibiting the secretion of another, as well as examples of mutual inhibition (Weiner and Mudge, 1964). In general these phenomena have been taken to demonstrate competition for a common transport mechanism (e.g., Smith *et al.*, 1938). It should be emphasized that the complexity of the overall system is great and that the usual criteria for competition are not rigorous (Weiner, 1973). Indeed, it has been proposed that there are several secretory mechanisms for organic anions and that these mechanisms have overlapping specificities; i.e., a single substance may be transported by (or have affinity for) more than one transport system and thus be a "competitive" inhibitor of more than one (Bárány, 1972, 1974). A specific example will be considered below. Regardless of whether or not there is more than one mechanism for organic anion secretion, one is impressed by the great variety of chemical structures which may be secreted (Weiner, 1973). There have been attempts to deduce specific structural requirements (Hober, 1945; Taggart, 1958; Despopolous, 1965), but none seems completely satisfactory (Weiner, 1973).

The mechanism(s) under consideration is limited entirely to the proximal tubule. In the rabbit the last part of the proximal tubule, the pars recta, contains more secretory activity than does the convoluted portion (Tune *et al.*, 1969). Similarly in snake tubules, the late proximal tubule has a greater transporting activity than does the early proximal tubule (Dantzler, 1974a). Comparable data in other species are not available. There is general agreement that a major active step in secretion occurs at the peritubular border of the proximal tubular cells (Forster and Copenhaver, 1956; Foulkes and Miller, 1959; Tune *et al.*, 1969; Dantzler, 1974a; Watrous *et al.*, 1970). This step, which requires the presence of potassium ions (Hong and Forster, 1959; Puck *et al.*, 1952; Cross and Taggart, 1950; Dantzler, 1974b; Dantzler and Bentley, 1975), results in the cell water containing a higher concentration of the transported substance than does the surrounding medium. The high concentration of substance in the cell water provides a driving force for the passive egress of the anion into the tubular fluid. These phenomena have been observed in the tubules of rabbits (Tune *et al.*, 1969) and snakes (Datzler, 1974a) with PAH and in the flounder with iodopyracet (Burg and Weller, 1969). On the other hand, there may be a second active transport step at the luminal border of cells, at least in the transport of sulfonphthalein dyes by the flounder tubule (Hong and Forster, 1959; Puck *et al.*, 1952; Kinter, 1966) and PAH in the rat (Wedeen and Weiner, 1973). The operation of this second step in the flounder appears to require the presence of calcium ions.

Evidence in several species (Hook *et al.*, 1970; Horster and Lewy, 1970), including man (Calcagno and Rubin, 1963), indicates that the capacity to secrete organic acids is lower in the kidney of the neonate than the adult. In the species tested (Hirsch and Hook, 1970a; Johnson *et al.*, 1974), administration of exogenous organic acids in the immediate postnatal period enhance the organic acid transport capacity of the kidneys, as evidenced by *in vitro* accumulation in slices. This accelerated maturation of the system is probably associated with enhanced synthesis of specific transport proteins (Hirsch and Hook, 1970b).

The second major secretory system recognized in the proximal tubule effects the transport of organic cations (Peters, 1960). This mechanism appears to be completely independent of the system for organic anions; i.e., substrates for one do not compete for the other. The system exhibits the properties of saturation, competitive inhibition, and inhibition by metabolic poisons. A considerable variety of chemical structures are compatible with secretion (see Chapter 11). The question of multiple transport mechanisms for cations has thus far not been raised.

The existence of a third secretory mechanism for which uric acid is the prototypical substrate has been inferred from studies with mammalian kidneys and has been directly demonstrated in the snake. The renal disposition of urate is quite complex (see Chapter 9). In mammals there may be either net secretion or net reabsorption, depending on species and in certain instances upon experimental conditions within a single species; but in those mammals thoroughly studied so far both secretion and reabsorption coexist. The following remarks concern only the secretory component of the bidirectional transport mechanism. The inference that urate secretion is not mediated by the general anion system, described above, was made from consideration of the rank order of inhibitor effectiveness. Certain substances, i.e., pyrazinoate (Fanelli and Weiner, 1973) and m-hydroxybenzoic acid (May and Weiner, 1971), are very weak competitors for the general anion mechanism, and their secretion is readily inhibited by PAH. However, both pyrazinoate and m-hydroxybenzoate are powerful inhibitors of the urate secretory mechanism. On the other hand, PAH, a powerful competitor for the general mechanism is a weak inhibitor of the urate secretory system. In the snake, active secretion but not active reabsorption of urate has been recognized (Dantzler, 1973). In these animals the distinction between PAH and urate secretory mechanisms is even more clear. The systems differ in their distribution of activities along the proximal tubule and the response to inhibitors and other physiologic challenges (Dantzler, 1970, 1974a). Moreover, there appears to be no competition between urate and PAH. It is not known if the so-called urate secretory mechanism is one of the components of the group of systems proposed by Bárány (1972, 1974). It should be emphasized that the distinction between the general anion and the urate systems is not clear in all species (e.g., Møller, 1967).

There are some compounds whose secretion is difficult to assign to any one of the preceding mechanisms. The secretion of creatinine, for example, is partially inhibited by organic anions or organic cations or both (see Arendhorst and Selkurt, 1970, for references). The complexity of catecholamine secretion is discussed in Chapter 11.

Thus far we have considered only compounds secreted in the proximal tubule by active mechanisms. There is one example of an organic compound secreted in the distal nephron: ascorbic acid (Kleit *et al.*, 1965). The mechanism is incompletely characterized. With the possible exception of secretion by nonionic diffusion, secretion of organic compounds by passive mechanisms has not been suggested, despite the fact that there are electrical potential differences across certain segments of the nephron (Giebish and Windhager, 1973) which could conceivably maintain high concentration differences of organic ions.

C. Reabsorption

The normal operation of the nephron to reabsorb inorganic electrolytes, and consequently water, tends to concentrate organic compounds in tubular fluid above the level in glomerular filtrate (plasma water). This concentration provides a driving force for reabsorption of the organic components, such reabsorption being limited by the permeability of the tubular wall to the substance in question. There may be superimposed on this passive mechanism special mechanisms which either enhance the permeability to a specific solute or actually cause the active reabsorption of the solute and thereby reduce its concentration in tubular fluid to below that in the surrounding plasma. Active transport mechanisms for the reabsorption of a number of endogenous organic substances are recognized, e.g., glucose and other sugars, amino acids, vitamins, urate, and acids of the tricarboxylic acid cycle (Mudge *et al.*, 1973). There are as yet, no clearcut examples of organic substances reabsorbed by specific mechanisms which do not involve active transport. Such mechanisms, known as carrier-mediated or facilitated-diffusion mechanisms, are well known in other systems such as the erythrocyte (Wilbrandt and Rosenberg, 1961).

The reabsorption of drugs or their metabolites by such specific systems, be they active or not, has not been well studied. In every instance of which we are aware (specific examples will be given later), the drug in question is probably both secreted and reabsorbed by specific mechanisms, making the separate study of the reabsorptive system difficult. Those examples of specific reabsorptive mechanisms which have been studied occur at least in major part in the proximal tubule (May and Weiner, 1970; Weiner and Tinker, 1972; Corr and May, 1975). In the case of oxypurinol, the metabolite of allopurinol, it is believed that the compound is entrained by the reabsorptive mechanism for uric acid (Elion *et al.*, 1968). Oxypurinol is an analog of urate. It is not known if the other substances are reabsorbed by the urate mechanism or some other mechanism(s).

Reabsorption of drugs by passive nonspecific mechanisms has been more extensively studied. It is widely held that small molecules such as urea, which are known to penetrate other cells in the body, also penetrate the membranes of tubules through aqueous channels. However, most drug molecules are of considerably larger size and the most frequent mode of passive reabsorption is probably a mechanism in which the drug dissolves in lipid phase of the membrane in the course of its passage (Milne *et al.*, 1958; Weiner, 1973). This mechanism is frequently called nonionic diffusion because in the case of weak electrolytes it is the nonionized form of the molecule which is more permeant. For the sake of simplicity we will assume that transmembrane movement is an exclusive property of the nonionized form.

Several major factors determine the extent of reabsorption by nonionic diffusion. One of these factors is the permeance of the nonionized species, i.e., its ability to dissolve in and thereby penetrate the cell membranes. This property is roughly reflected in the partition of the compound between aqueous solutions and various organic solvents. The other factors control the concentration of the nonionized species in tubular fluid. They are: the pK_a of the compound, the pH of the fluid, and the volume of the fluid (related to the rate of flow of tubular fluid). For an organic acid, the nonionized concentration [N] is given by the following form of the Henderson–Hasselbach equation:

$$[N] = [I] \cdot 10^{(pK_a - pH)}$$

where [I] is the concentration of the ionized form. For a base the equation is

$$[N] = [I] \cdot 10^{(pH - pK_a)}$$

Thus for any given acid the proportion of molecules in the reabsorbable (nonionized) form is greater the more acid the urine. For a base the proportion of molecules in the reabsorbable form is greater the more alkaline the urine. Because of their particular values of pK_a, some acids and bases are so little ionized in the pH ranges of blood and urine that they behave entirely as neutral compounds; i. e., their excretions are not influenced by changes in the pH of urine. Provided that the permeance of the nonionized form is sufficiently high, the greatest effect of changes in urinary pH will be observed with acids whose pK_a is below the range of urinary pH and with bases whose pK_a is above the range of urinary pH. A fairly extensive treatment of nonionic diffusion in this context has been published recently (Weiner, 1973), and an important extension of the concept has been provided by Mudge *et al.* (1975).

D. Drug Metabolism

The kidneys of various species contain enzymes which carry out a variety of oxidative, hydrolytic, and synthetic reactions characteristic of drug metabolism in the liver. Some examples are: oxidation of choline (Acara and Rennick, 1972), acetylation of aromatic amines (Gyrd-Hansen and Rasmussen, 1970), formation of glycine conjugates (Williams, 1959), oxidation of serotonin (Sanner and Wortman, 1962), formation of morphine sulfate (Watrous *et al.*, 1970), synthesis of phenolic glucuronides (Quebbemann and Anders, 1973) and acylglucuronides (Knoefel *et al.*, 1959), and hydrolysis of cyclic AMP and subsequent formation of urate (Coulson, personal communication). The metabolites thus formed may or may not be secreted into the urine. In some instances it has been possible to exploit the combined operation of renal transport and metabolism to make certain inferences about the site of action of transport inhibitors. Specific examples will be given in a later section.

E. Accumulation of Drugs in the Kidney

This subject has received recent impetus as a result of interest in drug-induced nephrotoxicity and the distribution of antibiotics used in the treatment of pyelonephritis (Whelton and Walker, 1974; Schreiner, 1972).

It has already been noted that secreted substances may reach a higher concentration in tubular cells than in either plasma or tubular fluid. With at least one substance (cephaloridine) there seems to be a severe limitation in its egress across the luminal cell membrane, resulting in very high intracellular concentrations (Tune and Fernholt, 1973). In other instances very high intracellular concentrations are achieved as a result of the combined operation of active transport and binding to intracellular components (e.g., Duggan, 1966). In the proximal tubules of *Necturus* very high concentrations of certain substances are achieved in proximal tubular cells as a result of bidirectional transport. Material is pumped into the cells from both lumen and plasma by transport mechanisms on both luminal and contraluminal membranes (Kinter, 1959; Kinter *et al.*, 1960; Tanner and Kinter, 1966; Tanner, 1967). It is not known to what extent this phenomenon occurs in mammals.

In addition to the foregoing types of intrarenal accumulation which depend in part on active transport, it seems that certain substances may accumulate in the medullary–papillary region by passive mechanisms analogous to those which operate for urea (Bluemle and Goldberg, 1968).

III. TECHNIQUES OF INVESTIGATION

A. Renal Clearance

This classic technique provides information on whether or not a compound undergoes tubular transport, the direction of net transport (secretion or reabsorption), the rate of net transport (mass/time), and apparent maximal rates of transport (Smith, 1951). Under appropriate conditions inferences may be made about the nature of transport mechanisms, active vs. passive, and the role of nonionic diffusion.

The direction of net transport is given by a comparison of the clearance (C) of the substance in question (x) with that of a substance used to measure glomerular filtration rate, usually inulin (In). Renal clearance is calculated as $U_x V / P_x$ where U_x and P_x are the concentrations of the substance in urine and plasma, respectively, and V is the volume of urine formed per minute. When $C_x / C_{In} < 1$, x is reabsorbed and when $C_x / C_{In} > 1$, x is secreted. Note that C_x / C_{In} = excreted/filtered.

The foregoing ignores the Donnan factor which, strictly speaking, should be applied when charged molecules are considered (see prior section). When a drug is partially bound to plasma proteins, other factors come into play. A rough and often satisfactory approach is calculation of $U_x V / F_x$, where F_x is the concentration of the substance in an ultrafiltrate of plasma. The most correct refinement is:

$$\text{Excreted/filtered} = U_x V / F_x \times W \times C_{In}$$

where W is the fraction of plasma occupied by water, usually 0.93. The latter factor derives from the fact that inulin is distributed in only the aqueous phase of plasma and measurement of inulin in ultrafiltrates is not practical.

The magnitude of net transport (T_x) is calculated as the difference between filtration and excretion of a substance. For a secreted substance, $T_x = U_x V - (F_x \times W \times C_{In})$ and for a reabsorbed substance, $T_x = (F_x \times W \times C_{In}) - U_x V$.

The following experimental manipulations and results are usually considered diagnostic. If the clearance of a substance is equal to C_{In} when studied over a wide range of concentrations in plasma and is unaffected by changes in urine flow and composition, such a substance is excreted largely by filtration with little or no contribution by transtubular transport.

If the clearance of a drug is very sensitive to changes in urine flow it is probable that passive reabsorption occurs. Theoretically, substances which are reabsorbed by active transport are also somewhat sensitive to changes in urine flow (Walser, 1966), and there is experimental evidence for this (e.g., Weiner and Tinker, 1972). However, such changes are relatively small. Enhanced clearance of an organic acid when urine is alkaline or of a base when urine is acid is presumptive evidence for reabsorption by nonionic diffusion (Milne *et al.*, 1958). However, reabsorption by this process is not excluded by a lack of effect of change in urinary pH (see previous discussion on the influence of pK_a).

All other factors being constant, a fall in the clearance of a secreted substance or a rise in the clearance of a reabsorbed substance when plasma level is increased is suggestive of a saturable (probably active) transport mechanism (Smith, 1951). Similarly, enhanced excretion of a reabsorbed substance or diminished excretion of a secreted substance following the introduction of a presumed inhibitor of transport is suggestive of active transport, provided that the inhibitor does not cause changes in other variables such as urinary pH and flow.

The clearance technique may be profitably complemented by measurements of arteriovenous differences in drug concentration. For substances which are not metabolized in the kidney, renal plasma flow is given by $C_x A_x / (A_x - V_x)$ where A and V are the arterial and venous plasma concentrations of drug, respectively. The application of the principle requires that diffusion of x from red cells into venous plasma be taken into account (Wedeen and Weiner, 1969). If there is an independent estimate of renal plasma flow, one can recognize disparities between the quantity of drug removed by the kidney and that appearing in the urine. Such disparities may be due to renal drug metabolism or accumulation.

B. The Sperber Technique

This technique, which is applicable in birds and other animals with renal portal circulations, is described in Chapter 11. Briefly, the method consists of presenting a substance to the renal tubules of one kidney via its portal circulation and estimating net secretion as the difference in excreted quantity between the infused and control kidneys. This difference divided by the rate of infusion gives the apparent tubular excretion fraction (ATEF). The method is convenient and allows the study of secreted substances which are too toxic for systemic administration. The method also allows large increases in the load presented for secretion without great changes in filtered load.

C. Stop-Flow

This procedure is of considerable value in the localization of transport processes along the length of the nephron (Malvin and Wilde, 1973). In brief, the ureter of an animal undergoing intense osmotic diuresis is clamped for several minutes allowing a relatively static column of urine to remain in contact with the various tubular segments for longer than usual periods of time. Thus the operation of each segment on the tubular fluid is exaggerated. After release of the ureteral occlusion, small serial samples are collected rapidly, the earliest sample representing fluid which had been in contact with the most distal nephron segments. Since the column of urine is not completely static and since nephrons vary appreciably in length and behavior, there is some slurring of the stop-flow patterns and only fairly gross differences in localization can be appreciated. Users of this technique must also appreciate that tubular segments downstream from the proximal segments may modify the tubular fluid during its egress. Despite these limitations a fairly large body of useful information has resulted from the application of this method.

In the conventional application of the method the substances examined are present along with inulin before the application of ureteral occlusion. Consequently, the ratio $U_x:P_x::U_{In}:P_{In}$ in the various samples has the qualitative connotation of the clearance ratios C_x/C_{In}. Thus, for a substance secreted in the proximal tubule, samples of urine derived from tubular fluid in long contact with proximal segments will give values of $U_x:P_x::U_{In}:P_{In}$ which are higher than those obtained during free flow. The converse obtains with materials which are reabsorbed. The tubular sites represented by the various samples are defined by the concentrations of substances such as PAH, sodium, and potassium, whose patterns of tubular handling are well defined.

An interesting variant of the stop-flow technique involves injecting intravenously or infusing into the renal artery the drug under study along with inulin after several minutes of ureteral occlusion (e.g., Rennick and Moe, 1960). The precession of the drug compared to inulin in the subsequently collected samples is evidence for transtubular permeability. The technique has been of value with compounds subject to bidirectional transport in demonstrating the secretory component when it is normally masked by reabsorption of greater magnitude (Zins and Weiner, 1968a,b).

D. Retrograde Intraureteral Injection

In this procedure a solution containing the test substance, inulin, and other appropriate markers is forced into the tubules in a retrograde fashion, allowed to remain for a brief time, and upon release of the ureter serial samples are collected. In one such study it was possible to demonstrate a reabsorptive flux of PAH in the proximal tubule which could be inhibited by probenecid (Cho and Cafruny, 1970). Samples which had been in contact with the proximal epithelium were identified by the loss of glucose which is known to be reabsorbed in the proximal tubule.

E. Tubular Micropuncture, Microinjection, and Microperfusion

These techniques are designed for the study of phenomena at the level of the single nephron (Gottschalk and Lassiter, 1973). In the free-slow micropuncture technique the ratio of concentrations $TF_x:P_x::TF_{In}:P_{In}$, where TF refers to concentration in tubular fluid, has the same connotation as the corresponding clearance ratio. Because it is possible to collect all of the fluid passing a given point and thus determine single nephron C_{In}, one may also determine net transport (T), and this can be related to the surface area of the tubular segment. A major advantage of the technique is its potential for precise localization of tubular functions. For the most part studies are limited to surface nephrons (which may not be representative of the total population) and to the specific regions of the nephron which appear on the surface, the convoluted part of the proximal tubule, and the distal tubule. There are special techniques which allow study of other nephrons and nephron segments, but these have not yet been applied to the study of drug excretion. Free-flow micropuncture studies of excretion of foreign chemicals (e.g., Cortney *et al.*, 1965; Ross *et al.*, 1975) are scarce. One reason may well be the difficulty in developing specific ultramicroanalytical methods for drugs.

The microperfusion technique involves perfusing a segment of tubule *in situ* with a solution of known composition. The rat is the most frequently used animal. The substance in question may be present in the lumen or in the circulation depending on whether secretion or reabsorption is being considered. Of particular relevance in the present context are studies on secretion and reabsorption of furosemide by proximal tubules (Deetjen, 1966) and fairly extensive studies on the passive reabsorption of several compounds in proximal and distal tubules (Sonnenberg*et al.*, 1965; Oelert *et al.*, 1969). The latter studies demonstrated that the proximal tubule is much more permeable to a variety of organic acids than is the distal.

In the microinjection technique known quantities of test substance and inulin are delivered into specific regions of the nephron, and the fraction of material escaping reabsorption is determined in serial samples of ureteral urine. The method has been applied with an organic acid (Baines *et al.*, 1968) and an organic base (Ross *et al.*, 1975).

F. Microperfusion of Isolated Tubules

This technique consists of mounting freshly dissected tubular segments between two pipet systems, one for perfusion and one for collection (Burg and Orloff, 1973). The compound under study may be introduced into the perfusion fluid, into the bath surrounding the tubule, or both. Since the composition of both perfusate and bath may be rigorously defined, this technique is eminently suited for study of the effects of various ions and other constituents on transport of organic compounds and for the study of transport kinetics. In addition, it is possible to get information on the concentration of transported materials in intracellular water. Of particular relevance in the present context are studies of PAH secretion by proximal tubules of rabbits (Tune *et al.*, 1969) and snakes (Dantzler, 1974a) and iodopyracet secretion by isolated tubules of the flounder (Burg and Weller, 1969).

G. Accumulation of Drugs by Renal Tissue *in Vitro*

The preparations which have been used include cultures of embryonic tissue (Chambers and Kempton, 1933), teased tubules of fish, slices of kidney from a variety of mammalian and nonmammalian species (Forster, 1948; Cross and Taggart, 1950), and suspension of separated tubules (Burg and Orloff, 1962b). The tissue-culture preparation and flounder teased-tubule preparation differ from the others in that patent tubular lumina are readily observed and thus transepithelial transport can be assessed by visual or spectrometric means (Kinter, 1966). In this respect such preparations resemble the isolated perfused tubules discussed in the preceding section. The flounder tubule has been especially useful for kinetic studies.

The incubated cortical-slice preparation and the tubule-suspension preparation have been widely used for kinetic studies of the secretory systems located on the antiluminal membrane based on measurements of the steady-state concentration difference between tissue and medium or on the rate of accumulation in tissue. For the latter purpose the separated-tubule preparation is superior since the rate of uptake is not influenced by diffusion through interstitial space (Burg and Orloff, 1962b). These preparations have also been widely used for studies on competitive inhibition (e.g., Huang and Lin, 1965), metabolic poisons (e.g., Farah et al., 1953), the influence of metabolic substrates (e.g., Koishi, 1959), and the influence of changes in the ionic environment (e.g., Chung et al., 1970; Gerenscer et al., 1973).

H. Tissue Analysis; in Vivo Experiments

The gross distribution of a drug in renal tissue is frequently determined as part of general distribution studies and is of interest with respect to regional toxicity and therapeutic potential (Whelton and Walker, 1974). It is often difficult to interpret such data in terms of mechanisms because of the heterogeneity of renal tissue, the drug being distributed in the water of cells, tubular lumina, interstitial space, and plasma. The problem is compounded further by lack of a suitable extracellular marker. Substances such as inulin, which can be used as extracellular markers in other tissues, are concentrated in tubular fluid and thus the apparent volume of distribution is larger than the actual extracellular space. In certain instances, however, the concentration of drug in renal cortex is large relative to concentrations in plasma and urine, and it may be reasonably inferred that the substance is accumulated within kidney cells. Ingenuous use has been made of such measurements (Tune and Fernholt, 1973; Tune, 1972; Foulkes and Miller, 1959; Whelton et.al., 1971).

The interpretation of drug distribution data in the inner medulla and papilla is particularly difficult. Attempts have been made to calculate the quantity of drug contained within collecting duct fluid, based on an apparent volume of distribution with urinary concentration as the reference (Whelton et al., 1971). The latter estimation is critical if one is to make inferences about the distribution of drug in other components of the tissue. However, it is clear that neither urinary nor systemic plasma concentration is a satisfactory reference (Mudge et al., 1975; Mudge and Duggan, personal communication). In antidiuresis the concentration of substances in collecting ducts tends to be high, and the changes in concentration along the length of the duct tend to be great. With intense diuresis the volume contained in the collecting ducts is much greater than in antidiuresis, but relative changes in intratubular volume (and thus concentration of solutes) along the length of the duct are smaller. Thus urinary concentration seemingly becomes a more satisfactory reference. However, the problem of quantifying the amount of drug in the vascular compartment remains. Moreover, during diuresis corticopapillary gradients tend to be minimal, and this provides a poor experimental setting for studying tissue concentration in relation to local toxicity.

The technique of freeze-dry autoradiography seems to offer an approach which eliminates some of the problems associated with tissue analysis, since it allows localization and quantification of drugs in the various compartments of tissue (Bordier *et al.*, 1970).

IV. PATTERNS OF DRUG EXCRETION: EXAMPLES

A. Filtration Only

There are relatively few foreign compounds which follow this simplest of patterns. Examples are certain triarylmethane dyes including lissamine green (Popa *et al.*, 1974), and the radiologic contrast medium iodipamide (Berndt and Mudge, 1968) (the latter in the dog but not rabbit). With compounds adhering to this pattern, excreted/filtered = 1 at all concentrations of drug in plasma, at all rates of urine flow, and at any value of urinary pH.

B. Filtration and Active Net Secretion

Prototypes of this kind of behavior are PAH among the anions and *N*-methylnicotinamide (Farah and Frazer, 1961) and tetraethylammonium ion (Rennick and Farah, 1956) among the cations. With such compounds clearances may be very high, approaching the rate of renal plasma flow. However, because the secretory mechanisms are saturable at high concentrations of drug in plasma, clearance diminishes and excreted/filtered approaches unity with increasing concentration. Clearance is independent of urine flow rate and pH, but can be considerably diminished by competitive inhibitors of secretion. Stop-flow experiments demonstrate prominent secretory peaks in samples corresponding to the proximal tubule (Malvin and Wilde, 1973).

A particularly complex factor is the role of binding on plasma proteins as a limiting factor in drug secretion. Certain compounds, e.g., chlorothiazide, are extensively bound yet their clearances are nearly at the level of plasma flow (Baer *et al.*, 1959). Conversely with other compounds, e.g., furosemide, binding on protein definitely hinders secretion. An edifying discussion of these phenomena is given by Bowman (1975).

C. Filtration and Passive Reabsorption

In such instances excretion will always be less than filtration, clearance will be independent of the concentration of drug in plasma water, clearance will be enhanced by increases in urine flow rate, and clearances may or may not be influenced by changes in urinary pH.

Nonelectrolytes or weak electrolytes which are largely nonionized in the pH range of urine will have clearances insensitive to changes in urinary pH (Waddell and Butler, 1957a). Within this group two patterns of behavior can be discerned. In one the molecules are extremely permeant with respect to the tubular epithelium, and no appreciable concentration difference can exist between tubular fluid (or urine) and plasma water. As a consequence clearance is virtually equal to rate of urine flow. Compounds in this category include some short-acting barbiturates (Bloomer, 1966), pyrazinamide (Weiner and Tinker, 1972), and zoxazolamine (Maroske and Weiner, 1968). On the other hand, with less permeant compounds, U_x/P_x will exceed unity and there will be a curvilinear relationship between U_x and urine flow, U_x being great at low flow. Barbital (Giotti and Maynert, 1951) and paracetamol (Duggan and Mudge, 1975) provide examples of such behavior.

The principles underlying the influence of urinary pH on the clearance of certain compounds have been outlined in a preceding section. Phenobarbital (Waddell and Butler, 1957a) and DMO, the metabolite of trimethadione (Waddell and Butler, 1957b), are examples of compounds in this group. It should be emphasized that the extent of change of renal clearance with changes in urinary pH may be sufficiently great as to alter the overall disposition of a drug and thus its therapeutic and toxic effects. A striking example of this phenomenon is provided by amphetamine (Davis et al., 1971).

D. Filtration and Passive Secretion

There are no clear examples of this pattern for either organic acids or bases, nor are such examples likely to be found. According to current concepts of renal physiology, the passive net secretion of an organic acid by nonionic diffusion is virtually impossible because of the small maximal pH difference between plasma and alkaline urine, about 0.6 units. This pH difference can account for a urinary concentration of drug which is no more than four times that of plasma.

On the other hand, the pH difference between acid urine and plasma may be as much as 3 units; theoretically this might allow the U_x/P_x ratio for an organic base to achieve 1000 by nonionic diffusion. However, the site at which urine reaches its maximum acidity is exposed to only a small fraction of renal plasma flow, and even total extraction of the compound from this fraction is not likely to result in overall net secretion. A more extensive consideration of this topic is given elsewhere (Weiner, 1973).

E. Filtration, Active Secretion, and Passive Reabsorption

This is a fairly common pattern of drug excretion. Among the acids, salicylate (Weiner et al., 1959) and probenecid (Weiner et al., 1960; Dayton et al., 1963) provide examples; among the bases there are mecamylamine and quinine (Torretti et al., 1962). The excretion patterns are quite complex, and they depend in large measure on which of the two transtubular process predominates in a given setting. Since the overall patterns for acids and bases are analogous except for direction of the effect of pH change on clearance, we will confine discussion to acids only.

With low concentrations of drug in plasma, alkaline urine, and sufficiently high urine flow, net secretion, i.e., excreted > filtered, may occur. Clearance may be further enhanced by increasing urine flow, suggesting that despite the condition of net secretion, passive reabsorption is occurring simultaneously. This suggestion is confirmed by the administration of competitive inhibitors of secretion; net secretion is converted to net reabsorption. As plasma concentration of the drug is raised, there is a tendency for net secretion to be converted to net reabsorption (Weiner *et al.*, 1961; Knoefel *et al.*, 1962). The latter phenomenon results from the secretory mechanism, which is saturable, being opposed by a passive, nonsaturable, reabsorptive process. The phenomenon provides additional evidence that secretion and reabsorption occur simultaneously.

With acid urine, the reabsorptive process may be so favored as to result in net reabsorption regardless of the concentration of drug in plasma. With this group of compounds as well as those reabsorbed by nonionic diffusion without active secretion, the critical pH range for demonstrating large changes in clearance is between 6 and 8. This follows from the fact that over most of the nephron from glomerulus to the end of distal convoluted tubule, pH falls within that range regardless of acid–base status (Gottschalk *et al.*, 1960).

It should be stressed that in experiments of the type discussed in this section, the administration of $NaHCO_3$ is a far more satisfactory method of urinary alkalinization than is the administration of carbonic anhydrase inhibitors. The common carbonic anhydrase inhibitors are organic anions capable of competing for the secretory process (Weiner *et al.*, 1959). Moreover, they may cause a fall in proximal tubular pH despite simultaneous alkalinization of the voided urine (Rector *et al.*, 1965).

F. Filtration and Active Reabsorption

This is a classic pattern for the disposition of endogenous substances such as sugars and amino acids (Mudge *et al.*, 1973). Many of the foreign compounds with this pattern are close analogs of naturally occurring substances. We are unaware of any clear example of a drug which follows this pattern. The most probable candidate is oxypurinol which may well be reabsorbed by the urate mechanism (Elion *et al.*, 1968). However, the possibility has not been excluded that oxypurinol, like urate, is also secreted.

The usual criteria for the existence of this pattern are: excreted/filtered < 1, clearance increases toward GFR with increasing concentration of substance in plasma, clearance is only modestly altered by changes in urine flow rate or urinary pH, special techniques do not give evidence for simultaneous secretion, and competitors for reabsorption enhance clearance.

G. Filtration and Bidirectional, Specifically Mediated Transport

A variety of patterns are possible in this category. At one extreme are compounds such as PAH. Although we characterized PAH as exhibiting the filtration and secretion pattern for heuristic purposes, the work of Cho and Cafruny (1970) establishes that it undergoes bidirectional transport, but secretion is dominant to the extent that the bidirectional transport is difficult to appreciate.

In contrast, pyrazinoate in the dog behaves as if it follows the filtration–active reabsorption pattern, and its secretory component is revealed only by special procedures (Weiner and Tinker, 1972). It is of interest that in certain primates the disproportion between secretion and reabsorption is not so great, and the bidirectional nature of pyrazinoate transport is more easily appreciated (Weiner and Tinker, 1972; Fanelli and Weiner, 1973). Fanelli et al. (1972) suggested that secretion is in general a more prominent process in herbivorous primates. In the chimpanzee secretion of pyrazinoate predominates. There is a tendency for lower clearance at high concentrations of compound in plasma. The administration of a competitor for secretion causes conversion of net secretion to net reabsorption. Under the influence of a competitive inhibitor the low clearance is not sensitive to large changes in urine flow.

A somewhat similar pattern has been observed with M-hydroxybenzoate in the *Cebus* monkey (May and Weiner, 1971). In this situation there is net secretion at low plasma concentrations of compound and net reabsorption at higher concentrations. The compound does not display the characteristics expected were it to undergo passive reabsorption. The latter and other evidence led to the conclusions that there is active, bidirectional transport, that both processes occur in the proximal tubule, and that the reabsorptive process has a greater capacity but lower efficiency than the secretory process.

In summary, the existence of bidirectional, specifically mediated transport may or may not be easily demonstrated depending on the degree of disparity in the magnitudes of the two transport processes. When the disparity is not great it is possible to determine whether or not both processes are capable of active (uphill) transport. With great disparity in magnitude it is much more difficult to ascertain the active or passive nature of the smaller process.

H. More Complex Patterns

In the previous section we suggested that PAH is handled by filtration and bidirectional, specifically mediated tubular transport. In addition, certain findings reported in the literature have been interpreted as suggesting a minor degree of passive nonionic diffusion for PAH, thus raising the possibility that PAH participates in all of the transtubular processes considered thus far (Weiner, 1973). A similar suggestion has been made for salicylate (May and Weiner, 1971). There is no a priori reason why a single compound might not participate in all of the foregoing processes and one or more of the processes to be considered subsequently.

I. Filtration and Sequestration in Cells by Active Transport

As already indicated the sequestration of certain anions by proximal tubular cells of *Necturus* is accomplished by bidirectional active transport. Another mechanism has been proposed for cephaloridine in the mammalian nephron. In this instance the drug is taken up by the active transport mechanism on the peritubular aspect of the proximal cells and, because of its low permeance to the luminal membrane, the efflux of the drug into tubular fluid is hindered (Tune, 1972). Thus, although the drug is rapidly cleared from plasma by a secretory mechanism of the kidney, the conventionally measured renal clearance is not very different from GFR. The cyanine dye, #863, is an organic base with similar overall behavior, but in this instance sequestration may be due to binding to intracellular elements in addition to poor permeance (Rennick et al., 1956).

J. Filtration, Passive Reabsorption, and Sequestration in the Medulla

The basic mechanism in this instance is one of recycling: the substance is reabsorbed in the medullary collecting duct, diffuses into the ascending limb of the loop of Henle, and is thereby reintroduced into the collecting duct. The only direct demonstrations of this mechanism have been made with urea by micropuncture techniques (see Kokko and Rector, 1972, for references). It has been proposed that phenacetin (Bluemle and Goldberg, 1968) is subject to the same mechanism on the basis of finding a corticomedullary concentration gradient of the compound. The pitfalls in interpretation of gross analysis of medullary tissue have been discussed in an earlier section.

K. Filtration, Secretion, and Metabolism with Ready Excretion of the Metabolite

The best examples of this pattern come from work in the chicken with the Sperber technique. For example, morphine, an organic base, is converted to its ethereal sulfate (MES), an anion, in the kidney of this species (Watrous et al., 1970). When the free base is presented to the tubules for secretion, a fraction of the material appearing in urine is unchanged drug, the rest being the sulfated compound. Inhibitors of the cation secretory mechanism diminish the excretion of both the free drug and the conjugate. This depression of MES excretion is presumably a reflection of the fact that morphine uptake by the secretory mechanism is inhibited and consequently there is less substrate for conjugation. Probenecid, an inhibitor of anion secretion, does not inhibit the excretion of either morphine or MES, formed intracellularly, despite the fact that the latter is an anion. On the other hand, when MES is infused into the portal circulation, i.e., it is presented from the peritubular side of the cells, probenecid inhibits its secretion. Apparently, in this situation probenecid competes with the anion for secretion at the peritubular membrane but not at the luminal membrane.

The excretory pattern for serotonin, which is converted to 5-hydroxyindole acetic acid is quite analogous to that just described (Sanner and Wortman, 1962; Hakim et al., 1970). The study of the excretion of phenol and p-nitrophenol and their intrarenal metabolites is particularly interesting since competitive phenomena at the level of metabolism, as well as at the level of transport, were demonstrated (Quebbemann and Anders, 1973).

L. Filtration, Secretion, and Metabolism with Minimal Excretion

A most striking example of this pattern is provided by the renal disposition of cyclic AMP in the rat. The isolated perfused rat kidney has the capacity to secrete, by a probenecid-sensitive mechanism, and to degrade cyclic AMP (Coulson and Bowman, 1974). In the course of traversing the tubular cells a large fraction of the nucleotide is degraded. *In vivo* the renal cortex is the principal tissue involved in the removal of cyclic AMP from the circulation. Despite this, only a small fraction of cyclic AMP and its metabolites was found in urine (Coulson *et al.*, 1974).

REFERENCES

Acara, M. and Rennick, B. R. 1972. Renal tubular transport of choline; modifications caused by intrarenal metabolism. *J. Pharmacol. Exp. Ther., 182*:1.

Arendhorst, W. J. and Selkurt, E. E. 1970. Renal tubular mechanisms for creatinine secretion in the guinea pig. *Am. J. Physiol., 218*:1661.

Baer, J. E., Leidy, H. L., Brooks, A. V., and Beyer, K. H. 1959. The physiological disposition of chlorothiazide (Diuril) in the dog. *J. Pharmacol. Exp. Ther., 125*:295.

Baines, A. D., Gottschalk, C. W., and Lassiter, W. E. 1968. Microinjection study of *p*-aminohippurate excretion by rat kidneys. *Am. J. Physiol., 214*:703.

Bárány, E. H. 1972. Inhibition by hippurate and probenecid of *in vitro* uptake of iodipamide and *o*-iodiohippurate. A composite uptake system for iodipamide in choroid plexus, kidney cortex and anterior urea of several species. *Acta Physiol. Scand., 86:*12.

Bárány, E. H. 1974. Bile acids as inhibitors of the liver-like anion transport system in the rabbit kidney, uvea and choroid plexus. *Acta Physiol. Scand., 92*:195.

Berndt, W. O. and Mudge, G. H. 1968. Renal excretion of iodipamide, comparative study in the dog and rabbit. *Invest. Radiol., 3*:414.

Beyer, K. H., Woodward, R., Peters, L., Verwey, W. F., and Mattis, P. A. 1944. The prolongation of penicillin retention in the body by means of *para*-aminohippuric acid. *Science, 100*:107.

Bloomer, H. A. 1966. A critical evaluation of diuresis in the treatment of barbiturate intoxication. *J. Lab. Clin. Med., 67*:898.

Bluemle, L., Jr. and Goldberg, M. 1968. Renal accumulation of salicylate and phenacetin: Possible mechanisms in the nephropathy of analgesic abuse. *J. Clin. Invest., 47*:2507.

Bordier, B., Ornstein, O., and Wedeen, R. P. 1970. The intrarenal distribution of tritiated *para*-aminohippuric acid determined by a modified technique of section freeze-dry radioautography. *J. Cell Biol., 46*:518.

Bowman, R. H. 1975. Renal secretion of [^{35}S]furosemide and its depression by albumin binding. *Am. J. Physiol., 229*:93.

Brenner, B. M., Troy, J. L., Dougharty, T. M., Deen, W. M., and Robertson, C. R. 1972. Dynamics of glomerular ultrafiltration in the rat. II. Plasma-flow dependence of GFR. *Am. J. Physiol., 223*:1184.

Burg, M. B. and Orloff, J. 1962a. Effect of strophanthidin on electrolyte content and PAH accumulation of rabbit kidney slices. *Am. J. Physiol., 202*:565.

Burg, M. B. and Orloff, J. 1962b. Oxygen consumption and active transport in separated renal tubules. *Am. J. Physiol., 203*:327.

Burg, M. B. and Orloff, J. 1973. Perfusion of isolated renal tubules. In: *Handbook of Physiology, Renal Physiology,* pp. 145–159. Ed. by Orloff, J. and Berliner, R. W. American Physiological Society, Washington, D.C.

Burg, M. and Weller, P. 1969. Iodopyracet transport by isolated perfused flounder proximal renal tubules. *Am. J. Physiol., 217*:1053.

Calcagno, P. L. and Rubin, M. I. 1963. Renal extraction of PAH in infants and children. *J. Clin. Invest., 42*:1632.

Chambers, R. and Kempton, R. T. 1933. Indications of function of the chick mesonephros in tissue culture and phenol red. *J. Cell. Comp. Physiol., 3*:131.

Cho, K. C. and Cafruny, E. J. 1970. Renal tubular reabsorption of *p*-aminohippuric acid (PAH) in the dog. *J. Pharmacol. Exp. Ther., 173*:1.

Cho, K. C., Kim, J. H., Hong, S. K., and Lee, W. C. 1960. Kinetic studies on the competition between *para*-aminohippuric acid (PAH) and Diodrast for renal transport in the dog. *Yonsei Med. J., 1*:25.

Chung, S. T., Park, Y. S., and Hong, S. K. 1970. Effect of cations on transport of weak organic acids in rabbit kidney slices. *Am. J. Physiol., 219*:30.

Corr, P. B. and May, D. G. 1975. Renal mechanisms for the excretion of nicotinic acid. *J. Pharmacol. Exp. Ther., 192*:195.

Cortney, M. A., Mylle, M., Lassiter, W. E., and Gottschalk, C. W. 1965. Renal transport of water, solute and PAH in rats loaded with isotonic saline. *Am. J. Physiol., 209*:1199.

Coulson, R. and Bowman, R. H. 1974. The excretion and degradation of exogenous adenosine 3',5'-monophosphate by the isolated perfused rat kidney. *Life Sci., 14*:545.

Coulson, R., Bowman, R. H., and Roch-Ramel, F. 1974. The effects of nephrectomy and probenecid on *in vivo* clearance of adenosine-3',5'-monophosphate from rat plasma. *Life Sci., 15*:877.

Cross, R. J. and Taggart, J. V. 1950. Renal tubular transport: Accumulation of *p*-aminohippurate by rabbit kidney slices. *Am. J. Physiol., 161*:181.

Dantzler, W. H. 1970. Comparison of renal tubular transport of urate and PAH uptake in water snakes: Evidence for differences in mechanisms and sites of transport. *Comp. Biochem. Physiol., 34*:609.

Dantzler, W. H. 1973. Characteristics of urate transport by isolated perfused snake proximal tubules. *Am. J. Physiol., 224*:445.

Dantzler, W. H. 1974a. PAH transport by snake proximal renal tubules: Differences from urate transport. *Am. J. Physiol., 226*:634.

Dantzler, W. H. 1974b. K^+ effects on PAH transport and membrane permeabilities in isolated snake renal tubules. *Am. J. Physiol., 227*:1361.

Dantzler, W. H. and Bentley, S. K. 1975. High K^+ effects on PAH transport and permeabilities in isolated snake renal tubules. *Am. J. Physiol., 229*:191.

Davis, J. M., Kopin, I. J., Lemberger, L., and Axelrod, J. 1971. Effects of urinary pH on amphetamine metabolism. *Ann. N.Y. Acad. Sci., 179*:493.

Dayton, P. G. and Perel, J. M. 1971. Physiological and physicochemical bases of drug interactions in man. *Ann. N.Y. Acad. Sci., 179*:67.

Dayton, P. G., Yü, T. F., Chen, W., Berger, L., West, L. A., and Gutman, A. B. 1963. The physiological disposition of probenecid, including renal clearance, in man, studied by an improved method for its estimation in biological material. *J. Pharmacol. Exp. Ther., 140*:278.

Deetjen, P. 1966. Micropuncture studies on site and mode of diuretic action of furosemide. *Ann. N.Y. Acad. Sci., 139*:408.

Despopolous, A. 1965. A definition of substrate specificity in renal transport of organic ions. *J. Theor. Biol., 8*:163.

Duggan, D. E. 1966. The accumulation of chlorothiazide and related saluretic agents by isolated renal tubules. *J. Pharmacol. Exp. Ther., 152*:122.

Duggan, G. G. and Mudge, G. H. 1975. Renal tubular transport of paracetamol and its conjugates in the dog. *Brit. J. Pharmacol., 54*:359.

Elion, G. B., Yü, T. F., Gutman, A. B., and Hitchings, G. H. 1968. Renal clearance of oxipurinol, the chief metabolite of allopurinol. *Am. J. Med., 46*:69.

Fanelli, G. M., Jr. and Weiner, I. M. 1973. Pyrazinoate excretion in the chimpanzee. Relation to urate disposition and the actions of uricosuric drugs. *J. Clin. Invest., 52*:1946.

Fanelli, G. M., Jr., Bohn, D. L., and Reilly, S. S. 1972. Effects of mercurial diuretics on the renal tubular transport of *p*-aminohippurate and Diodrast in the chimpanzee. *J. Pharmacol. Exp. Ther., 180*:759.

Farah, A. and Frazer, M. 1961. Studies on the renal tubular secretion of N'-methylnicotinamide. *J. Pharmacol. Exp. Ther., 134*:245.

Farah, A., Graham, G., and Koda, F. 1953. The action of sodium fluoroacetate on the renal tubular transport of *para*-aminohippurate and glucose in the dog. *J. Pharmacol. Exp. Ther., 108*:410.

Forster, R. P. 1948. Use of thin kidney slices and isolated renal tubules for direct study of cellular transport kinetics. *Science, 108*:65.

Forster, R. P. and Copenhaver, J. H., Jr. 1956. Intracellular accumulation as an active process in a mammalian renal transport system *in vitro*. Energy dependence and competitive phenomena. *Am. J. Physiol., 186*:167.

Foulkes, E. C. and Miller, B. F. 1959. Steps in *p*-aminohippurate transport by kidney slices. *Am. J. Physiol., 196*:83.

Gerenscer, G. A., Park, Y. S., and Hong, S. K. 1973. Sodium influence upon the transport kinetics of *p*-aminohippurate in rabbit kidney slices. *Proc. Soc. Exp. Biol. Med., 144*:440.

Giebisch, G. and Windhager, E. E. 1973. Electrolyte transport across renal tubular membranes. In: *Handbook of Physiology, Renal Physiology*, pp. 315–376. Ed. by Orloff, J. and Berliner, R. W. American Physiological Society, Washington, D.C.

Giotti, A. and Maynert, E. W. 1951. The renal clearance of barbital and the mechanism of its reabsorption. *J. Pharmacol. Exp. Ther., 101*:296.

Goldstein, A. 1949. Interactions of drugs and plasma proteins. *Pharmacol. Rev., 1*:102.

Gottschalk, C. W. and Lassiter, W. E. 1973. Micropuncture methodology. In: *Handbook of Physiology, Renal Pharmacology*, pp. 129–143. Ed. by Orloff, J. and Berliner, R. W. American Physiological Society, Washington, D.C.

Gottschalk, C. W., Lassiter, W. E., and Mylle, M. 1960. Localization of urine acidification in the mammalian kidney. *Am. J. Physiol., 198*:581.

Gyrd-Hansen, N. and Rasmussen, F. 1970. Acetylation of *p*-aminohippuric acid in the kidney. Renal clearance of *p*-aminohippuric acid and *N*-acetylated *p*-aminohippuric acid in pigs. *Acta Physiol. Scand., 80*:249.

Hakim, R., Watrous, W. M., and Fujimoto, J. M. 1970. The renal tubular transport and metabolism of serotonin (5-HT) and 5-hydroxyindoleacetic acid (5-HIAA) in the chicken. *J. Pharmacol. Exp. Ther., 175*:749.

Hirsch, G. H. and Hook, J. B. 1970a. Maturation of renal organic acid transport: Substrate stimulation by penicillin and *p*-aminohippurate (PAH), *J. Pharmacol. Exp. Ther., 171*:103.

Hirsch, G. H. and Hook, J. B. 1970b. Stimulation of renal organic acid transport and protein synthesis by penicillin. *J. Pharmacol. Exp. Ther., 174*:152.

Hober, R. 1945. *Physical Chemistry of Cells and Tissues*. Blakiston, Philadelphia.

Hong, S. K. and Forster, R. P. 1959. Further observations on the separate steps involved in the active transport of chlorphenol red by isolated renal tubules of the flounder *in vitro*. *J. Cell. Comp. Physiol., 54*:237.

Hook, J. B., Williamson, H. E., and Hirsch, G. H. 1970. Functional maturation of renal PAH transport in the dog. *Can. J. Physiol. Pharmacol., 48*:169.

Horster, M. and Lewy, J. E. 1970. Filtration fraction and extraction of PAH during neonatal period in the rat. *Am. J. Physiol., 219*:1061.

Huang, K. C. and Lin, D. S. T. 1965. Kinetic studies on transport of PAH and other organic acids in isolated renal tubules. *Am. J. Physiol., 208*:391.

Johnson, J. T., Holloway, L. S., Heisey, S. R., and Hook, J. B. 1974. Substrate stimulation of organic anion transport in newborn dog kidney and choroid plexus. *Biochem. Pharmacol., 23*:754.

Kiil, F. 1961. Dynamics of proximal tubular secretion. *Nature, 189*:927.

Kinter, W. B. 1959. Renal tubular transport of Diodrast-I[131] and PAH in *Necturus*: Evidence for simultaneous reabsorption and secretion. *Am. J. Physiol., 196*:1141.

Kinter, W. B. 1966. Chlorophenol red influx and efflux: Microspectrophotometry of flounder kidney tubules. *Am. J. Physiol., 211*:1152.

Kinter, W., Leape, L. L., and Cohen, J. J. 1960. Autoradiographic study of Diodrast I[131] transport in *Necturus* kidney. *Am. J. Physiol., 199*:931.

Kleit, S., Levin, D., Perenich, T., and Cade, R. 1965. Renal excretion of ascorbic acid by dogs. *Am. J. Physiol., 209*:195.

Knoefel, P. K., Huang, K. C., and Despopoulos, A. 1959. Conjugation and excretion of amino and acetamido benzoic acids. *Am. J. Physiol., 196*:1224.

Knoefel, P. K., Huang, K. C., and Jarboe, C. H. 1962. Renal disposal of salicyluric acid. *Am. J. Physiol., 203*:6.

Koishi, T. 1959. Studies on renal tubular transport. I. Accumulation of *p*-aminohippurate by kidney slices. *Jpn. J. Pharmacol., 8*:101.

Kokko, J. P. and Rector, F. C., Jr. 1972. Countercurrent multiplication system without active transport in inner medulla. *Kidney Int., 2*:214.

Maddox, D. A., Bennett, C. M., Deen, W. M., Glassock, R. J., Knutson, D., Daugharty, T. M., and Brenner, B. M. 1975. Determinants of glomerular filtration in experimental glomerulonephritis in the rat. *J. Clin. Invest., 55*:305.

Malvin, R. L. and Wilde, W. S. 1973. Stop-flow technique. In: *Handbook of Physiology, Renal Physiology*, pp. 119–128. Ed. by Orloff, J. and Berliner, R. W. American Physiological Society, Washington, D.C.

Maroske, D. and Weiner, I. M. 1968. The renal handling of zoxazolamine (Flexin). *J. Pharmacol. Exp. Ther., 159*:409.

May, D. G. and Weiner, I. M. 1970. Bidirectional active transport of *m*-hydroxybenzoate in proximal tubule of dog. *Am. J. Physiol., 218*:430.

May, D. G. and Weiner, I. M. 1971. The renal mechanisms for the excretion of *m*-hydroxybenzoate in *Cebus* monkeys: Relationship to urate transport. *J. Pharmacol. Exp. Ther., 176*:407.

Milne, M. D., Scribner, B. H., and Crawford, M. A. 1958. Nonionic diffusion and the excretion of weak acids and bases. *Am. J. Med., 24*:709.

Møller, J. V. 1967. The relation between secretion of urate and *p*-aminohippurate in the rabbit kidney. *J. Physiol., 192*:505.

Mudge, G. H., Berndt, W. O., and Valtin, H. 1973. Tubular transport of urea, glucose, phosphate, uric acid, sulfate and thiosulfate. In: *Handbook of Physiology, Renal Physiology,* pp. 587–652. Ed. by Orloff, J. and Berliner, R. W. American Physiological Society, Washington, D.C.

Mudge, G. H., Silva, P., and Stibitz, G. R. 1975. Renal excretion by non-ionic diffusion. The nature of the disequilibrium. *Med. Clin. N. Am., 59*:681.

Oelert, H., Baumann, K., and Gekle, D. 1969. Permeabilitäts Messungen einiger schwacher organischer Säuren aus dem distalen Konvolut der Rattenniere, *Pfluegers Arch., 307*:178.

Peters, L. 1960. Renal tubular excretion of organic bases. *Pharmacol. Rev., 12*:1.

Popa, G., Parekh, N., and Steinhausen, M. 1974. Renal test dyes. II. Renal handling of dyes suitable for renal passage time measurement. *Pfluegers Arch., 350*:273.

Puck, T. T., Wasserman, K., and Fishman, A. P. 1952. Some effects of inorganic ions on the active transport of phenol red by isolated kidney tubules of the flounder. *J. Cell. Comp. Physiol., 40*:73.

Quebbemann, A. J. and Anders, M. W. 1973. Renal tubular conjugation and excretion of phenol and p-nitrophenol in the chicken: Differing mechanisms of renal transfer. *J. Pharmacol. Exp. Ther., 184*:695.

Rector, F. C., Jr., Carter, N. W., and Seldin, D. W. 1965. The mechanism of bicarbonate reabsorption in the proximal and distal tubules of the kidney. *J. Clin. Invest., 44*:278.

Renkin, E. M. and Gilmore, J. P. 1973. Glomerular filtration. In: *Handbook of Physiology, Renal Physiology*, pp. 185–248. Ed. by Orloff, J. and Berliner, R. W. American Physiological Society, Washington, D.C.

Rennick, B. R. and Farah, A. 1956. Studies on renal tubular transport of tetraethylammonium ion in the dog. *J. Pharmacol. Exp. Ther., 116*:287.

Rennick, B. R. and Moe, G. K. 1960. Stop-flow localization of renal tubular excretion of tetraethylammonium. *Am. J. Physiol., 198*:1267.

Rennick, B. R., Kandel, A., and Peters, L. 1956. Inhibition of the renal tubular excretion of tetraethylammonium and *N'*-methylnicotinamide by basic cyanine dyes. *J. Pharmacol. Exp. Ther., 118*:204.

Ross, C. R., Diezi-Chomety, F., and Roch-Ramel, F. 1975. Renal excretion of N'-methylnicotin-amide in the rat. *Am. J. Physiol., 228:*1641.

Sanner, E. and Wortman, B. 1962. Tubular excretion of serotonin (5-hydroxytryptamine) in the chicken. *Acta Physiol. Scand., 55:*319.

Schreiner, G. E. 1972. Toxic nephropathy due to drugs, solvents and metals. In: *Drugs affecting Kidney Function and Metabolism,* pp. 248–284. Ed. by Edwards, K. D. G. Karger, Basel.

Seely, J. F. and Chirito, E. 1975. Studies of the electrical potential difference in rat proximal tubule. *Am. J. Physiol., 229:*72.

Shannon, J. A. 1939. Renal tubular excretion. *Physiol. Rev., 19:*63.

Smith, H. W. 1951. *The Kidney: Structure and Function in Health and Disease.* New York, Oxford.

Smith, H. W., Goldring, W., and Chasis, H. 1938. The measurement of the tubular excretory mass, effective blood flow, and filtration rate in the normal human kidney. *J. Clin. Invest., 17:*263.

Sonnenberg, H., Oelert, H., and Baumann, K. 1965. Proximal tubular reabsorption of some organic acids in the rat kidney *in vivo. Arch. Ges. Physiol., 286:*171.

Taggart, J. V. 1958. Mechanisms of renal tubular transport. *Am. J. Med., 24:*774.

Tanner, G. A. 1967. Micropuncture study of PAH and Diodrast transport in *Necturus* kidney. *Am. J. Physiol., 212:*1341.

Tanner, G. A. and Kinter, W. B. 1966. Reabsorption and secretion of *p*-aminohippurate and Diodrast in *Necturus* kidney. *Am. J. Physiol., 210:*221.

Torretti, J., Weiner, I. M., and Mudge, G. H. 1962. Renal tubular secretion and reabsorption of organic bases in the dog. *J. Clin. Invest., 41:*793.

Tune, B. M. 1972. Effect of organic acid transport inhibitors on renal cortical uptake and proximal tubular toxicity of cephaloridine. *J. Pharmacol. Exp. Ther., 181:*250.

Tune, B. M. and Fernholt, M. 1973. Relationship between cephaloridine and *p*-aminohippurate transport in the kidney. *Am. J. Physiol., 255:*1114.

Tune, B. M., Burg, M. B., and Patlak, C. S. 1969. Characteristics of *p*-aminohippurate transport in proximal renal tubules. *Am. J. Physiol., 217:*1057.

Vogel, G. and Kroger, W. 1966. Das Tm_{PAH} der Niere als Na$^+$-abhängige Grösse. *Arch. Ges. Physiol., 286:*317.

Vogel, G. and Stoekert, I. 1966. Die Bedeutung des Anions für den renal tubulären Transporte von Na$^+$ und die Transporte von Glucose und PAH. *Arch. Ges. Physiol., 292:*309.

Waddell, W. J. and Butler, T. C. 1957a. The distribution and excretion of phenobarbital. *J. Clin. Invest., 36:*1217.

Waddell, W. J. and Butler, T. C. 1957b. Renal excretion of 5,5-dimethyl-2,4-oxazolidinedione (product of demethylation of trimethadione). *Proc. Soc. Exp. Biol. Med., 96:*563.

Walser, M. 1966. Mathematical aspects of renal function: The dependence of solute reabsorption on water reabsorption and the mechanism of osmotic natriuresis. *J. Theor. Biol., 10:*307.

Watrous, W. M., May, D. G., and Fujimoto, J. M. 1970. Mechanism of the renal tubular transport of morphine and morphine ethereal sulfate in the chicken. *J. Pharmacol. Exp. Ther., 172:*224.

Wedeen, R. P. and Weiner, B. 1969. Extraction of hippuran-^{131}I and PAH-^{3}H from red blood cells and plasma in the rat. *Am. J. Physiol., 217:*838.

Wedeen, R. P. and Weiner, B. 1973. The distribution of *p*-aminohippuric acid in rat kidney slices. I. Tubular localization. *Kidney Int., 3:*215.

Weiner, I. M. 1973. Transport of weak acids and bases. In: *Handbook of Physiology, Renal Physiology,* pp. 521–554. Ed. by Orloff, J. and Berliner, R. W. American Physiological Society, Washington, D.C.

Weiner, I. M. and Mudge, G. H. 1964. Renal tubular mechanism for excretion of organic acids and bases. *Am. J. Med., 36:*743.

Weiner, I. M. and Tinker, J. P. 1972. Pharmacology of pyrazinamide: Metabolic and renal function studies related to the mechanism of drug-induced urate retention. *J. Pharmacol. Exp. Ther., 180:*411.

Weiner, I. M., Washington, J. A., II, and Mudge, G. H. 1959. Studies on the renal excretion of salicylate in the dog. *Bull. Johns Hopkins Hosp., 105:*284.

Weiner, I. M., Washington, J. A., II, and Mudge, G. H. 1960. On the mechanism of action of probenecid on renal tubular secretion. *Bull. Johns Hopkins Hosp., 106:*333.

Weiner, I. M., Garlid, K. D., Romeo, J. A., and Mudge, G. H. 1961. Effects of tubular secretion and reabsorption on titration curves of tubular transport. *Am. J. Physiol., 200*:393.

Whelton, A. and Walker, W. G. 1974. Intrarenal antibiotic distribution in health and disease (editorial). *Kidney Int., 6*:131.

Whelton, A., Sapir, D. G., Carter, G. G., Kramer, J., and Walker, G. W. 1971. Intrarenal distribution of penicillin, cephalothin, ampicillin and oxytetracycline during varied states of hydration. *J. Pharmacol. Exp. Ther., 179:*419.

Wilbrandt, W. and Rosenberg, T. 1961. The concept of carrier transport and its corollaries in pharmacology. *Pharmacol. Rev., 13*:109.

Williams, R. T. 1959. *Detoxication Mechanisms*, 2nd ed. Chapman and Hall, London.

Zins, G. R. and Weiner, I. M. 1968a. Bidirectional urate transport limited to the proximal tubule in dogs. *Am. J. Physiol., 215*:411.

Zins, G. R. and Weiner, I. M. 1968b. Bidirectional transport of taurocholoate by the proximal tubule of the dog. *Am. J. Physiol., 215*:840.

Index